*T*his Fourth Edition of Uppers, Downers, All Arounders is dedicated to all those who provide drug abuse treatment, aftercare, education, and prevention services. May you find continued fulfillment and joy in your work. The authors also acknowledge a debt of gratitude to those clients of the Haight-Ashbury Detox Clinic and other treatment facilities who so generously shared their stories of addiction and recovery so that others may learn from their experiences.

Uppers, Downers, All Arounders, Fourth Edition has been designed to emphasize the most important themes and concepts in the field of substance abuse and treatment. The **CHAPTER PROFILE,** the **HEADINGS** within the body of the chapter, and the **CHAPTER SUMMARY** consistently emphasize these themes, so although there is a wealth of information, focusing on the principle concepts will make the task of learning easier.

The information and quotations in this book are based on the experience and clinical expertise of the 130 staff members of the Haight-Ashbury Detox Clinic in San Francisco, California and on the experiences of more than 100,000 clients who have been treated at the clinic over the past 34 years.

The Haight-Ashbury Drug Detox Clinic's treatment program has one of the highest caseloads and best success rates in the country due in part to its success in drug education. The Clinic has found that objective nonjudgmental information about drugs and their effects are important in treatment and crucial in drug abuse prevention.

The most important changes in the Fourth Edition are

◊ comprehensive and detailed **CITATIONS** and **REFERENCES** in every chapter to aid in research and confirm the accuracy of the information;

◊ an extensive **GLOSSARY** that is directly related to information presented;

◊ the most **CURRENT STATISTICS, DATA,** and **RESEARCH** to keep up with advances in the field;

◊ an interactive **WEB SITE (www.addictionology.com)** to provide practice questions, case studies, articles from the *Journal of Psychoactive Drugs,* supplementary information, and links to other sources.

Note: In order to distinguish between trade (brand) names and chemical (generic) names of prescription and over-the-counter drugs, we have included the trademark symbol (®) after all trade names.

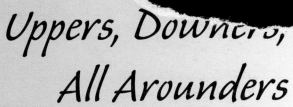

Uppers, Downers,
All Arounders

Physical and Mental Effects
of Psychoactive Drugs

Fourth Edition

Darryl S. Inaba, Pharm.D.
Chief Executive Officer, Haight-Ashbury Free Clinics
Associate Clinical Professor of Pharmacology,
University of California Medical Center, San Francisco

William E. Cohen
Communications and Education Consultant,
Haight-Ashbury Detox Clinic

CNS Publications, Inc.™
Ashland, Oregon

Publisher

P.O. Box 96
Ashland, OR 97520
Tel: (541) 488-2805   Fax: (541) 482-9252
Email: cns@mind.net
Web Site: www.cnspublications.com

Uppers, Downers, All Arounders
Fourth Edition
© 2000, William E. Cohen and Darryl S. Inaba
First Edition   ©1989
Second Edition   ©1993
Third Edition   ©1997

Editor: **Carol A. Caruso**

Book Design: **Data Management, Inc./Connie Wolfe**, Cedar Rapids, Iowa

Illustrations: **Impact Publications/David Ruppe**, Medford, Oregon

Cover Design: **Lightbourne Images**, Ashland, Oregon

Printing and Color Separations: **Cedar Graphics**, Cedar Rapids, Iowa

Special thanks to:
Michael Aldrich, Ph.D., Curator, Fitz Hugh Ludlow Memorial Library, San Francisco, California
Daniel Amen, M.D., Founder, Amen Clinic for Behavioral Medicine, Fairfax, California
BASN Treatment Unit of the Haight-Ashbury Clinics, San Francisco, California
Sterling K. Clarren, M.D., Children's Hospital, Seattle, Washington
Greg Hayner, Pharm.D., Chief Pharmacist, Haight-Ashbury Detox Clinic, San Francisco, California
Michael E. Holstein, Ph.D. School of Social Science, Education, Health, and Physical Education, Southern Oregon University, Ashland, Oregon
Kerry J. Redican, MPH, Ph.D., College of Human Resources, Virginia Tech, Blacksburg, Virginia
Ryther Clinic, Seattle, Washington
William P. Rockwood, Ph.D., Professor of Biology, Director Chemical Dependency Treatment Program, Russell Sage Colleges, Albany/Troy, New York
Rick Seymour, M.A., Managing Editor, Journal of Psychoactive Drugs, Director of Training and Education, Haight-Ashbury Free Clinics, San Francisco, California
David E. Smith, M.D., Founder and Medical Director, Haight-Ashbury Free Clinics, San Francisco, California
Nanda Sonpatki, consultant/photographer, Portland, Oregon

Disclaimer: Information in this book is in no way meant to replace professional medical advice or professional counseling and treatment.

Publisher's Cataloging-in-Publication
(Provided by Quality Books, Inc.)
Inaba, Darryl.
    Uppers, downers, all arounders / Darryl S.
Inaba, William E. Cohen. — 4th ed.
    p. cm.
    Includes bibliographical references and index.
    LCCN: 00-105811
    ISBN: 0-926544-26-8

    1. Psychotropic drugs—Side effects. 2. Drug
abuse—Complications. I. Cohen, William E.,
1941- II. Title

RM332.153 2000   616.86
            QB100-500089

Printed in the United States of America

CONTENTS

Psychoactive Drugs:
History & Classification

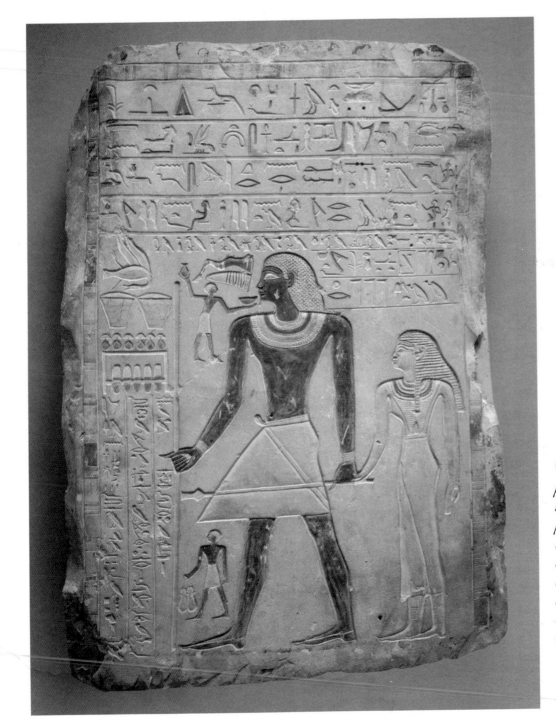

A stylized miniature physician dispenses beer to his noble patient. Egyptian physicians dissolved herbal medications in beer and even prescribed the carbohydrate and vitamin B-rich sediment for a variety of ailments including digestive disorders and boils.

Reprinted, by permission, Metropolitan Museum of Art, Rogers Fund, New York.

INTRODUCTION

- **Five themes of drug use become apparent when studying history:**
  1. a basic need of human beings to cope with their environment,
  2. the natural susceptibility of brain chemistry to psychoactive drugs,
  3. business and government involvement in the drug trade,
  4. technological advances in refining and synthesizing drugs,
  5. development of more efficient and faster methods of putting drugs in the body.

HISTORY OF PSYCHOACTIVE DRUGS

- **Prehistory & the Neolithic Period (8500–4000 B.C.):** The earliest human use of psychoactive drugs was plants and fruits whose mood-altering qualities were accidentally discovered and then cultivated.
- **Ancient Civilizations (4000 B.C.–A.D. 400):** Sumerian, Egyptian, Vedic Indian, Chinese, Mesoamerican Olmec, South American Chavin, and other ancient cultures used opium, alcohol, marijuana, peyote, psilocybin mushrooms, and coca.
- **Middle Ages (400–1400):** Psychoactive plants, such as belladonna, mandrake, and psilocybin mushrooms, were used by witches, shamans, and medicine men for healing and spiritual purposes.
- **Renaissance & the Age of Discovery (1400–1700):** Tobacco, coffee, tea, distilled alcohol beverages, and opium smoking spread along the trade routes. Governments and merchants controlled much of the trade for economic gain.
- **Age of Enlightenment & the Early Industrial Revolution (1700–1900):** New refinement techniques (e.g., heroin from opium), new delivery methods (e.g., hypodermic needle), and new manufacturing techniques (e.g., cigarette-rolling machine) increased use, abuse, and addiction liability. Temperance and prohibition movements spread.
- **Twentieth Century & the Electronic Revolution:** Wider distribution channels, improved refinement technology, and new synthetic drugs increased legal and illegal use. Government control of drugs led to criminal syndicate activity. New definitions of addiction as a disease and as a biochemical imbalance helped expand treatment options.
- **Today & Tomorrow:** After a decline in the 1980s, use of illegal drugs increased in the '90s. Expensive marijuana, plentiful methamphetamines, and cheaper heroin took their turns as the current drug of choice. As the twenty-first century begins, alcohol and tobacco continue to cause the most health and social problems but hard-core drug abuse is also on the rise.
- **Conclusions:** Psychoactive drugs have always influenced human behavior because they affect the old brain and disrupt communication with the new brain. The current drugs of choice change but the reasons for use remain the same.

CLASSIFICATION OF PSYCHOACTIVE DRUGS

- **What Is a Psychoactive Drug?** Psychoactive drugs can be identified by their chemical name, trade name, or street name. This book classifies most drugs by their general effects.
- **Major Drugs**
  - ◊ **Uppers:** Stimulants, such as cocaine, amphetamines, caffeine, and nicotine, force the release of energy chemicals. The strongest stimulants, cocaine and amphetamines, can produce an intense rush and ecstatic feelings.
  - ◊ **Downers:** Depressants include opioids (e.g., heroin), sedative-hypnotics, and alcohol. They depress circulatory, respiratory, and muscular systems; they lower inhibitions; they can induce euphoria.
  - ◊ **All Arounders:** Psychedelics, e.g., marijuana, LSD, "ecstasy," can cause some stimulation but mostly they alter sensory input and can cause illusions, delusions, and hallucinations.
- **Other Drugs & Addictions**
  - ◊ **Inhalants** include organic solvents, volatile nitrites, and nitrous oxide (laughing gas) and can induce the full range of upper, downer, or psychedelic effects depending on the specific substance and the amount used.
  - ◊ **Anabolic Steroids** and other sports drugs are used to enhance athletic performance by increasing endurance, muscle size, and/or aggression.
  - ◊ **Psychiatric Medications** include antidepressants, antipsychotics, and antianxiety drugs. They are prescribed to rebalance brain chemistry when there are mental problems.
  - ◊ **Compulsive Behaviors,** such as overeating, anorexia, bulimia, compulsive gambling, sexual compulsion, Internet addiction, compulsive shopping, and even codependency, affect many of the same areas of the brain influenced by psychoactive drugs.
- **Controlled Substances Act of 1970:** This Act consolidated and updated most drug laws. Its aim is to reduce the availability, use, and abuse of psychoactive drugs.

1921

HARDING'S PEN SPEEDS DRIVE AGAINST DRUGS

President Signs Congress Re-solution to Join with Other Nations in Limiting Supply

Negotiations to Open at Once with Lands That Grow the Bases of Opium and Cocaine

WASHINGTON, March 2 - President Harding today signed the joint Congressio[...] tion arguin[...] United Stat[...] with certa[...] government[...] the produc[...] tain drugs.

1989

1929

COOLIDGE SIGNS BILL FOR DOPE-CURE FARMS

NEW U.S. LAW WILL HELP END NARCOTIC EVIL, SAVE ADDICTS

JANUARY, 20, 1929
All Drug Slave" Convicts Will Be Sent to Farms First for Rehabilitation

Washington, Jan. 19 - President Coolidge today signed the Porter Bill [...] two [...] otic d o

1931

HOOVER BACKS U.S. IN DOPE WAR

WASHINGTON, Jan 21 - President Hoover today sent a message to Congress recommending $35,000 be appropriated for American participation in the International Conference on Limitation of the manufacture of narcotic drugs, to be held at Geneva,

Political Jockeying

Reagan, Congress Call for Drug War

1986

Washington

House and Senate leaders and President Reagan called for bipartisan cooperation against drugs yesterday while all sides continued to maneuver for the political spotlight on what is becoming a major issue of the 1986 Congressi[...]

Bush to unveil drug strategy

By Carolyn Skorneck
Of the Associated Press

WASHINGTON — President Bush's national drug strategy envisions sending up to $260 million in [...] sions and military aid to Colom[...] [...] Peru in an effort to [...]

American nations to subsidize the withdrawal of farm land from producing coca crops, which are refined to produce cocaine.

A U.S. investment of $400 million in such a plan could free enough funds to subsidize the withdrawal of every acre in Bolivia, Columbia and [...] duction, said Biden, [...]

1998 ## Clinton to Announce New Drug Plan

Los Angeles Times

Washington

The White House, in what may be the most ambitious anti-drug effort the nation has undertaken, has devised a plan that is intended to cut illicit drug supply and demand in half over the next decade.

volved in educating youths about narcotic abuse and reducing drug use in the workplace.

It's the first time the government has issued specific targets for such sharp reductions in drug use.

However, its lofty goals are not

gress, Clinton's budget for the 1999 fiscal year calls for spending $1.1 billion more for drug-control measures across all departments, representing slightly less than a 7 percent increase over the current year. The total spending would amount to $17.1 billion.

Although drug use has de-

INTRODUCTION

FIVE HISTORICAL THEMES OF DRUG USE

Drug use in contemporary life is by no means a new or unique phenomenon. For much of history, humans have searched for ways to alter their states of consciousness. Whether it has been to reduce pain, forget harsh surroundings, alter a mood, explore feelings, promote social interaction, escape boredom, treat a mental illness, stimulate creativity, or enhance the senses, some people have chosen to change their perception of reality chemically rather than by nondrug methods, such as fasting, dancing, and meditating. Which drugs are to be used, how they are to be used, what constitutes abuse, and how abuse is punished, treated, or prevented have varied from culture to culture and from century to century but certain themes transcend time and cultural makeup.

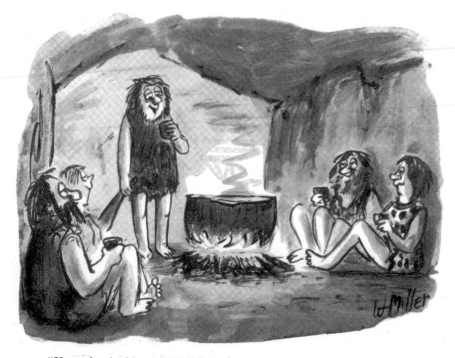

"Hey, what is this stuff? It makes everything I think seem profound."

The New Yorker Collection from Warren Miller, 1978. From Cartoonbank.com. Reprinted, by permission. All rights reserved.

• •

1. A basic need of human beings to cope with their environment

Early man lived in a dangerous and mysterious world that could inflict pain and death in an instant. Brutal weather, harsh surroundings, carnivorous animals, aggressive enemies, and life-threatening diseases could wound, maim, or kill. Primitive and eventually civilized human beings searched for ways to control these dangers. They drew cave pictures of animals 40,000 years ago in France to help in the hunt. They built the city of Jericho 10,000 years ago so they could grow and control their supply of food and protect themselves from their enemies. They worshipped hundreds of gods, praying for divine intervention that would let them find food, protect them from death, ease their pain, or increase their pleasure. They fasted, danced incessantly, practiced self-hypnosis, chanted, inflicted pain on themselves, went without sleep, meditated, and used other nondrug methods so they could receive revelations from the gods (Furst, 1976; La Barre, 1979). By chance and by

experimentation, they found that ingesting or smoking certain plants could help them communicate directly with their gods or at least help them believe they were. They also found these plants could ease fear and uncertainty, reduce pain and anxiety, and even treat some illnesses. Our modern environment has other uncertainties, pains, illnesses, insecurities, and fears (including boredom) that can cause a person to experiment with and possibly abuse drugs.

2. A susceptible brain chemistry that can be affected by psychoactive drugs (to induce an altered state of consciousness or mood, control pain, or treat illness)

If psychoactive drugs did not affect human brain chemistry in a desirable manner, then they would not be used to change consciousness. All psychoactive drugs affect the primitive brain that controls emotions, natural physiological functions (e.g., breathing, heart rate), emotional memories, sensory perception, physical and emotional pain, and instincts. They also affect the

reasoning and memory centers of the new brain called the "neocortex." Parts of these survival mechanisms and neurochemicals in the brain evolved hundreds of millions of years ago in invertebrate creatures, such as insects and snails, and grew in complexity in vertebrate creatures, especially Homo sapiens (Nesse & Berridge, 1997).

3. Business and government involvement in growing, manufacturing, distributing, taxing, and prohibiting drugs

The intensity of the demand for substances that could relieve pain and induce pleasure has matched the struggles for control of the supplies. The supplies of those substances have always been limited since effective agricultural, manufacturing, and distribution techniques have only existed for the last few hundred years. Some of the results of the desire for control of the supply have been

◇ use of opium by the medicine men of ancient Sumeria for their secret medicines;

◇ doling out of beer by the pharaohs to keep their slaves building pyramids;

◇ keeping secret the recipe for preparing mandrake and belladonna potions by shamans, Greek oracles, and witches in the Middle Ages;

◇ monopolization of coca leaf growing by the Conquistadors in Peru to increase tax revenues for Spain;

◇ exportation and taxation of rum, hemp, and tobacco to finance the American Revolution;

◇ sale of opium in China by Britain, Japan, and other imperial powers to support their colonies;

◇ and prohibition or restriction of gin, tobacco, opium, cocaine, and most every other psychoactive drug by virtually every country at one time or another, to control excessive drug use.

4. Technological advances in refining and synthesizing drugs

Over the centuries, various cultures have learned how to

◊ distill alcohol to higher potency (China, 600, Holland, 1600);

◊ refine morphine from opium (Germany, 1803);

◊ refine cocaine from coca leaves (Germany, 1855);

◊ refine heroin from morphine (England, 1874);

◊ create alcohol sedation in pill form by synthesizing sedative barbiturates (Germany, 1868 and 1908);

◊ create synthetic cocaine in the form of amphetamines (Germany, 1887 and 1932);

◊ increase the THC content of marijuana through the sinsemilla-growing technique (1960–1980);

◊ create synthetic and designer drugs to avoid the law, get high, and make money (1960–present).

These and other techniques have enabled drug users to put larger and more potent amounts of a substance in their bodies.

5. Development of more efficient and faster methods of putting drugs in the body

Technological and pragmatic discoveries have taught researchers and/or users to

◊ mix alcohol and opium for stronger effects (Sumeria, 4000 B.C.);

◊ inhale marijuana for greater absorption (Scythia, 500 B.C.);

◊ chew coca leaf with charred oyster shells to increase drug absorption (Peru, 1450);

◊ smoke opium to intensify the high (Arabia, 1600);

◊ inject morphine to put the drug directly into the bloodstream (England, 1855);

◊ mix wine and cocaine to make stimulant wines (France, 1885);

◊ snort cocaine to absorb the drug more quickly (Europe, 1900);

◊ dissolve LSD onto blotter paper so it can be absorbed on the tongue (United States, 1960s);

◊ smoke cocaine freebase and "crack" (United States, 1975);

◊ modify the amphetamine molecule to produce a street drug called "ice," which is twice as powerful as regular methamphetamine (United States, 1989);

◊ dissolve heroin into a water-based nasal spray for a quick yet safe (no IV-induced HIV or hepatitis C virus) access to the brain (United States, 1990s).

These techniques and others enabled users to shorten the time from ingestion of the drug until it reached the brain. When the history of substance use is closely examined, the five themes identified above appear time and time again. If we study the use of drugs in the past, then current drug problems become more comprehensible.

"Most of the crime in our city is caused by cocaine."
Police Chief of Atlanta, GA, 1911

HISTORY OF PSYCHOACTIVE DRUGS

PREHISTORY & THE NEOLITHIC PERIOD (8500–4000 B.C.)

Many of the drugs available today are of recent refinement or synthesis but they have antecedents in plants that have been around for hundreds of millions of years. It has been estimated that 4,000 plants yield psychoactive substances. About 150 have been used for their hallucinatory properties while only about 60 have been in constant use throughout history, with opium, *Cannabis,* coca, tea, coffee, tobacco, and plants that yield alcohol predominating (Austin, 1979).

Evidence exists that Neanderthals used medicinal plants 50,000 years ago and spread their use to neighboring locales. For example, one hypothesis maintains that mind-altering or psychoactive drugs were used by prehistoric shaman healers throughout Eurasia and that the earliest Native Americans were Eurasians who brought their interests in these drugs, such as the hallucinogenic mescal bean and sophora seeds, with them as they migrated to the Americas about 10,000 to 15,000 years ago (Furst, 1976; LaBarre, 1979).

Alcohol has been with us since Prehistoric times. Perhaps hunger, thirst, or curiosity made early humans eat or drink naturally growing substances that had begun to ferment (chemically change

into alcohol due to airborne yeast). Liking the taste, the nutrition, and the psychoactive effects, particularly the drunken states that made them feel closer to their gods, they learned how to make fermented beverages themselves (O'Brien & Chafetz, 1991). They collected honey to ferment into an alcoholic beverage called "mead"; they cultivated grains and used a more complex process to ferment starchy foods into beer; and finally they cultivated grapes and other fruits to make wine. These are the earliest signs of organized efforts to guarantee a steady supply of a desirable psychoactive substance. For example, jars found in a Neolithic kitchen in Iran, dating to 5000 B.C., contained a residue of reseinated wine (McGovern, Gluskee, Exner, & Voight, 1998).

ANCIENT CIVILIZATIONS (4000 B.C.–A.D. 400)

Civilizations arose where the land was fertile, usually next to rivers, such as the Tigris and Euphrates in the Middle East and the Nile in Egypt. The earliest crops were wheat and barley, used to make bread and beer (beer was much more nutritious than it is today) (Ganeri, Martell, & Williams, 1998). Asian civilizations used rice to make wine. Some ancient cultures also cultivated the opium poppy and hemp (marijuana). Nevertheless, despite the value and sometimes reverence placed on psychoactive substances, the reaction of the human brain and body to these drugs caused problems, particularly with beer and wine. Civilizations have differed in the religious and social controls placed on alcohol and other drug use.

In ancient times geographic isolation kept the customs of different peoples localized but migration, exploration, conquest, and trade made various psychoactive substances more widely available. The spread of *Cannabis* (also referred to as hemp and marijuana) along ancient trade routes is one example. The more contact people had with other cultures, the more drugs and drug practices there were to choose from.

ALCOHOL

The first written references to alcohol are 6,000-year-old Sumerian clay tablets found in ancient Mesopotamia, now known as Iraq and Iran. They contained recipes for using wine as a solvent for medications including opium. Wine was so prized that important citizens were buried with their own personal drinking cup (O'Brien, 1991).

Many ancient cultures looked on alcohol, particularly wine, as a gift from the gods. In legends Osiris gave alcohol to the Egyptians, as did Dionysus to the Greeks, and Bacchus to the Romans. In ancient Egypt alcohol (a barley beer called "hek") was given as a reward to slaves building the great pyramids. The value of hek was such that

This Egyptian hieroglyphic from 1500 B.C. advised moderation in barley beer drinking as well as avoidance of other compulsive behaviors.

Translation from Precepts of Ani, World Health Organization

bureaucrats were appointed to control its production. In a medical papyrus, about 15% of the prescriptions contained beer or wine.

In China about 180 B.C., a gift of grape wine was sufficient to serve as a bribe to get a civil service job (Lee, 1987). The Jewish people have historically used wine as part of their religious and secular celebrations including circumcisions, weddings, and the Sabbath. Though the Hebrews had eight different wines for various rites and the highest percentage of drinkers, historically they had one of the lowest rates of alcoholism because drunkenness was frowned upon (Keller, 1984). In the Old Testament of the Bible, in the story of the Adam's and Eve's expulsion from the Garden of Eden, one can translate the tree of knowledge as a grapevine and eating the apple as eating fermented grapes. Even the story of Noah has him getting drunk and lying about naked. In fact there are 150 biblical references to alcohol, often warnings.

"Wine gives life
if drunk in moderation.
What is life worth without wine?
It came into being to make people happy.

Drunk at the right time and in the right amount,
wine makes for a glad heart and a cheerful mind.
Bitterness of soul comes of wine drunk to excess
out of temper or bravado.
Drunkenness excites the stupid to a fury to his own harm,
it reduces his strength while leading to blows."

(The Bible, Ecclesiasticus, 31, 27)

All cultures have understood the dangers of heavy drinking. An early documented attempt to regulate and control alcohol use dates back to the Babylonian Code of Hammurabi in 1770 B.C. This code set forth standards of measurement for drink and outlined the responsibilities of tavern owners. (It also showed the status of women in ancient times.)

"If a 'sister of a god' open a tavern, or enter a tavern to drink, then shall this woman be burned to death."
Code of Hammurabi, Babylonia, 1770 B.C.

Another early attempt at temperance (limiting drinking) occurred in

China around 2200 B.C. when the legendary Emperor Yu levied a tax on wine in order to curtail consumption. Centuries later, during the Chu dynasty (1122–249 B.C.), the penalties for drunkenness were severe but at least the upper classes were given a chance at recovery (Cherrington, 1924).

"As to the ministers and officers who have been … addicted to drink, it is not necessary to put them to death; let them be taught for a time …. If you disregard my lessons, then I … will show you no pity."
Emperor Wu Wang, Founder of Chu dynasty, 1120 B.C.

Heavy drinking was recognized as a problem by the Egyptians in 1500 B.C. when their hieroglyphics recommended the moderate consumption of beer. As early as the fourth century B.C., the great philosopher Aristotle wrote about the tendency of alcohol abuse to run in families.

"… women who drink wine excessively give birth to children who drink excessively of wine."
Aristotle, 350 B. C.

Greek society appreciated the dangers of heavy drinking and so recommended diluting wine with water. Warnings abounded, reinforced with cautionary tales of battles lost due to drunkenness (O'Brien, 1991). Unfortunately the temperance of Greek society and the god Dionysus (god of wine and ecstasy) gave way to binge drinking in Roman society, encouraged by Bacchus, a more liberal version of Dionysus. Orgiastic drinking became such a problem that in A.D. 81, the Emperor Comitian destroyed half the nation's vineyards and prohibited the planting of new ones (Keller, 1984). The conflict between heavy consumption and temperance continued. By the fourth century A.D., heavy drinkers were led through town by a cord strung through their noses. Habitual offenders were tied with the nose cord in the public square and left for ridicule.

OPIUM

Around 4000 B.C. the Sumerians, in addition to barley and wheat, cultivated the opium poppy. They named it, *Hul Gil*, the plant of joy. The milky white fluid from the dried bulb was boiled to a sticky gum and chewed, burned and inhaled, or mixed with fermented liquids and drunk. It was used for both its medicinal properties of pain relief or diarrhea control and its mental

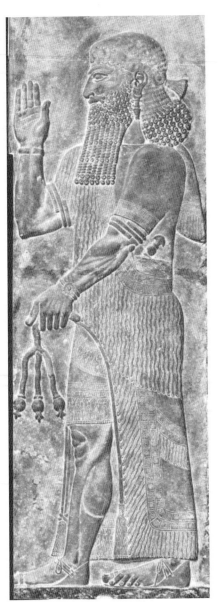

An Assyrian priest carries opium poppies as part of a ceremony to sacrifice a gazelle to the gods, circa eighth century B.C.
The Louvre Museum. Courtesy of Simone Garlaund

properties of euphoria and sedation (Hoffman, 1990). Its bitter taste and the moderate concentration of active ingredients limited the abuse potential. The stalk of the poppy was used as fodder for the animals and the seeds were used in breads and other foods but its main use was as a drug.

Opium was used in many ways. Ancient Egyptian medical texts referred to it as both medicine and as poison. In Egypt it was also a remedy for crying babies. About 700 B.C. in the *Odyssey*, Homer spoke about an opium mixture called "nepenthe," given by Helen of Troy to Telemachus.

"Then Jove's daughter Helen bethought her of another matter. She drugged the wine with an herb that banishes all care, sorrow, and ill humour. Whoever drinks wine thus drugged cannot shed a single tear all the rest of the day, not even though his father and mother both of them drop down dead, or he sees a brother or a son hewn in pieces before his very eyes."
Homer, 850 B.C., Odyssey, IV, 221-226

Greek statues and paintings often show Greek gods and heroes, including Jason and Theseus, holding poppies, which they often used to sedate their enemies (Hoffman, 1990).

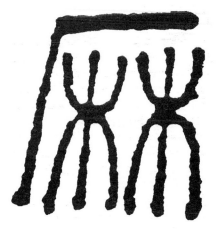

The Chinese ideogram for Cannabis *from the* Pen-tsao *shows two marijuana plants drying in the shed.*
Courtesy of the Fitz Hugh Ludlow Memorial Library

CANNABIS (marijuana)

According to legend, in 2737 B.C., the Chinese emperor Shen-Nung studied, experimented on himself, and recorded his efforts to use *Cannabis* (Ma-fen) as a medicine. In a medical herbal encyclopedia called the "*Pentsao*," written in A.D. 100 but referring back to Shen-Nung and his study of 364 drugs (including ephedra and ginseng), marijuana is not only referred to as a medication but as substance with stupefying and hallucinogenic properties (Schultes & Hoffman, 1992). Over the centuries, marijuana has been recommended for constipation, rheumatism, absent-mindedness, female disorders, malaria, beriberi, and for the treatment of wasting diseases. The Chinese physician Hua T'o, in A.D. 200, recommended *Cannabis* as an analgesic or painkiller for surgery (Li, 1974).

In India almost 1,500 years before the birth of Christ, the *Atharva-Veda* (sacred psalms) sang of *Cannabis* (bhang) as one of five plants that give freedom from distress or anxiety. Other texts listed dozens of medicinal uses for the drug (Aldrich, 1977, 1997).

About 500 B.C. the Scythians, whose territory ranged from the Danube to the Volga River in Eastern Europe, threw *Cannabis* on hot stones placed in small tents and inhaled the vapors. The Greek historian Herodotus wrote,

"The Scythians then take the seed of this hemp and, crawling in under the mats, throw it on the red-hot stones, where it smoulders and sends forth such fumes that no Greek vapor bath could surpass it. The Scythians, transported with the vapor, shout for joy."

(Herodotus, 500 B. C., The Histories, 4.75.1)

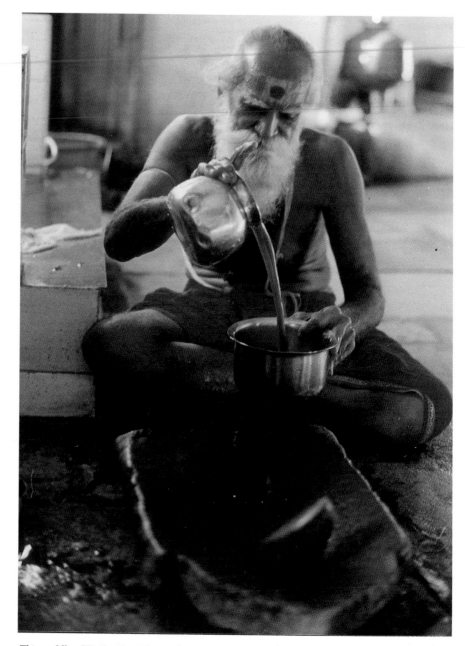

This saddhu (Hindu ascetic) is making a beverage from Cannabis indica. *He grinds the leaves into a paste, filters out the remains of the plant by pouring water through cheesecloth, then drinks the resulting infusion. He uses the drink as part of his religious belief system, for meditation, and concentration. He is a follower of the Hindu God Shiva. Shivaites believe in the use of this intoxicant while many other Hindus do not believe in the use of* Cannabis. *The use of* Cannabis *for spiritual purposes in India goes back at least 3,500 years.*
Courtesy of Simone Garlaund

Most often though, *Cannabis* was prized as a source of fiber and oil, for its edible seeds, and as a medicine. Archaeologists have found traces of its use for the fiber in clothes, shoes, paper, and rope 10,000 years ago in China (Stafford, 1982).

PEYOTE & MESCALINE IN MESOAMERICA

A specimen of the San Pedro cactus, which contains the hallucinogen mescaline and dates back to 1300 B.C., was found in the Peruvian Highlands at a Chavin temple. The cacti were boiled and drunk to produce hallucinations to facilitate communications with supernatural beings (La Barre, 1979). Evidence of use of the peyotl or peyote cactus, which also contains mescaline, dates back 3,000 years. Ceremonial use of these plants was widespread but its foul taste and nauseating effect kept it from everyday use.

COCA LEAF & TOBACCO IN MESOAMERICA

The development of plants containing stimulant alkaloids, such as those found in tobacco and coca leaves, occurred 65–250 million years ago. The bitter alkaloids were the plants' way to keep dinosaurs, other herbivores, and insects away. It wasn't until approximately 5000 B.C., however, that humans, on a regular basis, started drinking, chewing, snorting, and possibly smoking tobacco for religious ceremonies and for the stimulation. About the same time, they started chewing the coca leaf for stimulation, for nutrition, and to control their appetite when food was not available (Siegel, 1982). Burial sites unearthed on the north coast of Peru and dating back to 2500 B.C. contained bags that held coca leaves, flowers, and occasionally a chewed ball of coca leaves called "*cocada.*" The coca was probably used to facilitate the dead one's journey through death. The word "coca" comes from the ancient South American Aymara Indian word, *khoka,* meaning "the tree" (Karch, 1996).

PSYCHEDELIC MUSHROOMS IN INDIA & SIBERIA

The Vedas of ancient India also sang of various psychedelic drugs. Aryan tribes drank an extract of the *Amanita muscaria* mushroom, also called the "fly agaric." In fact "Soma," their name for the hallucinogen, was also the name of one of their most important gods. Over 100 holy hymns from the Rig-Veda are devoted to Soma.

"It is drunk by the sick man as medicine at sunrise; partaking of it strengthens the limbs, preserves the legs from breaking, wards off all disease and lengthens life. Then need and trouble vanish away."
Rig-Veda, 1500 B.C., (McKenna, 1992)

The name "Soma" has been used to represent such diverse drugs as a mythical psychedelic in Aldous Huxley's novel *Brave New World* and a modern prescription muscle relaxant. The intoxication, hallucinations, and delirium produced by psychedelic mushrooms have been employed over the centuries in religious ceremonies by native tribes from India and Siberia. A totally different species of mushroom, *Psilocybe,* was used in Aztec and Mayan cultures in pre-Columbian Mexico (Schultes, 1992).

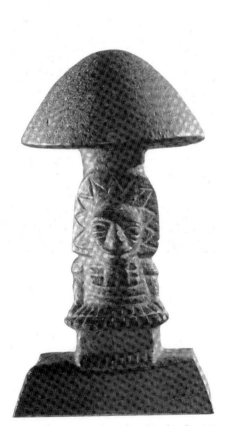

A Mayan stone god, sculpted in the shape of a mushroom (circa A.D. 5), is one of many sculptures of the psychedelic Psilocybe *mushroom. Some date back to A.D. 100.*

Courtesy of Archives Sandoz, Basel

MIDDLE AGES (400–1400)

PSYCHEDELIC "HEXING HERBS"

Other psychedelics used over the centuries include members of the nightshade family *Solanaceae* that contain the psychedelic chemicals atropine and scopolamine. Commonly abused plants in this family are belladonna, henbane, mandrake root, and jimson weed or datura (thornapple). They were sometimes used by medicine men and women accused of witchcraft. Henbane had been referred to as early as 1500 B.C. in Egyptian medical texts. It was used as a poison and a painkiller. It was also used to mimic insanity, produce hallucinations, and generate prophecies. Delirium-inducing datura, another botanical hallucinogen, was taken into the body through skin absorption as a salve or ointment (McKenna, 1992). Belladonna, known as "witch's berry" and "devil's herb," dilates pupils and inebriates the user. Mandrake or mandragora, a root occasionally shaped like a human body, was used in ancient Greece as well as in medieval times. Its properties, similar to those of belladonna and henbane, cause disorientation and delirium.

"... and then, after binding and stupefying the worthy shipmaster with mandragora or intoxication or otherwise, they take command of the ship, consume its stores and, drinking and feasting, make such a voyage."
Plato, 380 B.C., The Republic

PSYCHEDELIC MOLD– ERGOT (St. Anthony's Fire)

Another psychedelic that has persisted through the ages is found in ergot, a brownish purple fungus, *Claviceps purpurea,* that grows on rye or wheat plants and contains lysergic acid diethylamide, the natural form of synthetic LSD. This drug is referred to in ancient Greek and medieval European literature. *Claviceps paspali* was suspected of being used to communicate with the gods. It was recognized as a poison as early as 600 B.C. and as a possible medication in the Middle Ages to induce childbirth (Schultes, 1992).

Over the centuries there have been numerous outbreaks of ergot poisoning when whole towns, particularly in rye-consuming areas of Eastern Europe, seemed to go mad, occasionally with great loss of life. In France in A.D. 944, 40,000 people are estimated to have died from an ergotism epidemic (Seigal, 1985). There were outbreaks as recently as 1953 in France and Belgium. Hallucinations, nervous convulsions, possibly permanent insanity, a burning sensation in the feet and hands, and gangrene that occasionally caused a loss of extremities—toes, feet, fingers, noses—were common. One of the outbreaks in 1039 probably gave the name "St. Anthony's Fire" to the affliction when a wealthy French citizen and his son who were afflicted with the disease, prayed to St. Anthony, a fourth century saint who protects supplicants against fire, epilepsy, and infection. His and his son's recoveries inspired the father to build a hospital in Dauphiné, France (where St. Anthony was buried) for the care of sufferers of ergotism.

MEDICINE, TO PSYCHOACTIVE DRUG, TO POISON

It is important to remember that the same substance (e.g., ergot) can be a medicine at a low dose, a psychoactive drug at a moderate dose, and a deadly poison at a high dose. Healers and shamans would experiment with various substances to find the correct dose to heal a patient or induce a trance state and probably lost a few patients in the process. Another example of dose-dependent effects is the coca leaf. Chewing a few coca leaves releases enough cocaine to keep a chewer awake and working. A large amount of chopped coca leaves mixed with lime to increase absorption will cause a mild high, keep the chewer chewing and awake for days while suppressing ap-

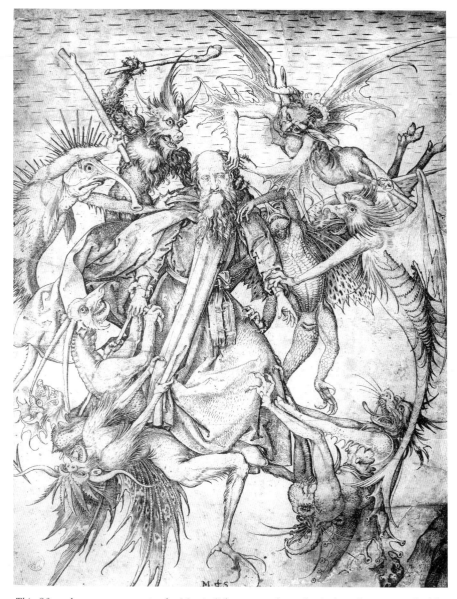

This fifteenth century engraving by Martin Schongauer shows St. Anthony being assaulted by visions of sexual licentiousness and savage animals, visions similar to those caused by the ergot fungus found on spoiled rye or wheat cereal grasses. The chemical produced by the fungus is a natural source for lysergic acid, a naturally occurring form of LSD. St. Anthony's success in battling his demons and hallucinations associated him with ergotism and so St. Anthony's Fire became a synonym for the ergot-caused affliction. Ergotism was often fatal because it led to gangrene and extreme delirium.

petite. A high dose of cocaine, refined from the coca leaf and injected or smoked, can freeze the heart and cause a fatal overdose.

ALCOHOL DISTILLATION

Alcoholic beverage consumption continued throughout the Middle Ages with cultural attitudes bouncing between abstention and bingeing. Technical advances in cultivation and purification also made a difference in consumption. In China about A.D. 400, the Chinese Alchemist Ko Hung wrote about wine purification. His description has been taken to mean distillation, that is, raising the alcohol content of beverages from 14% up to 40% or more through an evaporation process (McKenna, 1992). Even though techniques for distillation of seawater and alcohol had been around for thousands of years (e.g., boiling mead under a cloth that catches the evaporating alcohol and is wrung out), it wasn't until the eighth to fourteenth centuries that knowledge of the techniques became widespread. An Arabian alchemist named Geber is credited with perfecting a wine distillation method in the eighth century A.D. Distillation of whiskey in Ireland was popular by the twelfth century, particularly because the cold damp climate was bad for grape cultivation (O'Brien, 1991). In the thirteenth century two chemists in Switzerland, Arnaldus de Villanova and Raymone Lully, promoted distilled alcohol or *aqua vitae* (water of life) as a marvelous cure-all and longevity enhancer.

In the Middle Ages European monasteries and feudal lords used the *sirah* grape, imported during the Crusades, to cultivate their own vineyards and assure a supply of wine for their thirst, for their meals, for passing thirsty travelers, and for the Eucharist (sacrament) of the Catholic Church. Since alcohol also killed bacteria and microorganisms that lived in water, alcoholic beverages, along with boiled beverages, were often the only safe liquids to drink.

ISLAMIC SUBSTITUTES FOR ALCOHOL

After wine was condemned by the Koran in the seventh century, many Islamic countries banned its use. Since the reasons that people were drawn to psychoactive substances remained, some Muslims searched for alternatives. Opium for the relief of pain, both physical and mental, was seen as an acceptable substitute. Later coffee, tobacco, and hashish (concentrated marijuana) were employed as substitutes for alcohol in order to provide stimulation, induce sedation, and alter consciousness.

Khat, a stimulant, was permissible in Islamic cultures. It was originally cultivated in the southern Arabian Peninsula and the Horn of Africa. It was used during long prayer ceremonies to help the people stay awake. Khat also seems to have paved the way for coffee among Islamic peoples. In A.D. 1238 the Arab physician Naguib Ad-Din distributed khat to soldiers to prevent hunger and fatigue. In the fourteenth century another Arab king, Sabr Ad-Din, gave it freely to subjects he had recently conquered to placate them and quell their revolutionary tendencies (Giannini, Burge, Shaheen, & Price, 1986).

COFFEE (caffeine)

Centuries after the coffee plant *Coffea Arabica* was found growing wild in Ethiopia about A.D. 850, it was imported and intensely cultivated in Arabia around the fourteenth century. It was popularized by those who liked the stimulation but condemned by Orthodox Muslims because it was intoxicating although, like khat, it helped worshippers stay awake during long prayer ceremonies (Coste, 1984). The stimulating chemical, caffeine, made many ignore the mosque's condemnation. At first, coffee was consumed by chewing the beans or by infusing them in water. It was also used for medicinal purposes (e.g., diuretic, asthma treatment, headache relief). Then during the later Middle Ages, coffee, like alcohol, was made even more potent once people learned how to roast and grind the beans, producing a tastier version. It took 500 more years (1820) until caffeine, the active alkaloid in coffee and tea, was finally identified.

Tea was supposedly used in China thousands of years before the discovery of coffee but the first written evidence of its use didn't appear until approximately A.D. 350. The fact that boiling water killed germs made it a popular drink. Cultivation of tea in Japan and development of tea ceremonies occurred about A.D. 800 and remained the heart of social and religious ceremonies to the present day (Harler, 1984). There are also approximately 60 other plants that contain caffeine, such as guarana, mate, yoco, kola nut, and cocoa.

COCA IN THE NEW WORLD

Almost eight centuries ago in South America, the legendary Inca Emperor Manco Capac, worshipped as the divine son of the Sun god, was supposed to have brought the coca leaf to earth to satiate the hungry, strengthen the weak, and help them to forget their misfortunes (Scrivener, 1871). All the nobility carried their precious supply of

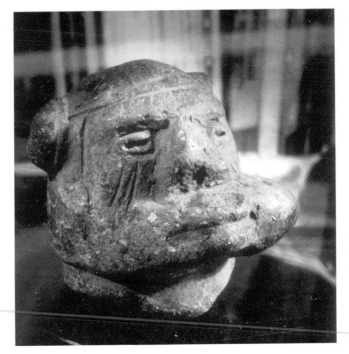

Colombian stone head depicting user's cheek stuffed with cocada, coca leaf mixed with powdered lime.
Courtesy of the Fitz Hugh Ludlow Memorial Library

coca leaves in ornate bags strapped to their wrists. A plentiful supply of the drug, which was considered divine, was buried with the nobility. Coca use was started by pre-Inca cultures about A.D. 600 but previous cultures, such as the Valdivia, began their use of coca leaf as early as 1500 B.C. (White, 1989).

PSYCHEDELIC FUNGI & PLANTS IN THE AMERICAS

To the north of the Inca Empire, about the time Columbus arrived in the Americas, the Aztec, Huichol, Cora, and Tarahumare Indians of Mexico were digging up the peyote cactus (containing mescaline), "magic" mushrooms (containing psilocybin), and the ololiuqui or morning-glory seed (containing LSD-like ergot alkaloids). They celebrated the hallucinogenic effects of these plants in sacred ceremonies. Later, missionaries wrote that the North American Indians used the drug to communicate with the devil (Diaz, 1979). They were rarely used recreationally like alcoholic beverages, tobacco, or coca leaves.

RENAISSANCE & THE AGE OF DISCOVERY (1400–1700)

Two general trends continued the spread of psychoactive substances. Beginning with Portuguese, Spanish, British, and Dutch exploration, trade, and colonization, Europeans encountered diverse cultures and unfamiliar psychoactive plants. The most notable substances were coffee from Turkey and Arabia, tobacco and coca from the New World, tea from China, and the kola nut from Africa. Similarly, European explorers, soldiers, merchants, traders, and missionaries carried their own culture's drug-using customs and drugs (mainly alcohol) to the rest of the world. Greater secularization of life (less control by churches), urbanization, spreading wealth, and growing personal freedom increased use.

ALCOHOL

It is important to note that it was the actual overuse and subsequent toxic effects of alcoholic beverages, particularly high-potency distilled beverages that led to most laws limiting use. Switzerland and England passed closing time laws in the thirteenth century. Even Scotland and Germany limited sales on religious days in the fifteenth century (O'Brien, 1991). But since the medicinal and recreational values of drinking were well established, laws were aimed more at temperance than prohibition, particularly since the increasing availability of distilled beverages produced hefty tax revenues. There was a belief in alcohol's curative properties and it was given for many ailments. Even monasteries used to dispense alcoholic beverages to visitors. The French Benedictine Monk Dom Bernardo Vincelli invented Benedictine®, a high-potency liqueur (43% alcohol), in 1510. The liqueur, which contained 30 different aromatic substances besides sugar, fruit rinds, honey, and brandy, helped support the religious order and gladden visitors until 1793 when the monastery was destroyed in the French Revolution. The recipe for the liqueur was preserved and is still manufactured today (O'Brien, 1991).

COCA & THE CONQUISTADORS

One example of how the economic and political needs of a country transformed the way a substance was used is the interaction between the Spanish Conquistadors who colonized Peru in the 1500s and the native Indians' use of coca leaf. Until the explorers/invaders arrived, coca leaf was used as a mild stimulant, as a reward, and as a way to suppress hunger and thirst.

"They carry them from some high mountains, to others, as merchandise to be sold, and they barter and change them for mantillas, and cattle, and salt, and other things."

(Monardes, 1577)

As the Incas cultivated a larger supply, some people chewed throughout the day, much as Americans drink coffee nowadays, but since the leaf was only 0.5% cocaine, it was never toxic. When the Conquistadors started to exploit the silver mines they discovered at extremely high altitudes in the Andes mountains, they needed to find ways to keep the subjugated Indians working. The Spanish started appropriating the Incan coca plantations and planted thousands of acres more so they could keep the natives supplied with the stimulant. They planted so much that at times there was a glut on the market (Cleza de Leon, 1959). Coca chewing increased dramatically as did revenue from the trade. About eight percent of the Spaniards living in Peru were involved in the coca trade (Gagliano, 1994). They even had their own lobby back in Spain. Although the tax revenues from the coca trade helped pay for the colony, there were also many Spaniards who opposed the use of coca (Acosta, 1588). But even the church was split between needing the revenue to pay for their missionary activities vs. revulsion at the way the Incas were exploited and doubt that someone chewing coca could be converted to Christianity. Native workers at the silver mining towns spent twice as much on coca leaves as they did for food (Karch, 1997).

TOBACCO CROSSES THE OCEANS

Along with coca, tobacco was also cultivated in the Western Hemisphere by various Native Americans. In 1492 after Christopher Columbus had crossed the Atlantic and landed in Hispaniola in the Caribbean, he noted the natives' use of tobacco. They used it as a medicine for a wide variety of ailments including headache, snakebite, stomach and heart pains, skin diseases, and toothaches. It was also widely used for rituals including planting, fertility, good fishing, consulting the spirits, and preparing magical cures. Shamans in South America used the toxicity of tobacco to induce comas and trance-like states to awe their tribesmen (Benowitz &

Fredericks, 1995). Columbus also noted that the Caribbean natives snuffed cohoba, a potent hallucinogenic substance. The chronicler Monardes wrote about the use of tobacco in South America.

"When they used to travel byways, where they find no water nor meat, they take a little ball of these (tobacco balls), and they put it between the lower lip and the teeth, and they go chewing it all the time that they do travel, and that which they do chew, they do swallow it down."

Monardes, 1574

(Most historians point out that there is absolutely no evidence that the Inca used tobacco. Thus they feel that Monardes' quotes about tobacco use by the Inca were a mistake. He misidentified coca leaf as tobacco leaf and what he is really chronicling is the Inca use of coca.)

Soon the Spaniards and the British were exporting tobacco to Europe where it was received enthusiastically, originally as a medicine and later as a stimulant, mild relaxant, and mild euphoriant. Sir Walter Raleigh brought "tobacco smoking for recreation" to the court of Queen Elizabeth (Benowitz, 1995). In France tobacco was called "nicotiana" after Jean Nicot who described its medicinal properties. Portuguese sailors introduced tobacco to Japan where its cultivation began about 1605. The Portuguese also introduced tobacco to China where it was also highly regarded as a medicine. It was carried throughout China by soldiers, then banned, then taxed. It was in vogue at the Emperor's court, then among the people, and then actively propagated throughout Asia. Despite sporadic attempts at prohibition by rulers, governments, and churches that thought tobacco use to be wrong or harmful to society, its use spread.

"The use of tobacco is growing greater and conquers men with a certain secret pleasure, so that those who have once become accustomed thereto can later hardly be restrained therefrom."

Sir Francis Bacon, 1620

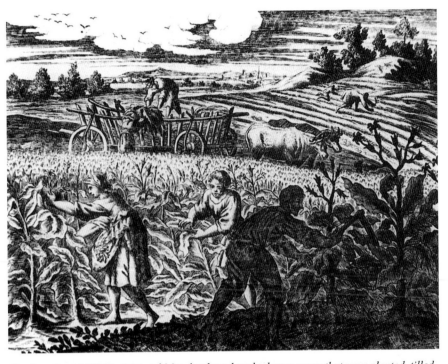

Starting about 1610 Virginia and Maryland produced tobacco crops that were planted, tilled, and picked by slave labor and which supported the Chesapeake Colonies for two centuries.
Courtesy of The National Library of Medicine, Bethesda

Back in Europe, the dangers of fire, the congregation of smokers in tobacco houses or tobacco taverns where ideas and politics were discussed, and the abuse of tobacco by the clergy led to vigorous attacks by various authorities including King James I of England.

"[Smoking is] a custome lothsome to the eye, hatefull to the Nose, harmefull to the braine, dangerous to the Lungs, and the blacke stinking fume thereof, neerest resembling the horrible Stigian smoke of the pit that is bottomless."

(James I, 1604)

Pope Urban VIII forbade smoking under pain of excommunication. It was also forbidden in Turkey by sultans under pain of torture and death and banned by Czars Michael and Alexis in Russia under similar penalties (Benowitz, 1995). But smuggling and widespread covert use by clergy, by commoners, and by people at court defeated all attempts at prohibition. Over the centuries, the craving for tobacco and the addictive qualities of nicotine have overwhelmed most calls for prohibition.

From the beginning the economic power of trade in a substance that was both pleasurable and habit forming was recognized. Eventually tobacco became a large source of revenue for many governments, especially for Spain and later for England.

COFFEE & TEA

Coffee drinking became widespread in Europe, first among wealthy classes, then, as quantities increased and prices declined, among middle and lower classes. Coffee became a favorite drink as an alternative to alcohol use and abuse. In cities, such as Amsterdam, London, and later on Paris, New York, and Boston, it was drunk in coffeehouses that became popular centers of intellectual, political, and literary discussion and news circulation. The truth was they were popular because Lloyds of London and others started taking bets (insurance) on ships. They were also popular in both Turkey and

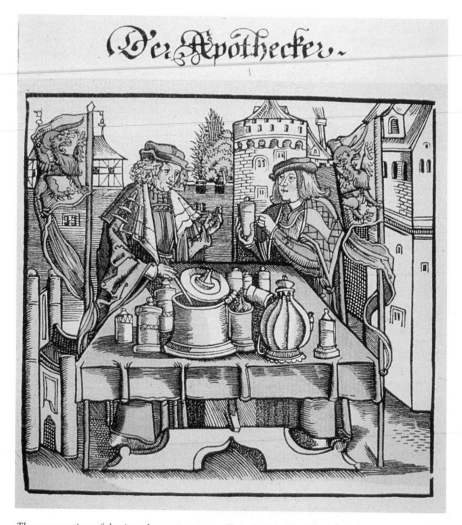

Der Apothecker

The preparation of theriac, the ancient cure-all, is depicted in this sixteenth century woodcut. From H. Brunschwig, Das Neu Distiller Buch, *Strassburg, 1537.*

Courtesy of the National Library of Medicine, Bethesda

pearls, coral, amber, musk, and essential oils added). It was employed as a panacea or cure-all medication and, for many, a simple way to soothe a crying child. It was readily available, inexpensive, and soon was widely used (and abused) in all strata of society. Laudanum, like both nepenthe and theriac (opium preparations) before it, was found in most home remedy chests. Parcelsus believed and widely promoted the idea that pain relief and sleep were part of the cure for any disease and so he medicated many of his patients with medicines containing opium (Karch, 1997).

AGE OF ENLIGHTENMENT & THE EARLY INDUSTRIAL REVOLUTION (1700–1900)

The development of refined forms of psychoactive drugs, new methods of use, and improved production techniques, along with governments' and merchants' economic motives, led not only to greater and greater numbers of users but also to a greater proportion of users who developed mental and physical problems including abuse and addiction.

DISTILLED LIQUORS & THE GIN EPIDEMIC

Beer and wine had long been part of the European diet. Ancient beer, much thicker than modern beer, was a food contributing B vitamins and other nutrients to European diets. Wine, used moderately, was beneficial to health and had some food value. Some people then began to drink distilled spirits (40% alcohol concentration) having virtually no nutritional content just to get drunk. Distilled spirits are often said to provide "empty calories," that is caloric food value with no real nutrition.

Gin, first made in Holland during the 1600s from fermented mixtures of

England where coffeehouses were closely watched by authorities as possible hotbeds of political dissent, sedition, and revolution.

Tea wasn't popular outside Asia until Dutch traders introduced it in Europe in 1610 and in America 40 years later. Then its popularity grew until it became the center of social interaction and a ritualistic part of family life.

OPIUM RETURNS

During the Renaissance in the fifteenth and sixteenth centuries, the use of opium in medicinal concoctions came back into favor when the works of

the second-century physician Galen and the Moorish physician Avicenna became widely taught in medical education (Acker, 1995). Theriac, one of the opium preparations that came into favor again, was used in the Middle East and in Europe. It originally contained more than 70 ingredients in addition to opium and Galen added over 30 more. It was prescribed for an incredible variety of illnesses including inflammation, diarrhea, headaches, anything involving pain, and even pestilence.

In 1524 Paracelsus (Theophrastus von Hohenheim) returned from Constantinople to Western Europe with the secret of laudanum, a tincture of opium in alcohol (with henbane juice, crushed

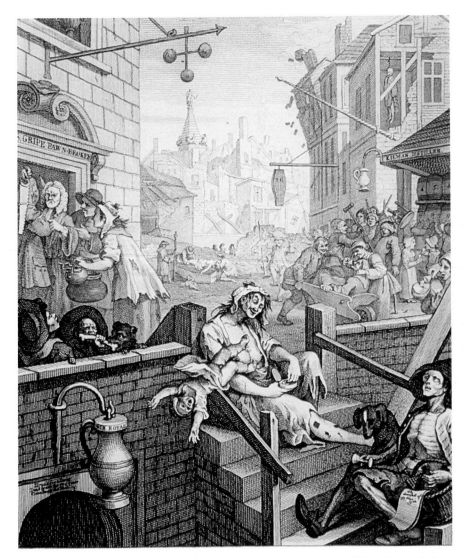

The gin epidemic devastated London from 1710 to 1750. Engraving by William Hogarth depicts "Gin Lane."

Courtesy of the National Library of Medicine, Bethesda

During the latter half of the eighteenth century, rum was the chief medium of exchange in the slave trade and one of the mainstays of the economy of colonial America producing probably the highest level of alcohol consumption in American history. A farmer using a 25¢ bushel of corn could produce two and a half gallons of whiskey valued at $1.25 that could be shipped easily and not spoil (Skolnick, 1997). Around 1790 per capita consumption was three times what it is today. Similarly, white trappers and settlers trading whiskey ("firewater") to Native Americans for furs in the late eighteenth and early nineteenth centuries led to epidemics of alcoholism among both settlers and indigenous peoples.

TOBACCO, HEMP, & THE AMERICAN REVOLUTION

Tobacco was introduced to the Jamestown colony in 1612. *Nicotiana tabacum* (Virginia leaf) became a mainstay for the southern colonies as much of it was exported to England. Virtually all of it was chewed or smoked in cigars and pipes. Tobacco was so important to America that sculptures of tobacco leaves and flowers were used to decorate the columns supporting the dome of the U.S. Capitol building which was built in 1818 (Slade, 1989). Tobacco, along with rum (and continental currency or "continentals" that weren't worth much), helped finance much of the U.S. Revolutionary War.

King George III of England sent a proclamation to America in 1764 to encourage the planting of hemp, another important crop in the new American colonies, to send to England. "Hemp" is the word used to describe *Cannabis sativa* plants that are high in fiber content and generally low in psychoactive components. "Marijuana" is used to describe *Cannabis sativa* plants that are high in psychoactive ingredients. George III wanted to monopolize the hemp trade and required the Americans to buy back their own hemp from England. George Washington directed

grains flavored with juniper berries, became popular throughout Europe. When the English Parliament encouraged production and consumption, urban alcoholism and the mortality rate skyrocketed. During the London Gin Epidemic from 1710 to 1750, the novelist Henry Fielding said that gin was the principal sustenance of more than 100,000 Londoners, and he predicted that

"... should the drinking of this poison be continued at its present height, during the next 20 years, there will be

by that time very few of the common people left to drink it."
Fielding, 1740

It was estimated that one house in six in London was a gin house. Production went from ¹/₂ million gallons in 1684 to 19 million gallons in 1742, and when distillation was banned in 1742, back to 4 million. It showed how unlimited production of a desirable substance causes excess use. Only stiff taxes and the strict regulation of sales brought the epidemic under control (Lichine, 1990).

colonists to comply but to retain much of their own hemp in America. His purpose was to establish an American textile and rope industry so the colonies could depend on a local supply. George Washington cultivated hemp at his Mount Vernon plantation and he too encouraged its production as a domestic source of rope and sails for the fledgling navy of the United States. Until the Civil War, hemp was the South's second largest crop behind cotton. But because hemp was dependent on slave labor, it was no longer profitable after the slaves were freed.

NITROUS OXIDE, OTHER ANESTHETICS, & OTHER INHALANTS

The first anesthetic called "anodyne" (a liquid form of ether) was discovered in 1730 by Frederick Hoffmann, a German physician. It was used as a medicine, a drink, and an inhalant, often for intoxication because it was thought to be less harmful than alcohol.

Inhaling a gas (as opposed to smoking a drug) became more popular after Joseph Priestly discovered nitrous oxide or "laughing gas" in 1776. Its popularity was encouraged by Sir Humphry Davy in the early 1800s who noted its use as an anesthetic, analgesic, and euphoriant. A nitrous oxide tavern was even suggested by Davy as an alternative to saloons since it had none of the brutalizing effects of alcohol (Agnew, 1968).

"It is a clearly time-saving, exhilarating, angelizing ether; whereas spirituous liquors are besotting, brutalizing, devil-inspiring draughts which in the end clog the ideas whereas the etherial oxide sets them free."

(Chemical Experimentalist, circa 1810. In Lynn, Walter, Harris, et al., 1972)

Several other gases used for anesthesia were also developed during the century including chloroform in 1831. Both men and women participated in "gas frolics" in the 1830s. Later in the nineteenth century, the synthesis of various hydrocarbons (fossil fuels) into solvents increased the range of substances that could be inhaled.

OPIUM TO MORPHINE TO HEROIN

Several areas of development led to the increased use and addiction to opium: technical developments and economic/political developments. The technical developments were the spread of smoking as a means of using opium, the refinement of morphine from opium, the refinement of heroin from morphine, and the invention of the hypodermic needle to inject drugs directly into the body. The economic/political developments stemmed from recognition that huge profits could be made from the drug trade. That money could then finance other activities (e.g., excise taxes to finance exploration or wars of conquest).

Opium Smoking

Opium smoking was first introduced to China about A.D. 1500 by Portuguese traders but didn't become popular for 200 more years. Smoking put greater amounts of the opium into the blood, via the lungs, more quickly and therefore into the brain more quickly, increasing the intensity of the effects. Since the lungs had such a large surface area, large amounts could be absorbed rapidly. Dependence and addiction were therefore more likely to develop.

Morphine

The next development occurred in 1804 when a German pharmacist, Frederick W. Serturner, discovered how to refine *morphium* (morphine) from opium. Morphine is much more powerful than opium and therefore a more effective pain reliever. Given the proliferation of wars in the nineteenth century, the need for effective painkillers for wounded soldiers was high. Morphine was first used in the Crimean War and most notably in the U.S. Civil War. Unfortunately the higher potency of the preparation caused greater changes in the human body leading to more rapid development of a tolerance to the drug and therefore greater dependence on the drug. When opium was ingested (not smoked) and partly metabolized before reaching the brain, overdose was rarely a problem. The potency of morphine made overdose and addiction more common (Karch, 1996; Hoffman, 1990).

Hypodermic Needle

With the development of the hypodermic needle in 1855 by a Scottish physician, Alexander Wood, drugs could be put directly into the bloodstream and therefore reach the brain more quickly causing much more intense effects. It also made it easier to overload the brain. Unfortunately Wood, through self-experimentation, managed to addict himself and his wife to morphine (Karch, 1998). Morphine kits with hypodermic needles were widely distributed by the early twentieth century in the United States. The other result of Serturner's discovery of morphine was the discovery of active alkaloids in many other plants leading to more concentrated forms of a number of drugs.

Heroin

In 1874 diacetyl morphine, better known as heroin, was refined from morphine at St. Mary's Hospital in London by C. R. Alder Wright but it wasn't until 1898 that the German Bayer Company began marketing Heroin® as a remedy for coughs, chest pains, and tuberculosis. At one time it was considered a possible cure for morphine addiction and alcoholism. Of course the greater intensity of the heroin high caused a more rapid progression to abuse and addiction but it wasn't until the twentieth century that heroin became such a large problem on the world stage.

Opium Wars

Economic and political changes were the other factors that increased the use of drugs. The spread of opium in China is a prime example. Opium use in China was mostly medicinal but with the introduction of smoking, many more developed a need for the substance and an addiction. By the late 1700s China was known to be a lucrative trading partner with many national riches like silk, jade, porcelains, and tea, all ripe for exploitation. However, the Chinese didn't seem to be interested in trading their riches for anything except opium that came under the control of the West. Colonial powers vied for the right to sell opium in China. At the same time England had developed an addiction to tea that in the eighteenth century mainly grew in China. Since the Chinese did not want to buy anything that the English sold, the British government grew opium in India to trade for tea with China in order to balance their trade. In the early 1800s the Chinese had banned opium use and imports because of the terrible costs of crime, corruption, and addiction but the British insisted on their "right" of free trade. "The Wars for Free Trade," as the British called them, or the "Opium Wars" (1839–42, 1856–60), as the rest of the world called them, were fought to enforce the British right to sell opium to Chinese merchants who, in turn, sold it to the peasants, creating one of the world's worst drug problems (Wallbank & Taylor, 1992). Later in the century, the French as well as the English both owned a monopoly on the distribution of opium throughout their empires. The resulting addiction of many Chinese, the indignities of China's defeat, and the unequal treaties imposed by Western countries after the Opium Wars continue to complicate China's relations with the West even today (McCoy, 1972; Latimer & Goldberg, 1981).

By midcentury, morphine tablets were being dispensed and by the time of the Civil War, it began to be used by injection. By 1868 both opium and morphine had become cheaper than drinking alcohol and use had spread.

FROM COCA TO COCAINE

One of the most powerful examples of how refinement of a substance changed its use and addiction liability is the history of the coca leaf's transfor-

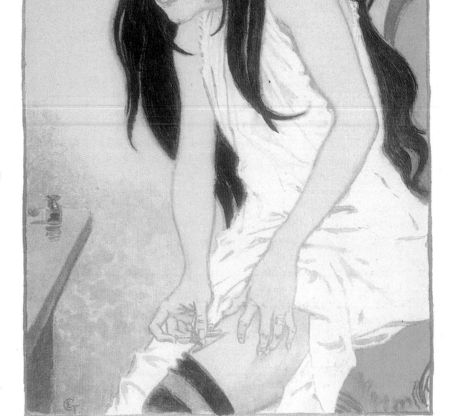

Morphinomanie. *Color lithograph by Eugene Samuel Grasset, 1897.*
Philadelphia Museum of Art. Reprinted, by permission, SmithKline Beecham Corporation Fund for The Ars Medica Collection

mation from mild stimulant to a powerful stimulating drug. Until 1859 when Albert Nieman isolated cocaine, the chief alkaloid of the coca leaf, the drug was chewed or chopped and kept on the gums so the stimulatory effect was similar to several cups of coffee consumed over several hours. The Conquistadors increased the cultivation of the coca bush and spread its use to the masses. They made large quantities available for sale and even as wages to the workers of their fields and silver mines, which increased their work perfor-

mance and endurance. This level of use remained until the late 1800s when three events occurred:

◇ the physician Karl Koller found that cocaine was a great topical anesthetic that made eye surgery possible;

◇ a French chemist, Angelo Mariani, popularized his cocaine wine as a medicinal tonic (Vin Mariani);

◇ Freud published his treatise, *Über Coca,* and suggested its use for a number of ailments.

"Here we would like to recapitulate the indications that Dr. Freud proposed for cocaine in July of last year; these are:
Coca as stimulant;
Coca in the treatment of gastric disorders;
Coca in cachexia [weight loss and wasting caused by illness];
Coca for the treatment of morphine and alcohol addicts;
Coca for the treatment of asthma;
Coca as an aphrodisiac; and
The local application of coca [local anesthetic]."

Guttmacher, 1885

Freud and others also used cocaine to feel better. There is no evidence that he became addicted, only that he experimented extensively.

"During the first hours of the coca effect one cannot sleep, but this sleeplessness is in no way distressing. I have tested this effect of coca, which wards off hunger, sleep, and fatigue and steels one to intellectual effort, some dozen times on myself."

Sigmund Freud, 1884

Because cocaine had been refined and was 200 times stronger than the coca leaf, the mild stimulation produced by chewing the leaf became an intense rush and subsequent ecstatic feeling when injected or smoked and a very powerful stimulant when snorted, absorbed on the gums, or drunk. Though the manufacture and sale of coca wine and patent medicines spread, along with widespread binge use and dependency, the possibility of negative consequences was minimized.

"As, at present, many authorities seem to harbor unjustified fears with regard to the internal use of cocaine, it is not out of place to stress that even subcutaneous injections—such as I have used with success in cases of long-standing sciatica [pinched sciatic

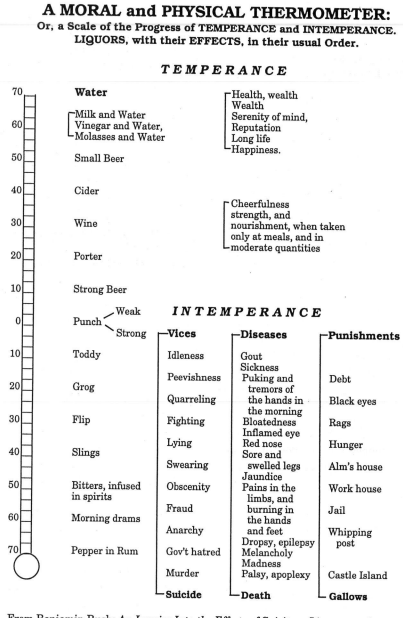

A MORAL and PHYSICAL THERMOMETER:
Or, a Scale of the Progress of TEMPERANCE and INTEMPERANCE. LIQUORS, with their EFFECTS, in their usual Order.

T E M P E R A N C E

70	Water	⎰Health, wealth
60	Milk and Water	Wealth
	Vinegar and Water,	Serenity of mind,
	Molasses and Water	Reputation
50	Small Beer	Long life
		⎱Happiness.
40	Cider	
30	Wine	⎰Cheerfulness
		strength, and
		nourishment, when taken
20	Porter	only at meals, and in
		⎱moderate quantities
10	Strong Beer	

I N T E M P E R A N C E

Punch ⎰Weak
⎱Strong

		Vices	Diseases	Punishments
10	Toddy	Idleness	Gout	
			Sickness	Debt
20	Grog	Peevishness	Puking and tremors of the hands in the morning	Black eyes
		Quarreling	Bloatedness	Rags
30	Flip	Fighting	Inflamed eye	
		Lying	Red nose	Hunger
40	Slings	Swearing	Sore and swelled legs	Alm's house
			Jaundice	
50	Bitters, infused in spirits	Obscenity	Pains in the limbs, and burning in the hands and feet	Work house
		Fraud		Jail
60	Morning drams	Anarchy	Dropsy, epilepsy	Whipping post
		Gov't hatred	Melancholy Madness	
70	Pepper in Rum	Murder	Palsy, apoplexy	Castle Island
		Suicide	Death	Gallows

From Benjamin Rush: *An Inquiry Into the Effects of Spiritous Liquors on the Human body,* 1790

Published in 1790, A Moral and Physical Thermometer *by Dr. Benjamin Rush, an early temperance pioneer, allowed for the moderate and medicinal use of alcohol but warned that excess use would eventually lead to the stocks, insanity, death, jail, or the gallows. His booklet* An Inquiry into the Effects of Ardent Spirits upon the Human Mind and Body *was widely distributed in post-Revolutionary America.*

(Armstrong & Armstrong, 1991)

nerve]—are quite harmless. For humans the toxic dose is very high, and there seems to be no lethal dose."

Sigmund Freud, 1884

It was only been through the hindsight of a generation of abuse that the addictive nature of cocaine was seen and its widespread availability curtailed. Unfortunately the next generation often forgets the lessons of the past.

TEMPERANCE & PROHIBITION MOVEMENTS

The first temperance movement in the United States had been started about 1785 by Dr. Benjamin Rush, a noted physician and reformer who warned against overuse of alcohol but praised limited amounts for health reasons. The disease concept of alcohol was suggested by the early writings of Rush (Goodwin & Gabrielli, 1997). The first national temperance organization, the American Temperance Society, was created in 1826. It was supported by businessmen who needed sober and industrious workers (Langton, 1995). The growth of these societies to more than 1,000 four years later did not stem the increased use of alcohol. Consumption peaked in 1830 in the United States with a per capita consumption of 7.1 gallons of pure alcohol vs. 1.8 gallons today. In fact at Andrew Jackson's inauguration in 1833, the new President's staff stopped serving alcohol because they were afraid drunken revelers would destroy the White House. But it wasn't until 1851 that Maine passed the first prohibition law. Within four years, 1/3 of the states had laws controlling the sale and use of alcohol, and consumption fell to 1/3 of pre-Prohibition and temperance levels. The Civil War stalled and in some cases reversed the prohibition movement but after the war the Women's Crusade, the Women's Christian Temperance Union, and the Anti-Saloon League led the temperance movement, which later became the prohibition movement, into the twentieth century. The first facility that treated alcoholics was a hospital that opened in 1841 in Massachusetts.

FROM PIPES & SMOKELESS TOBACCO TO CIGARETTES

By the middle of the nineteenth century, both men and women used snuff and smoked pipes. In addition men smoked cigars, chewed tobacco, and spat tobacco juice where and when they pleased. One of the changes that propelled tobacco to a grave health problem was the invention of the automatic cigarette-rolling machine in 1884. Historically only small amounts of tobacco had been used—a pinch of snuff or some chopped leaf in the cheek or in a pipe although even at those levels it was addicting. It wasn't until later in the century that automation, advertising, and a more plentiful supply of tobacco vastly expanded the use of cigarettes and smoking.

HEROIN & COCAINE IN PATENT MEDICINES & PRESCRIPTION DRUGS

Over-the-counter medicines sold at the turn of the century had imaginative names, such as Mrs. Winslow's Soothing Syrup, Roger's Cocaine Pile Remedy, Lloyd's Cocaine Toothache Drops, and McMunn's Elixir of Opium, all loaded with opium, morphine, cocaine, and usually alcohol. Needless to say, patent medicines were very popular in all strata of society and were used to cure any illness from lumbago to depression, much like nepenthe, theriac, and laudanum centuries before.

"It may strike you as strange that I who have had no pain—no acute suffering to keep down from its angles—should need opium in any shape. But I have had restlessness till it made me almost mad.... So the medical people gave me opium—a preparation of it, called morphine, and ether—and ever since I have been calling it my amreeta... my elixir."

Elizabeth Barrett Browning, 1837, (Aldrich, 1994)

One of the finest poets of the nineteenth century, Elizabeth Barrett Browning became dependent on opium and morphine in much the same way that other middle and upper class European and American women of that era did, through prescriptions from their physicians. In fact the majority of addicts in the Victorian era were women

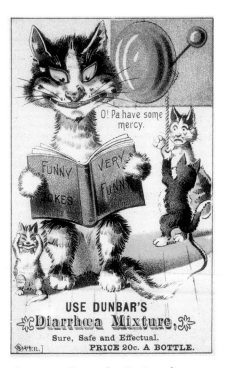

USE DUNBAR'S **Diarrhœa Mixture,**
Sure, Safe and Effectual.
PRICE 20c. A BOTTLE.

Opium was the usual active ingredient on diarrhea medications. It was also prescribed for almost every other illness because it could relieve pain. It was mostly used to treat symptoms rather than correct the disease state.

Courtesy of the National Library of Medicine, Bethesda

(Courtwright, 1982). Some of the more well-known female addicts were the writers Louisa May Alcott, Charlotte Bronte, George Sand, and the actress Sarah Bernhardt. Laudanum compounds and patent medicines, prescribed for nervousness, depression, and menopause, were dispensed by the medical profession and available over-the-counter. Male doctors prescribed hypodermic morphine for almost every complaint presented to them including anemia, angina, and asthma (Aldrich, 1994).

Cocaine was very popular in America by 1885. In 1887 the Hay Fever Association declared cocaine to be its official remedy. It was offered for sale in drug stores, by mail order, and in catalogues. From its formulation in 1886 until 1903, Coca-Cola® contained about five milligrams of cocaine or 1/3 to 1/2 of a "line." Today the beverage contains

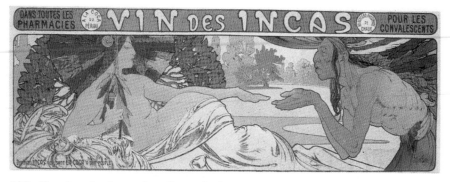

Ad for French tonic wine made with coca leaf extract. It promised to help the user's digestion and disposition (circa 1896 by Charles Levy).

Courtesy of the estate of Timothy C. Plowman

a denatured coca leaves and caffeine (Karch, 1998). In fact Coca-Cola® continues to this day to be the largest single buyer of Trujillo coca extract.

TWENTIETH CENTURY & THE ELECTRONIC REVOLUTION

THE BUSINESS OF TOBACCO

A variety of factors increased the use of cigarettes and decreased the cigar smoking and tobacco chewing that had marked the nineteenth century: public health campaigns against chewing tobacco and spitting; better cigarette paper and machinery for producing more cigarettes at a cheaper cost; development of a milder strain of tobacco that enabled smokers to inhale deeply; and encouragement of women and children to learn to smoke (O'Brien, Cohen, Evans & Fine, 1992).

The pioneer of the "mild" cigarette was the Camel® brand produced by R.J. Reynolds. During the 1920s this brand began to be actively marketed to women (as a symbol of female emancipation), to young people, and to those on diets. Inspired by the success of Prohibition, antismoking efforts redoubled. State laws were passed prohibiting cigarettes but they were largely unenforceable and were repealed by the late 1920s. By the '30s, taxes on cigarettes provided a rich source of revenue

for federal and state governments during the Depression and World War II. Cigarette packs were distributed free to soldiers during World War II and the Korean War. By the end of the war, demand for cigarettes sometimes exceeded supply and smoking was considered socially acceptable.

By midcentury smoking was entrenched in American society. It was a source of revenue for advertisers, retailers, tobacco farmers, the media, and government treasuries. Warnings of the

health hazards of smoking were issued as early as 1945 by the Mayo Clinic. Warnings continued throughout the early 1950s from the American Cancer Society and various heart and physicians' associations. The tobacco industry ridiculed health concerns and responded to health warnings with slogans, such as "Old Golds: For a treat instead of a treatment," and with the formation of The Tobacco Institute, the chief political lobbying group of the industry. In 1964 the Surgeon General issued a report that concluded, "Cigarette smoking is a health hazard." Smoking in the United States generally decreased through the '60s, then began rising during the '70s, and finally went into a long decline that continues into the present.

DRUG REGULATION

Heroin/cocaine kits were advertised in newspapers and sold in the best stores. Even though by the 1890s physicians understood the addictive and health liabilities of opiates and cocaine, it took another two decades before regulation began. The Pure Food and Drug Act (1906) prohibited inter-

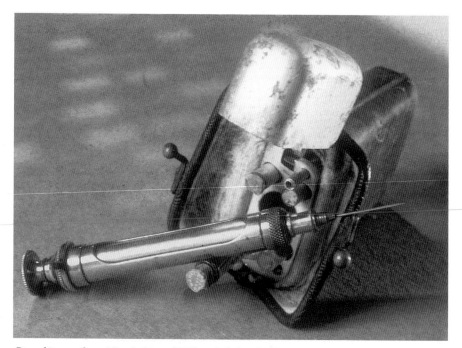

Drug kit on sale at Macy's (circa 1908) included vials of cocaine, heroin, and a reusable syringe. Sears Roebuck also sold a drug kit.

Courtesy of the Fitz Hugh Ludlow Memorial Library

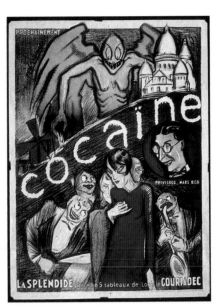

Cocaine regained some popularity in the 1920s and again elicited a backlash about abuse. Posters, plays, books, and films were popular.

Courtesy of the National Library of Medicine, Bethesda

. . . .

state commerce in misbranded and adulterated foods, drinks, and drugs. It required accurate labeling of the ingredients. The Opium Exclusion Act (1909) encouraged the gradual reduction in worldwide opium production and an eventual ban on smoking. Congress banned the importation of opium not intended for medical use the

same year. The Harrison Narcotic Act (1914) controlled the sale of opium, opium derivatives, and cocaine in the United States by requiring all distributors to pay a tax on these drugs that could then be monitored by the federal government (Acker, 1995). These acts and others did, in fact, eliminate the over-the-counter availability of opiates and cocaine in the United States. Unfortunately the tight control of all supplies encouraged prescription drug diversion and the development of a huge illicit drug trade.

ALCOHOL PROHIBITION & TREATMENT

In spite of the fact that between 1870 and 1915, from 1/2 to 2/3 of the U.S. budget came from the tax on liquor, in 1920 it took just 13 months to ratify the Eighteenth Amendment prohibiting the manufacture and sale of any beverage with an alcohol content greater than 0.5%. This was called "the noble experiment" but it wasn't only the United States that tried prohibition. Shorter noble experiments were tried in Iceland, Russia, parts of Canada, India, and Finland among others (Heath, 1995). Thirteen years later it only took 10 months to repeal that same amendment. Americans hadn't changed their feelings about the benefits or liabilities of alcohol. They had simply found out that

Prohibition created other serious problems for America in spite of the fact that it did help control a number of serious health and social problems: cirrhosis of the liver and other alcohol-related diseases declined dramatically; domestic violence fell; and public drunkenness almost disappeared even though people still disregarded the law and drank in speakeasies or made bathtub gin and beer.

Unfortunately, during tenure of the eighteenth amendment, along with the Volstead Act that implemented it, a new coalition of smugglers, strong-arm thieves, Mafia members, corrupt politicians, and crooked police had developed a lucrative trade in the distribution and sale of illicit alcohol. With the return of alcohol to legal status, this coalition turned to other illicit drugs, like heroin and cocaine, which eventually gave rise to a multibillion dollar business that continues to make illegal drugs the leading cause of crime and corruption in the world today.

With the end of Prohibition, alcoholism increased again, though it took 20 years for per capita drinking to reach pre-Prohibition levels. Higher levels of alcoholism were answered by the creation of an organization to help alcoholics recover. Alcoholics Anonymous (AA), a spiritual program that teaches alcoholics 12 steps to recovery, was founded in 1934 by two alcoholics,

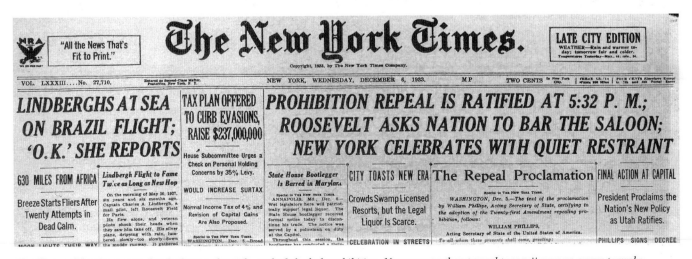

Headlines of the time seemed to be happy about the end of alcohol prohibition. Newspapers then turned to marijuana as a way to make headlines.

. . . .

Bill Wilson and Doctor Bob Smith (AA, 1934). Over the years AA and its offshoots, such as Narcotics Anonymous, have proved themselves to be the most successful drug treatment programs in history (Trice, 1995). Other addictions used the 12-step model to help narcotics addicts, marijuana addicts, overeaters, gamblers, adult children of alcoholics, and even sexual addicts.

The success of Alcoholics Anonymous encouraged the medical community to examine addiction in a new light—as a medical condition rather than as a moral failure.

MARIJUANA: FROM DITCHWEED TO SINSEMILLA

In 1937 *Cannabis sativa* (marijuana) was banned, despite its use in numerous medicines for over 5,000 years. However, the discovery of newer medications lowered its medicinal value. Although marijuana was banned, its sterilized seeds could still be sold for birdseed under the Marijuana Tax

Act. The growing of *Cannabis* in the United States for other economic uses of hemp fiber, rope, paper, and oil were also effectively prohibited in the United States except for a brief period during World War II when hemp fiber was needed by the military. Banning medicinal uses of marijuana was unusual since opiate-based medications, which are stronger than marijuana, were never banned, only controlled through prescription. One reason that marijuana was banned was an antimarijuana campaign by the Hearst newspapers. Publisher William Randolph Hearst had his papers popularize the Spanish word "marijuana" to make the drug sound more foreign and menacing. In addition alcohol prohibition had ended and so there were a large number of federal drug-regulatory employees who needed a new mission. Marijuana seemed a likely target.

During the 1950s marijuana use was confined mainly to specific rural areas, jazz musicians, and residents of urban ghettos. It was celebrated in the

novels and poetry of the "beat" generation poets and writers, chiefly Allen Ginsberg, Jack Kerouac, and Gregory Corso. By the 1960s a new generation began to defy prohibitions against marijuana use, in part because they discovered it was not the demonic drug portrayed in pulp fiction.

It was also a symbol of youthful rebellion against parents, against authority, and even against the war in Vietnam. Once it became popular, people started practicing different growing techniques. Window garden boxes and growing lights became a hot item. The price of marijuana was low ($50 to $100 a pound) as was the concentration of THC, the active psychedelic ingredient, although stronger concentrations were available, along with hashish. It wasn't until the '70s that the sinsemilla-growing technique (which increased the concentration of THC) was widespread and the price skyrocketed. Worldwide, in the 1960s, it was estimated that 250 million people were using marijuana (Fort, 1968).

AMPHETAMINES IN WAR & WEIGHT LOSS

Amphetamine was first synthesized in 1887 and methamphetamine in 1919 but it wasn't until the 1930s when they began to be used medically. Amphetamine was marketed as a decongestant and blood pressure medication under the trade name Benzedrine®. It was during this period when its stimulating effects on the central nervous system were recognized and the drug was used nonmedically as a stimulant to help performance and recreationally for the stimulation and the euphoria. Its appetite suppressant qualities were recognized, along with its calming and focusing effect on children with hyperactivity or attention deficit disorders.

During World War II, in an attempt to improve the physical performance of soldiers, American, British, German, and Japanese army doctors routinely prescribed amphetamines ("speed") to fight fatigue, heighten endurance, and "elevate the fighting spirit" (Marnell, 1997). Illicit amphetamine abuse also

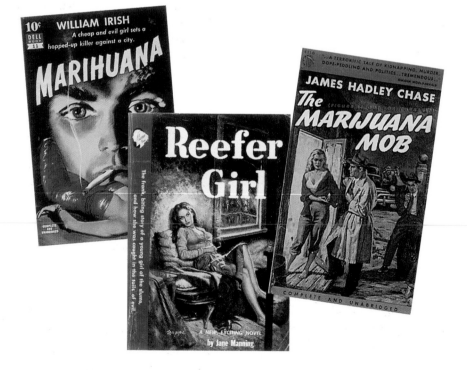

The 1950s saw dozens of pulp novels warning of the dangers of marijuana. The "beat" poets and counterculture writers of the '60s reversed this trend.

increased greatly during the 1940s and '50s among civilian truck drivers and workers engaged in monotonous factory jobs, or college students who needed to cram for their exams.

The appetite suppressant qualities led to the massive use of amphetamines as diet drugs in the '50s and '60s. Ten billion tablets, e.g., Dexedrine® and Dexamyl®, were manufactured worldwide in 1970. In 1970 it is estimated that six percent to eight percent of the American population were using legal amphetamines, mostly for weight loss (Balter, 1972).

Simultaneously with the weight-loss use of amphetamines were their use as the chemical fuel, along with LSD, for the "hippie movement" and the "Summer of Love" in 1967. As a reaction to the suddenly expanded use of amphetamines, LSD, and marijuana, The Controlled Substances Act of 1970 was passed, which initially made it harder to illegally manufacture amphetamines in the United States. (The Controlled Substances Act also controlled the manufacture, sale, and use of all psychoactive drugs.) In addition prescription use of the drugs was more tightly regulated. The street market expanded to fill the need. "Crosstops," smuggled in from Mexico, were the most popular but methamphetamine in powder or crystal form ("crank," "crystal") were also available. In the late '80s a new and more powerful smokable methamphetamine, called "ice," came onto the scene. Also called "L.A. glass" and "rose quartz," it was stronger and its effects lasted longer than regular methamphetamines. The initial center of "ice" abuse was Hawaii. By the beginning of the '90s, its use hadn't spread nearly as rapidly as had been feared although other forms of illegally manufactured amphetamine abuse reached epidemic proportions in western states.

SPORTS & DRUGS

The cold war inflamed athletic competition between the Free World and the Communist block countries. This was very evident at the Olympics and other international sporting events during the years. The use of stimulants, anabolic androgenic steroids, and other performance-enhancing drugs became widespread during the cold war era.

"The athletes themselves came out and told that their coaches and scientists forced these drugs on them. And then they found the records that proved it. I've seen these German girls; swimmers with their beards growing out. We used to dance with them after the meet. And their great strength— you didn't want to mess with any of them. They had muscles. They could knock you out."
Former 1972 Olympic athlete

By 1968 the IOC (International Olympic Committee) had defined doping, made a list of banned substances, and began drug testing (ADF, 1999). The NCAA (National Collegiate Athletic Association) began drug testing 18 years later. By that time the proliferation of various steroids, the expansion of an underground steroid network in weightlifting gyms, the growing sophistication of street chemists, and the growth of over-the-counter nutritional supplements, including andrestondione, GHB, and creatine, had multiplied.

SEDATIVE-HYPNOTICS & PSYCHIATRIC MEDICATIONS

The first barbiturate, marketed in 1903, was Veronal® (barbital). Phenobarbital came 10 years later and eventually 50 barbiturates were used to induce sleep and calm anxiety. They replaced bromides, chloral hydrate, ether, paraldehyde, and opioids used for the same purpose. Their use peaked the 1930s and '40s. Unfortunately the over prescribing of these drugs, plus their addiction and overdose liability, led to the development of Miltown® and other supposedly milder tranquilizers in the '50s and '60s (Hollister, 1983). Benzodiazepines, such as Librium®, Valium®, and later Xanax®, Klonopin®, and Halcion®, came to dominate the prescrip-

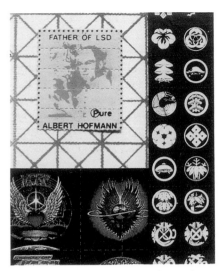

The hallucinogen LSD is manufactured as a liquid and dropped onto perforated blotter paper. A small square is swallowed for the effect. The designs varied from cartoon characters to a picture of Albert Hoffman, the Sandoz Pharmaceuticals® chemist who first synthesized LSD.

tion downer market. At one point in the 1980s, 100 million prescriptions were written for sedative-hypnotics.

The recognition of chemical brain imbalance as a cause of certain mental illnesses led to the development of medications other than antianxiety drugs to treat mental illnesses. The development of tricyclic antidepressants, antipsychotic drugs, and later, selective serotonin reuptake inhibitors (SSRIs) such as Prozac® led to a clearer understanding of both addictive processes and mental illnesses. The use of psychiatric medications and other drugs to aid in detoxification, long-term abstinence, and relapse prevention of drug addicts became much more common.

LSD & THE NEW PSYCHEDELICS

"Since my illumination of August, 1960, I have devoted most of my energies to try to understand the revelatory potentialities of the human nervous system and to make these insights available to others."
Timothy Leary (Leary, 1970)

Dr. Timothy Leary encouraged the youth of the '60s to turn on, tune in, and drop out. The so-called guru of LSD advocated drug experimentation to alter the mind. Psychedelics, such as LSD, marijuana, and psilocybin mushrooms, were the most popular. LSD had been synthesized in 1943 in Switzerland by Albert Hoffman of Sandoz Pharmaceuticals. Various groups experimented with LSD including the psychiatric community, seeing it as a potential treatment for schizophrenia, while the army experimented with it for mind control and disruption of the enemy's thought processes. In the years to come, a flood of new psychedelic drugs, like MDA, MDMA, DOB, DMT, PCP, 2CB, CBR (nexus), and others, combined with the new experimental attitude of the times, made many believe in the slogan, "better living through chemistry."

LEGAL & MEDICAL RESPONSES

The increase in drug use was met with attempts to address the problem of abuse, addiction, and crime brought on by the misuse of drugs. The methods tried were interdiction plus stricter laws concerning use (supply reduction) and prevention coupled with treatment (demand reduction).

As research findings, including the discovery of brain chemicals (endorphins) that acted like psychoactive drugs (heroin), were compiled, understanding of the process of addiction grew and treatment facilities expanded. Alcoholism and other addictions were slowly being defined and, to a certain extent, accepted as illnesses. The treatment of compulsive use became a medical as well as a social science. Some of the treatment protocols tried were therapeutic communities, treatment hospitals, free clinics, 12-step fellowships, and methadone maintenance.

METHADONE & HEROIN

Developed during the 1960s in New York, methadone maintenance treatment programs substituted the legal narcotic methadone for heroin. They spread throughout the country. Methadone maintenance programs attempted to bring the heroin addict population under control. The idea was that if addicted people didn't have to steal for their drug, crime would go down, needle infections would be greatly reduced, and heroin addicts could get some control over their lives. It was an early example of a harm reduction goal that was targeted to benefit society as well as the addict. Methadone maintenance continues today as the medical treatment model for opiate or opioid addiction.

In the 1970s an unpopular war in Vietnam, along with a flood of opium from the Golden Triangle (Burma, Laos, and Thailand), encouraged the use of downers, such as heroin, Valium®, Quaalude®, and the barbiturates. A new group of heroin addicts was created during the years of America's involvement in the war. Only a small percentage of Vietnam veterans continued their heroin use after the war. The bulk of this new wave of heroin abusers was composed of counterculture and inner-city youth.

COCAINE & THE "CRACK" EPIDEMIC

From the 1930s to the 1960s, cocaine use was limited primarily to the inner city, underworld, jazz musicians, and some high-society types. During the late '70s and early '80s, an excess of publicity surrounding cocaine use promoted the drug. Cocaine became the fashionable drug. Restricted to the wealthy and elite at first, cocaine use became widespread as supplies increased and prices dropped (Siegal, 1985).

Snorting, the traditional method for using cocaine, gave way to smokable cocaine, known most commonly as "freebase," "crack," or "rock." Use went from after-hours clubs, to freebase parlors, to "crack" houses and individuals' apartments, and finally to street dealers (Hamid, 1992). The ensuing "crack" epidemic in the mid- and late '80s, was partly fueled by the media's heavy-handed news coverage. Mostly smokable cocaine became widely used because of the low cost of a "hit," the incredibly addictive prop-

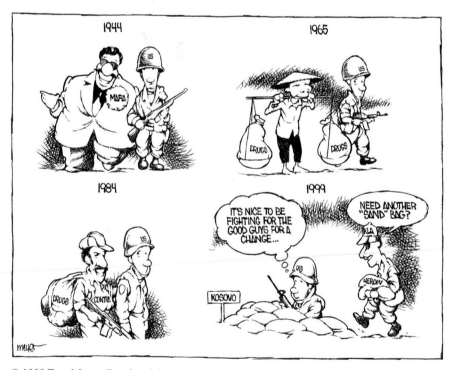

The use of drug profits to finance civil wars and insurrections is well documented. It is also the source of many myths. The full truth will probably never be known.

erties of this form of cocaine, and various socioeconomic forces in the inner city including dissolution of family structures and lack of economic opportunities that led to its spread (Dunlop & Johnson, 1992). Experimentation and binge use was common in the suburbs. At the beginning of the 1990s, "crack" was firmly entrenched in the drug culture but at least its glamorization had faded.

UPPER-DOWNER CYCLE

Beginning in the mid-nineteenth century, the United States saw a cycle of alternating depressant and stimulant abuse eras (Musto, 1997).

◊ Renewed heavy use of alcohol and a generation of morphine abusers populated America after the Civil War.

◊ The widespread use and abuse of cocaine and energy tonics was spurred by Freud and Vin Mariani less than a generation later.

◊ The opium dens and opium-based tonics at the start of the twentieth century were halted by federal and international legislation while heavy alcohol use continued.

◊ Renewed cocaine use, along with expanded cigarette smoking and coffee drinking, marked the Roaring Twenties.

◊ The end of Prohibition expanded alcohol use again, along with use of barbiturates, symbolically coinciding with the Great Depression.

◊ During World War II amphetamines and cigarettes (stimulants) were dispensed to troops freely.

◊ The abuse of depressants like Miltown®, benzodiazepines, and alcohol ("three-martini lunches") followed in the downer years of the '50s and early '60s.

◊ Along with psychedelics and marijuana (all arounders), illegal "speed" or "meth" and legal diet pills became fashionable in the 1960s and '70s.

◊ Some troops brought back their heroin use from Vietnam but the

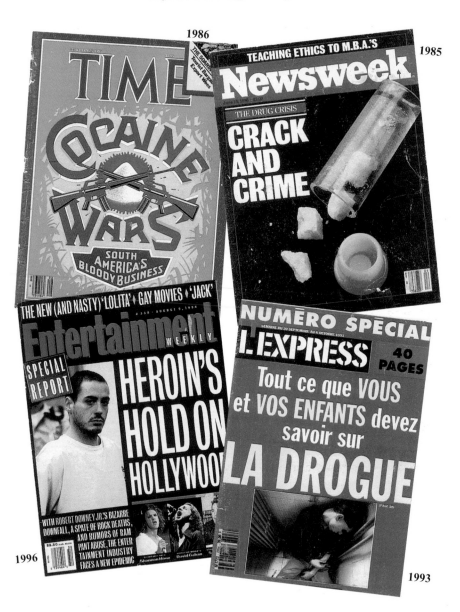

The hundreds of cover stories and headlines about cocaine that deluged the public in the mid-'80s gave the impression that everyone used cocaine. Surveys, however, indicated that only two percent or three percent of the adult population used the drug on a regular basis. In the 1990s the headlines featured heroin because of the growth in use.

drug-seeking counterculture took up heroin, Quaaludes®, benzodiazepines, and alcohol.

◊ The '80s saw the spread of cocaine, particularly smokable "crack" cocaine, and a resurgence of methamphetamines by the late 1980s and into the 1990s.

◊ The '90s saw continued use of amphetamines but heroin has recently made a comeback, along with the continued heavy use of alcohol,

which carried through into the second millennium.

The reasons for these cycles are related to people's desire to experiment with psychoactive drugs, the drugs' shifting patterns of availability, changing political climates, the exigencies of war, general economic conditions, and especially by a social amnesia about the damage done in previous generations by abuse of certain substances.

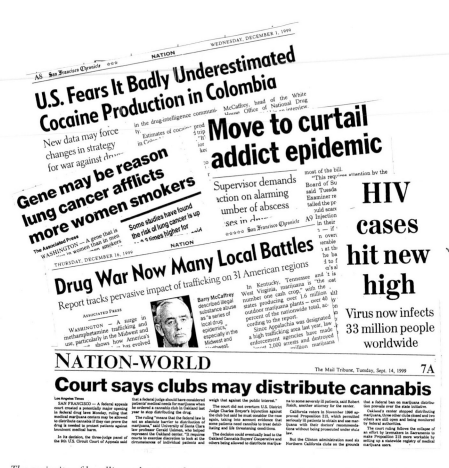

The majority of headlines about psychoactive drugs focus on their negative effects. The positive headlines focus mostly on the heart benefits of moderate alcohol consumption, scientific breakthroughs involving drugs and their neural mechanisms, or the progress of medical marijuana through the courts and ballot box.

TODAY & TOMORROW

Overall, drug use has declined since its peak in 1979 and 1980. The major difference is that the age of first use of almost all psychoactive drugs has gone down. Younger and younger people are using drugs experimentally and socially and are getting into habituation, abuse, and addiction. There has been a slight increase in drug abuse since 1990 but there is a much greater increase in hard-core drug users over the past two decades.

COCAINE

From years of peak use in the early and mid-1980s, cocaine use has generally trended lower, the exact levels of use depending on the age group. Hard-core use hasn't dropped quite so dra-

matically and has spread more to the inner cities. By the late 1990s, "crack" use was declining and cocaine use remained lower, whether by itself (snorted, smoked or injected), or in combination with other drugs. The *U.S. Household Survey* documented that at least 3.8 million Americans had used cocaine during 1998. In 1999 the government reassessed its estimates of the level of cocaine importation when some highly publicized drug busts yielded very high tonnage—it was estimated that a single Colombian cocaine network alone was responsible for 30 metric tons a month (ONDCP, 1999).

METHAMPHETAMINES

The mid-1990s saw street chemists developing newer and more effective ways of manufacturing illicit methamphetamines sold as "crank," "crystal,"

"meth," and "speed." Some of the drugs are produced on small stovetop operations but most of the manufacture and wholesaling is done by Mexican gangs. They either manufacture the drugs in Mexico and smuggle them into the United States or they supply raw materials and personnel to set up labs in the United States, mostly in California. In addition an increase in smoking as the route for methamphetamine has also promoted this resurgence of "speed" abuse (NIDA, 1998).

PSYCHEDELICS & "RAVE" CLUBS

There has also been a modest upsurge in the use of psychedelics, particularly MDMA, and high potency marijuana. LSD is sold in lower dosages than in the '60s and '70s and acts more like a stimulant than a psychedelic. It is one of the drugs used in "rave" clubs, a '90s version of the psychedelic rock clubs of the '60s. At these parties, sometimes held in legitimate clubs, sometimes in hastily rented warehouses, dancing, partying, and drug use are the rule. MDMA, GHB, LSD, amphetamines, Rohypnol® (a sedative), alcohol, Ketamine® ("special k"), 2CB (nexus), and "smart" drinks (drinks containing substances that supposedly help brain function), used individually or in combination with each other, are the most common substances taken at "raves."

MDMA, also known as "ecstasy," "X," "Adam," and "rave," is a stimulatory psychedelic. It has become more widely used in the '90s, much as MDA, a similar drug, was in the '60s. Users claim it is mellower than its chemical kin, amphetamines. MDMA users claim that it promotes closeness and empathy, along with a loss of inhibitions that can trigger a strong urge to dance.

INHALANTS

Another disturbing '90s trend is the use of spray can solvents and their propellants as inhalants. Younger and younger students are inhaling ("huffing") anything from fabric stain protectors to ethyl chloride. Metallic paints and glue are even more common. Young people use inhalants alone or at "huffing" parties. Current trends include formaldehyde and embalming fluid, gasoline additives (STP®), and even Raid Ant and Roach Killer®. Up to 1,200 deaths from inhalant abuse are reported in the United States annually.

HEROIN

Heroin use witnessed a huge resurgence in the late 1990s. Not only are there the traditional "China white" (from the Golden Triangle in Asia) and "Mexican brown" types of heroin, but also "Persian brown," "Mexican or black tar," "Afghani," "Colombian," "African tar," and even an American domestic opium in limited quantities. Because of the money involved and the growing number of users, Chinese tongs (criminal societies) in the early '90s tried to wrest control of a part of the heroin trade in the United States from the Mafia. Indeed, for the first time, federal reports listed the Golden Triangle in Asia as the primary source of street heroin sold in the United States instead of Turkey and Mexico though much of this "China white" enters the United States from the west coast of Canada and is quickly moved to the East Coast where it can be sold at higher prices. The west coast of the United States is left with mostly "black tar." However, the Mexican gangs are fighting back and spreading into distribution of not only heroin but cocaine, marijuana, and methamphetamine as well. The biggest change has been the spread of Colombian heroin. More than 60% of DEA heroin seizures in 1997 were Colombian heroin. The Colombian drug cartels have used their cocaine distribution channels to make their inroads into the heroin market.

MARIJUANA (*Cannabis*) & HEALTH

In a 1999 study of marijuana commissioned by the White House Office of National Drug Control Policy, researchers at the National Academy of Sciences concluded that

◇ cannabinoids have a natural role in pain modulation, control of movement, and memory;

◇ the brain develops a tolerance to cannabinoids;

◇ cannabinoids have a potential for dependence and mild withdrawal symptoms;

◇ cannabinoids have a mild therapeutic value for pain relief, nausea, and appetite stimulation but more studies are required and there are more effective medications;

◇ clinical trials should be conducted to develop rapid-onset, reliable, and safe delivery systems;

◇ the psychological effects, such as anxiety reduction, sedation, and euphoria, influence the therapeutic value;

◇ smoking should not be the method of delivery;

◇ the research data on marijuana as a gateway drug is inconclusive (Institute of Medicine, 1999).

Marijuana is one of the drugs that has never been out of favor and is still popular at the start of the twenty-first century. Internationally marijuana is the most widely used illicit drug in countries such as Canada, Mexico, Costa Rica, El Salvador, Panama, Australia, and South Africa (NIDA, 1998). The biggest change in this drug is the increase in the availability of highly potent marijuana (up to 14 times as strong as varieties available in the '70s) and the increase in price which has gone up 10- to 30-fold since the early '70s. (Higher potency marijuana was always available but it was just not very plentiful.) Just as the refinement of coca leaves into cocaine and opium into heroin led to greater abuse of those drugs, so have better cultivation techniques increased the compulsive liability of marijuana use. There is also an increase in the practice of mixing marijuana with other drugs like cocaine, amphetamine, and PCP. Some users even smoke marijuana "joints" that have been soaked in formaldehyde and embalming fluid or even sprayed with Raid Roach Killer®, called "canonaide," for a bigger kick.

In recent years there has been a drive to legalize marijuana for medical purposes. NORML (National Organization for the Reform of Marijuana Laws) and other groups have also pressed for legalization of marijuana, citing, among other reasons, the use of hemp to make paper or other products. Opponents contend that legalization is a cover for use of marijuana as a euphoriant, that there is not enough sound medical evidence of the drug's usefulness in medical treatment, and that other drugs are medically more effective. The controversy is likely to continue well into the future.

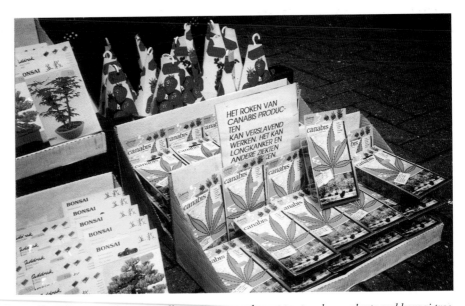

In Amsterdam, a garden store sells marijuana seeds next to strawberry plants and bonsai tree seeds. The Netherlands has Europe's most liberal drug laws.
Courtesy of Simone Garlaund

TOBACCO, HEALTH, & THE LAW

From the peak smoking year of 1962, tobacco use in the United States has been gradually declining. This decline resulted in part from the U.S. Surgeon General's Report on the dangers of smoking in 1965, continuing research on dangerous health effects from smoking, antismoking information campaigns, warnings printed on packaging and advertising, legislation prohibiting smoking on aircraft and in public places, an acceptance by the public of the dangers of smoking, lawsuits against tobacco companies, and restrictions placed on tobacco advertising on radio and television. Between 1962 and 1998, per capita tobacco use declined by 30% (SAMHSA, 1998).

Statistics in 1998 documented about 3,500 cigarette smokers who quit each day and 1,178 who die each day in the United States. The tobacco companies responded by developing generic brands, cutting prices, developing foreign markets, as well as targeting females, minorities, and younger smokers. The biggest change has been the rash of lawsuits against the tobacco companies claiming that they knew tobacco caused disease and premature deaths and that it was addictive. Many states and the federal government joined in these lawsuits to recover the money spent on health care for smokers.

In 1998, in the biggest class-action lawsuit settlement ever, the major tobacco companies agreed to pay $246 billion over a period of 25 years to the various states to prevent teenagers from smoking and to help defray the medical costs associated with diseases caused by smoking or chewing tobacco. Unfortunately many of the states used the largest percentage of the money to defray the costs of other programs rather than for the stated purposes.

In 1999 in Florida, big tobacco lost its second class-action lawsuit. The first class-action lawsuit was filed by 60,000 flight attendants who claimed injury from secondhand smoke. Their settlement was $300 million. The tobacco companies had begun losing individual

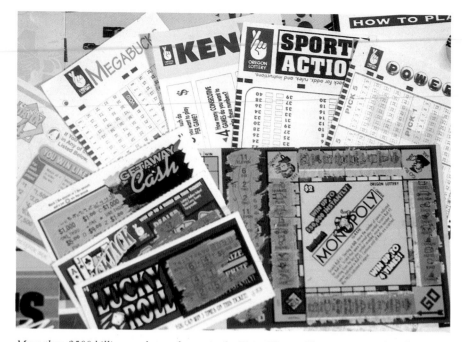

More than $500 billion are bet each year in the United States. The games vary from keno and state-run lotteries to scratch-off games, sports betting, slot and poker machines, and casino table games.

lawsuits, e.g., an $81 million judgment in Oregon and a $51.5 million lawsuit in California. Most of the verdicts are under appeal but obviously the number of cases will mushroom dramatically. Ironically, despite the heavy negative publicity and multiple court losses, tobacco company stocks remain fairly stable and have actually increased in value during the late 1990s.

ALCOHOL HANGS ON

The other drug that has never been out of favor is alcohol. It is still widely used in every age group and in every country (except Muslim nations). It is used for a dozen different reasons from supplementing meals, reducing the risk of heart attacks, lowering inhibitions, being social, getting high, or becoming drunk. But, as in the past, used separately or in combination with other psychoactive drugs, alcohol kills over 130,000 persons a year in the United States, compared to only 8,000 killed by all other illicit psychoactive drugs combined. There were an estimated 10–12 million Americans suffering from alcoholism in 1998.

BEHAVIORAL ADDICTIONS, e.g., EATING DISORDERS, COMPULSIVE GAMBLING

Research in the 1990s has strongly suggested that addiction is not limited to psychoactive drugs. Compulsive behaviors, including gambling, compulsive overeating, bulimia, anorexia, sexual addiction, Internet addiction, and even compulsive shopping have many of the same signs and symptoms. Research has even suggested similar hereditary indications for these behavioral addictions (Blum, Braverman, Cull, et al., 2000). The proliferation of fast-food restaurants with high-fat foods and the explosion of gambling establishments, Native American casinos, and state-sponsored gambling have greatly added to the environmental component of these addictions.

CONCLUSIONS

The history of civilization is intertwined with the continuous use and abuse of mind-altering substances. Some historians have even suggested that the drive to alter states of consciousness is as essential to human nature as the drive to survive and procreate (Siegal, 1985). There is even a theory that some civilizations arose as a direct result of the desire to have a continued, uninterrupted access to substances that alter perceptions of the world. For example, agriculture in the Mesopotamian River Valley in the Middle East may have evolved some 10,000 years ago to cultivate the opium poppy (which offered no food value) to provide a reliable supply of opium for medicinal, cultural, and ritualistic uses. Theories such as these are tenable if one understands that the use of psychoactive substances can create a drive or compulsion to continue using, which supersedes many survival instincts. Botanical, pharmacological, and technological advances have increased the concentration and delivery methods of these drugs such that they overwhelm the brain's ability to rebalance itself more quickly than with the original substances.

Attempts to address this problem of the addictive potential of psychoactive substances are also well documented throughout the millennia but most methods have failed to prevent abuse or addiction. Partly, the problem of compulsion lies in the configuration of the human brain. We have evolved the neocortex that allows us to reason and to make more complex decisions than other creatures. Yet, because the action of drugs affects the neocortex thereby disrupting reasoning and distorting judgment, compulsive use continues despite negative consequences once addiction has developed. More importantly, addictive drugs cause compulsive use in the more primitive brain or meso cortex. This is the automatic, instinctive, non-thinking, survival part of our brain. It is not surprising that addiction continues to be our society's major public health and social problem. Psychoactive drugs, particularly alcohol and tobacco, kill more Americans every year than any

other medical problem. Thus, it now seems that what may have stimulated the development of human civilization is now a major threat to its members.

If one then couples the drive to overuse these substances with economic, political, and spiritual motives—e.g., increased tax and trade revenues, control of a substance desired by the populace, and control of a substance used in religious and shamanistic rituals—then the influence of drugs on our development as human beings can be better understood.

The basic reasons for wanting to change one's perception of reality and consciousness will probably stay the same in succeeding generations and psychoactive drugs are one way that people will choose to try to bring about that change. It is, therefore, crucial to understand psychoactive drugs because they will affect us directly (physically and mentally) or indirectly (economically and socially) for the rest of our lives.

CLASSIFICATION OF PSYCHOACTIVE DRUGS

The top shelf of this medicine cabinet has the stronger uppers (stimulants): amphetamines on the left and cocaine on the right. The next shelf on the left contains the weaker stimulants: amphetamine congeners (diet pills, Ritalin®), tobacco, and caffeine. Below are the downers (depressants): alcohol, sedative-hypnotics, and the opioids, including heroin. On the door are some of the all arounders (psychedelics): blotter "acid" (LSD), psilocybin mushrooms, mescaline capsules, a dried peyote button, and "Sherms," cigarettes laced with PCP. On the second shelf on the right is the other major psychedelic, marijuana.

WHAT IS A PSYCHO-ACTIVE DRUG?

◇ In ancient Egypt, the Pharaoh Ramses might have defined a psychoactive drug as the beer he gave his pyramid workers to keep them happy.

◇ In second century Greece, the physician Galen would have defined it as theriac, an opium-based cure-all he prescribed for his patients.

◇ About A.D. 1550, Spanish Conquistadors in Peru would have defined it as the coca leaves they gave to the native laborers to keep them working in the silver mines.

◇ A pilot in World War II would have defined it as the amphetamine the medic gave him to stay awake on a night bombing run.

◇ In the 1990s, an AIDS patient might define a psychoactive drug as a joint of marijuana that he/she smokes to control nausea.

◇ A law enforcement officer might define a psychoactive drug by its legal classification as a schedule I, II, III, or IV substance whose illegal use and sale carry legal penalties.

◇ A counselor working at a drug treatment center might define a psychoactive drug as any substance whose compulsive use keeps the client from functioning in a normal manner.

◇ A member of Gambler's Anonymous might define a psychoactive drug as a video poker machine available at the local tavern.

"A psychoactive drug is any substance that when injected into a rat gives rise to a scientific paper."
Darryl Inaba, Pharm.D., CEO, Haight-Ashbury Free Clinics

Each culture, each generation, each profession, and particularly each user have a definition of what constitutes a psychoactive drug. Most people who take psychoactive drugs on a regular basis use more than one drug.

DEFINITION

Our definition of a psychoactive drug is **any substance that directly alters the normal functioning of the central nervous system.** In our modern society there are any number of drugs that fit this definition. Today there are more psychoactive drugs to choose from than at any time in history. Modern transportation, a more open society, greater and more rapid Internet communication, greater financial incentives for drug dealing, easy access to legal psychoactive drugs like tobacco, alcohol, caffeine, and prescription medications, new refinement techniques, along with the development of new drugs in sophisticated or street laboratories, have all come together to increase availability of these chemicals to all strata of society.

CHEMICAL, TRADE, & STREET NAMES

The difficulty in studying, defining, and categorizing psychoactive drugs is that they have chemical names, trade names, and street names. For example, street names like "blunts," "illusion," "rave," "ice," "snot," "flip flop," "crack," "junk," "angel dust," "loads," "crank," "base," "window pane," "roofies," "chronic" (strong marijuana), "bammer" (weak marijuana), "Adam," "hubba," "rock," "horse," "ecstasy," and "U4Euh" continue to evolve almost daily among drug users. Each commonly used and abused substance may have 10 or more informal names. Just as confusing is the continued synthesis of new psychoactive drugs with chemical names such as methylenedioxymethamphetamine and alpha-methyl-fentanyl. Trade names, such as Prozac® instead of its chemical name fluoxetine, or Xanax® instead of alprazolam, further confuse the issue of how to classify psychoactive drugs. Lawmakers have to be careful when outlawing a drug since they must describe its exact chemical formula. Customs officials have to examine imported herbal medicines carefully because some of them contain natural forms of restricted psychoactive substances.

CLASSIFICATION BY EFFECTS

A more practical way of classifying these substances is to distinguish them by their overall effects. Thus the terms "uppers" for stimulants, "downers" for depressants, and "all arounders" for psychedelics have been chosen to describe the most commonly abused psychoactive drugs. Then there are other drugs, drugs such as inhalants, steroids, psychiatric medications, and a few more that don't fit one of these categories but that can be defined by their purpose for use, such as performance-enhancing sports drugs, antidepressants, or antipsychotics.

Caution: *Since drug effects depend on amount, frequency, and duration of use as well as the makeup of the user*

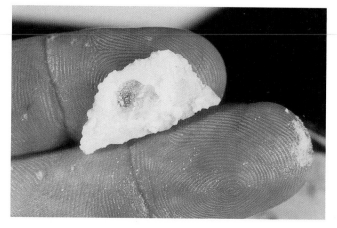

This piece of "crack" cocaine can be called "rock," "boulya," "hubba," or a dozen other street names.

and the setting in which the drug is used, reactions to psychoactive substances can vary radically from person to person and even from dose to dose. Our information about the action of drugs on the body should be used as a general guideline and not as an absolute guide to the effects.

MAJOR DRUGS

UPPERS (stimulants)

Uppers, central nervous system stimulants, include cocaine ("freebase," "crack"), amphetamines ("meth," "crystal," "speed," "crank," "ice"), diet pills, Ritalin®, khat, lookalikes, nicotine, and caffeine.

Physical Effects

The usual effect of a small to moderate dose is excessive stimulation of the nervous system creating energized muscles, increased heart rate, increased blood pressure, insomnia, and decreased appetite. Strong stimulants, like methamphetamines or cocaine, can also cause jitteriness, anger, aggressiveness, and dilated pupils. If large amounts are used or if the user is extrasensitive, heart, blood vessel, and seizure problems can occur. Frequent use over a period of a few days will deplete the body's energy chemicals and exhaust the user. Although tobacco is a weak stimulant, its long-term health effects can be dangerous, causing such diseases as cancer, emphysema, and heart disease.

Mental/Emotional Effects

A small to moderate dose of the stronger stimulants can make someone feel more confident, outgoing, eager to perform, and excited. It can also cause a certain rush or ecstatic feeling depending on the physiology of the user and the specific drug. Larger doses or prolonged use of the stronger stimulants can cause anxiety, paranoia, anhedonia (inability to experience pleasure), and mental confusion. Overuse of strong stimulants can even mimic a psychosis.

DOWNERS (depressants)

Downers (central nervous system depressants) are divided into four main categories:

Opiates and Opioids: Opium, morphine, codeine, heroin, oxycodone (Percodan®), hydrocodone (Vicodin®), methadone, morphine, hydromorphone (Dilaudid®), meperidine (Demerol®), propoxyphene (Darvon®)

Sedative-Hypnotics: Benzodiazepines, e.g., alprazolam (Xanax®), diazepam (Valium®), lorazepam (Ativan®), flunitrazepam (Rohypnol®), barbiturates, e.g. butalbital, zolpidem (Ambien®), meprobamate (Miltown®)

Alcohol: Beer, lite beer, wine, wine coolers, hard liquors, and mixed drinks

Others: Antihistamines, skeletal muscle relaxants, lookalike sedatives, and bromides

Physical Effects

Small doses of downers slow heart rate and respiration, relax muscles, decrease coordination, induce sleep, and dull the senses (e.g., diminish pain). Opiates and opioids can also cause constipation, nausea, and pinpoint pupils. Excessive drinking or sedative-hypnotic use can slur speech and cause digestive problems. Sedative-hypnotics and alcohol in large doses can cause dangerous respiratory depression and coma. Large-dose use or prolonged use of any depressant can cause sexual dysfunction and tissue dependence.

Mental/Emotional Effects

Initially, small doses (particularly with alcohol) seem to act like stimulants because they lower inhibitions but as more of the drug is taken, the overall depressant effect begins to dominate, relaxing and dulling the mind, diminishing anxiety, and controlling some neuroses. Certain downers can also induce euphoria or a sense of well-being. Long-term use of any depressant can cause psychic and physical dependence.

ALL AROUNDERS (psychedelics)

All arounders, or psychedelics, are substances that can distort perceptions and induce illusions, delusions, or hallucinations: LSD, PCP, psilocybin mushrooms, peyote (mescaline), MDA, MDMA ("ecstasy"), marijuana, 2CB, methylpemoline ("U4Euh"), ayahuasca, and DMT.

Physical Effects

Most hallucinogenic plants, particularly cacti and some mushrooms, cause nausea and dizziness. Marijuana increases appetite and makes the eyes bloodshot. LSD raises the blood pressure and causes sweating. MDMA and even LSD act like stimulants. Generally, except for PCP and ketamine that act as anesthetics, the physical effects are not as dominant as the mental effects.

Mental/Emotional Effects

Most often, psychedelics overload or distort messages to and from the brain stem, the sensory switchboard for the mind, so that many physical stimuli, particularly visual ones, are intensified or distorted. Imaginary messages (hallucinations) can also be created by the brain.

OTHER DRUGS & ADDICTIONS

In this category, there are three main groups that can stimulate, depress, or confuse the user: inhalants, anabolic steroids and other sports drugs, and psychiatric medications.

INHALANTS

Inhalants are gaseous or liquid substances that are inhaled and absorbed through the lungs. They include organic solvents, such as glue, gasoline, metallic paints, gasoline additives (STP®) and household sprays; volatile nitrites, such as amyl or butyl nitrate (also called "poppers"); and nitrous oxide (laughing gas).

Physical Effects

Most often there is central nervous system depression. Dizziness, slurred speech, unsteady gait, and drowsiness are seen early on. Some inhalants lower the blood pressure, causing the user to faint or lose balance. The solvents can be quite toxic to lung, brain, liver, and kidney tissues, and even blood cells.

Mental/Emotional Effects

With small amounts, impulsiveness, excitement, and irritability are common. Eventually delirium with confusion, some hallucinations, drowsiness, and stupor or even coma can occur.

ANABOLIC STEROIDS & OTHER SPORTS DRUGS

Performance-enhancing drugs, such as anabolic-androgenic steroids, are the most common. Others include stimulants (e.g., amphetamines), therapeutic drugs, such as painkillers, human growth hormones, HCG, caffeine, beta-blockers, and even diuretics.

Physical Effects

Anabolic steroids increase muscle mass and strength. Prolonged use can cause acne, high blood pressure, shrunken testes, and masculinization in women.

Mental/Emotional Effects

Anabolic steroids often cause a stimulant-like high, increased confidence, and increased aggression. Prolonged large-dose use can be accompanied by outbursts of anger, known as "rhoid rage."

PSYCHIATRIC MEDICATIONS

These medications are used by psychiatrists and others in an expanding field known as psychopharmacology to try to rebalance brain chemistry that causes mental problems, drug addiction, and other compulsive disorders. The most common are antidepressants (e.g., Tofranil®, Prozac®, Zoloft®), antipsychotics (e.g., Thorazine®, Haldol®), antianxiety drugs (e.g., Xanax®, BuSpar®), and panic disorder drugs (e.g., Inderal®). These drugs are being prescribed more and more frequently despite the fact that the national inci-

dence of the disorders has remained fairly constant over the past 30 years.

Physical Effects

Psychiatric medications are accompanied by a wide variety of physical side effects, particularly on the heart, blood, and skeletal-muscle systems, but their mental and emotional effects are the most important. Side effects, adverse reactions, and toxic effects are especially severe with antipsychotic drug use (also called "neuroleptic drugs").

Mental/Emotional Effects

Antidepressants counteract depression by manipulating brain chemicals, such as serotonin, that elevate mood. Antipsychotics manipulate dopamine action in the brain to control schizophrenic mood swings and hallucinations. Antianxiety drugs also manipulate brain chemicals, such as GABA, to inhibit anxiety-producing thoughts.

COMPULSIVE BEHAVIORS

Behaviors such as compulsive overeating, anorexia, bulimia, compulsive gambling, sexual compulsion, Internet addiction, compulsive shopping, and even codependency affect many of the same areas of the brain impacted by compulsive use of psychoactive drugs.

Physical Effects

The major physical effects of compulsive behaviors are generally confined to neurologic changes in the

brain's reward pathway except with eating disorders when excess or extremely limited food intake can lead to cardiovascular problems, diabetes, nutritional diseases, and obesity.

Mental/Emotional Effects

The development of tolerance, psychological dependence, and even withdrawal symptoms exist with compulsive behaviors as does abuse and addiction. The compulsion to gamble or overeat is every bit as strong as drug-seeking behavior.

CONTROLLED SUBSTANCES ACT OF 1970

The Comprehensive Drug Abuse Prevention and Control Act of 1970 better known as the Controlled Substances Act was enacted to reduce the burgeoning availability and use of psychoactive drugs that occurred in the 1960s in the United States. The Act consolidated and brought up to date most drug laws that had been passed in the twentieth century. The Drug Enforcement Administration (DEA) was made responsible for enforcing the provisions of the Act. The key provisions were to classify all psychoactive drugs, to control their manufacture, sale and use, to limit imports and exports, and to define criminal penalties. Five levels or schedules of drugs were defined based on abuse liability, its value as a medica-

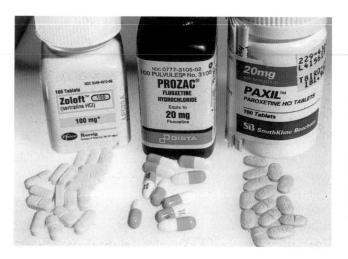

In the last few years, the number of available psychiatric drugs has increased. The most popular have been the new selective serotonin reuptake inhibitors (SSRIs) (e.g., Prozac®, Zoloft®, and Paxil®).

tion, its history of use and abuse, and the risk to public health.

◇ Schedule I includes heroin, LSD, marijuana, peyote, psilocybin, mescaline, and MDMA. These drugs have a high abuse potential and no accepted medical use (although recent activity with medical marijuana might make some people call for its rescheduling).

◇ Schedule II substances have a high abuse potential with severe psychic or physical dependence liability even though there are medical uses for the drugs. It includes cocaine, methamphetamine, opium, morphine, hydromorphone, codeine, meperidine, oxycodone, and methylphenidate (Ritalin®).

◇ Schedule III substances have less abuse potential and include schedule II drugs when used in compounds with other drugs. Schedule III drugs include Tylenol® with codeine, some barbiturate compounds, and paregoric.

◇ Schedule IV drugs have even less abuse potential including chloral hydrate, meprobamate, fenfluramine, diazepam (Valium®) and the other benzodiazepines, and phenobarbital.

◇ Schedule V substances have very low abuse potential because they contain very limited quantities of certain narcotic and stimulant drugs. Examples of schedule V are Robitussin AC® and Lomotil®. Some of these drugs are sold over the counter.

CHAPTER SUMMARY

INTRODUCTION

1. Psychoactive drugs and drug-seeking behaviors have always been extremely influential in all aspects of human endeavors. Historically five themes have affected the use and abuse of these substances:

◇ a basic need of human beings to cope with their environment;

◇ a brain chemistry that can be affected by certain substances to induce an altered state of consciousness, control pain, or treat illness;

◇ business and government involvement in growing, manufacturing, distributing, taxing, and prohibiting drugs;

◇ technological advances in refining and synthesizing drugs;

◇ development of more efficient and faster methods for putting drugs into the body.

HISTORY OF PSYCHOACTIVE DRUGS

Prehistory & the Neolithic Period (8500–4000 B.C.)

2. More than 4,000 plants yield psychoactive substances. Their use dates back 50,000 years or more.

3. Psychoactive drugs have been used throughout history as a shortcut to an altered consciousness, to relieve pain, and for spiritual rituals.

Ancient Civilizations (4000 B.C.–A.D. 400)

4. Drugs and methods of use gradually spread as contact among different cultures increased.

5. Alcohol (beer and wine), opium, *Cannabis,* and psychedelic mushrooms were the earliest psychoactive drugs employed by various civilizations.

6. Six historical uses of opium have been to stop pain, control diarrhea, stop coughs, lessen anxiety, promote sleep, and induce euphoria.

7. Two of the psychoactive drugs available in ancient Egypt were beer (as a reward for pyramid builders) and opium (medicine).

8. Two of the drugs used in ancient India were *Cannabis* (as a medicine and vision-inducing drug) and amanita mushrooms (called "Soma" and used for visions and sacred ceremonies).

9. Wine was mentioned numerous times in the Bible, along with warnings about overindulgence.

10. The peyote and San Pedro cacti (mescaline), the coca leaf (cocaine), the psilocybe mushroom (psilocybin), and tobacco (nicotine) were used in Mesoamerica before the birth of Christ and that use continues to this day.

Middle Ages (400–1400)

11. Several psychedelic plants that have been employed in religious, magic, or social ceremonies throughout history and especially in the Middle Ages are datura, belladonna, henbane, and mandrake. Their active ingredients include scopolamine and atropine.

12. Psychedelic mold on rye plants (which produced natural LSD) caused poisonings in the Middle Ages and beyond.

13. During the Middle Ages, distillation was discovered. It increased the alcoholic content of beverages through evaporation but caused widespread alcoholism.

14. In many Islamic countries, tobacco, hashish, and especially coffee were employed as substitutes for alcohol that was forbidden by the holy book of the Islamic religion, the *Koran.*

15. The use of coffee and tea spread to Europe and became extremely popular.

16. The *psilocybe* mushroom, peyote cactus, and coca leaf were used in the Americas in pre-Columbian times, mostly by the ruling classes.

17. Regulation of psychoactive drugs was one way political and religious leaders kept control of their people.

Renaissance & the Age of Discovery (1400–1700)

18. European explorers brought back various drugs to Europe and carried European drugs, principally alcohol and the newly discovered tobacco, to other peoples they encountered. In Europe various attempts were made to control use of alcohol and tobacco.

19. Spanish Conquistadors conquered the Incas and took control of coca leaf production. They used it to make money, as wages, and to stimulate the peasants who worked the silver mines, so they could work longer.

20. Tobacco was introduced to Europe and the Americas in the 1500s. Tobacco and hemp helped support many colonies. Coffee and tea drinking continued to spread.

21. Opium was used as a cure-all throughout history. Avicenna reintroduced theriac made from opium and many other ingredients. Laudanum, made from opium and alcohol, was also formulated and popularized.

Age of Enlightenment & the Early Industrial Revolution (1700–1900)

22. During this period new refinement techniques and new methods of using were developed.

23. Consumption of distilled liquors like rum, gin, and whiskey increased alcohol abuse, sometimes to epidemic proportions as in the Gin Epidemic in London (1710–1750).

24. The American Revolution was supported by tobacco and rum, as exports and for taxes.

25. In the nineteenth century nitrous oxide (laughing gas) was used as an anesthetic and intoxicant. Other anesthetics developed were chloroform and ether.

26. The refinement of morphine from opium (1804), the invention of the hypodermic needle (1855), the refinement of heroin (1874), and the use of morphine in wartime to control pain expanded the addictive use of opiates.

27. The Opium Wars between England and China in the early to mid-1800s were fought for economic reasons: one was the right of the British to sell opium to China in order to improve the British balance of trade.

28. In the second half of the nineteenth century, the refinement of cocaine from coca, the invention of the hypodermic needle, the popularization of cocaine by Freud, and the manufacture of stimulant wines such as Vin Mariani led to the first cocaine epidemic.

29. The temperance movement, begun in the eighteenth century in the United States, led to state prohibition laws and temperance societies.

30. The invention of the cigarette-rolling machine and milder strains of tobacco vastly expanded the use of tobacco.

31. Patent medicines at the turn of the century frequently contained opium, cocaine, and alcohol as their active ingredients.

Twentieth Century & the Electronic Revolution

32. Cigarettes gradually replaced cigars and chewing tobacco as the most popular method of nicotine consumption. Use increased through the first half of the century and then began to decline following public health campaigns. Recognition of the health problems caused by smoking gradually became known.

33. In 1914 the Harrison Narcotic Act was passed to control opiates and cocaine. Marijuana was banned in 1937.

34. The alcohol prohibition amendment (Volstead Act) lasted from 1920 to 1933. It helped create the multi-billion dollar illegal drug business. The widespread abuse of alcohol encouraged the creation of Alcoholics Anonymous in 1934, the most successful drug treatment program in history.

35. Marijuana became popular in the '60s. It became a symbol of the beat generation and of the hippie generation and as a symbol of rebellion.

36. Amphetamines, first popularized in the '30s, were used by soldiers on both sides in World War II. They became popular and eventually abused as a diet medication and marked the "Summer of Love" in 1967. Methamphetamines became the amphetamines of choice.

37. Steroids and other performance-enhancing drugs became popular due to the cold war and subsequent Olympic and other sports competitions.

38. Sedative-hypnotics started with bromides and barbiturates and switched to benzodiazepines such as Valium® and Xanax® starting in the 1960s. Psychiatric medications, including antidepressants and antipsychotics, also became popular starting in the '50s and vastly expanding in the '90s.

39. LSD and other designer psychedelics, including MDA, MDMA, and DMT, were developed.

40. Supply reduction and demand reduction were tried in order to limit the growth of illegal drug use.

41. Methadone use and maintenance was developed as a harm-reduction technique to control heroin use. The Vietnam War expanded heroin use although not as much as experts thought it would.

42. Regular cocaine use and smokable cocaine ("crack") use became popular in the late '70s and '80s.

43. An upper-downer cycle has been occurring in the United States, e.g., the downer alcohol in the '30s; stimulants like amphetamines in the '40s; sedative-downers like Miltown® in the '50s; amphetamine uppers in the '60s; heroin and Valium® downers in the '70s; cocaine (including "crack") and amphetamine (including

"ice") uppers in the '80s; and heroin or sedative-downers in the late-1990s.

Today & Tomorrow

44. Overall drug use has declined since 1979 and 1980 although the age of first use has gotten younger and hard-core users have increased. Cocaine and "crack" cocaine remain in decreased levels of use, methamphetamines are growing in popularity, while GHB, LSD, ketamine ("special-K"), and MDMA ("ecstasy") are making a comeback often in "rave" clubs. Inhalant abuse has increased a little. Heroin use also made a comeback in the late '90s. Marijuana use has remained fairly constant, although the potency of commonly available "pot" has greatly increased and there is a battle over its legalization for medical purposes. Tobacco remains the target of numerous lawsuits while smoking in the United States has declined. Alcohol remains the number one drug problem in most of the world.

45. There is growing recognition that behavioral addictions, such as eating and gambling, are very similar to drug addictions in the way they affect the reward-pleasure center.

Conclusions

46. Stronger psychoactive drugs can overwhelm the brain's ability to naturally rebalance itself resulting in increased hard-core drug users

despite the fact that overall drug use has declined in recent years.

CLASSIFICATION OF PSYCHOACTIVE DRUGS

What Is a Psychoactive Drug?

47. The major classes of psychoactive drugs are uppers (stimulants), downers (depressants), and all arounders (psychedelics).

Major Drugs

48. Uppers include cocaine, amphetamines, diet pills, and the plant stimulants (e.g., khat, caffeine, and tobacco). Major effects are increased energy, feelings of confidence, and raised heart rate and blood pressure. Euphoria occurs initially with stronger stimulants. Overuse can cause jitteriness, anger, depletion of energy, anhedonia (lack of ability to feel pleasure), and paranoia, along with damage to the heart, lungs, and blood vessels.

49. Downers include opiates (e.g., heroin, codeine), sedative-hypnotics (e.g., benzodiazepines, barbiturates), and alcohol (beer, wine, and distilled liquor). These drugs depress circulatory, respiratory, and muscular systems. The stronger opiates and sedative-hypnotics can initially cause euphoria. Prolonged use can cause health problems and dependence.

50. All arounders include marijuana, LSD, MDMA, PCP, psilocybin mushrooms, and peyote. Major

mental effects are illusions, hallucinations, and confused sensations. Physically, many psychedelics cause stimulation but marijuana usually causes relaxation.

Other Drugs & Addictions

51. Other psychoactive drugs include inhalants, which are depressants but also cause dizziness and delirium accompanied by confusion; steroids and other sports drugs, which are used to enhance performance, such as muscle growth or relief from pain; and psychiatric drugs, which help rebalance brain chemistry disrupted by mental illness (e.g., antidepressants, antipsychotics, and antianxiety drugs).

52. Certain addictive behaviors, including gambling, compulsive eating, anorexia, bulimia, sexual compulsivity, compulsive shopping, and even Internet addiction, affect the human brain in the same way as many drug addictions.

Controlled Substances Act of 1970

53. The Controlled Substances Act of 1970 was enacted to limit the availability, use, and abuse of psychoactive substances. It categorized dangerous substances into five schedules. Schedules I and II include the major psychoactive drugs, e.g., heroin, cocaine, marijuana, and methamphetamine (drugs with a high abuse potential) and define criminal penalties for possession, intent to sell, and use.

REFERENCES

AA (Alcoholics Anonymous). (1934, 1976). *Alcoholics Anonymous*. New York. Alcoholics Anonymous World Services, Inc.

Acker, C. J. (1995). Opioids and opioid control: History. In *Encyclopedia of Drugs and Alcohol* (Vol. 2, pp. 763–769). New York: Simon & Schuster Macmillan.

Acosta, J. (1588). *Historia Natural y Moral de las Indias*. English translation by C. R. Markham. London: Hakluyt Society, 1880.

ADF (Australian Drug Foundation). (1999). *The History of Drug Use in Sport. http:// www.adf.org.au/archive/asda/history.html*.

Agnew, L. R. (1968). On blowing one's mind (19th century style). *JAMA* (pp. 61–62).

Aldrich, M. R. (1977). Tantric cannabis use in India. *Journal of Psychoactive Drugs, 9*(3), 227–233.

Aldrich, M. R. (1994). Historical notes on women addicts. *Journal of Psychoactive Drugs, 26* (1), 61–64.

Aldrich, M. R. (1997). History of therapeutic cannabis. In M. L. Mathre (Ed.), *Cannabis in Medical Practice* (pp. 35–55). Jefferson, NC: McFarland & Company, Inc.

Armstrong, D., & Armstrong, E. M. (1991).

The Great American Medicine Show. New York: Prentice Hall.

Austin, G. A. (1979). *Perspectives on the History of Psychoactive Substance Use.* DHEW Publication No. (ADM) 79–81.

Benowitz, N., & Fredericks, A. (1995). History of tobacco use. *Encyclopedia of Drugs and Alcohol* (Vol. 3, pp. 1032–1036).

Blum, K., Braverman, E. R., Cull, J. G., Holder, J. M., Luck, R., Lubar, J., Miller, D., & Comings, D. E. (2000). Reward deficiency syndrome (RDS): A biogenetic model for the diagnosis and treatment of impulsive, addictive, and compulsive behaviors. *Journal of Psychoactive Drugs, 32*(1).

Cherrington, E. H. (Ed.). (1924). *Standard Encyclopedia of the Alcohol Problem,* (Vol. II). Westerville, Ohio: American Issue Publishing.

Cleza de Leon. (1959). The Incas. Translated by Harriet de Onis. *The Civilization of the American Indian Series* (Vol. 53). Tulsa: University of Oklahoma Press.

Coste, R. (1984). Coffee production. *Encyclopaedia Britannica* (Vol. 4, pp. 818–820). Chicago: Encyclopaedia Britannica.

Courtwright, D. (1982). *Dark Paradise: Opiate Addiction in America Before 1940.* Cambridge, MA: Harvard University Press.

Diaz, J. L. (1979). Ethnopharmacology and taxonomy of Mexican psychodysleptic plants. *Journal of Psychoactive Drugs, 11*(1–2), 71–101.

Dunlop, E., & Johnson, B. D. (1992). The setting for the crack era: Macro forces, micro consequences (1960–1992). *Journal of Psychoactive Drugs, 24*(4), 307–322.

Fort, J. (1968). A world view of marijuana. *Journal of Psychoactive Drugs, 2*(1), 1–14.

Freud, S. (1884). Uber Coca. In R. Byck (1974), *The Cocaine Papers: Sigmund Freud.* New York: Stonehill.

Furst, P. T. (1976). *Hallucinogens and Culture.* San Francisco: Chandler & Sharp Publishers, Inc.

Gagliano, J. (1994). *Coca production in Peru, the historical debates.* Tucson & London: University of Arizona Press. In S. B. Karch (1998), *A Brief History of Cocaine.* Boca Raton: CRC Press.

Ganeri, A., Martell, H. M., & Williams, B. (1998). *World History Encyclopedia.* New York: Barnes & Noble.

Giannini, A. J., Burge, H., Shaheen, J. M., & Price, W. A. (1986). Khat: Another drug of abuse. *Journal of Psychoactive Drugs, 18*(2), 155–158.

Goodwin, D. W., & Gabrielli, W. F. (1997). Alcohol: clinical aspects. In J. H. Lowinson, P. Ruiz, R. B. Millman, & J. G. Langrod (Eds.), *Substance Abuse: A Comprehensive Textbook* (3rd ed., pp.142–147). Baltimore: Williams & Wilkins.

Guttmacher, H. (1885). New medications and therapeutic techniques concerning the different cocaine preparations and their effects. Vienna Medical Press. In R. Byck, (1974), *The Cocaine Papers Sigmund* (p. 123). New York: Stonehill.

Hamid, A. (1992). The developmental cycle of a drug epidemic: The cocaine-smoking epidemic of 1981–1991. *Journal of Psychoactive Drugs, 24*(4), 337–348.

Harler, C. R. (1984). Tea production. *Encyclopaedia Britannica* (Vol. 18, pp. 16–19). Chicago: Encyclopaedia Britannica.

Heath, D. B. (1995). Alcohol: History. *Encyclopedia of Drugs and Alcohol* (Vol.1, pp. 70–78). New York: Simon & Schuster Macmillan.

Herodotus. (450 B.C.). *The Histories. 1.202,* 4.75.1.

Hoffman, J. P. (1990). The historical shift in the perception of opiates: From medicine to social medicine. *Journal of Psychoactive Drugs, 22*(1), 53–62.

Hollister, L. E. (1983). The Pre-Benzodiazepine Era. *Journal of Psychoactive Drugs, 15*(1–2), 9–13.

Institute of Medicine. (1999). *Marijuana and Medicine: Assessing the Science Base.* Washington, DC: National Academy Press.

James I. (1604). *A Counter-Blaste to Tobacco.* Reprinted in 1954. London: The Rodale Press.

Karch, S. B. (1997). *A Brief History of Cocaine.* Boca Raton, FL: CRC Press.

Karch, S. B. (1998). *Drug Abuse Handbook.* Boca Raton, FL: CRC Press.

Karch, S. B. (1996). *The Pathology of Drug Abuse.* Boca Raton, FL: CRC Press.

Keller, M. (1984). Alcohol consumption. *Encyclopaedia Britannica* (Vol. 1, pp. 437–450). Chicago: Encyclopaedia Britannica.

La Barre, W. (1979). Shamanic origins of religion and medicine. *Journal of Psychoactive Drugs, 11*(1–2), 7–11.

La Barre, W. (1979). Peyotl and mescaline. *Journal of Psychoactive Drugs, 11*(1–2), 33–39.

Langton, P. A. (1995). Temperance movement. *Encyclopedia of Drugs and Alcohol* (Vol.3, pp. 1019–1023). New York: Simon & Schuster Macmillan.

Latimer, D., & Goldberg, J. (1981). *Flowers in the Blood: The Story of Opium.* New York: Franklin Watts.

Leary, T. (1970). The religious experience: Its production and interpretation. *Journal of Psychoactive Drugs, 3*(1), 76–86.

Lee, J. A. (1987). Chinese, alcohol and flushing: Sociohistorical and biobehavioral considerations. *Journal of Psychoactive Drugs, 19*(4), 319–327.

Li, H. L. (1974). An archeological and historical account of *Cannabis* in China. *Economic Botany, 28,* 437–438.

Lichine, A. (1990). Distilled Spirits. *Encyclopedia Americana* (Vol. 11, pp. 188–190).

Lynn, E. J., Walter, R. G., Harris, L. A., Dendy, R., & James, M. (1972). Nitrous oxide: It's a gas. *Journal of Psychoactive Drugs, 5*(1), 1–7.

Marnell, T. (Ed.). (1997). Drug Identification Bible. Denver: Drug Identification Bible.

McCoy, A. W. (1972). *The Politics of Heroin in Southeast Asia.* New York, Harper & Row, Publishers.

McGovern, P., Gluskee, D. L., Exner, L. J., & Voight, M. M. (1998). Archeology: Neolithic resinated wine. *Nature: 381,* 480–481.

McKenna, T. (1992). *Food of the Gods.* New York: Bantam Books.

Monardes, N. (1577). *Joyfull Newes Out of the Newe Founde Worlde.* Translated by J. Frampton. Reprinted in 1967. New York: AMS Press, Inc.

Musto, C. F. (1997). Historical perspectives. In J. H. Lowinson, P. Ruiz, R. B. Millman, & J. G. Langrod, (Eds.), *Substance Abuse: A Comprehensive Textbook* (3rd ed., pp.142–147). Baltimore: Williams & Wilkins.

Nesse, R. A., & Berridge, K. C. (1997). Psychoactive drug use in evolutionary perspective. *Science, 278,* 63–65.

NIDA (National Institute of Drug Abuse). (1998). Current trends in drug use worldwide. *NIDA Notes, 13*(2).

O'Brien, R., & Chafetz, M. (1991). *The Encyclopedia of Alcoholism,* (2nd ed.). New York: Facts on File.

O'Brien, R., Cohen, S., Evans, G., & Fine, J. (1992). *The Encyclopedia of Drug Abuse* (2nd ed.). New York: Facts On File.

ONDCP (Office of National Drug Control Policy. (1999). *National Drug Control Strategy, 1999.* Rockville, MD: National Drug Clearinghouse.

SAMHSA (Substance Abuse and Mental Health Services Administration). (1999). *National Household Survey on Drug Abuse: Population Estimates 1998.* Rockville, MD: SAMHSA.

Schultes, R.E., & Hofmann, A. (1992). *Plants of the Gods.* Rochester, VT: Healing Arts Press.

Scrivener (1871). On the coca leaf and its use in diet and medicine. *Medical Times and Gazette.* In R. Byck, *The Cocaine Papers.* New York: Stonehill.

Skolnik, A. A. (1997). Lessons from US history of drug use. *JAMA, 277*(24), 1919–1921.

Slade, J. (1989). The tobacco epidemic: lessons from history. *Journal of Psychoactive Drugs, 21*(3), 281–291.

Stafford, P. (1982). *Psychedelics Encyclopedia* (Vol. 1, p. 157). Berkeley, CA: Ronin Publishing.

The Bible. (1990) The New Jerusalem Bible Translation. *Ecclesiasticus, 31,* 27. New York: Doubleday.

Trice, H. M. (1995). Alcoholics Anonymous. *In J. H. Jaffe, Encyclopedia of Drugs and Alcohol* (Vol.1, pp. 85–92). New York: Simon & Schuster Macmillan.

Wallbank, T. W., & Taylor, A. M. (1992). A Short History of the Opium Wars. *Civilizations Past and Present: Chapter 29.* New York: Addison-Wesley Publishing Co.

White, P. T. (1989). Cocaine's deadly reach. *National Geographic, 175*(1).

CHAPTER 2

Heredity, Environment, Psychoactive Drugs

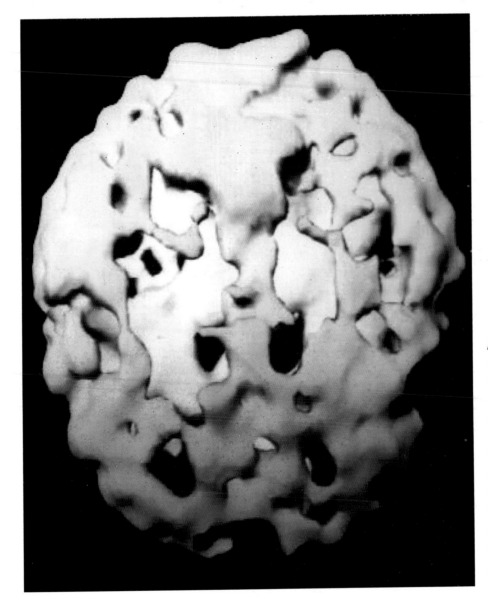

T his SPECT (single positron emission computerized tomography) scan of the brain of a long-time heroin addict shows an overall decrease in cerebral activity. The areas with a moth-eaten look are actually areas of the brain that are suppressed or inactivated by the drug. Normally the brain has a more even appearance.
Courtesy of the Amen Clinic for Behavioral Medicine

HOW PSYCHOACTIVE DRUGS AFFECT US

- **How Drugs Get to the Brain:** A psychoactive drug is absorbed into the body and distributed through the circulatory system.
  - ◊ **Routes of Administration & Drug Absorption:** Drugs can be absorbed through smoking, injecting, mucous membrane contact, ingestion, or direct contact.
  - ◊ **Drug Distribution:** Psychoactive drugs travel through the bloodstream and finally cross the blood-brain barrier to the central nervous system. The drugs will either cause an effect, be ignored, be absorbed, or be transformed.
- **The Nervous System:** The two parts of the nervous system are the peripheral nervous system (autonomic and somatic systems) and the central nervous system (brain and spinal cord).
  - ◊ **Peripheral Nervous System:** This two-part system controls involuntary functions, relays sensory information, and sends messages to muscles and organs.
  - ◊ **Central Nervous System (brain & spinal cord):** This system receives messages from the peripheral system, analyzes them, and then sends appropriate messages to the involved organs and muscles.
  - ◊ **Old Brain-New Brain:** Craving for psychoactive drugs resides mostly in the old brain.
  - ◊ **The Reward/Pleasure Center:** This part of the old brain gives a surge of satisfaction when a bodily or environmental need is met. Psychoactive drugs affect this center directly.
  - ◊ **Neuroanatomy:** Psychoactive drugs affect the nerve cells of the brain and spinal cord and alter the way nerves transmit messages.
  - ◊ **Neurotransmitters & Receptors:** Neurochemicals called "neurotransmitters" transmit messages across the tiny gap between nerve cells. When psychoactive drugs mimic or modify the way these neurotransmitters function, they cause physical and mental effects.
- **Physiological Responses to Drugs:** In addition to direct effects, phenomena such as tolerance, tissue dependence, and withdrawal determine a user's reaction to psychoactive drugs.
- **Basic Pharmacology:** Drug metabolization and elimination, along with molecular size, drug solubility, drug half-life, and dose-response relationships, help determine the effects a drug will have on the user.

FROM EXPERIMENTATION TO ADDICTION

- **Desired Effects vs. Side Effects:** People use psychoactive drugs to get high, to self-medicate, and for a dozen other reasons. Drugs also have undesired effects (side effects), adverse reactions, and toxic effects particularly with prolonged or high-dose use.
- **Levels of Use:** The amount, frequency, and duration of drug use help indicate levels of use: abstinence, experimentation, and social/recreational use up to habituation, abuse, and addiction.
- **Theories of Addiction:** Theories of addiction emphasize heredity, environment, psychoactive drugs, and compulsive behaviors or a combination of those factors as the basis for addiction.
- **Heredity, Environment, Psychoactive Drugs, & Compulsive Behaviors:** Four major factors determine at what level a person might use psychoactive drugs.
  - ◊ **Heredity:** Family history can indicate a genetic susceptibility to compulsive drug use.
  - ◊ **Environment:** The pressures and stress of growing up can make people more susceptible to addiction especially if there is a strong hereditary component. Dietary imbalances also contribute to drug dependency.
  - ◊ **Psychoactive Drugs:** Drugs can activate a genetic/environmental susceptibility to drug abuse and addiction. They also cause direct changes in brain chemistry, structure, activity, and function, which can lead to addiction.
  - ◊ **Compulsive Behaviors:** Compulsive gambling, eating, shopping, sexuality, and other uncontrolled behaviors cause changes in brain function and neurochemistry similar to those caused by psychoactive drugs.
- **Alcoholic Mice & Sober Mice:** Classic experiments with mice strongly suggest the interrelationship between heredity, environment, psychoactive drugs, and level of use.
- **Compulsion Curves:** The way heredity, environment, and drug use combine to increase susceptibility to addiction can be visualized with compulsion graphs.
- **Conclusions:** Any examination of drug or behavioral addiction should focus on the totality of one's life not just the specific drug problem.

8D · THURSDAY, MARCH 19, 1998 · USA TODAY

HEALTH AND EDUCATION

Strain of stress can be drain on brain

By Karen S. Peterson
USA TODAY

Dealing with stress effectively not only protects one's general health: It can help keep memory and mental abilities strong as we age, ers are learning.

Stress actually can dam hippocampus, an area of th governing learning and m says neurologist Richard Re *The Longevity Strategy: H Live to 100 Using the Brair Connection* (Wiley, $22.95).

"It is no longer just common to avoid stress, to reframe stre situations and see them in tern challenges" to reduce the feelin pressure, he says. Paying attentio stress is a necessity. "Stress cau brain damage."

Research reported this week the *Proceedings of the Nation Academy of Sciences* reinforces h analysis. A Princeton-Rockefelle University team finds the productior of new cells in the hippocampus or monkeys is diminished under stress.

The fact that new cells are produced in their brains at all may amaze some scientists.

"There has been enormous skepticism for several decades that this was possible," Princeton researcher beth Gould says. "Up to this point, there been a lot of resistance to the idea, but I t people are going to change their attitude

Earlier research established the growth new cells in the olfactory bulbs of rats, area used in the sense of smell, she says. "I ours is the first to demonstrate growth in t primate brain."

In her study, male monkeys that had a ways lived alone were placed in small cage

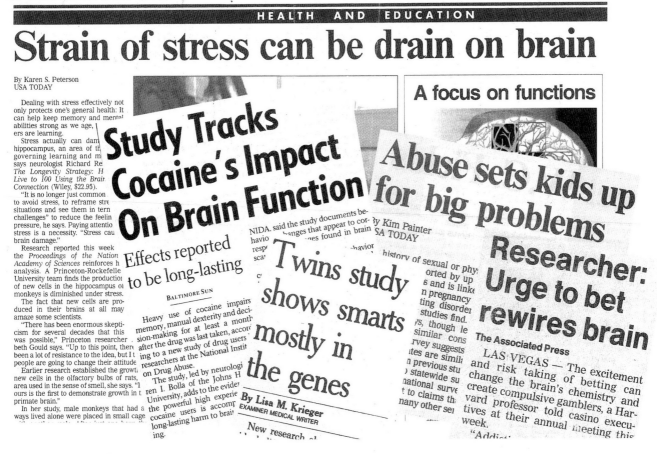

A focus on functions

Study Tracks Cocaine's Impact On Brain Function

Effects reported to be long-lasting

BALTIMORE SUN

Heavy use of cocaine impairs memory, manual dexterity and decision-making for at least a month after the drug was last taken, accor ing to a new study of drug users researchers at the National Instit on Drug Abuse.

The study, led by neurologi ren I. Bolla of the Johns H University, adds to the evide the powerful high experie cocaine users is accomp long-lasting harm to brain ing.

NIDA said the study documents be- hanges that appear to cor- es found in brain havio respi sca

Twins study shows smarts mostly in the genes

By Lisa M. Krieger
EXAMINER MEDICAL WRITER

New research

Abuse sets kids up for big problems

By Kim Painter
SA TODAY

havior history of sexual or phy orted by up s and is linke n pregnancy ting disorder studies find. /s, though le similar cons rvey suggests ites are simil: n previous stu) statewide su national surve t to claims th: nany other sei

Researcher: Urge to bet rewires brain

The Associated Press

LAS VEGAS — The excitement and risk taking of betting can change the brain's chemistry and create compulsive gamblers, a Harvard professor told casino executives at their annual meeting this week.

"Addict

HOW PSYCHOACTIVE DRUGS AFFECT US

"I don't think that a drug is evil in and of itself, but just as drugs can be used to help heal a person, they can result in destroying a life as they did to me. So it really depends on the individual—what and how he chooses, and how wisely he uses or chooses not to use medications and drugs."

28-year-old recovering sedative-hypnotic abuser

HOW DRUGS GET TO THE BRAIN

By definition, **psychoactive drugs** are substances that affect the central nervous system to cause physical and mental changes. Factors that determine

the effects they will have and their abuse potential include

◇ the methods that people use to put psychoactive drugs in their bodies,

◇ the speed of transit to the brain,

◇ and the affinity of that drug for nerve cells, neurotransmitters, and other brain chemicals.

ROUTES OF ADMINISTRATION & DRUG ABSORPTION

There are five common ways that drugs may enter the body: (1) inhaling, (2) injecting, (3) mucosal absorption, (4) oral ingestion, and (5) contact absorption (Fig. 2-1). The methods are arranged in the order of the speed with which they will reach the brain and spinal cord and begin to have an effect.

Inhaling

When a person smokes a marijuana joint, inhales freebase cocaine, or "huffs" airplane glue, the vaporized drug enters the lungs and is rapidly absorbed through a network of tiny blood vessels (**capillaries**) lining the air sacs (alveoli) of the bronchi. From the capillaries the drug-laden blood travels back to the veins and then to the heart where it is pumped directly to the brain and rest of the body. Smoking acts more quickly than any other method of use (7–10 seconds before the drug reaches the brain and begins to cause changes). Since the effects are felt so quickly and only a small amount of the drug is absorbed with each puff, the user can regulate the amount of drug they are receiving

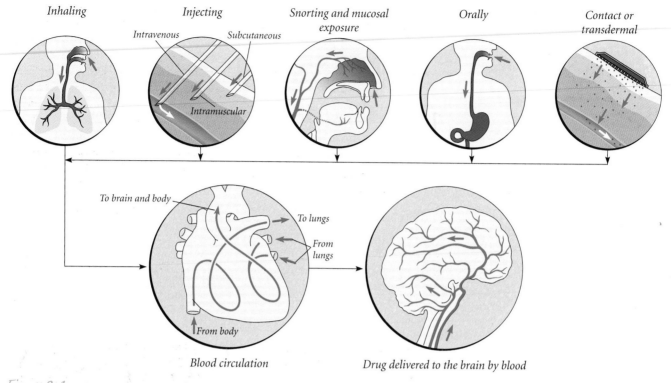

| Inhaling | Injecting | Snorting and mucosal exposure | Orally | Contact or transdermal |

Intravenous   *Subcutaneous*

Intramuscular

To brain and body

To lungs

From lungs

From body

Blood circulation

Drug delivered to the brain by blood

Figure 2-1 •

Whether inhaled (and absorbed in the lungs), injected (in a vein, muscle, or under the skin), snorted (through the nasal mucosa), drunk (and absorbed by the small intestine), or absorbed by contact (with the skin), the drug enters the bloodstream and eventually makes its way to the brain.

(titration). For example, cigarette smokers titrate the amount of nicotine they put in their bloodstream by controlling how many cigarettes they smoke and how deeply they inhale. Currently Roxanne Laboratories, the only maker of synthetic THC (Marinol®), the active ingredient in marijuana, is developing a deep lung aerosol spray and a nasal spray as delivery systems for medical marijuana that would avoid the hazards of smoking (Institute of Medicine, 1999).

Injecting (parenteral route)

Substances such as heroin, cocaine, and methamphetamine can be injected directly into the body with a needle by three methods:

◇ **intravenously (IV or "slamming"):** directly into the bloodstream by way of a vein,

◇ **intramuscularly (IM or "muscling"):** into a muscle mass, or

◇ **subcutaneously ("skin popping"):** under the skin.

Injection is a quick and potent way to absorb a drug (15–30 seconds in a vein compared to 3–5 minutes in a muscle or under the skin). Because a large amount of the drug enters the blood at one time, injecting is most likely to produce an intense "rush" or flash of ecstasy similar to a sexual orgasm. The slower routes of administration will produce euphoria but it will not arrive in a "rush." It will build up more slowly (Jaffe, Knapp, & Ciraulo, 1998). This is the main reason that IV use of heroin, cocaine, and methamphetamine is preferred. In addition none of the drug is wasted as occurs with side-stream smoke when a drug is smoked, or destruction by other body fluids when taken orally. This large bolus (amount)

of drugs can cause an overdose since the illicit user often does not know the purity of the drug or even which drug it is. Injecting is also the most dangerous method of use because it bypasses most of the body's natural defenses thereby exposing the user to many health problems, such as hepatitis, abscesses, septicemia, or HIV infection. Finally many psychoactive drugs do not dissolve fully and contain additives that can cause infections, embolisms, or other illnesses.

"I'm addicted to needles. Like sticking any needle in my vein will pretty much alleviate my dope sickness even if it's like 'speed' or even water. That would make it go away for a little while—just the part of my brain that would make me think that everything is all right."

17-year-old heroin addict

Snorting & Mucosal Absorption

Certain drugs, such as cocaine and heroin, can be snorted into the nose (**insufflation**) and absorbed by the capillaries enmeshed in the mucous membranes lining the nasal passages. The effects are usually more intense and occur more quickly than with the oral route because the drug initially bypasses digestive acids, enzymes, and the liver. A similar method involves placing a drug, such as crushed coca leaves (mixed with ash or soda lime), on the mucous membranes under the tongue (**sublingual**). Chewing tobacco or other medications can be absorbed by the mucosa sublingually or **buccally** (between the gums and the cheek: 3–5 minutes for effects to begin). Trials with a marijuana nasal gel or sublingual preparation for mucosal absorption are under review. In hospices for terminally ill patients, morphine suppositories are used for patients too weak for an oral dose of a painkiller (10–15 minutes for effects to begin). The drug is absorbed through mucosal tissues lining the rectum. Vaginal absorption of drugs is also occasionally employed.

Oral Ingestion

When someone swallows alcohol or a codeine tablet, the drug passes through the esophagus and stomach to the small intestine where it is absorbed into the capillaries. The drug enters the veins and then the liver where it is partly metabolized (**first-pass metabolism**). It is then pumped back to the heart and subsequently to the rest of the body. Since drugs taken by this route also have to pass through mouth enzymes and stomach acids besides the liver before they can get to the brain, effects are delayed (20–30 minutes). Some drugs are absorbed on the way to the small intestines. Alcohol (beer, wine, and distilled liquor) is partially absorbed by the stomach and can therefore reach the brain more quickly (10–15 minutes for effects to begin) though the majority of the alcohol is still absorbed by the small intestines.

Drugs are generally passively absorbed in the small intestine. This occurs because many drugs move from an area of high concentration of a drug to areas of low concentration of that same drug. Fat-soluble drugs, which include most psychoactive drugs, move readily across most biological barriers (membranes) through passive absorption.

Contact & Transdermal Absorption

LSD in a liquid form can be absorbed as eye drops when it is placed on the eye where it is rapidly absorbed by ocular capillaries. LSD can also be somewhat absorbed if placed on a moist part of the body. Skin creams and ointments are absorbed through the skin, as is DMSO, a penetrating solvent that enhances the absorption of drugs. Drugs can also be applied to the skin through saturated adhesive patches that allow measured quantities of the drug to be passively absorbed over a long period of time (up to seven days). It often takes one to two days for effects to begin. This noninvasive **transdermal** method of use includes nicotine patches to help smokers quit, fentanyl patches to control pain, clonidine patches to dampen drug withdrawal symptoms, and heart medication patches to control angina (heart pain).

DRUG DISTRIBUTION

No matter how a drug enters the circulatory system, it eventually ends up in the bloodstream and is distributed to the rest of the body. In the bloodstream the drug may be carried inside

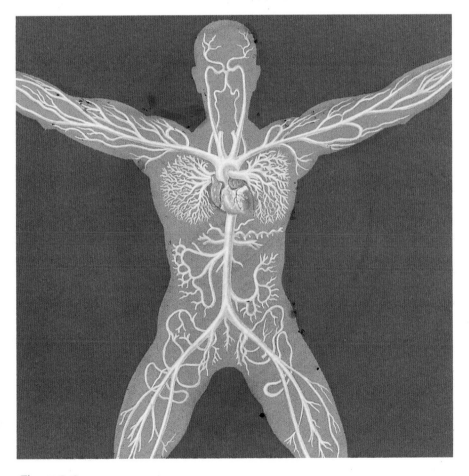

Figure 2-2 •

This drawing shows a fraction of the veins and arteries of the circulatory system that in an adult carry an average of 5 liters of blood to every part of the body. Miles of tiny capillaries then deliver blood to tissues, especially the nerve cells of the central nervous system. The circulatory system also carries the drug and its metabolites away from the brain by running 500 gallons of blood a day through the kidneys.

the blood cells, in the plasma outside the cells, or it might hitch a ride on protein molecules. Drug molecules then circulate and travel to and through every organ, fluid, and tissue in the body where they will either be (1) **ignored,** (2) **stored** (usually in fat cells), (3) **biotransformed** into metabolites or chemical variations of the original drug, some of which can cause effects, or (4) **cause an effect** directly.

The distribution of a drug within the body depends not only on the characteristics of the drug but on blood volume as well. The lighter the person, the less blood volume there is, so a child of 12 might only have three to four quarts of blood to dilute the drug instead of the six to eight quarts in an adult circulatory system. The effect of a drug on a specific organ or tissue is also dependent on the number of blood vessels reaching that site. For example, veins and arteries saturate the heart muscles, and since all drugs pass through these vessels, a drug such as cocaine can have a direct effect on heart function. Bones and muscles have fewer blood vessels, so most drugs will have less effect at these sites.

Most important, within only 10–15 seconds after entering the bloodstream, the drug will reach the gateway to the central nervous system, the blood-brain barrier. On the other side of the barrier, the drug will have its greatest effects on the brain and spinal cord.

The Blood-Brain Barrier

The drug-laden blood flows through the internal carotid arteries toward the central nervous system, also called the CNS (the brain and spinal cord). The walls of the capillaries enmeshed in the nerve cells of the CNS consist of tightly sealed cells that allow only certain substances to penetrate. Normally substances such as toxins, viruses, and bacteria can't cross this barrier. One class of drugs that can infiltrate this blood-brain barrier is psychoactive drugs (stimulants, depressants, psychedelics, inhalants). Psychotropic drugs, such as antipsychotics or antidepressants, also cross this barrier as do most steroids and some muscle relaxants.

One reason why many psychoactive drugs, including cocaine, nicotine, alcohol, and marijuana, cross this barrier is that they are **fat-soluble (lipophilic)** and since the brain is essentially fatty, it has an affinity for lipophilic substances. For example, morphine is partly fat-soluble, so it takes somewhat longer to cross the barrier than the more fat-soluble drug heroin. Even though a number of clinical studies say that people who were injected with morphine or heroin could not tell the difference, street users claim that the heroin crosses to the brain more quickly and gives a more intense "rush" (Jaffee, Knapp, & Ciraulo, 1977). "Crack" cocaine is more fat-soluble than cocaine hydrochloride, so it too crosses the barrier more quickly and gives the user a faster and often more intense reaction. Most substances that are **water-soluble (hydrophilic)**, such as antibiotics, are prevented from entering the brain. Alcohol is both lipophilic and hydrophilic.

THE NERVOUS SYSTEM

Since the principal target of psychoactive drugs is the central nervous system, it is important to understand how this network of 100 billion nerve cells and 100 trillion connections functions.

◇ The **central nervous system (CNS)** is half of the complete nervous system. It contains the brain and spinal cord. It is better protected by the skull and spine than most of the peripheral nervous systems.

◇ The **peripheral nervous system (PNS)** is the other half. It connects the central nervous system with its internal and external environments. The peripheral system is further divided into the **autonomic** and the **somatic** systems.

The Blood–Brain Barrier

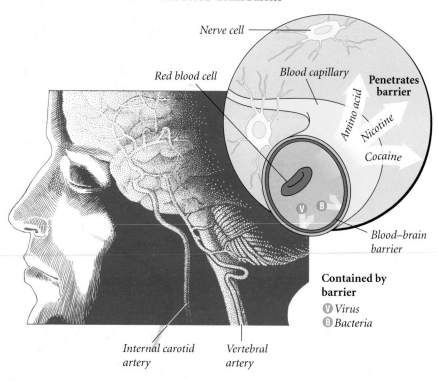

Nerve cell

Red blood cell

Blood capillary

Penetrates barrier

Amino acid

Nicotine

Cocaine

Ⓥ Ⓑ

Blood–brain barrier

Contained by barrier
Ⓥ *Virus*
Ⓑ *Bacteria*

Internal carotid artery

Vertebral artery

Figure 2-3 •

The inset shows the wall of a capillary in the brain whose tightly sealed cells, with no clefts, pores, or gaps, act as a barrier to most substances. Psychoactive substances, which are fat-soluble, cross this barrier.

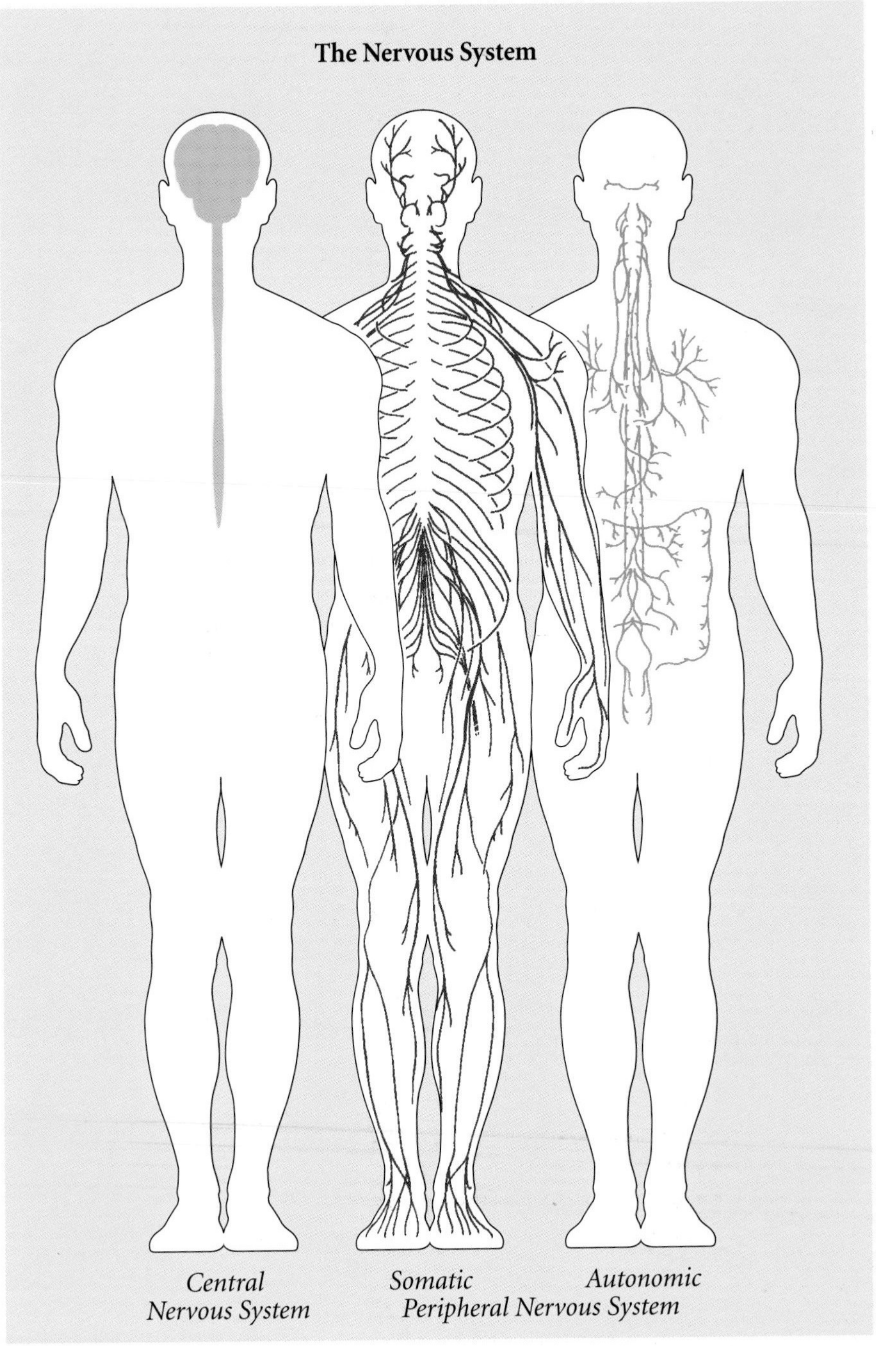

The Nervous System

Central
Nervous System

Somatic
Peripheral Nervous System

Autonomic

Figure 2-4 •

The three parts of the complete nervous system function together to transmit, interpret, store, and respond to information from the environment and from other parts of the body.

PERIPHERAL NERVOUS SYSTEM

The **autonomic nervous system** controls involuntary internal functions such as circulation, digestion, respiration, glandular output, and genital reactions. It consists of the sympathetic division, which helps the body respond to stress, the parasympathetic division, which conserves the body's resources and restores homeostasis (physiological balance), and the enteric division, which controls smooth muscles in the gut. This system automatically helps us breathe, sweat, pump blood, release adrenaline, and so forth, to preserve a stable internal environment. For example, sympathetic nerves speed up the heart in response to stress while parasympathetic nerves slow it down when the threat is passed (Kandel, Schwartz, & Jessell, 1991).

Though many cell bodies of the autonomic nervous system are located in the brain (hypothalamus) and spinal cord, their axons reach out to the affected organs and muscles. This means that since psychoactive drugs cross the blood-brain barrier, they can also speed up, slow down, or disrupt these involuntary functions in addition to triggering emotional and mental effects. This is why cocaine raises the heart rate, constricts blood vessels, and causes heightened sexual reactions. This is why heroin slows respiration, lowers blood pressure, and dulls sexual desire.

The **somatic nervous system,** which includes sensory neurons that reach the skin, muscles, and joints, transmits sensory information about the environment and about limb and muscle position to the central nervous system. It then transmits instructions back to skeletal muscles, allowing us to respond voluntarily rather than involuntarily as the autonomic system does.

CENTRAL NERVOUS SYSTEM (brain & spinal cord)

The central nervous system, especially the brain, acts as a combination switchboard and computer, receiving messages from the peripheral nervous system, analyzing those messages, and then sending a response to the appropriate system of the body: nervous (CNS and PNS), muscular, skeletal, circulatory, respiratory, digestive, excretory, endocrine, and reproductive. The CNS also enables us to reason and make judgments.

A psychoactive drug, being a powerful external agent, can alter information sent to our brain from our environment. It can also disrupt messages sent back to the various parts of the body; and it can disrupt our ability to think, reason, and interpret sensory input. A psychoactive drug not only affects the nervous system, it can affect

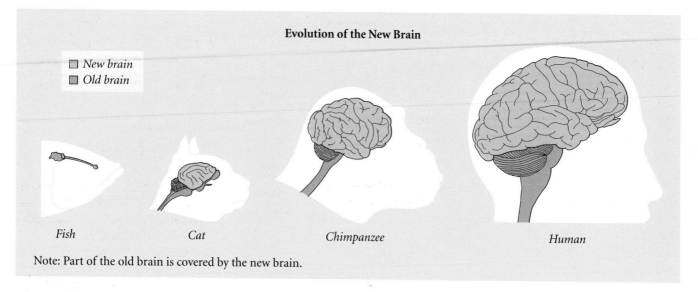

Evolution of the New Brain

☐ *New brain*
☐ *Old brain*

Fish   Cat   Chimpanzee   Human

Note: Part of the old brain is covered by the new brain.

Figure 2-5 •

On the evolutionary scale, from a fish, to a cat, to a chimpanzee, and finally to a human being, the new brain has grown in proportion to the old brain. However, though the new brain is much larger, the old brain tends to override it, particularly in times of stress.

other systems of the body as well. It can affect them directly while passing through the organ or tissue and it can affect them indirectly by manipulating nerve cell chemistry in the brain that then sends messages back to that organ. For example, alcohol can irritate the lining of the stomach and alter liver cells directly. It can also slow respiration and muscular reflexes indirectly through the CNS.

OLD BRAIN-NEW BRAIN

The brain can be described several ways.

◇ It can be anatomically divided into its component parts (spinal cord, medulla, pons and cerebellum, midbrain, diencephalon, and the cerebral hemispheres).

◇ It can be described by function, (e.g., vision center, motor cortex, somatosensory cortex, hearing centers).

◇ It can be divided by location (hindbrain, midbrain, forebrain).

For the purposes of understanding how psychoactive drugs work and what causes addiction, we have found it valuable to look at the brain in an evolutionary sense (Nesse & Berridge, 1997; Nesse, 1994). The evolutionary perspective looks at physiological changes in the brain as survival adaptations. For example, the evolutionary development of a desire for sweet-tasting substances helped survival by identifying food that could supply quick energy for fight or flight reactions. The instinctual desire for sex assured offspring that could guarantee survival of the species.

The evolutionary perspective also theorizes that psychoactive drugs have an affinity for natural survival mechanisms and initially cause desirable effects. The problem is that since refined and potent psychoactive drugs are so new in the evolutionary time scale and are more powerful than naturally occurring substances, the body has not had time to adapt to their effects. The net effect is that they end up being antisurvival.

Using the evolutionary perspective, the two major parts of the brain are defined as the old brain and the new brain.

Old Brain

The old brain, also called the primitive brain, consists of the brain stem, cerebellum, and mesocortex or midbrain that contains the limbic system (the emotional center). The spinal cord can be considered part of this system. The old brain exists in all animals from a fish to a human being (Fig. 2-5). The two main functions of the old brain are

◇ regulation of physiologic functions of the body (e.g., respiration, heartbeat, body temperature, hormone release, muscle movement),

◇ experiencing basic emotions and cravings (e.g., anger, fear, hunger, thirst, lust, and pleasure).

The emotions experienced by a person occur when the old brain responds to internal changes and memories or external influences from the environment. For example, if a person has not had enough liquid, the old brain feels the body's thirst and triggers a craving for water. If a deer hears a twig snap in the woods, the old brain feels fear and triggers a desire to escape from that danger. If a man and woman are in a sensual situation, they might have a desire for sex.

When anyone uses psychoactive drugs, it is most often the old brain that is involved in craving and addiction.

New Brain

The new brain, also called the **neocortex** (cerebrum and cerebral cortex), processes information that comes in from the old brain, from the other areas of the new brain, or from the senses via the peripheral nervous system. So, if a human being is thirsty and craves water, the new brain can help locate the nearest source of water. If there is danger, the new brain might figure out a smarter way of avoiding that danger instead of just running away. The new brain allows us to speak, reason, and create. Over millions of years, but particularly the last 200,000 years, the new brain has grown over the old brain until, in humans, it has folded in on itself to make room for all the billions of new cells (Suzuki, 1994). The higher up on the evolutionary ladder, the larger the new brain (Fig. 2-5). The new brain tries to make sense of the feelings and emotions coming from its more primitive half.

One would think that since the old brain is smaller, the new brain rules, but that's not the case. The old brain is the senior partner. It was there first and the new brain is the latecomer. Whenever the two brains are challenged by a crisis, such as fear or anger, there's an automatic tendency to revert to old brain function. And since the craving to use a psychoactive drug often resides in the old brain, the desire for the pleasure, pain relief, and excitement that drugs promise can be very powerful. That craving can override the new brain's rational arguments that say, "Too expensive," "Bad side effects," or "There's a midterm exam in the morning, so no partying tonight."

"The impact of that drug, the impact of that sensation and how it immobilized me and made me incapable of dealing with the simplest realities of walking to the bus, of going into my office, of

getting on the phone, and of picking up my children was so frightening to me that I did not want to repeat it. I was, however, very compelled to repeat the use of methamphetamine, which I did for years."

Recovering methamphetamine abuser

If a person is to live a balanced life, there has to be good communication between the old brain and new brain. Communication can be disrupted by psychoactive drugs.

"What brought me to the conclusion to completely get all the way sober was my perception of my sober picture vs. my high picture. When you're on drugs, you're just seeing through that vision. It's all kind of fuzzy and blurry or whatnot and that blurriness and fuzziness was blending into my sober

picture and if I wouldn't have 60 days clean today, I'd be listening to you and I'd be concentrating on you completely as hard as I could but I still wouldn't be able to react."

17-year-old recovering addict

THE REWARD/PLEASURE CENTER

The specific area of the old brain that encourages a human being to repeat an action that promotes survival is called the reward/pleasure center. It is also the part of the brain that is most affected by psychoactive drugs. Technically it is referred to as the **mesolimbic dopaminergic reward pathway** (Fig. 2-6). The most important part is a small group of nerve cells called the "medial forebrain bundle" that contains the nucleus accumbens septi (aka **nucleus accumbens**). This area of the brain was first pinpointed

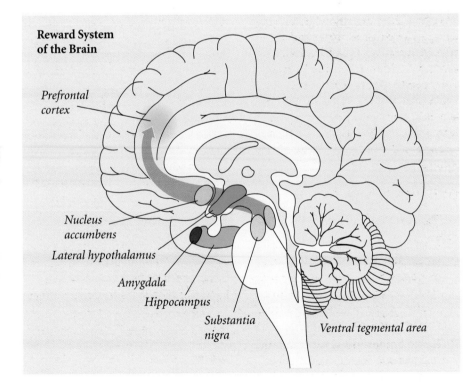

Reward System of the Brain

Prefrontal cortex
Nucleus accumbens
Lateral hypothalamus
Amygdala
Hippocampus
Substantia nigra
Ventral tegmental area

Figure 2-6 •

The reward/pleasure center is really a combination of several structures in the old brain that are activated when the person fulfills some emotion or feeling that has arisen, such as hunger, thirst, or sexual desire. The principle parts are the ventral tegmental region, nucleus accumbens septi, lateral hypothalamus, and the prefrontal cortex.

Courtesy of Kenneth Blum, John Cull, Eric Braverman, and David Comings

in 1954 by Canadian biologist Dr. James Olds (Olds & Milner, 1954). What Dr. Olds and others have hypothesized and, to a large extent, proven is that the reward/pleasure center in the brain is a powerful motivator. Experimentally when a rat had its nucleus accumbens connected to an electrical switch and was allowed to activate that part of its brain, it kept pressing the switch to keep stimulating this center. In fact it was so powerful a reinforcer, the rat would press the switch 5,000 times an hour. It wouldn't eat, it wouldn't sleep, it would just keep pushing the lever. Dr. Olds and other researchers found that many psychoactive drugs also stimulate this same reward/pleasure center (Olds, 1956). For example, when they had the rat push a lever which gave it a shot of cocaine, the rat would push that lever in much the same way it pushed the lever for the electrical stimulation of the nucleus accumbens, only this time it was drug-induced stimulation.

The other major parts of the **mesolimbic reward pathway** are the VTA or ventral tegmental area, the lateral hypothalamus, and the prefrontal cortex (Blum, Braverman, Cull, et al., 2000). This network gives animals and eventually human beings a feeling of pleasure or satisfaction when they fulfill a craving or even anticipate fulfilling a craving that has been triggered by an instinct, a physical imbalance, or an emotional memory. And, just as important, it gives a sense of relief, similar to the euphoria of reward, when pain was moderated or eliminated (Goldstein, 1994). The reward pathway can be activated at a variety of locations and through different mechanisms depending on the drug used. Alcohol might activate the nucleus accumbens via the globus palladus, heroin through the VTA, and cocaine directly through the nucleus accumbens.

When repetition of the action finally satisfies the hunger, thirst, sex drive, or other desire, the craving is turned off until the need arises again. This **satiation switch** is crucial in keeping craving and satiation in balance. In actuality, there seem to be

fewer areas involved in satiation and they vary somewhat depending on the type of craving. For example, thirst seems to involve 22 areas of the brain whereas satiation seems to involve 3 areas in the cingulate gyrus (Denton, Shade, Zamarippa, et al., 1999).

Animals can't control the cravings of their instincts or the messages from the reward/pleasure center on their own. They can only keep trying to satisfy them until the satiation switch kicks in. This **reward/satiation network** involving several kinds of neurotransmitters (brain chemicals), particularly dopamine and endorphins, was developed over millions of years in all animals as a way to reinforce survival instincts, such as quenching thirst, satisfying hunger, or having sex. Recent research has suggested that when this system is activated, the memory of the action that caused the reward is more strongly imprinted. The more intense the reward, the more ingrained the memory and so the more likely the action will be repeated (Wicklegren, 1998). Refined psychoactive drugs are so strong that they can imprint the emotion associated with the subsequent euphoria or pain relief more deeply than most natural memories. The triggering of these deeply imprinted memories can more easily induce craving and other drug-using behaviors and disrupt communication with the reasoning new brain.

"When I started drinking, everything went blank in my mind as far as thinking, feelings, emotions. So I like kind of started getting used to it. I said, 'Well that numbed me the first time.' I didn't think of the abuse or the sexual molestation, so I just continued on, everyday, and then I got used to the alcohol."
42-year-old recovering polydrug abuser

Since the reward/pleasure center in the old brain is tightly intertwined with the physiologic regulatory centers of the body (autonomic nervous system), when drugs are used for intoxication or

pleasure, especially stimulants and depressants, they necessarily affect physiologic functions, especially heart rate and respiration. Psychedelics seem to have a greater affect on the new brain although they will affect physiologic functions in the old brain (e.g., LSD stimulates, marijuana sedates). Most drugs also affect memory in one way or another because emotionally tinged memories often involve the amygdala and hippocampus in the old brain.

What makes human beings unique is that starting around the age of three or four years old, their neocortex (new brain) becomes stronger. Its strength comes from survival lessons and problem-solving skills taught from the day they were born by parents, schoolteachers, neighbors, and friends.

"I was doing things like driving around with my children in the car and not remembering how I got home in blackouts. And I thought I didn't really care much about myself but I don't think I could have lived with hurting my children. So I realized I had to do something. I had a problem."
42-year-old recovering polydrug abuser

In most cases, as people continue to grow up, they learn how to integrate the drives of the old brain and the common sense of the new brain. Unfortunately some people lose full use of this ability (usually due to genetic abnormalities, a chaotic or abusive childhood, and/or psychoactive drugs (often leading to mental illness or addiction). These people come to rely on one part of the brain to the exclusion of the other. For example, someone with a mood disorder, such as major depression or bipolar disease, is buffeted by the emotional memories of their old brain. Another person with an obsessive-compulsive disorder could be stuck in their new brain where an obsessive idea is repeated constantly by the prefrontal cortex (Pepper, 1991). Psychoactive drugs disrupt this integration when they essentially commandeer or hijack the survival mechanism because they are often more powerful than natural influences (Hyman, 1998).

"I don't like being stuck on stupid, like tweaking all the time. When I'm doing 'speed,' I'm just in this whole little world (can't get me out of it), finding something, nothing, and everything in the dirt."
24-year-old polydrug addict

There are a number of theories or ideas about how psychoactive drugs disrupt the reward/pleasure center and the satiation switches.

◇ One concept is that the on-off switch of the satiation center becomes stuck. The mechanism that normally informs the brain that a craving has been satisfied becomes damaged by the use of refined powerful substances. It becomes stuck in the on position so the person never reacts to the fact that the task has been completed. The use of the drug then continues until the drug runs out or the user hits bottom (Koob & Le Moal, 1997).

"'Crack' tastes like more, that's all I can say. You take one hit, it's not enough, and a thousand is not enough. You just want to keep going on and on because it's like a 10-second head rush right after you let the smoke out and you don't get that effect again unless you take another hit."
32-year-old recovering "crack" addict

Another theory postulates that the satiation switch is not damaged but it is ignored because the user wants to continue the euphoria or pain relief experiences from the psychoactive drug's effect on the reward/pleasure center.

A third concept is that users become so busy practicing the addiction, they have no time to learn and practice alternate behaviors. They don't learn how to solve problems.

◇ Another idea is that psychoactive substances disrupt and even sever communication between the two brains directly (Hyman, 1996). They turn off the new brain (thinking and insight) and disconnect it from trying to control the instinctive or automatic old brain.

"You keep thinking your best thinking got you into this. So then you start to question your own thinking and then you think, 'Well, I think I'm pretty smart. My best thinking got me to do this.' So that's pretty scary for you right there."
38-year-old compulsive gambler

And finally the desire to act out certain behaviors, such as compulsive sex, gambling, and risk-taking, also originate in the primal brain and so are subject to addictive behavioral patterns (Hyman, 1998). In addition the disruption of the reward pathway and satiation switches due to behavior can feed into a drug addiction. Further, potent psychoactive drugs can shut down the new brain (rationality, inhibitions, intellect) increasing compulsive behaviors.

The longer the drug or behavior is practiced, the more the brain changes and the harder it becomes to restore it to full functioning.

Morality & the Reward/ Pleasure Center

"It was like it was two people. My inner self would try to communicate to me that 'This is not you.' You know what I mean? My outer self would communicate to me, 'This is who you have to be.' So I was caught in between two entities, you know, the entities of what is good to you or what is good for you."
44-year-old recovering heroin addict

The Trappist Monk Thomas Merton wrote about the conflict be-

tween desire and common sense in more poetic terms than old brain vs. new brain.

"As long as pleasure is our end, we will be dishonest with ourselves and with those we love. We will not seek their good but only our own pleasure. Authentic love requires times of self-sacrifice. It requires that people monitor the sensations and feelings and moods of others, not just those of themselves."
(Merton, 1955)

"Get addicts together and everyone's like, 'Me first.' Even me. You know, we fight about who's going to go first. It's always about me, me, me, you know. It's just about the selfishness of it and wanting to feel good."
19-year-old polydrug abuser

Since the reward/pleasure center and the rest of the primal brain is normally much stronger than the neocortex, it takes a conscious effort to override cravings and desires from the old brain even when they are antisurvival. The Greek Philosopher Plato wrote almost 2,400 years ago that

"Passions, and desires, and fears make it impossible for us to think."
Plato, 400 B.C.

Christian, Buddhist, Islamic, and almost all theologies teach that one must resist most primal cravings in order to live a moral or fulfilling life. Freud wrote about how the ego and superego try to rein in the primal urges of the id (Freud, 1995). So throughout human history, this battle that pits primal urges, intense emotional memories, and desires against reason, common sense, and morality has raged unabated.

NEUROANATOMY

Nerve Cells

Understanding the precise way messages are transmitted by the ner-

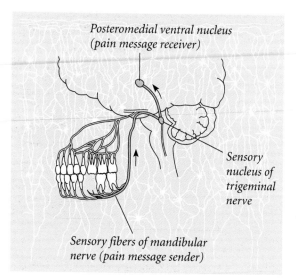

Figure 2-7 •

Posteromedial ventral nucleus
(pain message receiver)

Sensory
nucleus of
trigeminal
nerve

Sensory fibers of mandibular
nerve (pain message sender)

Figure 2-7 •

View of the nerves that would transmit a message of pain from a drilled left molar through the trigeminal nerve to the thalamus.

vous system is crucial to understanding how psychoactive drugs affect a user's physical, emotional, and mental functioning. For example, if a dentist drills a lower left molar, the damaged sensory fibers of the mandibular nerve (Fig. 2-7) send tiny electrical pain signals via the trigeminal nerve to the sensory nucleus in the spinal cord. The message is immediately relayed to the primal brain and cerebellum where a reflex action might jerk the head away from the drill. A slower signal continues to the postero ventral nucleus in the thalamus at the top of the brainstem. The thalamus identifies the signals as painful and then forwards them to the sensory cortex where intensity and location of the pain is identified. The signal is also forwarded to the frontal cortex where the cause of the pain is identified and a possible course of action decided. The brain might tell the patient's neck muscles to continue to move the head away from the drill, it might instruct the jaw to bite the dentist's finger, or it might tell the vocal muscles to ask the dentist to prescribe a painkiller. Nerve impulses might fire up to 1,000 pulses a second at speeds approaching 270 miles per hour depending on the size of the nerve (Diagram Group, 1991).

The building blocks of the nervous system, the nerve cells, are called **neurons** (Fig. 2-8). Each neuron has four essential parts: **dendrites,** which receive signals from other nerve cells and relay them through the cell body; the **cell body** (soma), which nourishes the organism and keeps it alive; the **axon,** which carries the message from the cell body to the **terminals,** which then relay the message to the dendrites, cell body, or even terminals of the next nerve cell. A single cell might have anywhere from a few contacts up to 150,000 contacts with other cells' dendrites. For example, a spinal motor cell would receive 8,000 contacts on its dendrites and 2,000 on its cell body. A Purkinje cell in the cerebellum might have as many as 150,000 contacts (Fig. 2-9). It is estimated that there are 100 trillion connections among nerve cells. Of course only a

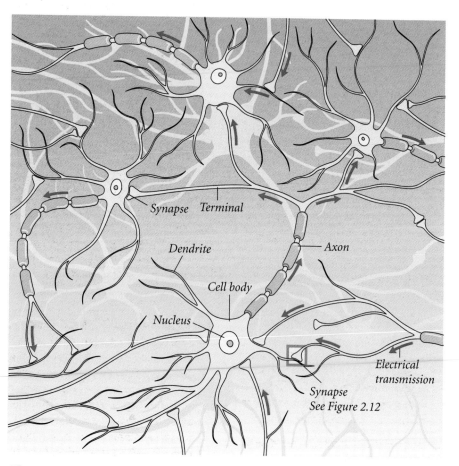

Synapse   Terminal

Dendrite

Axon

Cell body

Nucleus

Electrical
transmission

Synapse
See Figure 2.12

Figure 2-8 •

Stylized depiction of how nerve cells connect with each other. The dendrites receive signals from the terminals of other nerve cells. The transmitted signal then travels through the axon to the next set of terminals and the message is retransmitted. The process continues until the appropriate part of the nervous system is reached.

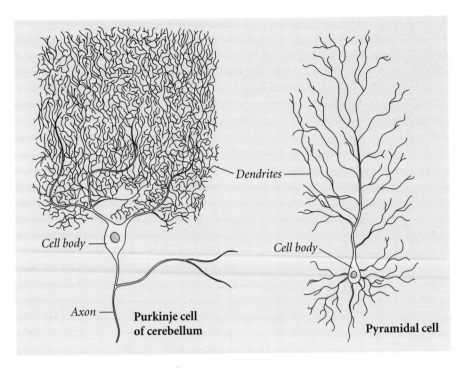

Dendrites

Cell body

Axon

**Purkinje cell
of cerebellum**

Cell body

Pyramidal cell

Figure 2-9 •

A tracing of a Purkinje cell shows just a fraction of the dendrites that receive signals from other cells. A three-dimensional view of the cell would show tens of thousands of connections.

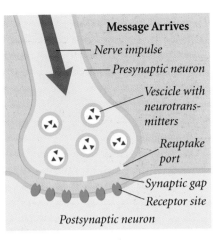

Message Arrives

Nerve impulse

Presynaptic neuron

Vescicle with neurotrans-mitters

Reuptake port

Synaptic gap

Receptor site

Postsynaptic neuron

Figure 2-10 •

This is a simplified version of the synapse between nerve cells. The electrical message (nerve impulse) arrives at the junction of two nerve cells, the synaptic gap.

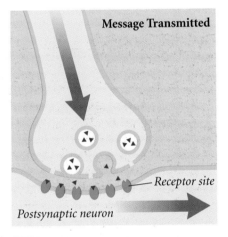

Message Transmitted

Receptor site

Postsynaptic neuron

Figure 2-11 •

The electrical message is retriggered in the postsynaptic neuron by neurotransmitters slotting into specialized receptors.

fraction of the synapses will fire at any given time.

The length of a neuron is determined by the length of the cell body, dendrites, terminals, and particularly the axon which varies from a fraction of a millimeter between brain cells, to a foot between the tooth and brain, to several feet between the spinal cord and toe. Terminals of one nerve cell do not touch dendrites of the adjoining nerve cell because a microscopic gap (**synaptic gap**) exists between them. This gap is 15–50 nm wide. A nanometer (nm) is one billionth of a meter. A million synaptic gap widths added together barely total about one inch.

The message jumps this synaptic gap, from the presynaptic terminal to the postsynaptic dendrite, not as an electrical signal but as microscopic bits of messenger chemicals called "**neurotransmitters**" (Fig. 2-11). These bits of chemicals have been synthesized within the neuron and stored in tiny sacs called **vesicles**. This chemical signal is then converted back to an electrical signal and travels to the next synapse where it's converted to a neu-

rochemical signal. This transmission process across the gap between nerve cells is called a **synapse**. Electrical and chemical signals alternate until the message reaches the appropriate section of the brain. (Some synaptic gaps are one-tenth the width of normal synapses. At these junctures the signal is transmitted electrically. Our focus is on the synapses that need neurotransmitters to jump the gap.)

NEUROTRANSMITTERS & RECEPTORS

This part of the chapter focuses on neurotransmitters and receptors because they are the parts of the central nervous system most affected by psychoactive drugs. Some of the names of the neurotransmitters most involved in psychoactive drug effects are

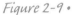 acetylcholine: the first known neurotransmitter, it is mostly active at nerve-muscle junctions; it also affects mental acuity, memory, and learning. Acetylcholine imbalance has been implicated in Alzheimer's disease;

norepinephrine (NE) and epinephrine (E): the second set of neurotransmitters to be discovered, they are classified as catecholamines and function as stimulants when activated by a demand from the body for energy. Besides stimulating the autonomic nervous system, they also affect motivation, hunger, attention span, confidence, and alertness;

dopamine (D): discovered in 1958, this catecholamine helps regulate fine motor muscular activity, emotional stability, satiation, and the reward/pleasure center. Parkinson's disease destroys dopamine-producing areas of the brain thereby inducing erratic motor movements. Too much dopamine causes many of the effects of schizophrenia;

◊ enkephalin: these neuropeptides act on opiate receptors to deaden pain and trigger the reward/pleasure center when pain is relieved. Enkephalins are just part of the more than 24 neuropeptides that have been discovered;

◊ serotonin: this neurotransmitter helps control mood stability including depression and anxiety, appetite, sleep, and sexual activity. Many antidepressants drugs, including Prozac® and Paxil®, are aimed at increasing the amount of serotonin in the system to elevate mood;

◊ GABA (gamma amino butyric acid): GABA, an inhibitory neurotransmitter, is involved in 25% to 40% of all synapses in the brain. It controls impulses, muscle relaxation, and arousal. It is the brain's main inhibitory neurotransmitter;

◊ substance "P": found in sensory neurons, this peptide conveys pain impulses from the peripheral nervous system to the central nervous system. Enkephalins and opiate drugs block release of substance "P";

◊ anandamide: this neurotransmitter discovered in 1995 has an affinity for receptor sites discovered three years earlier which accommodate THC, the main active ingredient in marijuana. It is found in the limbic system and the areas responsible for integration of sensory experiences with emotions as well as those controlling learning, motor coordination, and memory;

◊ glycine: this inhibitory neurotransmitter is found mostly in the spinal cord and brain stem. It is also prominent in protein synthesis;

◊ histamine: besides controlling inflammation of tissues and allergic response, histamine helps regulate emotional behavior and sleep;

◊ nitric oxide: this recently identified neurotransmitter is involved in message transmission to the intestines and other organs including the penis (erectile function). It also has a part in regulation of emotions. When mice are bred without nitric oxide, they exhibit aggression, along with bizarre and excessive sexual behavior (Snyder, 1996);

◊ glutamic acid: this principal excitatory neurotransmitter is one of the major amino acids;

◊ cortisone (corticotrophin): these neurochemicals aid the immune system, healing, and stress.

Besides the 13 listed above, at least 80 more neurotransmitters have been discovered. Researchers have also discovered hundreds of receptors, each one with a different shape. A single neurotransmitter may have multiple receptors; serotonin has at least seven (e.g., 5-HT1A, 5-HT4), each one causing a slightly different effect. Although each nerve cell produces only one type of neurotransmitter, a single neuron might receive messages from several neurotransmitters. A pain message will release substance "P" at one synapse and enkephalin at another. In addition the release of one neurotransmitter usually has a cascade effect. For example, the release of serotonin will trigger the release of enkephalin that then triggers dopamine that will result in a feeling of well-being in the brain's emotional center.

Message transmission (Fig. 2-12) occurs when the incoming electrical signal (1) forces the release of neurotransmitters (2) from the vesicles (3) and sends them across the synaptic gap (4). On the other side of the gap, the neurotransmitters will slot into precise and complex receptor sites (5). These **receptor sites** are structural protein molecules that when activated by a neurotransmitter cause an ion molecular gate (6) to open allowing sodium (7), potassium, or chloride ionic electrical charges in or out. Neurotrans-

mitters that open the gate and allow positive sodium ions in, thus increasing cell firings, are called **excitatory**. Those that allow negative chloride ions in and push positive potassium ions, thus reducing cell firings, are called **inhibitory**.

When enough excitatory neurotransmitters cause sufficient movement of the positively charged sodium ions and the total voltage reaches a certain action potential (about 40–60 mv or millivolts), it fires the signal (8). If enough inhibitory neurotransmitters allow sufficient negative chloride ions in and positive potassium ions out, the electrical potential is kept below the action potential level and the cell is inhibited from firing. The process just described is called the "**first messenger system**." There is also a **second messenger system** where the slotting in of neurotransmitters makes it more likely that other neurotransmitters will stimulate or inhibit a signal. The same neurotransmitter can be a first messenger in one part of the nervous system and a second messenger in another.

Each receptor site is specific for a certain neurotransmitter but a single nerve cell can have receptor sites for a variety of neurochemicals. For example, a serotonin receptor will not accommodate dopamine but a single nerve cell can contain dopamine and serotonin receptors. It is the electral-charge sum of all the activated receptor sites that can cause the cell to reach its action potential and fire off the signal.

As neurotransmitters do their job, they are released back into the synaptic gap and are reabsorbed by the sending nerve cell membrane (reuptake ports [9]) and returned to the vesicles, ready to fire again. Some of the neurotransmitters don't make it back to the reuptake ports of the sending neurons and are metabolized by enzymes surrounding the nerve cells.

The amount of neurotransmitters available for message transmission is constantly monitored by an autoreceptor (10) on the sending neuron. If there are too many neurotransmitters, the cell slows their synthesis and release. If there are too few, it speeds up the

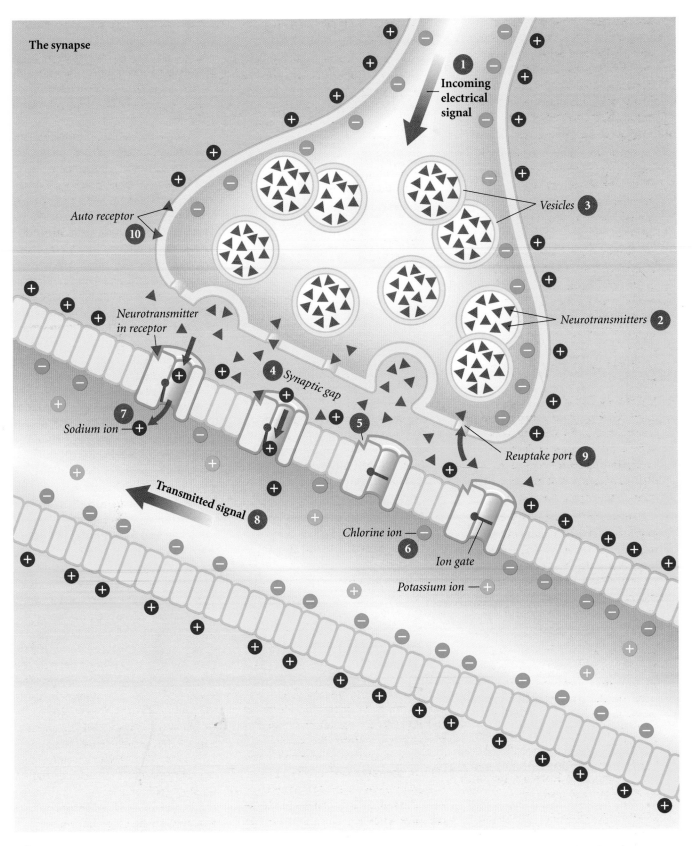

Figure 2-12 •

This is a more complex illustration of what occurs neurochemically and electrically at the synaptic gap. In fact to truly depict the complexity of what happens at the synaptic gap would require dozens of illustrations.

process. In addition the number of receptor sites is altered to compensate for variations in the number of neurotransmitters. If the cell senses there are too many neurotransmitters, it will decrease the number of receptor sites to slow message transmission (**down regulation**). If there are too few neurotransmitters available to trigger the message, the receiving neuron will increase the number of receptor sites so the few neurotransmitters remaining can be more active (**up regulation**). This information will be crucial later in this section to understanding how tolerance, dependence, withdrawal, and addiction occur.

This description of the process of neural transmission is greatly simplified but it is possible to see that it would be easy to induce significant changes in human functioning by making changes at a molecular level. Besides disease states and environmental influences, psychoactive drugs have profound effects at this level.

Agonist & Antagonist

Psychoactive drugs are used because they disrupt the process of message transmission. Generally drugs that enhance the activity of neurotransmitters and receptor sites are called **agonists** and drugs that block the activity are called **antagonists** (somewhat similar to neurotransmitters that are excitatory and inhibitory).

Drugs can act in a variety of ways. They can

◇ chemically imitate part of a neurotransmitter and fool the receptor site into accepting it, thus triggering a false message (e.g., morphine imitates endorphins, thus blocking transmission of substance "P," the neurotransmitter that transmits the sensations of pain);

◇ prevent neurotransmitters from being reabsorbed into the sending neuron, thereby causing more intense effects of that neurochemical (e.g., tricyclic antidepressants prevent the reuptake of serotonin, thus elevating mood);

◇ force the release of neurotransmitters by entering the vesicles and crowding out the natural neurotransmitter, thus causing an exaggerated effect. Cocaine works this way on norepinephrine and dopamine;

◇ inhibit an enzyme that helps synthesize neurotransmitters to slow the nerve cell's production of neurotransmitters, (e.g., heart medications that lower blood pressure by blocking production of norepinephrine which can raise blood pressure);

◇ block the release of neurotransmitters from the vesicles;

◇ interfere with the storage of neurotransmitters allowing them to seep out of vesicles where they are degraded, thus causing a shortage of those neurotransmitters;

◇ inhibit enzymes that metabolize neurotransmitters in the synaptic gap, thus increasing the number of active neurotransmitters. Methamphetamine inhibits monamine oxidase and catechol-O-methyltransferase enzymes that metabolize norepinephrine and epinephrine;

◇ do a combination of these interactions (Snyder, 1996).

A drug will sometimes disrupt communication in more than one of the above ways, e.g., acting as an agonist at low doses and an antagonist at high doses. Sometimes the disruption of neurotransmitters is useful (blocking pain messages), sometimes desirable (releasing stimulatory chemicals), and sometimes it is extremely dangerous (blocking inhibitory neurotransmitters that control violent behavior). For example, a stimulant, such as cocaine, will force the release of norepinephrine (a stimulatory chemical) and dopamine (a pleasure-inducing chemical) from the vesicles and then prevent them from being reabsorbed. The net result is that there are then more of both those neurotransmitters available to exaggerate existing messages and stimulate new ones (Fig. 2-13). The user will stay up past normal exhaustion and feel alert until the neurotransmitters are depleted.

A depressant, such as heroin, will act like a second messenger by mimicking enkephalins and slot into opioid (enkephalin) receptors, thus inhibiting the release of substance "P," a pain-transmitting neurotransmitter (Fig. 2-14). This is the reason that heroin and opioids lessen pain. Heroin also slots into substance "P" receptor sites on the receiving neurons without causing pain

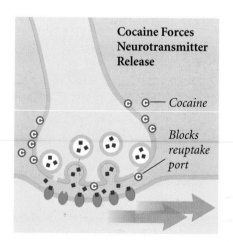

Figure 2-13 •
Cocaine forces the release of extra neurotransmitters and blocks their reabsorption, thus increasing the frequency and therefore the intensity of the electrical signal in the postsynaptic neuron.

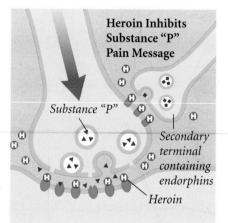

Figure 2-14 •
Heroin inhibits the release of substance "P" and helps block most of the neurotransmitters that do get through. So the electrical signal is greatly weakened each time it crosses a substance "P" synapse.

and acts like an antagonist, further blocking pain transmission. Finally it attaches itself to certain receptor sites in the reward/pleasure center inducing a euphoric sensation. This too is a desired effect. Unfortunately it attaches itself to the breathing center, thereby depressing respiration. This is a dangerous effect.

An all arounder (psychedelic or hallucinogen), such as LSD, will release some stimulatory neurotransmitters but mostly it will alter messages from the external environment; sounds become visual distortions and visual images become distorted sounds. This intermixing of senses is known as **synesthesia**. Other hallucinogens create images that don't exist at all in the external world by blocking the action of acetylcholine. These imaginary images are called **hallucinations**.

Naturally Occurring Substances

Although the first neurotransmitters were discovered in the 1920s (acetylcholine) and 1930s (norepinephrine), it was the discovery in the mid-1970s of endorphins and enkaphlins, neurotransmitters that produce the same effects as opioid drugs, that finally gave an understanding of how psychoactive drugs work in the body. For the first time, reaction and addiction to psychoactive drugs could be described in terms of specific naturally occurring chemical and biologic processes.

Once the existence of endorphins and enkephalins was confirmed, the search for other natural neurochemicals that mimic other psychoactive drugs began in earnest. Over the next 20 years, researchers were able to correlate dozens of psychoactive drugs with the neurotransmitters they affect (Table 2-1).

Besides more than 90 known substances such as neurotransmitters and neuromodulators, it is estimated that eventually several hundred brain chemicals will be identified.

One implication of the research implies that virtually any psychoactive drug works because it mimics or disrupts naturally occurring chemicals in the body that have specific receptor sites. It means that **psychoactive drugs cannot create sensations or feelings that don't have a natural counterpart in the body.** It also implies that human beings can naturally create virtually all of the sensations and feelings they try to get through drugs, although many of them are not as intense as those received through highly concentrated drugs. Here are some examples.

◇ A genuine scare will force the release of adrenaline that will mimic part of an amphetamine rush.

◇ Prolonged running produces a runner's high through the release of endorphins and enkephalins, similar to a modified heroin rush.

◇ Sleep or sensory deprivation can produce true hallucinations through the same neurotransmitters affected by peyote.

◇ Relaxation and stress-reduction exercises can calm restlessness through glycine and GABA modulation, similar to the effects of benzodiazepines, such as Xanax®.

◇ Shock can depress respiration and body functions in a similar fashion as a heroin overdose.

A big difference between natural sensations and drug-induced sensations is that drugs have side effects, particularly if used to excess, and the natural methods of producing the desired effects usually have no side effects. In addition, the more a drug is used, the weaker the effects become (due to tolerance) and the harder it becomes to reproduce the desired sensations. With natural sensations, the opposite is true. The desired effects become easier to reproduce over time.

Neurotransmitter research seems to indicate that some people are drawn to certain drugs because they have an imbalance in one or more neurotransmitter and they discovered through experimentation that a specific drug or drugs would help correct that imbalance. For example, people who are born with low endorphin/enkephalin levels or who have damaged their ability to make these chemicals have a propensity for opioid and alcohol use. Similarly those with low epinephrine and norepinephrine (which can cause attention deficit disorder) may be predisposed to amphetamine or cocaine abuse. This is because those drugs mimic the deficient neurotransmitters and make the user feel normal, satisfied, and in control.

TABLE 2–1   PSYCHOACTIVE DRUG/NEUROTRANSMITTER RELATIONSHIPS

Drug	Neurotransmitters Directly Affected
Alcohol	GABA (gama amine butyric acid), met-enkephalin, serotonin
Benzodiazepines	GABA, glycine
Marijuana	Anandamide, acetylcholine
Heroin	Endorphin, enkephalin, dopamine
LSD	Acetylcholine, dopamine, serotonin
Nicotine	Epinephrine, endorphin, acetylcholine
Cocaine and amphetamines	Epinephrine, norepinephrine, serotonin, dopamine, acetylcholine
MDA, MDMA	Serotonin, dopamine, epinephrine, norepinephrine
PCP	Dopamine, acetylcholine, alpha-endopsychosin

PHYSIOLOGICAL RESPONSES TO DRUGS

It is the way in which psychoactive drugs interact with neurotransmitters, nerve cells, and other tissues that helps determine how drugs affect people and why it is difficult to control their levels of use. Factors such as tolerance, tissue dependence, psychic dependence, withdrawal, and drug metabolism can moderate or intensify these effects.

TOLERANCE

"When I first started, I remember having a huge reaction to a small amount of 'speed.' Inside of a year I could shoot a spoon of it easily, which is a pretty fair amount, and it finally got to a point where I couldn't even sleep unless I'd done some."

Recovering 34-year-old methamphetamine user

The body regards any drug it takes as a toxin. Various organs, especially the liver and kidneys, try to eliminate the chemical before it does too much damage. But if the use continues over a long period of time, the body is forced to change and adapt to develop **tolerance** to the continued input of foreign substances. The net result is that the user has to take larger and larger amounts to achieve the same effect. In experiments with rats, one hour of access to self-administered cocaine per session did not increase intake or tolerance. However, six hours of access escalated tolerance and increased the **hedonic set point** that is defined as an individual's preferred level of pharmacological effects from a drug (Ahmed & Koob, 1998). For example, the body adapts to an upper, such as methamphetamine, in order to minimize the stimulant's effect on the heart and other systems, so the drug appears to weaken with each succeeding dose if it's used frequently. More has to be taken just to achieve the same effect. One amphetamine tablet on the first day of use will energize a user and trigger a euphoria that can only be matched by 20 tablets on the 100th day of use.

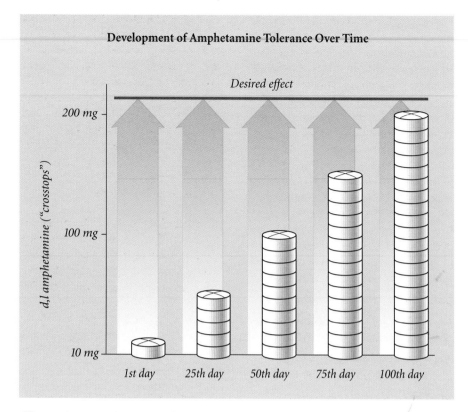

Development of Amphetamine Tolerance Over Time

Desired effect

d,l amphetamine ("crosstops")

200 mg
100 mg
10 mg

1st day   25th day   50th day   75th day   100th day

Figure 2-15 •

This graph shows the gradually increasing amounts of amphetamine needed to produce stimulation or euphoria over time.

Some degree of tolerance develops with all psychoactive drugs. One dose of LSD on the 1st day, three on the 7th day, and nine on the 30th day might be needed to give the same psychedelic effect if the drug were taken daily. A glass of whiskey at the beginning of one's drinking career might give the same buzz as a five drinks on New Year's Eve 4 years later.

The development of tolerance varies widely depending mostly on the qualities of the drug itself. But it also depends on the amount, frequency, and duration of use, the chemistry of the user, and the psychological state of mind of the user. There are several different kinds of tolerance.

Kinds of Tolerance

Dispositional Tolerance. The body speeds up the breakdown (metabolism) of the drug in order to eliminate it. This is particularly the case with barbiturates and alcohol. An example of this biological adaptation can be seen with alcohol. It increases the amount of cytocells and mitochondria in the liver that are available to neutralize the drug, therefore more has to be drunk to reach the same level of intoxication.

Pharmacodynamic Tolerance. Nerve cells become less sensitive to the effects of the drug and even produce an antidote or antagonist to the drug. With opioids, the brain will generate more opioid receptor sites and produce its own antagonist, cholecystokinin. Further, down regulation of receptor sites results in pharmacodynamic tolerance.

Behavioral Tolerance. The brain learns to compensate for the effects of the drug by using parts of the brain not affected. A drunk person can make himself appear sober when confronted by police but might be staggering again a few minutes later.

Reverse Tolerance. Initially one becomes less sensitive to the drug but as it destroys certain tissues and/or as one grows older, the trend is suddenly reversed and the user becomes less able to handle even moderate amounts. This is particularly true in alcoholics when, as the liver is destroyed, it loses the ability to metabolize the drug. An alcoholic with cirrhosis of the liver can stay drunk all day long on a pint of wine because the raw alcohol is passing through the body repeatedly, unchanged.

"At first I could drink a lot, for about eight or nine years. They'd say I finished 10 or more highballs in the bar but I'd never get falling-down drunk. I'd be pretty high but never passed out. Now, especially since my liver is only slightly smaller than a Volkswagen and not doing its job, if I drink over about 4 drinks, I can't walk one of those white lines a cop makes you walk if he thinks you're DUI."
43-year-old alcohol user

Acute Tolerance (tachyphylaxis). In these cases, the body begins to adapt almost instantly to the toxic effects of the drug. With tobacco, for example, tolerance and adaptation begin to develop with the first puff. Someone who tries suicide with barbiturates can develop an acute tolerance and survive the attempt. They could be awake and alert even with twice the lethal dose in their systems even if they've never taken barbiturates before.

Select Tolerance. If increased quantities of a drug are taken to overcome this tolerance and to achieve a certain high, it's easy to forget that tolerance to the physical side effects also continues to escalate but not at the same rate. The dose needed to achieve an emotional high comes closer and closer to the lethal physical dose of that drug (Fig. 2-16).

"As many pills as I had, I would take. I didn't really care about overdose, which I did many times."
Former barbiturate user

Thus people develop different rates of tolerance to different effects of the same drug. Codeine kills pain but causes nausea on the first day it is taken. Within a week it still kills pain but no longer causes nausea.

Inverse Tolerance (kindling). The person becomes more sensitive to the effects of the drug as the brain chemistry changes. A marijuana or cocaine user, after months of getting a minimal effect from the drug, will all of a sudden get an intense reaction.

"At first I couldn't understand what people got out of methamphetamine. I'd shoot some and it gave me a little lift but that was it. Then one time I got a 1/4 gram, all for myself, and did it all in one shot and the effect was unlike anything I'd ever had before, like liquid fire. My brain was all of a sudden trained to recognize the effects. Then after that, when I'd use a smaller amount, I would experience those same effects though never quite as intense."
Recovering methamphetamine abuser

A cocaine or methamphetamine addict develops a greater risk of heart attack or stroke after prolonged use due to the toxic effects of those drugs. Thus they become more sensitive to the toxic effects after continued use.

TISSUE DEPENDENCE

Tissue dependence is the **biological adaptation** of the body due to prolonged use of drugs It is often quite extensive, particularly with downers. In fact with certain drugs, the body can change so much that the tissues and organs come to depend on the drug just to stay normal. If the body doesn't have the drug, its biological adaptations can cause a series of side effects. For example, the increased number of cytocells and mitochondria in the liver of an alcoholic depends on repeated use of alcohol to maintain their existence. When alcohol is discontinued, their numbers return to nor-

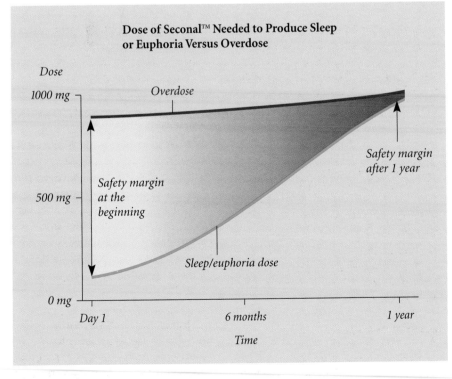

Figure 2-16 •

With many drugs, tolerance to mental effects develops at a different rate than tolerance to physical effects.

mal levels. Enzymatic changes in the liver of a heroin addict trigger the need for regular doses of heroin to maintain the new chemical balance.

"I would start to feel very abnormal after two or three hours and it was like trying to maintain until I could begin to feel normal. And that was the only kind of normal that I knew, Darvon® -induced normality."
Recovering Darvon® user

In the past a drug was called addicting only if clear-cut tissue dependence developed as evidenced by objective physical signs of withdrawal, but with breakthroughs in modern neurochemical research, more subtle changes in body chemistry can be measured. In addition psychological dependence has been recognized in recent years as an important factor in the development of addictive behavior. Researchers, such as Dr. Anna Rose Childress at Veterans Hospital in Philadelphia, have shown that psychological dependence actually produces many physical effects, meaning that defining drug dependence as strictly physical or strictly mental is not accurate (Childress, McElgin, Mozley, et al., 1996).

PSYCHIC DEPENDENCE & THE REWARD-REINFORCING ACTION OF DRUGS

Psychic dependence and the positive reward-reinforcing action of drugs result from the direct influence of drugs on brain chemistry. Drugs cause an altered state of consciousness and distorted perceptions pleasurable to the user. These reinforce the continued use of the drug. Psychic dependence can therefore result from the continued misuse of drugs to deal with life's problems or from their continued use to compensate for inherited deficiencies in brain-reward hormones.

Drugs also have the innate ability to guide and virtually hypnotize the user into continual use (called the **"positive reward-reinforcing action of drugs"**). In the animal experiments in which rats were trained to press a lever that would feed them heroin or other drugs intravenously, they would continue to press the lever even before physical dependence had developed, showing that a psychoactive drug, in and of itself, can reinforce the desire to use.

"I have a choice about the first snort of cocaine I take. I have no choice about the second."
Recovering cocaine user

WITHDRAWAL

When the user stops taking a drug that has created tolerance and tissue dependence, the body is left with an altered chemistry. There might be an overabundance of enzymes, receptor sites, or neurotransmitters. Without the drug to support this altered chemistry, the body all of a sudden tries to return to normal. **Withdrawal** is defined as the body's attempt to rebalance itself after prolonged use of a psychoactive drug. All the things the body was kept from doing while taking the drug, it does to excess while in withdrawal. For example, consider how the desired effects of heroin are quickly replaced by unpleasant withdrawal symptoms once a long-time user stops taking the drug (Table 2-2).

In fact with many compulsive users, the fear of withdrawal is one reason they keep using. They don't want to go through the aches, pains, insomnia, vomiting, cramps, and occasional convulsions that accompany withdrawal.

"The rush I would get from shooting up again was all of a sudden my body wouldn't be sick anymore from withdrawal. That was the high."
32-year-old recovering heroin user

Because the withdrawal as well as the fear of withdrawal can be so severe, many treatment programs use mild drugs to temper these symptoms. Withdrawal from opiates, alcohol, many sedatives, and even nicotine seems to be triggered by an area of the brainstem known as the locus cereleus. Drugs like Catapres®, Vasopressin®, and Baclofen®, which act on this part of the brain, block out the withdrawal symptoms of these drugs.

Kinds of Withdrawal

There are three distinct types of withdrawal symptoms: nonpurposive, purposive, and protracted.

TABLE 2–2 OPIOID EFFECTS VS. WITHDRAWAL SYMPTOMS

(Withdrawal effects are often the opposite of the drug's direct effects.)

Effects	Withdrawal Symptoms
Numbness	becomes pain
Euphoria	becomes anxiety
Dryness of mouth	becomes sweating, runny nose, tearing, and increased salivation
Constipation	becomes diarrhea
Slow pulse	becomes rapid pulse
Low blood pressure	becomes high blood pressure
Shallow breathing and suppressed cough	become coughing
Pinpoint pupils	become dilated pupils
Sluggishness	becomes severe hyper-reflexes & muscle cramps

Nonpurposive Withdrawal. Nonpurposive withdrawal consists of objective physical signs that are directly observable upon cessation of drug use by an addict. These include seizures, sweating, goose bumps, vomiting, diarrhea, and tremors that are a direct result of the tissue dependence.

"When I ran out, it was severe. I mean, body convulsions, long memory lapses, cramps that were just enough to— you couldn't stand them. And it lasted for about five days; the actual convulsions, the cramps, and the pain and stuff. And then it took another couple of weeks before I ever felt anywhere near normal."
Recovering 18-year-old heroin user

Purposive Withdrawal. Purposive withdrawal results from either addict manipulation (hence purposive or with purpose) or from a psychic conversion reaction from the expectation of the withdrawal process. **Psychic conversion** is an emotional expectation of physical effects that have no biological explanation. Since a common behavior of most addicts is malingering or manipulation in an effort to secure more drugs, sympathy, or money, they may claim to have withdrawal symptoms that are very diverse and difficult to verify, e.g., "My nerves are in an uproar. You've got to give me something, Doc!" Physicians and pharmacists have to be very aware of these kinds of manipulations.

"It takes a doctor 30 minutes to say no but it only takes him 5 minutes to say yes. We used to share doctors that we could scam. We called them 'croakers.'"
Recovering 33-year-old heroin user

Within the past few decades, the portrayal of drug addiction by the media, books, movies, and television has resulted in another kind of purposive withdrawal. When they run out of drugs, younger addiction-naive drug users expect to suffer withdrawal symptoms similar to those portrayed in the media. This expectation results in a neurotic condition whereby they experience a wide range of reactions even though tissue dependence has not truly developed. Treatment personnel need to avoid overreacting to these symptoms.

Protracted Withdrawal (environmental triggers & cues). A major danger to maintaining recovery and preventing a drug overdose during relapse is protracted withdrawal. This is a flashback or recurrence of the addiction withdrawal symptoms and triggering of a heavy craving for the drug long after an addict has been detoxified. The cause of this reaction (similar to a posttraumatic stress phenomenon) often happens when some sensory input (odor, sight, noise) stimulates the memories experienced during drug use or withdrawal and evokes a desire for the drug by the addict. For instance, the odor of burnt matches or burning metal (smells that occur when cooking heroin) several months after detoxification may cause a heroin addict to suffer some withdrawal symptoms. Any white powder may cause craving in a cocaine addict; a blue pill may do it to a Valium® addict; and a barbecue can cause a recovering alcoholic to crave a drink.

"I had just got a disability check and that check was like a trigger for me. It just sent me into a state of nervousness or anxiety and I didn't know what to do. Today, I may not even walk on the same block that I used to walk on because I know if I'm feeling shaky, there could be a possibility that I'll run into somebody I want to use with, so I have to stay away from those areas."
Recovering 32-year-old "crack" cocaine abuser

Protracted withdrawal often causes users to try their drug again, generally leading to a full relapse. Unfortunately these slips are associated with a greater chance of drug overdose since users are prone to use the same dose they were injecting, smoking, or snorting when they quit. They often forget that their last dose was probably a very high one that they could handle because tolerance had developed. They don't remember that abstinence allowed their bodies to return to a less tolerant state.

"We cleaned up because we didn't have any connections when we moved. We had about 15 clonidine pills to help us through and I was drinking. Then we shared one bag, one $20 bag of 'cut,' and both of us were on the floor."
33-year-old husband and wife heroin users

Strangely, research with animals and interviews with addicts demonstrates that once abstinence is interrupted, both tolerance and tissue dependence develop at a much faster rate than before.

BASIC PHARMACOLOGY

METABOLISM & EXCRETION

"If you want to explain any poison properly, then remember, all things are poison. Nothing is without poison; the dose alone causes a thing to be a poison."
Theophrastus von Hohenhein, aka Paracelsus, 1535

Metabolism is defined as the body's mechanism for processing, using, and inactivating a foreign substance, such as a drug or food in the body, while **excretion** is the process of eliminating those foreign substances and their metabolites from the body.

As a drug exerts its influence upon the body, it is gradually neutralized, usually by the liver. It can also be metabolized in the blood, in the lymph fluid, by brain enzymes and chemicals, or by most any body tissue that recognizes the drug as a foreign substance. Drugs can also be inactivated by diverting them to body fat or proteins that hold the substances to prevent them from acting on body organs.

The **liver,** in particular, has the ability to break down or alter the

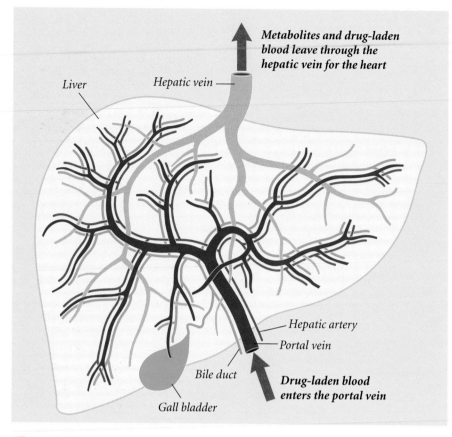

Metabolites and drug-laden blood leave through the hepatic vein for the heart

Liver

Hepatic vein

Hepatic artery

Portal vein

Bile duct

Drug-laden blood enters the portal vein

Gall bladder

Figure 2-17 •

The liver deactivates a portion of the drug with each recirculation through the circulatory system.

chemical structure of drugs, making them less active or inert. The **kidneys,** on the other hand, filter the metabolites, water, and other waste from the blood and the resulting urine through the ureter, bladder, and urethra. Drugs can also be excreted out of the body by the lungs, in sweat, or in feces.

Metabolic processes generally decrease (but occasionally increase) the effects of psychoactive drugs. For instance, the liver's enzymes help convert alcohol to water, oxygen, and carbon dioxide that are then excreted from the body through the kidneys, sweat glands, and lungs. Some drugs, such as Valium®, are known as prodrugs because they are transformed by the liver's enzymes into three or four other drugs that are more active than the original drug.

If a drug is eliminated slowly, as with Valium®, it can affect the body for hours, even days. If it is eliminated quickly, as with smokable cocaine or nitrous oxide, the major actions might last just a few minutes, though other subtle side effects last for days, weeks, or even longer. Following are some other factors that affect the metabolism of drugs.

◊ Age: After the age of 30 and with each subsequent year, the body produces fewer and fewer liver enzymes capable of metabolizing certain drugs, thus the older the person, the greater the effect. This is especially true with drugs like alcohol and sedative-hypnotics.

◊ Race: Different ethnic groups have different levels of enzymes. Over 50% of Asians break down alcohol more slowly than do Caucasians. They suffer more side effects, such as redness of the face, than many other ethnic groups.

◊ Heredity: Individuals pass certain traits to their offspring that affect

the metabolism of drugs. They can have a low level of enzymes that metabolize the drug; they can have more body fat that will store certain drugs like Valium® or marijuana; or they can have a high metabolic rate that will usually eliminate drugs more quickly from the body.

◊ Sex: Males and females have different body chemistry and different body water volumes. Drugs such as alcohol and barbiturates generally have greater effects in women than in men.

◊ Health: Certain medical conditions affect metabolism. Alcohol in a drinker with severe liver damage (hepatitis, cirrhosis) causes more problems than in a drinker with a healthy liver.

◊ Emotional State: The emotional state of the drug user also has a major influence on the drug's effects. LSD in people with paranoia can be very dangerous because it can further disrupt the chemical imbalance of the brain and increase their paranoia.

◊ Other Drugs: The presence of two or more drugs can keep the body so busy metabolizing one that metabolism of the second drug is delayed. For example, the presence of alcohol keeps the liver so busy that a Xanax® or Seconal® will remain in the body two or three times longer than normal. Other drug interactions also cause increased or decreased effects and toxicity.

◊ Other Factors: In addition factors such as the weight of the user, the level of tolerance, the state of mind, and even the weather can affect metabolism of a psychoactive drug.

◊ Exaggerated Reaction: In some cases the reaction to a drug will be out of proportion to the amount taken. Perhaps the user has an allergy to the drug in much the same way a person can go into shock from a single bee sting. For example, a person who lacks the enzyme which metabolizes cocaine can die from exposure to just a tiny amount.

FROM EXPERIMENTATION TO ADDICTION

DESIRED EFFECTS VS. SIDE EFFECTS

"Let's not kid ourselves. People initially do get something from drugs. They don't say, 'Well, I want to feel miserable so I think I'll swallow this.' They don't think, 'I'm gonna make myself cough by smoking a joint until my eyes become bloodshot.' They don't plan to get hepatitis or AIDS from a shared needle. They get something out of the drug, something desirable enough to throw caution to the wind."

Darryl S. Inaba, CEO, Haight-Ashbury Free Clinics

DESIRED EFFECTS

People take psychoactive drugs for the mental, emotional, and even physical effects they induce. In some cases they are specific about the effect they want and in other cases they are more abstract about their desires.

Curiosity & Availability

"I would be doing a lot better in school if I didn't get stoned. But marijuana is always around and everybody was doing it so I said, 'Why not?'"

16-year-old marijuana smoker

To Get High

"It's kind of like life without a coherent thought. It's kind of like an escape. It's like when you go to sleep, you kind of forget about things in your sleep. It's like everything's dreamlike and there's no restraints on anything."

17-year-old heroin user

Self-Medication

"I was very hyperactive, you know. Just always getting into trouble doing things, getting hurt, falling off of things, getting in fights, getting in arguments. And the more I smoked as the years went on, the mellower I got. I stopped getting into trouble."

23-year-old marijuana user

Confidence

"I felt like I was on top of the world and I could accomplish anything. I was self-confident. Just the physical part of staying up so long and being able to feel the freedom of staying up so long was great."

22-year-old recovering methamphetamine addict

Energy

"I felt really tingly, excited, sexy. I felt that I had all this energy. I felt like I could do anything. I felt really powerful and I enjoyed that feeling. It made me feel good."

19-year-old recovering male methamphetamine addict

Pain Relief

"I'm always in pain. I have bad shoulders, arthritis, and all these things, so it was my excuse 'cause I knew this stuff would get me high, so I would take it. I would say, 'Oh, I'm just killing my pain.'"

26-year-old opioid user

Anxiety Control

"It relieved certain anxieties. It alleviated depression, which I had. Lots of depression. You tell the doctor, 'I'm depressed.' 'Okay, take some Valium".' Now they try to give you antidepressant medications prescribed by the doctor. I'll take the Valium®"

44-year-old Valium® user

To Oblige Friends (internal & external peer pressure)

"If your friends are all getting stoned, then you don't want to just sit there, you know, they're all going to be like having supposedly even more fun because they're stoned, you know. And then they make you look stupid because you feel stupid if you're not."

15-year-old marijuana smoker

Social Confidence

"Somebody walks in the room and what do you do, you offer them a drink. It's cordial. That's how you break the ice. You ask, 'Would you like a drink?' And I frankly don't know anyone who says no. I like to drink. Drink is good. It makes me happy. It makes everybody else I know happy. It's a social event."

42-year-old alcohol user

Boredom Relief

"They tell you you're going to school to get an education so you can get a good job, okay? They told me how to get a job, so that's eight hours a day. I knew how to sleep, that's eight hours a day. I had another eight hours a day that I didn't know how to fill and I used marijuana to fill those eight hours. Period."

35-year-old recovering marijuana user

Altered Consciousness

"I was really into the literature of the time—The Politics of Ecstasy, or something like that, by Timothy Leary, High Priest of the LSD movement. It was more like an adventure, looking for things in it. I think people doing it

at that time were trying to find out what it was like to have some sort of spiritual experience."
48-year-old LSD user

To Deal with Isolation or Life Problems

"When I got addicted to the cocaine, it was because I was being battered and I used that to hide. When I left the cocaine, I used the drinking to hide. When I left the drinking, the cigarettes kicked in. When I left the cigarettes, I began to overeat. It was like I had to fill up that hole with something."
28-year-old recovering compulsive overeater

Oblivion

"I would sit there with a nice little metal pipe and a sack of big 'chronic bud' and try to see how much of it I could smoke and basically I'd get to the point where I realize I'm laying on the floor. I've got the pipe in my hand; I can barely keep my eyes open and I'm trying to light the pipe with a child-proof lighter that just doesn't work, so I assume that that's as high as I'm going to get."
22-year-old marijuana user

Competitive Edge

"I was 125 pounds. Not big enough for the team. I started taking steroids I got from a weightlifter friend so I could bulk up. I also started eating like a hungry hog."
19-year-old steroid user

SIDE EFFECTS

If drugs did only what people wanted them to and they weren't used to excess, they wouldn't be much of a problem. But drugs not only generate desired emotional and physical effects; they also trigger side effects that can be mild, moderate, dangerous, or sometimes fatal. This competition between the emotional/physical effects that users want and those they don't want is one of the main problems with using psychoactive drugs. For example, a psychoactive drug such as codeine (an opioid-downer) can be prescribed by a physician to relieve pain, to suppress a cough, or to treat severe diarrhea. It also acts as a sedative, gives a feeling of well-being, and induces numbness and relaxation. People who self-prescribe codeine just for the feeling of well-being or numbness will have slower reaction time and often become constipated. With moderate use they can also be subject to nausea, pinpoint pupils, dry skin, and slowed respiration. And if users keep using in order to recapture that feeling of well-being over a long period of time, they can become lethargic, lose sexual desire, and even become compulsive users of the drug.

Users try to learn ways to take enough of a drug or drugs to get the desired emotional and physical effects without too many side effects that might disrupt their lives. They also try to keep drug use from accelerating to the point where craving for the drug overwhelms common sense. And if drug use continues to accelerate, toxic effects begin to overwhelm the desired effects.

Other complications of drug use include legal problems, relationship problems, financial problems, emotional problems, health problems, control problems, and work problems. The more compulsively a person uses, the more severe the various complications.

POLYDRUG ABUSE

Virtually every client who comes in for treatment to a clinic has not confined drug use to just one drug or behavior. For this reason treatment is more complex than just getting a person off a drug. There are a number of reasons a person will resort to polydrug use.

◊ Replacement: using another drug when the desired drug is not available, e.g., drinking alcohol when heroin is not available.

◊ Multiple drug use: the use of several drugs of different types for different feelings, e.g., taking methamphetamine for stimulation and being bored with it; then using ketamine for a different effect, as long as it changes one's mood.

◊ Cycling: using drugs intensely for a period of time, abstaining or using another drug to rest the body or lower tolerance and then using again, e.g., taking an anabolic steroid for two weeks then a different steroid for two weeks, then nothing for two weeks, then back to the original steroid.

◊ Stacking: using two or more similar drugs at one time to enhance a specific desired effect, e.g., using a barbiturate and benzodiazepine to get to sleep; using MDMA ("ecstasy") with methamphetamine to enhance the "ecstasy" high.

◊ Mixing: somewhat similar to stacking, mixing uses drug combinations to induce different effects, e.g., "speedballs" (cocaine with heroin); lacing a marijuana joint with cocaine; X and L ("ecstasy" and LSD) to prolong the effects of each; methadone with klonopine to mimic the effect of heroin; an antihistamine and a sedative to intensify the downer effects. Some of these combinations are taken intentionally and some unintentionally when a dealer spikes his drug with a cheaper drug, e.g., PCP is used to spike a marijuana cigarette to mimic a high THC content.

◊ Sequentialing: using one drug in an abusive or addictive manner then later on switching to another addiction, e.g., a recovering heroin addict who starts using alcohol compulsively; a cocaine addict who switches to methamphetamines. The sequence can include behavioral addictions, e.g., a recovering alcoholic who becomes a compulsive gambler, a compulsive marijuana smoker who switches to compulsive eating, or a two-pack-a-day smoker who switches to marijuana.

◇ Morphing: the use of one drug to counteract the effects of another drug, e.g., a cocaine user so wired he/she has to drink alcohol to come down; the drunk who drinks coffee to try and wake up; the heroin addict who uses "meth" to function.

LEVELS OF USE

It is important to judge the level at which a person uses drugs and thereby have a benchmark by which to judge whether drug use is accelerating or becoming problematic. To judge a person's level of use, it is necessary to first know the amount, frequency, and duration of psychoactive drug use. These three factors by themselves are not enough to judge the level of use. The second key factor is to know the impact the use has on an individual's life. For example, a man might drink a six-pack of lager beer (amount) twice a week (frequency) and keep it up for 12 years (duration) without developing any problems. Another man might only drink on Fridays but doesn't stop until he passes out. The second man might have more problems regarding health, the law, or money than the first man who drinks every evening but functions well on the job and works at his relationships.

The categories we've chosen to help people judge the level of use are abstinence, experimentation, social use, habituation, drug abuse, and addiction. The levels of use are presented as distinct categories although the transition from experimentation to habituation or habituation to addiction does not happen in distinct phases. Rather it is a continuous process that can ebb and flow depending on whether the person is using, how much is being used, and what effect the use is having. Unfortunately with most psychoactive drugs, a point is passed where it becomes harder and harder for the person to choose the level at

which they want to continue to use. That point can vary radically from person to person.

ABSTINENCE

Abstinence means people do not use a psychoactive substance except accidentally, for example, when they drink some alcohol-laced punch, take prescribed medication that has a psychoactive component they don't know about, or are in an unventilated room with smokers. The important fact to remember about abstinence is that even if people have a very strong hereditary and environmental susceptibility to use drugs compulsively, they will never have a problem if they never begin to use. If they never use, there is no possibility of developing drug craving. They might, however, have a problem with compulsive behaviors, such as gambling, overeating, excessive TV watching, or obsessive sexual behavior. In addition exposure to family drug use often affects a person's behavior and life even if they remain abstinent from drugs. Adult children of addicts often have difficulty in maintaining relationships or holding a steady job.

Recent archival research by the Office of National Drug Control Policy has shown that those who experiment with alcohol, nicotine, and marijuana between the ages of 10–12 are tremendously more likely to become a heroin or cocaine addict than those who don't. Further, their research demonstrates that those individuals who never try nicotine before the age of 21 have almost zero addiction to tobacco later in life.

"My brother died of alcoholism, so I have never had a drink of alcohol or for that matter, a puff on a cigarette."
Donald Trump, 1999

EXPERIMENTATION

With experimentation, people become curious about the effects of a drug or are influenced by relatives, friends, advertising, or other media

and take some when it becomes available to satisfy that curiosity. The feature that distinguishes experimentation from abstinence is the curiosity about drug use and the willingness to act on that curiosity. With experimentation, drug use is limited to only a few exposures. No patterns of use develop and there are only limited negative consequences in the person's life except if

◇ large amounts are used at one time leading to accident, injury, or illness (e.g., drinking binge);

◇ the person has an exaggerated reaction to a small amount (e.g., cocaine allergy);

◇ a preexisting physical or mental condition is aggravated (e.g., schizophrenia);

◇ the user is pregnant;

◇ legal troubles arise (e.g., drug test, possession arrest);

◇ a high genetic and/or environmental susceptibility to compulsive use triggers abuse;

◇ a history of addictive behavior with other psychoactive drugs leads to a relapse.

Then experimentation can rapidly become a more serious level of drug use.

"A lot of my friends did heroin. I just wanted to try it. It was an experiment. I just wanted to see what it was like. It felt good for a little while; you nod off and you are half-dreaming."
22-year-old polydrug user

SOCIAL/RECREATIONAL

Whether it's a legal six-pack at a party, an illegal "joint" with a friend, or a couple of lines of cocaine at home, with social/recreational use, the person does seek out a drug and does want to experience a certain effect, but there is no established pattern. Drug use is irregular, infrequent, and has a relatively small impact on the person's life except if it triggers exaggerated reactions, preexisting mental and physical conditions, an existing addiction, genetic/

environmental susceptibility, or legal troubles. Social/recreational use is therefore distinguished from experimental use by the establishment of drug-seeking behavior.

"The friends I started hanging out with in school were pretty much the ones that were really rebelling and already knew about cigarettes and pot and so we just started sneaking off and someone would have the end of a joint or something that their dad left around."
24-year-old marijuana smoker

HABITUATION

With habituation, there is a definite pattern of use: the TGIF high, the five cups of coffee every day, or the 1/2-gram of cocaine most weekends. No matter what happens that day or that week, the person will use that drug. As long as it doesn't affect that person's life in a really negative way, it could be called habituation. This level of use clearly demonstrates that one has lost some control of use of the drug. Regardless of how frequently or infrequently a drug is used, a definite pattern of use indicates that the craving for the drug is now starting to control the user.

"You would say that I was a habitual user but I don't really think that's the case. So, it is a habit. I like a drink. And the question, you know, the question is could I go a day without having a drink? I think so but I've never had a reason to try."
42-year-old habitual drinker

DRUG ABUSE

Our definition of drug abuse is **the continued use of a drug despite negative consequences.** It's the use of cocaine in spite of high blood pressure; the use of LSD though there's a history of mental instability; the alcoholic with diabetes; the two-pack-a-day smoker with emphysema; or the user with a series of arrests for possession. No mat-

ter how often a person uses a drug, if negative consequences develop in relationships, social life, finances, legal status, health, work, school, or emotional well-being and drug use continues on a regular basis, then that behavior could be classified as drug abuse.

"I had an EEG and a CAT scan and I was told that I had lowered my seizure threshold by doing so many stimulants but that's not the reason I stopped using them. The reason I actually stopped was because I discovered heroin and I liked it better. I would probably have continued using 'speed' even with the seizures."
36-year-old "speed" user

ADDICTION

The step between abuse and addiction has to do with **compulsion.** If users

◇ spend most of their time either using, getting, or thinking about the drug;

◇ continue to use in spite of negative life and health consequences, mental or physical;

◇ often deny there's a problem or claim that they can stop anytime they want;

◇ and, after withdrawal, still have a strong tendency to relapse and start using again;

then that can be classified as addiction. The users have lost control of their use of drugs and those substances have become the most important things in their lives.

"The craving was just continuous. It was just like if I was coming off 'speed,' I wanted heroin. If I was coming off heroin, I wanted to snort cocaine. And if I was coming off that, I wanted to stay numb. I wanted to go from one drug to another. If I wanted to stay up all night, I would do 'speed.'"
38-year-old recovering polydrug addict

THEORIES OF ADDICTION

"It's just not a physical addiction. It's a spiritual and emotional problem too. It just doesn't encompass your body. Your mind is totally off key. You're just so involved in whatever the addiction is. You're not living your life. You're living for the addiction."
43-year-old recovering addict

In the past two decades, a tremendous amount of research has been done and many theories have been generated to help understand the process of drug addiction. These theories have a strong influence on drug abuse education, prevention, and treatment. Besides early and recent psychodynamic concepts of compulsive behaviors (Brehm & Khantzian, 1997), there have been three major schools of thought about addiction. One of the theories emphasizes the influence of heredity (Addictive Disease Model), another the influence of environment and behavior (Behavioral/Environmental Model), and the third the influence of the physiological effects of psychoactive drugs (Academic Model).

ADDICTIVE DISEASE MODEL

The addictive disease model, sometimes called the "**medical model,**" maintains that the disease of addiction is a chronic, progressive, relapsing, incurable, and potentially fatal condition that is mostly a consequence of genetic irregularities in brain chemistry and anatomy that may be activated by the particular drugs that are abused. It also maintains that addiction is set into motion by experimentation with the drug by a susceptible host in an environment that is conducive to drug misuse. The susceptible user quickly experiences a compulsion to use, a loss of control, and a determination to continue the use despite negative physical, emotional, or life consequences.

"The first time I tried it and I got high I said, 'I think I want to use some of

*this for the rest of my life if I could af-
ford it. If I could afford this, I would do
this everyday for the rest of my life.'"*
43-year-old recovering heroin addict.

Several studies of twins, along with other human and animal studies, strongly support the view that heredity is a powerful influence on uncontrolled compulsive drug use and behavioral addictions (Noble, Blum, Montgomery, Sheridan, 1991; Blum, Cull, Braverman, Comings, 1996; Clark, Moss, Kirisci, 1997; Schuckit, 1986; Eisen, et al., 1998). Under the Addictive Disease Model, addiction is characterized by

◊ impulsive drug abuse marked by intoxication throughout the day and an overwhelming need to continue use;

◊ loss of control over the use of a drug with an inability to reduce intake or stop use;

◊ repeated attempts to control use with periods of temporary abstinence interrupted by relapse into compulsive continual drug use;

◊ continuation of abuse despite the progressive development of serious physical, mental, or social disorders aggravated by the use of the substance;

◊ episodes or complications which result from intoxication, such as an arrest, heart attack, alcoholic blackout, opiate overdose, loss of job, breakup of a relationship, or any other disabling or impairing condition;

◊ pathological initial reaction to initial drug use such as increased initial tolerance, black- or brownouts, dramatic personality and lifestyle changes.

(APA, 1994)

BEHAVIORAL/ ENVIRONMENTAL MODEL

This theory emphasizes the overriding importance of environmental and developmental influences in leading a user to progress into addictive behavior. As seen in animal and human studies, **environmental factors can change brain chemistry** as surely as drug use or heredity (LeDoux, 1996). Many studies, supported by SPECT and PET scans that show brain function, suggest that physical/emotional stress, such as abuse, anger, peer pressure, and other environmental factors, cause people to seek, use, and sustain their continued dependence on drugs (Griffiths, Bigelow, & Liebson, 1978). For example, chronic stress can decrease brain levels of met-enkephalin (a neurotransmitter) in mice, making normal alcohol-avoiding mice more susceptible to alcohol use (Miczek, Hubbard, & Cantuti-Castelvetri, 1995). Other studies also cite environment as a critical influence (Swain, Oetting, Edwards, & Beauvais, 1989; Peel & Brodsky, 1991; Zinberg, 1984).

The behavioral/environmental model delineates six levels of drug use: abstinence, experimentation, social/recreational use, habituation, abuse, and addiction.

ACADEMIC MODEL

In this model, addiction occurs when the body adapts to the toxic effects of drugs at the biochemical and cellular level (Spragg, 1940; Tsai, Gastfriend, & Coyle, 1995; Wickelgren, 1998). The principle is that given sufficient quantities of drugs for an appropriate duration of time, changes in body/brain cells will occur that will lead to addiction. Four physiological changes characterize this process:

◊ tolerance: resistance to the drug's effects increase, necessitating larger and larger doses;

◊ tissue dependence: actual changes in body cells occur because of excessive use, so the body needs the drug to stay in balance;

◊ withdrawal syndrome: physical signs and symptoms of tissue dependence appear when drug use is stopped;

◊ psychic dependence: the effects of the drug are desired by the user and these reinforce the desire to keep using.

(Also see Physiological Responses to Drugs in this chapter.)

DIATHESIS-STRESS THEORY OF ADDICTION

All of the existing theories of addiction, including current psychodynamic theories, are true in their own right. It is beneficial however to integrate these theories and look at addiction as a process that often encompasses a user's life from birth to death.

The original diathesis-stress model of psychological disorders (not addictions) says that

◊ A **diathesis** is a constitutional predisposition or vulnerability to develop a given disorder under certain conditions. The genotype may provide a diathesis (predisposition) within the person that leads to the development of the disorder if the person encounters a level of stress that exceeds his or her stress threshold or coping abilities. The diathesis (the biological predisposition or vulnerability) may be so potent that the person will develop the disorder even in the most benign of environments (Nevid, Rathus, & Greene, 1997).

The above theory was originally developed to help explain the causes of schizophrenia (Meehl, 1962; Gottesman, McGuffin, & Farmer, 1987).

Our diathesis-stress theory of addiction is similar to the addictive-disease model but gives somewhat more flexibility in determining the influence of each of the factors: heredity, environment, and psychoactive drugs.

◊ A **diathesis** or **predisposition to addiction** is the result of genetic and environmental influences, such as stress. When a person is further stressed or challenged by the use of psychoactive drugs or the practice of certain behaviors, then neurochemistry and brain function are further changed to the point that a return to normal use or normal behavior is extremely difficult. The stronger the diathesis, the fewer drugs or less acting out is needed to push the person into addiction; conversely, the weaker the diathesis, the more drugs or behaviors are needed to force a person into addiction.

HEREDITY, ENVIRON-MENT, PSYCHOACTIVE DRUGS, & COMPULSIVE BEHAVIORS

Currently it is the belief of more and more researchers in the field of addictionology that the reasons for drug addiction are indeed a combination of the three factors of heredity, environment, and the use of psychoactive drugs (DuPont, 1997; Koob, 1998; Leshner, 1998). Because individual personalities, physiology, and lifestyles vary, each person's resistance or susceptibility to excessive drug use also varies. It is necessary therefore to study the determining factors more closely in order to understand why one person might remain abstinent, another might use drugs sparingly, a third will use for a lifetime and never have problems, and someone else will use and accelerate to addiction within a few months.

HEREDITY

For years scientists have known that many traits are passed on through generations by genes; features such as eye and hair color, nose shape, bone structure, and most important, the initial structure and chemistry of the nervous system. In recent years scientists have expanded that list of genetically influenced traits to include more complex physical reactions and diseases such as juvenile diabetes, some forms of Alzheimer's disease, schizophrenia, some forms of depression, and even a tendency to certain cancers. Most surprisingly many behaviors seem to have an inheritable component as well whether it's simply a brain chemistry that results in an exaggerated reaction to alcohol and other psychoactive drugs or a personality that gets a charge from gambling (Noble, Blum, Montgomery, & Sheridan, 1991; Shaffer, 1998).

Twin & Retrospective Studies

One set of proofs that a tendency to addiction has an inheritable component is twin studies that have been done in several countries over several decades. Dr. Donald Goodwin of Washington University School of Medicine in St. Louis looked at identical twins that were adopted into separate foster families shortly after birth. These studies strongly support genetics and heredity as the determining factors in alcohol use. Regardless of the foster parent family environment, adopted children developed alcohol abuse or abstinence patterns similar to their biologic parent's use of alcohol (Goodwin, 1976).

Other evidence of genetic alcoholism comes from reviewing the biologic family records of those alcoholics in various treatment programs across the United States (Cloninger, 1987). The statistics showed that if one biological parent was alcoholic, a male child was about 34% more likely to be an alcoholic than the male child of nonalcoholics. If both biological parents were alcoholic, the child was about 400% more likely to be alcoholic. If both parents and a grandfather were alcoholic, that child was about 900% more likely to develop alcoholism. About 28 million Americans have at least one alcoholic parent (Schuckit, 1986).

"I didn't like the way my father fought with my mother when he drank, so I never drank a drop, not a drop, until I was 27. Then it was like a light got turned on and I tried to make up for lost time."

37-year-old drinker

Alcoholism-Associated Gene

Another breakthrough in this line of inquiry came in 1990 when a specific gene associated with alcoholism was identified by Ernest Nobel and Ken Blum, researchers at UCLA and the University of Texas at San Antonio (Blum et al., 1990). Many researchers believe this gene helps indicate a person's susceptibility to compulsive drinking. In some studies this DRD_2A_1 Allele gene was found in more than 70% of severe alcoholics in treatment but in less than 30% of people who were assessed to be social drinkers or abstainers (Feingold, Ball, Kranzler, & Rounsaville, 1996). What the presence of this gene and other yet-to-be discovered ones means is that when people with these hereditary associations do use alcohol, they have a much higher chance of becoming alcoholics than drinkers in the general population (Anthenelli & Schuckit, 1998). However if they never drink, problems with alcohol can never occur.

"I think I really have like an addictive personality in terms of, I mean my parents are both alcoholics and I know that has something to do with it. It's a genetic part of it."

36-year-old recovering alcoholic

Kenneth Blum and fellow researchers believe this gene indicates a tendency to a number of compulsive behaviors, including gambling, psychoactive drug use, attention-deficit disorder, aberrant sexual behavior, overeating, antisocial personality, and even Tourette's syndrome, not just drinking. They refer to it as a compulsivity gene not just an alcoholic gene and call the process the **reward deficiency syndrome** (Blum et al., 1996).

In practical terms what genetic associations mean is that people who are susceptible to developing alcoholism (or other compulsive drug use) begin drinking or using other drugs at a more rapid rate than people without that susceptibility. Though many susceptible people receive an intense reaction from alcohol with their first drinking experience, they also seem to need larger amounts of alcohol than others do to get drunk. So when they reach that intoxicated state, it is much more intense and causes greater dysfunction (Cloninger, Bohman, & Sigvardsson, 1981; Cloninger, 1987). Many have blackouts starting with the first few times they use, where they don't remember what happened to them while drunk, or brownouts where they can remember only parts of their drunken experience.

ENVIRONMENT

The environmental influences that help determine the level at which a person uses drugs can be positive or negative and as varied as stress, love, violence, sexual abuse, nutrition, living conditions, family relationships, nutritional balance, health care, neighborhood safety, school quality, peer pressure, and television. The pressures and influences of environment, particularly home environment, actually shape and connect the nerve cells and neurochemistry a person is born with, thereby helping to determine how that person will use psychoactive drugs. Even one's diet affects brain chemistry.

Environment & Brain Development

Environmental influences have the greatest impact on the development of the brain. Though we are born with all the nerve cells we will ever have, about 100 billion in the brain alone, environment influences the 100 trillion connections that develop between nerve cells. In this way environment molds the brain's architecture and neurochemistry, thus altering the way the brain reacts to outside influences. The growth and alteration are especially widespread in the first 10 years of life.

"My mother was addicted to 'speed' and heroin and I grew up with it. Then I was taken away from her. I'd go and visit her, seeing her high, seeing her not high, seeing her high again, coming down the next, back and forth. And then when I was 11 years old, she was shot and killed on Valentine's Day. After that I didn't have anything to look forward to and so I didn't care anymore."
24-year-old heroin addict

The process of making new connections and altering brain chemistry continues after the first 10 years but at an increasingly slower rate. Current evidence indicates that it may take up to 20 years for the brain to get "hard wired" or form its major and vital connections.

"Every experience you have matters to your brain. And if you are being bathed with repetitive stress hormones and stress chemicals in your brain, it changes your brain in a negative way and can actually cause your brain to become more at risk for these disorders."
Daniel Amen, M.D., 1998

Through subtle chemical, structural, and biological changes, the brain keeps track of all that happens to a person in his or her lifetime. The stronger the environmental influences and the more often they are repeated, the more indelible the imprinting on the brain. For example, if a person uses a certain telephone number again and again, the person memorizes it because the area of the brain responsible for numbers has physiologically written that information in the brain. Because a traumatic experience, such as an accident, a war experience, or even addiction, is so intense, it can leave intense and lasting impressions on the brain (LeDoux, 1996).

"I broke down after about six months over in Vietnam and I was in charge of a gun crew. I didn't respond to my duty of opening up an M-60 and some people's lives were lost in my outfit and I'm responsible. They flew me out to the States, and I immediately jumped into alcohol and heroin."
46-year-old Vietnam veteran

Children who are subject to excessive emotional pain while growing up in a chaotic household remember that pain and may try different ways to deal with it. They can try to understand why it happened, learn how to face it, find people to help them, and accept what happened or they can run away, become hyperactive, make jokes, use drugs, gamble, or overeat; anything to temper the pain or discomfort. If stress continues long enough, the counter-behavior that the child learned also becomes ingrained in the brain (Nestler, 1995). The brain remembers that counter-behavior just as it remembered the stress and pain. Once connections are made and chemistry altered in response to environmental challenges, they are very difficult to change but not impossible (Bierman, 1995).

"My grandfather was a drunk, and my father was a drunk. That is who basically beat me up. I figured the more pain he caused me, the more 'pot' I could smoke. Being abused as a kid really scars you for life. So the more 'pot' I could smoke, the more relief I got from the pressure of being abused."
35-year-old male in recovery

Environment can make a person more liable to use and abuse psychoactive substances

◇ if stress is common in the home,

◇ if drinking or other drug use is common in the home,

◇ if different ways of reacting to stress or anger aren't learned and self-medication becomes the only solution,

◇ if there are mental health problems triggered by the home environment,

◇ or if their diet lacks sufficient vitamins and proteins needed for healthy brain chemistry.

People can also become more susceptible to use if society tells them in word and deed that drinking, smoking, and using drugs to solve all problems is a normal part of life. Massive advertising campaigns for tobacco or alcohol make people more likely to use. Belonging to a social, business, or peer group where excessive drinking or drug use is considered normal increases use. Living in a community where access to legal and illegal drugs is easy increases use (DuPont, 1997).

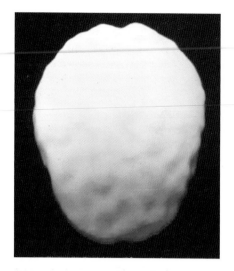

Figure 2-18 •

When the brain is functioning normally, there is an even distribution of function throughout the brain. When drugs are used, many parts of the brain become inactive or occasionally overactive.

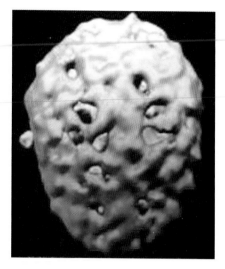

Figure 2-19 •

This is a SPECT scan of a person who has abused methamphetamine for about 8 years. What we see are multiple areas of decreased activity (not real holes in the brain tissue) across the cortical surface of the brain.

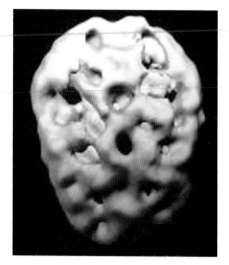

Figure 2-20 •

This SPECT scan shows someone who had been abusing alcohol for about 20 years and what is seen is a dramatic overall shutdown or decreased areas of activity across the brain.

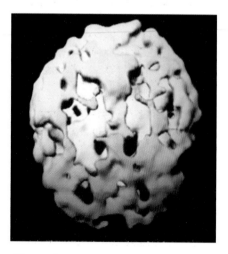

Figure 2-21 •

Heroin gives the classic brain-melt picture, dramatic suppression of overall cerebral activity. In the Amen Clinic for Behavioral Medicine's experience, people treated with methadone have the same brain dysfunction.

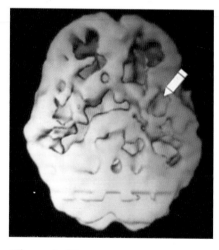

Figure 2-22 •

This SPECT scan shows the brain of a man who had been abusing marijuana heavily for about 12 years. There is a strong suppression of temporal lobe activity on both sides that strongly affect his memory and motivation. Given that he's used for such a long period of time, when he stops using he'll begin to get increased function in his lobes but his brain will never return to normal.

All scans are courtesy of the Amen Clinic for Behavioral Medicine, 1998

"My parents have a glass of wine after they come home from work to relax and unwind. I'm the same way, just with marijuana. It's just kind of a regular thing that I do instead of alcohol or anything else."

23-year-old marijuana smoker

And if, in addition to these environmental stressors and influences, people have a hereditary susceptibility to use, the chances that they will slide into compulsive use (if they start drinking or taking drugs) greatly increases (DuPont, 1997).

An often-overlooked environmental influence is nutrition. The food we ingest provides the proteins that brain cells use to produce their neurotransmitters. An unbalanced diet therefore impacts brain chemistry that can affect an individual's susceptibility to addiction.

PSYCHOACTIVE DRUGS

The hereditary and environmental influences mean nothing in terms of addiction unless the person actually uses psychoactive substances, so the final factor that determines the level at which a person might use drugs is the drugs themselves. Drugs can affect not only susceptible individuals but also those with no predisposing factors. This occurs because, by definition, psychoactive drugs are substances that affect the functioning of the central nervous system. Excessive, frequent, or prolonged use of alcohol or other drugs inevitably modifies many of the same nerve cells and neurochemistry that are affected by heredity and environment. This influences not only the person's reaction to those substances when they are used but also the level at which they are used (Hyman 1998). Compulsive behaviors also influence the progression to addiction.

The development of tolerance, tissue dependence, withdrawal, and psychic dependence are signs that the drugs themselves are causing physical and chemical changes in the body that tend to raise the level of use.

Psychoactive drugs and addictive behaviors cause temporary and permanent changes in various parts of the brain that can be imaged. For many years Dr. Daniel Amen has studied these changes in brain function at his clinic in Fairfield, California using **SPECT scans** of the brain. SPECT scans are very sophisticated nuclear medicine studies that look at blood flow and metabolic activity in the brain to show how the brain functions during a given activity, such as taking a psychoactive drug. A **CAT scan** (computerized axial tomography-x-rays) or **MRI** (magnetic resonance imaging) on the other hand produce anatomical studies of the brain but don't show brain function. **PET** (positron emission tomography) shows brain function.

SPECT scans and other brain studies indicate that psychoactive drug use on both an initial and chronic exposure basis decreases vital functioning of the brain's neocortex. Thus reason and thinking are impaired and this has a major influence on maintaining compulsive drug use.

Finally, animal studies confirm that some drugs have greater power to compel continued use than other drugs. This is called positive reinforcement. For example, cocaine and heroin have a more hypnotizing effect to continue their use than Thorazine® or Tofranil®.

COMPULSIVE BEHAVIORS

There is a growing belief among many researchers that certain behaviors that become compulsive, such as gambling, sexual activity, and eating disorders, also accelerate, supplant, or even cause compulsive drug use. For example, Dr. Howard Shaffer, director of Harvard Medical School's Division on Addictions told a group of Las Vegas casino executives that the excitement from gambling causes the brain to be rewired, particularly the reward/pleasure center. He stated that some people could limit their betting while others experience a loss of control plus craving and they continue to gamble despite adverse consequences (Shaffer, 1998). Gambling and other behaviors affect many of the same structures in the brain affected by psychoactive drugs. Behavioral compulsions often accompany or follow drug addictions. For example, 25% to 63% of all compulsive gamblers (depending on the study) have been alcohol or drug dependent (NRC, 1999). Many recovering addicts switched to gambling to pass the time because they thought it was harmless. It is now recognized that gambling and other compulsive behaviors (overeating, shoplifting, sexual addiction, Internet obsession, etc.) are actual dysfunctions of brain chemistry in the same way that drugs disrupt brain chemistry. Psychological and social treatment for these compulsive behaviors are evolving along the same lines and using the same interventions as used in the treatment of drug addiction. These compulsive behaviors are different from **obsessive-compulsive disorder** (OCD) such as repetitive hand washing, repeated and excessive checking to insure that the door is locked or

that the stove is turned off, and compulsive ordering like arranging magazines, books, or objects into a certain order and being upset if they are not in the expected place. OCD has been shown to occur along a different brain and neurotransmitter pathway than that associated with compulsive behaviors. With compulsive behaviors there is an experience of pleasure associated with the action whereas OCD actions are not associated with a pleasurable experience. (OCD is also different than **obsessive-compulsive personality disorder** where a person is preoccupied with details, rules, lists, order, organization, control, and doing things just right to the point that less gets done.)

ALCOHOLIC MICE & SOBER MICE

To better understand the close connection between heredity, environment, and psychoactive drugs/compulsive behaviors and to further visualize the diathesis-stress theory of addiction, it might be helpful to examine a series of classical animal studies done over the past 40 years by Gerald McLaren, T.K. Li, Horace Lo, Cannon, and other researchers (Li, Lumeng, McBride, Waller, & Murphy, 1986; NIDA, 1999). Animal experiments are often used to help us understand what the effects of a drug would be on human beings. They were first used scientifically by Johann Jakob Wepfer, a seventeenth century scientist.

The basic experiments are as follows: years ago researchers developed two genetic strains of mice (Fig. 2-23a) to help researchers understand alcoholism. One of the strains of mice loved alcohol. When given the choice between water and even 70% concentrations of alcohol, these mice went for the alcohol every time. If all they had was water, then they would grudgingly drink water. The other strain of mice hated alcohol. Given the same choice, even with concentrations as low as 2% alcohol, the mice always chose the pure water (Cannon & Carrell, 1987).

In one experiment researchers first took a group of the alcohol-hating mice and injected them with high levels of alcohol, the equivalent of what adult human beings would drink if they were heavy drinkers. Within a few weeks these once-sober mice came to prefer alcohol. In fact if not stopped, they would drink themselves to death (Fig. 2-23b).

Researchers then took another group of the alcohol-hating mice and subjected them to stress by putting them in very small constrictive tubes for intermittent periods. Within a few weeks this group of sober mice also came to prefer higher and higher concentrations of alcohol to pure water. In essence sober mice had been turned into alcoholic mice, first through applying stress (environment) and then allowing them access to alcohol (exposure to psychoactive drugs (Fig. 2-23c).

Furthermore researcher Dr. Jorge Madronis, a nutritionist, took another group of alcohol-hating mice and restricted their diet of vitamin B and some essential proteins. This also resulted in increasing alcohol use after several months (Madronis, 1951) (Fig. 2-23d).

Finally once the mice whose heredity made them prefer alcohol were given access to alcohol, they drank themselves to death (genetics). Even when they were subjected to electrical shocks aimed at preventing them from drinking the alcohol (aversive therapy), they continued to drink even when the shocks came close to being fatal (Fig. 2-23e). It is important to remember that none of the mice would become alcoholic if they were never given alcohol, even those mice with the highest susceptibility to compulsive drinking.

What was most interesting was that when the forced drinking, stress induction, and nutritional restrictions were stopped, the genetically sober alcohol-hating mice did not return to their normal nondrinking habits. They had been transformed into alcohol-loving mice and if given the chance to drink, they would be alcoholic mice.

When the brains of the four groups of mice were examined (the hereditary

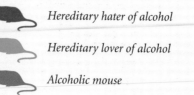

Hereditary hater of alcohol

Hereditary lover of alcohol

Alcoholic mouse

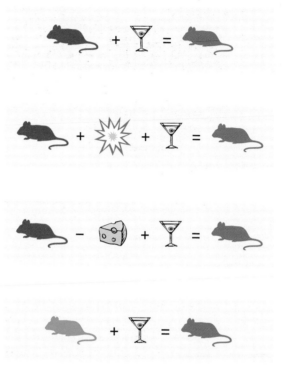

Figure 2-23a •

Two strains of mice have been bred to help test theories of addiction, an alcohol-hating mouse and an alcohol-loving mouse.

Figure 2-23b •

Alcohol-hating mouse is force fed large quantities of alcohol.

Figure 2-23c •

Alcohol-hating mouse is subjected to stress and alcohol is made available.

Figure 2-23d •

Alcohol-hating mouse is nutritionally deprived and alcohol is made available.

Figure 2-23e •

Alcohol is made available to alcohol-loving mouse.

alcoholic mice, the stress-induced alcoholic mice, the alcohol-induced alcoholic mice, and the nutritionally restricted alcoholic mice), all had similar brain cell changes and neurotransmitter imbalances that made them prefer alcohol even though they started with different neurochemical balances. This research suggests that whether the neurochemical disruption can be caused by heredity, environment, psychoactive drugs, nutritional deficiency, or a combination of several of the factors, they can all lead to serious addiction (Li et al., 1984, 1986).

COMPULSION CURVES

Human beings, of course, are different from mice. We are more com-

plex, our brains are more intricate, and our social patterns are much more complex. We have the power of reason, we have more control of our environment, we have self-awareness, and yet research, especially over the last 10 years, shows that the basic drug-craving mechanisms, which reside mostly in the old brain, are similar to those of most other mammals. The difference is that in humans, it usually takes a combination of heredity, environment, and psychoactive drug use to increase compulsive use. In addition since the environmental factors are much more complex than with simpler animals, the new brain has the ability to delay or divert activation of the old brain and human beings have the capacity to change. Addicts can learn to accept their condition and do all they can to avoid a relapse. But if they ex-

Researcher says he built intellectually better mouse

A Princeton scientist says his success in genetically enhancing the intelligence of mice could lead to applications for humans

By NICHOLAS WADE
NEW YORK TIMES NEWS SERVICE

In a major test of how learning works at the level of nerve cells, a scientist has created a smarter strain of mice by manipulating a gene involved in memory formation.

The scientist thinks his work lays the basis for doing the same in people, whether in helping patients with memory deficits, counteracting the loss of memory in older people, or making healthy individuals smarter.

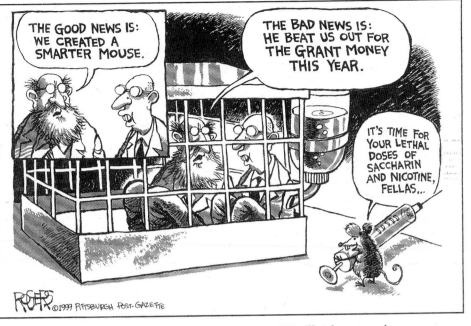

perience a slip and use, they will fall back into addictive use 95% of the time (O'Malley & Volpicelli, 1995).

To help understand the interrelationship of heredity, environment, and the use of psychoactive drugs in human beings, we have developed a graphic representation of the ways that a user might advance from experimentation to addiction.

Since every person is unique, every person starts with a different genetic susceptibility. Those with low genetic susceptibility or predisposition have more room for drug experimentation or environmental stressors than those with high genetic predisposition. The susceptibility is most often reflected by the brain's structure and neurochemical composition. The determining factor might be an inherited lack of dopamine receptors that can help signal pleasure making the person more likely to use drugs (Noble et al., 1991). The important point is that more and more studies confirm that there is at least some heredity influence to any addiction, even compulsive overeating, smoking, and gambling (Brownell &

Wadden, 1992; Carmelli, Swan, Robinette, & Fabstiz, 1992; Eisen et al., 1998). The contribution of heredity to drug addiction in our society is only an educated guess but researchers have estimated figures of anywhere from 10% to 60% (Fig. 2-24).

Once a person is born with their

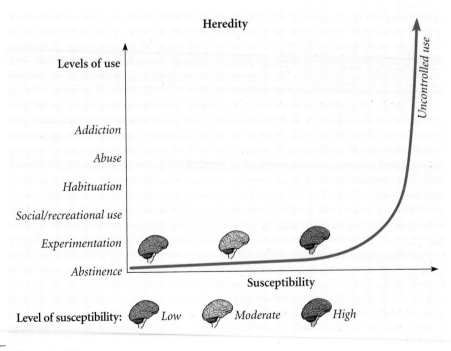

Figure 2-24 •

Initial susceptibility is inherited.

genetic makeup, environmental influences, particularly stressors, have the greatest effect. These influences include lack of bonding with a caregiver, physical/emotional/sexual abuse during adolescence, poor nutrition, or societal attitudes that permit drug use (Peele & Brodsky, 1991; Zinberg, 1984). Again, a person may have low, medium, or high environmental contributions towards drug addiction (Fig. 2-25).

The final factor that will push a person to addiction is the use of psychoactive drugs. The practice of compulsive behaviors, such as gambling, can also push one along the curve (Fig. 2-26). Therefore a person who starts with a low inherited susceptibility and low environmental stress might need intense use of drugs or behaviors to push him/her into addiction. The greater the environmental stress, the fewer drugs or behaviors needed. Drug use is not just measured by frequency or amount of drug used; drugs have different potencies (heroin vs. alcohol) and different routes of administration (crack cocaine vs. snorting cocaine).

The drugs that push the hardest and the quickest towards addiction are, in order from fastest to slowest,

smoking tobacco,
smoking "crack" cocaine,
smoking or injecting heroin,
injecting methamphetamines,
snorting cocaine,
ingesting opioid painkillers,
ingesting amphetamines,
ingesting sedative hypnotics,
drinking alcohol,
smoking marijuana,
ingesting PCP,
ingesting caffeine,
ingesting MDMA,
ingesting LSD,
ingesting peyote.

If a person starts with a low or even moderate level of inherited susceptibility, it takes a larger amount of environmental influences to push him/her close to the level of critical susceptibility and addiction than someone with a high inherited susceptibility (Fig. 2-27). Depending on the environ-

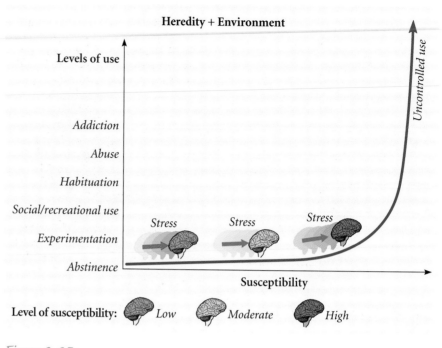

Figure 2-25 •
Susceptibility increases due to environmental stressors.

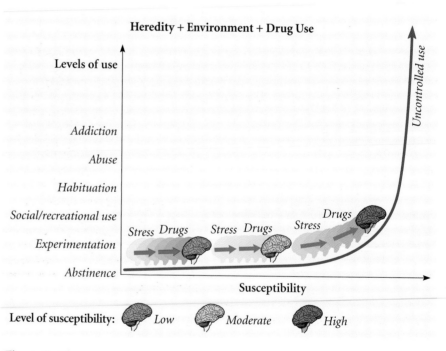

Figure 2-26 •
Susceptibility increases due to drug use. It can progress to abuse and addiction.

mental contribution, it then takes a lot more drug use or acting out to push them into uncontrolled use of drugs (or acting out of compulsive behaviors) than someone with high inherited susceptibility.

It might take those with low susceptibility 10 years of drinking to be-

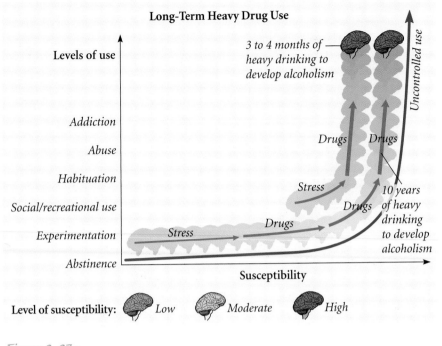

Long-Term Heavy Drug Use

Figure 2-27 •
Addiction develops at different rates.

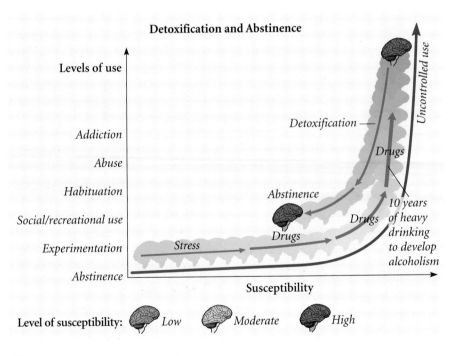

Detoxification and Abstinence

Figure 2-28 •
Susceptibility doesn't return to normal after detoxification and abstinence.

come alcoholics or it might never occur. It might take them 2 years of occasional injection to become a heroin addict or 6 months of smoking to get to a pack of cigarettes a day. People in the middle of the scale, with moderate inherited susceptibility, might need just 2 or 3 years of use to slip into alcohol addiction or 6 months of heroin use to graduate to a $200-a-day habit. People with a high susceptibility might slip into compulsive heavy drinking after just 3–4 months of bingeing or heavy drinking because their bodies are primed for compulsive use.

What happens to addicts when they stop using cocaine or stop gambling (Fig. 2-28)? They drop below critical susceptibility but not back to the level they were at before they started using drugs or practicing their behavior (Gold, 1998). This is because their addiction, aggravated by the development of tolerance and tissue dependence, has permanently altered their brain chemistry making them forever liable to redevelop uncontrolled use or behavior quicker than before. Note that their level of use may return to abstinence but their brain susceptibility remains extremely high.

So if their environment continues to pile stress on them, they will move to a level of susceptibility where they will return to uncontrolled addictive use or behavior with just one drink or just one bet (Fig. 2-29) (Clark et al., 1997). If however, they reduce stress in their environment by staying away from environmental cues, learning how to relax, having therapy, attending self-help groups, continuing to learn, and overcoming stressful thoughts, memories, and mental conflicts, then they have a chance at recovery.

CONCLUSIONS

The interrelations of heredity, environment, psychoactive drugs, and compulsive behaviors emphasize that any study of addiction should focus on the totality of people's lives: their personality, relationships, how they live, what they eat, and their family history. In succeeding chapters, this book will not only study stimulants, depressants, psychedelics, inhalants, and other drugs but also look at compulsive behaviors, including compulsive overeating and gambling, whose causes are similar to those that lead to drug use, abuse, or addiction.

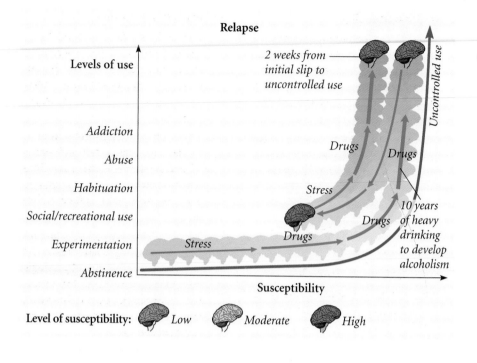

Figure 2-29 •
Users return to addictive use more quickly after relapse.

CHAPTER SUMMARY

HOW PSYCHOACTIVE DRUGS AFFECT US

How Drugs Get to the Brain

1. Drugs are absorbed into the body in five ways. In order of the speed with which they begin to exert their effects, they are: inhaling (including smoking), injecting (in a vein, muscle, or subcutaneously), mucosal absorption (snorting, under the tongue, next to the cheek, rectally), eating or drinking, and contact (on the skin, transdermal skin patches).

2. Drugs enter the body and are distributed through the bloodstream until they reach the central nervous system (CNS = brain and spinal cord) where they will have the greatest effect. They must cross the blood-brain barrier to reach the nerve cells of the brain.

3. Psychoactive drugs affect the rest of the body either directly or by acting on the nerves of the central nervous system.

The Nervous System

4. The nervous system, with 100 billion nerve cells and 100 trillion connections, consists of the central nervous system (brain and spinal cord) and the peripheral nervous system (autonomic and somatic systems) that connects the senses and organs to the outside world and to the central nervous system and that regulates involuntary functions and controls voluntary muscle movements.

5. The old brain controls physiologic functions, emotions, and feelings while the new brain controls reasoning, language, creativity, and other higher-order functions.

6. Depressants and stimulants work mostly on the old brain, psychedelics work more on the new brain.

7. Drug craving seems to reside mostly in the old brain.

8. A survival mechanism called the reward/pleasure center uses the nucleus accumbens and other structures to give a surge of pleasure and a craving to repeat an action that is favorable to the organism. Psychoactive drugs and compulsive behaviors can disrupt this mechanism and lead to craving, abuse, and addiction.

9. The conflict between doing what our old brain tells us and the common sense and morality of our new brain is found in the writings and beliefs of religions and social systems throughout history.

10. A nerve cell consists of dendrites, cell body, axon, and terminals.

11. Messages travel within a nerve cell as electrical signals. However between most nerve cells there is a synaptic gap. Messages cross this gap as chemical signals called "neurotransmitters" and are then converted back to electrical signals. This message transmission process that occurs at the synaptic gap is called a synapse.

12. Neurotransmitters are the neurochemicals (e.g., dopamine, GABA,

serotonin, norepinephrine, and enkephalin) that signal messages between nerve cells. Psychoactive drugs affect neurotransmitters thereby exerting their effect on the central and peripheral nervous systems.

13. Psychoactive drugs increase, mimic, block, or otherwise disrupt the release of these chemicals. In turn the neurotransmitters intensify signals (agonist) or inhibit signals (antagonist).

14. All psychoactive drugs mimic or disrupt naturally occurring neurotransmitters by slotting into their existing receptor sites.

Physiological Responses to Drugs

15. When a person takes certain drugs over a long period of time, the body becomes used to their effects, so more is needed to achieve the same high. The user develops a tolerance to the drug.

16. The tolerance to physical and psychological effects can develop at different rates.

17. The body tries to adapt to the increased quantities of drugs by changing its chemical balance and cellular composition of organs, such as the liver. This results in physical or tissue dependence.

18. The pleasurable effects of drugs reinforce the desire to continue use. The direct influence of drugs possess the innate ability to keep someone using. This is just part of the psychic dependence people develop to drugs.

19. When a user stops taking a drug after tissue dependence has developed (mostly with opiates, alcohol, and sedative-hypnotics), the body experiences many of the unpleasant sensations and physical changes it was kept from feeling while taking the drug. This backlash is known as "withdrawal."

20. Protracted withdrawal, which is a delayed psychic and physiological remembrance of drug experiences, is one of the main reasons for relapse.

Basic Pharmacology

21. The liver is the principal organ for neutralizing or metabolizing drugs in the body. The kidneys are the principal organs for filtering drugs from the blood and excreting them in the urine.

22. A variety of factors, such as age, race, health, and sex, help determine how fast a drug is metabolized.

FROM EXPERIMENTATION TO ADDICTION

Desired Effects vs. Side Effects

23. People take drugs for a variety of reasons including getting high, self-medicating, building confidence, increasing energy, satisfying curiosity, obliging friends (peer pressure), and avoiding problems. These are the desired effects.

24. The major problem with psychoactive drugs is that some people who take them focus on the desired mental and emotional effects and ignore the potentially damaging physical and mental side effects that can occur.

25. Virtually every person who abuses drugs is a polydrug user even though they have their drug of choice. They can use other drugs to enhance the effect of their primary drug, to counteract unwanted side effects, to act as a substitute, and for a variety of other reasons.

Levels of Use

26. The level of use is judged first by the amount, frequency, and duration of use, then by the effect use has on the individual's life.

27. The six levels of use are abstinence, experimentation, social/recreational use, habituation, abuse, and addiction.

28. The hallmark of drug abuse is continued use despite adverse consequences.

29. The hallmarks of addiction are loss of control and compulsion to use.

Theories of Addiction

30. The Addictive Disease Model says addiction is a chronic, progressive, relapsing, incurable, and potentially fatal condition that is mostly a consequence of genetic irregularities.

31. The Behavioral/Environmental Model says that certain influences of one's environment, including stress, nutrition, abuse, anger, and peer pressure, can induce addiction.

32. The Academic Model says that it's the use of drugs that causes the body to adapt through physiologic mechanisms, such as tolerance, tissue dependence, withdrawal, and psychic dependence that result in addiction.

33. The Diathesis-Stress Theory states that the combination of heredity and environment creates a susceptibility to addiction that can be triggered and advanced by using psychoactive drugs and/or by acting out certain behaviors.

Heredity, Environment, Psychoactive Drugs, & Compulsive Behaviors

34. Heredity gives people their starting point in life. They begin with a certain susceptibility to use or not use drugs. This susceptibility is reflected in certain neurochemical or neurostructural imbalances.

35. Environment, especially stress, then molds that basic architecture of the nervous system, further increasing or decreasing susceptibility to compulsive drug use. Dietary imbalances also affect the chemistry of the brain.

36. Psychoactive drug use itself triggers that existing hereditary/environmental susceptibility and through tolerance and other physiological mechanisms further pushes a user towards compulsive use.

37. Compulsive behaviors, such as compulsive gambling, overeating, compulsive sexual activity, and Internet obsession, add to the

stress and can become addictions in and of themselves.

large amounts of alcohol or other drugs.

recreational use towards habituation, abuse, and addiction.

Alcoholic Mice & Sober Mice

38. Animal experiments exhibit that compulsive use can be reached through heredity, stress, nutritional restriction, or ingestion of

Compulsion Curves

39. In humans it is the combination of heredity, environment, and/or drug use that can push a person out of experimentation and social/

Conclusions

40. To understand addiction, one has to look at the totality of people's lives not just their drug-seeking behavior.

REFERENCES

Ahmed, S. H., & Koob, G. F. (1998). Transition from moderate to excessive drug intake: Change in hedonic set point. *Science, 282,* 5387.

Amen, D. (1998). *Interview on May 18, 1998* with author.

APA (American Psychiatric Association). (1994). *Diagnostic and Statistical Manual of Mental Disorders* (4th ed.). Washington, DC: Author.

Anthenelli, R. M., & Schuckit, M. A. (1998). Genetic influences in addiction. In A. W. Graham, & T. K. Schultz (Eds.), *Principles of Addiction Medicine* (2nd ed., pp. 17-36). Chevy Chase, MD: American Society of Addiction Medicine, Inc.

Bierman, K. (11-3-95). Early Violence Leaves Its Mark on the Brain. *The New York Times,* pp. B5, B10.

Blum, K., Braverman, E. R., Cull, J. G., Holder, J. M., Luck, R., Lubar, J., Miller, D., & Comings, D. E. (2000). Reward deficiency syndrome (RDS): A biogenetic model for the diagnosis and treatment of impulsive, addictive, and compulsive behaviors. *Journal of Psychoactive Drugs, 32*(1).

Blum, K., Cull, J. G., Braverman, E. R., & Comings, D. E. (1996). Reward deficiency syndrome. *American Scientist, 84,* 132–145.

Brehm, N. M., & Khantzian, E. J. (1997). Psychodynamics. In J. H. Lowinson, P. Ruiz, R. B. Millman, & J. G. Langrod (Eds.), *Substance Abuse: A Comprehensive Textbook* (3rd ed., pp. 91–100). Baltimore: Williams & Wilkins.

Brownell, K. D., & Wadden, T. A. (1992). Etiology and treatment of obesity: Understanding a serious, prevalent, and refractory disorder. *Journal of Consulting and Clinical Psychology, 60,* 505–517.

Cannon, D. S., & Carrell, L. E., (1987). Rat strain differences in ethanol self-administration. *Pharmacology of Biochemical Behavior, 28,* 57–63.

Carmelli, D., Swan, G. E., Robinette, D., & Fabstiz, R. (1992). Genetic influences on smoking: A study of male twins. *The New England Journal of Medicine, 327,* 899–933.

Childress, A. R., McElgin, W., Mozley, D., Reivich, M., & O'Brien, G. (1996). Brain correlates of cue-induced cocaine and opiate craving. *Society for Neuroscience Abstracts 22,* 365-369.

Clark, D. B., Moss, H. B., Kirisci, L, Mezzich, A. C., Miles, R., & Ott, P. (1997). Psychopathology in preadolescent sons of fathers with substance use disorders. *Journal of the American Academy of Child and Adolescent Psychiatry, 36*(4), 495–502.

Cloninger, C. R., Bohman, M., & Sigvardson, S. (1986). Inheritance of risk to develop alcoholism. In M. C. Braude, & H. M. Chao (Eds.), *Genetic and Biological Markers in Drug Abuse and Alcoholism. NIDA Research Monograph 66.* Rockville, MD: Department of Health and Human Services.

Cloninger, C. R. (1987). Neurogenetic adaptive mechanisms in alcoholism. *Science, 236,* 410–416.

Denton, D., Shade, R., Zamarippa, F., Egan, G., Blair-West, J., McKinley, M., Lancaster, J., & Fox, P. (1999). Neuroimaging of genesis and satiation of thirst and an interceptor-driven theory of origins of primary consciousness. *Proceedings of the National Academy of Sciences, 96*(9), 5304–5309.

Diagram Group. (1991). *The Brain: A User's Manual.* Rockville Centre, NY: Berkley.

DuPont, R. L. (1997). *The Selfish Brain: Learning From Addiction.* Washington, DC: American Psychiatric Press, Inc.

Eisen, S. A., Lin, N., Lyons, M. J., Scherrer, J. F., Kristin, G., True, W. R., Goldberg, J., & Tsuang, M. T. (1998). Familial influences on gambling behavior. *Addiction Magazine, 93,* 1375–1384.

Feingold, A., Ball, S. A., Kranzler, H. R., & Rounsaville, B. J. (1996). Generalizability of the Type A/Type B distinction across different psychoactive substances. *American Journal of Drug and Alcohol Abuse, 22*(n3), 449–463.

Freud, S. (1995). *The Complete Letters of Sigmund Freud to Wilhelm Fliess* (p. 287). Cambridge, MA: Harvard University Press.

Gold, M. (1998). From documentary interview on PBS by *Bill Moyers: Close to Home.* PBS Online.

Goldstein, A. (1994). *Addiction: From Biology to Drug Policy.* New York: W.H. Freeman and Company.

Goodwin, D. W. (1976). *Is Alcoholism Hereditary?* New York: Oxford University Press.

Gottesman, I. I., McGuffin, P., & Farmer, A. E. (1987). Clinical clues to the "real" genetics of schizophrenia. *Schizophrenia Bulletin, 13,* 23–47.

Griffiths, R. R., Bigelow, C. E., & Liebson, I. (1978). Experimental drug self-administration: generality across species and type of drug. *National Institute of Drug Abuse Research. Monograph Series, 20,* 24–43.

Hyman, S. E. (1996). Shaking out the cause of addiction. *Science, 273*(5275), 611.

Hyman, S. E., Director of the National Institute of Mental Health. (March, 30, 1998). Interview with Bill Moyers,

Close to Home. *http://www.pbs.org/ wnet/ closetohome/science/html/hyman. html.*

Institute of Medicine. (1999). *Marijuana and Medicine: Assessing the Science Base.* Washington, DC: National Academy Press.

Jaffe, J. H., Knapp, C. M., & Ciraulo, D.A. (1997). Opiates: Clinical aspects. In J. H. Lowinson, P. Ruiz, R. B. Millman, & J. G. Langrod (Eds.), *Substance Abuse: A comprehensive Textbook* (3rd. ed., pp. 51–84). Baltimore: Williams & Wilkins.

Kandel, E. R., Schwartz, J. H., & Jessell, T. M. (Eds.). (1991). *Principles of Neural Science* (3rd ed.*).* New York: Elsevier.

Koob, G. F., & Le Moal, M. (1997). Drug abuse: Hedonic homeostatic dysregulation. *Science, 278,* 52–63.

Koob, G. F. (March 30, 1998). Interview with Bill Moyers. *http://www.pbs. org/wnet/ closetohome/science/html/ koob.html.*

LeDoux, J. E. (1996). *The Emotional Brain* (p. 68). New York: Simon and Schuster.

Leshner, A. (1998). Close to Home: Interview with Alan Leshner. Moyers on Addiction. *http://www.pbs.org/wnet/ closetohome/science/html.*

Li, T. K., & Lumeng, L. (1984). Alcohol preference and voluntary alcohol intakes of inbred rat strains and the National Institutes of Health heterogeneous stock of rats. *Alcoholism, 8,* 485–486.

Li, T. K., Lumeng, L., McBride, W. J., Waller, M.B., & Murphy, J. M. (1986). Studies on an animal model of alcoholism. In M. C. Braude, & H. M. Chao (Eds.). *Genetic and Biological Markers in Drug Abuse and Alcoholism. NIDA Research Monograph 66.* Rockville, MD: Department of Health and Human Services.

Madrones, R. J. (1951). On the relationship between deficiency of B vitamins and alcohol intake in rats. *Quarterly Journal of Studies on Alcoholism, 12,* 563–575.

Meehl, P. E. (1962). Schizotoma, schizolyphy, schizophrenia. *American Psychologist, 17,* 827–838.

Merton, T. (1955). *No Man Is an Island.* New York: Harcourt, Brace & Company.

Miczek, K.A., Hubbard, N., & Cantuti-Castelvetri, I. (1995). Increased cocaine self-administration after social stress. *Neuroscience Abstracts, 21.*

Nesse, R. M. (1994). An Evolutionary Perspective on Substance Abuse. *Etiology and Sociobiology, 15,* (339–348). New York: Elsevier Science, Inc.

Nesse, R. M., & Berridge, K. C. (1997). Psychoactive Drug Use in Evolutionary Perspective. *Science, 278,* 63–65.

Nestler, E. J. (1995). Molecular basis of addictive states. *Neuroscientist, 1,* 212–220.

Nestler, E. J. & Aghajanian, G. K. (1997). Molecular and Cellular Basis of Addiction. *Science, 278,* 58–63.

Nevid, J. S., Rathus, S. A., & Greene, B. (1997). *Abnormal Psychology in a Changing World.* Upper Saddle River, NJ: Prentice Hall.

Noble, E. P., Blum, K., Montgomery, A., & Sheridan, P. J. (1991). Allelic association of the D2 dopamine receptor gene with receptor-binding characteristics in alcoholism. *Archives of General Psychiatry, 48,* 648–654.

Noble, E. P., Blum, K., Sheridan, P. J., et al. (1990). Allelic association of human dopamine D2 receptor gene in alcoholism. *JAMA, 263,* 2055–2060.

NRC. (1999). *Pathological Gambling: A Critical Review.* Washington, DC: National Research Council.

Olds, J., & Milner, P. (1954). Positive reinforcement produced by electrical stimulation of septal area and other regions of rat brain. *Journal of Comprehensive Physiology and Psychology, 47,* 419–427.

Olds, J. (1956). Pleasure centers in the brain. *Scientific American, 195*(4), 105–116.

O'Malley, & Volpicelli. (1995). Slip vs. relapse (in-house study). *Haight-Ashbury Files.*

Peele, S., & Brodsky, A. (1991). *The Truth About Addiction and Recovery.* New York: Simon & Schuster.

Pepper, C. (1994). Interview. *Author's files.*

Schuckit, M. A. (1986). Alcoholism and affective disorders: Genetic and clinical implications. *American Journal of Psychiatry, 143,* 140–147.

Shaffer, H. (2-28-98). Lecture to casino executives, Las Vegas gaming convention. *Medford Mail Tribune.* Medford, OR.

Snyder, S. H. (1996). *Drugs and the Brain.* New York: Scientific American Library.

Spragg, S. D. S. (1940). Morphine addiction in chimpanzees. *Comparative Psychology Monograph, 15* (7), 1–132.

Suzuki, D. (1994). *The Brain* (TV show). Discover Channel.

Swain, R. C., Oetting, E. R., Edwards, R. W., & Beauvais, F. (1989). Links from emotional distress to adolescent drug use: A pathological model. *Journal of Consulting and Clinical Psychology, 57,* 227–231.

Tsai, G., Gastfriend, D. R., & Coyle, J. T. (1995). The glutamatergic basis of human alcoholism. *American Journal of Psychiatry, 152,* 332–340.

Wickelgren, I. (1998). Teaching the brain to take drugs. *Science, 280,* 2045.

Zinberg, N. (1984). *Drugs, Set and Setting.* New Haven: Yale University Press.

Uppers

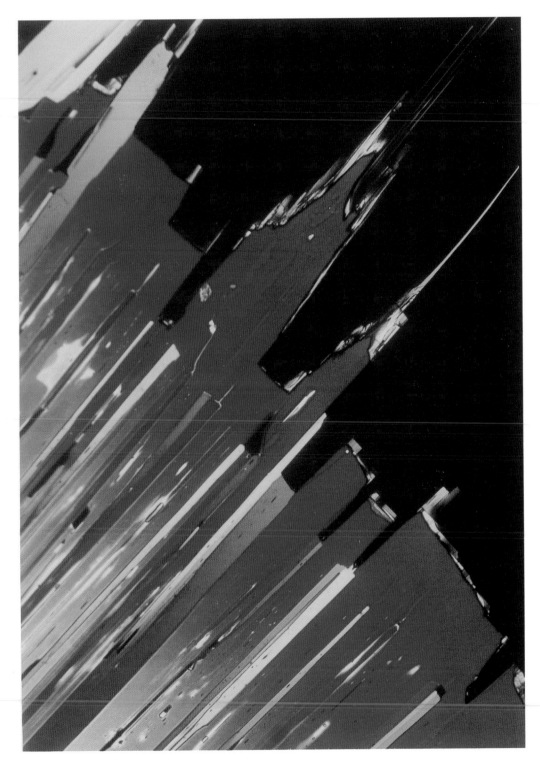

T he dynamic tension of this photomicrograph of cocaine hydrochloride crystal seems symbolic of the extreme stimulating properties of the drug.
Courtesy of Michael W. Davidson, © 1999, Institute of Molecular Biophysics, Florida State University, Tallahassee, FL

- **General Classification:** Uppers include very strong stimulants (cocaine and amphetamines), moderate stimulants, mostly from plants (e.g., khat and ephedra), and legal mild stimulants (caffeine and nicotine).

- **General Effects:** Stimulants force the release of the body's own energy chemicals and stimulate the brain's reward/pleasure center. They also constrict blood vessels, speed the heart, and raise blood pressure. Prolonged use of the stronger stimulants depletes energy resources, induces paranoia, and triggers intense craving.

- **Cocaine:** Usually injected, snorted, or smoked, cocaine, an extract of the coca leaf, causes the most rapid stimulation and subsequent severe comedown of all the stimulants.

- **Smokable Cocaine ("crack," freebase):** The effects of smoking cocaine are almost the same as snorting or injecting cocaine. It is the most rapid and, some say, intense method of use.

- **Amphetamines:** Longer lasting, slightly less intense, and usually cheaper than cocaine, these synthetic stimulants, including methamphetamine ("meth," "crank," and "ice"), saw a rapid increase of use in the 1990s.

- **Amphetamine Congeners:** Methylphenidate (Ritalin) is used to treat attention deficit/hyperactivity disorder (AD/HD) in children and adults whereas diet pills are used to control weight gain. A popular combination, "fen-phen," was banned because of dangerous cardiovascular effects and the potential for abuse.

- **Lookalike & Over-the-Counter (OTC) Stimulants:** Counterfeit stimulants often containing caffeine or other mild stimulants are falsely advertised as amphetamines or cocaine. Legal mild over-the-counter stimulants can have toxic cardiovascular effects to the system.

- **Miscellaneous Plant Stimulants:** Extracts of plants, like khat, yohimbe, betel nuts, and ephedra, are used worldwide in addition to coffee, tea, or colas. Synthetic versions of plant extracts, such as methcathinone, pseudoephedrine, and Pervitine , have many of the effects of methamphetamine.

- **Caffeine:** Coffee, tea, chocolate, and some soft drinks contain the alkaloid caffeine and can be mildly addicting. Many over-the-counter medications also contain caffeine.

- **Tobacco & Nicotine:** Nicotine is a toxic alkaloid found in tobacco. When tobacco is smoked or chewed, it first stimulates, then relaxes, then, at large doses, it depresses. Hundreds of other byproducts and additives in tobacco, like tar and nitrosamines, can cause cancer and respiratory or cardiovascular problems.

- **Conclusions:** Though stimulants initially boost many of the qualities we admire, they have a full share of side effects that cause damage when the substance is over used.

WEDNESDAY, MARCH 22, 2000
COPYRIGHT 2000/THE TIMES MIRROR COMPANY

DAILY 50 CENTS
AN EDITION OF THE LOS ANGELES TIMES

High Court Bars FDA From Regulating Tobacco as Drug

law: Despite calling ...rettes the 'single most ...ificant threat to public ...lth,' justices issue 5-4 ...ng that delivers a blow ...dministration efforts ...ontrol their sale.

...AVID G. SAVAGE
...TAFF WRITER

Su-
y that
...ve no
nufac-
, even
erica's
reat to

ngress
roducts
...der the
Act, the
...ne Clin-
...its

Meth use etches pain in Japan

Drug abuse growth alarms officials

Monday, March 27, 2000

TOKYO — Yoichi Tsubokura, 51, has spent two-thirds of his life addicted to methamphetamines. Speed had such a grip over him that be once used money earmarked for his mother's funeral to get high.

Three years ago, however, he entered counseling, kicked the habit and now works ...

drugs combined.

And recently, the drug has been landing on Japanese shores in chart-busting quantities, ringing alarm bells with police and ...

which accounts for an estimated 40 percent of the supply — Japan has little influence in North Korea and Southeast Asia's Golden Triangle.

As quantities increase, police say, ...al dealers have become more ...ept at marketing and distribu-...n. Speed ...ditionally was sold ...ectly by ...anese ...y moto ...eral) ... hire othe ...led (... the ...rs ...ta ...h ...e

This often means buyers and sellers never meet, making it tougher to engineer a bust. And a shift to pill and powder forms, rather than traditional injectable doses, has expanded the appeal among a middle class wary of contracting AIDS.

Unfortunately, the gangs also are finding young Japanese increasingly receptive. Arrests among senior and junior high school students have gone up several fold in recent ... small base.

Study to Look at Effects of Prozac, Ritalin on Kids

By NICK ANDERSON
TIMES STAFF WRITER

WASHINGTON—The White House said Monday that the federal government will intensify research on medications used to treat preschoolers for behavioral disorders, responding to growing concerns ab of youngste tion drugs Prozac.

The gove launch a $5-, ect over five dren who tak tention-defici efforts to stu age of psy youngsters; a ence on the is fall.

are being systematically misdiagnosed," said Donna Shalala, secretary of Health and Human Services.

Despite the potential political overtones, some health care experts said the event served a useful purpose.

ficant that ...ion to this we really ...at's goin ...in, an e ... disorde | Medi "Giv is a . ...rtici . B ...he n

2000

WHOLE TOWN MAD FOR COCAINE

Most Prominent Residents of Manchester, Conn, Afflicted with the General Craze for the Drug.

WANT LEGISLATIVE ACTION

Druggist Started the Habit a YearAgo by Preparing a SeductivePreparation of Drugs for use by townspeople.

1897

Cocaine Use Linked To Brain Hemorrhages

2000

By David Perlman
Chronicle Science Editor

When emergency room doctors at Detroit's major trauma center began seeing unusually large numbers of patients suffering from bursting blood vessels in their brains, it did not take them long to make the cocaine connection.

The patients seeking help were primarily inner-city men in their 30s, which was unusual because brain hemorrhages — the bleeding that results when weakened artery walls balloon and rupture — are far more common among people over 50, in whom they can cause major strokes.

COCAINE, BROUGHT TO U.S. AS BLESSING, SOON A CURSE

Addict Army Here Grew Rapidly as "Glorious Discovery" of 35 Years Ago Was Boughtfor Base Uses and Became Ally of Crime

by Winifred Black

San Francisco, Feb 12 - Cocaine came into America about 35 years ago.

It was hailed as a glorious discovery and for a long time, no one realized the insidious and cruel danger it brought with it.

1927

GENERAL CLASSIFICATION

"I took it for weight loss 'cause I have a weight problem but I also like the high. I liked how it made me feel. I liked the rush, the way that you could get everything done, boom, boom, boom. Just like that."

20-year-old female recovering from methamphetamine addiction

From powerful stimulants, including methamphetamine and "crack" cocaine, to milder ones, such as caffeinated soft drinks and cigarettes, uppers are a regular part of life for many human beings. The National Institute of Drug Abuse (NIDA) and other sources stated that during 1999 in the United States, approximately

◇ 1.7 million Americans used amphetamines ("speed," "meth," "ice") for nonmedical reasons;

◇ 4.2 million used cocaine, including "crack," at least occasionally;

◇ 68 million smoked cigarettes;

◇ 200 million drank coffee, tea, 100 billion caffeinated soft drinks, or took an over-the-counter medication containing caffeine.

Some stimulants are found naturally in plants: the coca bush (cocaine), the tobacco plant (nicotine), the khat tree (cathinone), the ephedra bush (ephedrine), and the coffee plant (caffeine). Other stimulants are synthesized in legal or "street" laboratories. Methamphetamines, diet pills, methylphenidate (Ritalin®), methcathinone, and lookalike stimulants are the most common.

TABLE 3–1 UPPERS (STIMULANTS)

Drug Name	Some Trade Names	Street or Slang Names
COCAINE (from coca leaf)		
Cocaine HCL (hydrochloride) (schedule II)	None, but it is manufactured and sold legally for medical purposes (anesthetic)	Coke, blow, toot, snow, flake, girl, lady, nose candy, big C, la dama blanca
Cocaine freebase (schedule II but extra legal penalties)	None	Crack, base, rock, basay, boulya, pasta, paste, hubba, basuco, pestillos, primo
AMPHETAMINES (synthetic)		
d,l amphetamine (schedule II)	Adderall®, Biphetamine®	Crosstops, whites, speed, black beauties, bennies, cartwheels, pep pills
Benzphetamine (schedule III)	Didrex®	
Dextroamphetamine sulfate (schedule II)	Dexedrine®	Dexies, Christmas trees, beans
Dextromethamphetamine base (schedule II)	none	Ice, glass, batu, shabu, yellow rock
Freebase methamphetamine (schedule II)	none	Snot
Levo amphetamine (no schedule)	Vick's Inhaler®	
Methamphetamine HCL (schedule II)	Desoxyn®	Crank, meth, crystal, peanut butter speed, pervitin (overseas)
AMPHETAMINE CONGENERS		
Dexfenfluramine (schedule IV)	Redux® (no longer sold in the United States)	The combination of dexfenfluramine and fenfluramine with phentermine HCL or phentermine resin is called "fen-phen"
Diethylpropion (schedule IV)	Tenuate®, Tepanil®	
Fenfluramine (schedule IV)	Pondimin®	Fen-phen (in combination)
Methylphenidate (schedule II)	Ritalin®	Pellets
Phendimetrazine (schedule III)	Bontril®, Plegine®, Prelu-2® Anorex®, Adipost®	Pink hearts
Pemoline (schedule II)	Cylert®	Popcorn coke
Phenmetrazine (schedule II)	Preludin®	
Phentermine HCL (schedule IV)	Fastin®, Adipex-P®, Banobese®, Obenix®, Zantryl®	Robin's eggs, black and whites, fen-phen (in combination)
Phentermine resin complex (schedule IV)	Ionamin®	Part of fen-phen
OTHER DIET PILLS		
Mazindol (schedule IV)	Mazanor®, Sanorex®	
Sibutramine (schedule IV)	Meridia®	
LOOKALIKE & OVER-THE-COUNTER STIMULANTS		
Can contain: caffeine, ephedrine, phenylephrine, phenylpropanolamine, pseudoephedrine	Lookalikes: Super Toot® OTCs: Dexatrim®, Acutrim®, Sudafed®	Legal speed, robin's eggs, black beauties
Herbal caffeine, herbal ephedra	Herbal Ecstasy®, Herbal Nexus®, Cloud Nine®, Nirvana®	Herbal X
MISCELLANEOUS PLANT STIMULANTS		
Arecoline (betel nut)	none	Areca, supai, pan parag, marg, maag, pinang
Cathinone, cathine (khat bush) (*Catha edulis*) (methcathinone is the synthetic version)	none	Cat, qat, chat, miraa, Arabian tea, catha, goob, ikwa, ischott, khat kaad, kafta, la salade, liss, bathtub speed, wild cat, mulka,
Ephedrine (ephedra bush)	Many commercial products:	Ma huang, marwath
Yohimbine (yohimbe tree)	Yohimbi 8®, Manpower®	

continued

TABLE 3–1 (continued)

Drug Name	Some Trade Names	Street or Slang Names
CAFFEINE (xanthines)		
Chocolate (cocoa beans)	Hershey®, Nestles®	
Coffee	Colombian, French, espresso	Java, Joe, mud, roast
Colas (from cola nut)	Coca Cola®, Pepsi®	Coke
Over-the-counter stimulants	No Doz®, Alert®, Vivarin®	
Tea	Lipton®, Stash®	Cha, chai
NICOTINE		
Chewing tobacco	Day's Work®, Beechnut®, Levi-Garrett®, Redman®	Chew, chaw
Cigarettes, cigars	Marlboro®, Kents®, Pall Mall®, American Spirit®	Cancer stick, smoke, butts, toke, coffin nails
Pipe tobacco	Sir Walter Raleigh®	
Snuff	Copenhagen®, Skoal®	Dip

GENERAL EFFECTS

Stimulants, particularly the stronger ones like cocaine, amphetamines, and amphetamine congeners, increase the chemical and electrical activity in the central nervous system. In low doses they increase energy, raise the heart rate and blood pressure, increase respiration, and reduce appetite and thirst. They also make the user more alert, active, confident, anxious, restless, and aggressive. Those effects allow some stimulants to be used clinically to treat narcolepsy, obesity, and attention deficit/hyperactivity disorder. Some stimulants are used illegally to keep the user awake and energized for long periods of time and to induce euphoria. The major effects of stimulants occur because of the way they manipulate energy chemicals and trigger the reward/pleasure center of the brain and central nervous system.

BORROWED ENERGY

Normally, day in and day out, the body releases energy chemicals, hormones, and neurotransmitters, such as epinephrine (adrenaline) and norepinephrine (noradrenaline). Epinephrine (E) has greater effects on physical energy while norepinephrine (NE) has greater effects on confidence, motivation, and feelings of well-being. Most NE and E neurons arise in a small area in the brainstem called the "locus coeruleus." The 3,000 neurons communicate to almost every part of the brain, communicating across synaptic gaps to 1/3 to 1/2 of all the cells in the brain (Snyder, 1996; King & Ellinwood, 1997). Remember that a single neuron can have thousands of dendrites and terminals. As expected, more of these chemicals are released while we are awake than when we are asleep but the average 24-hour output is fairly constant. These energy chemicals can increase heart rate, energize muscles, keep us alert and confident, and help us move and function. In time they are reabsorbed and rereleased when needed or they are metabolized and depleted, signaling the nerve cells to synthesize fresh neurotransmitters.

Sometimes, though, the body needs extra energy or a shot of confidence, e.g., when the person exercises, is scared and needs to flee, is making love, is participating in a sport, has to give a speech, or is in a fight. At these moments the nervous system automatically and naturally releases extra amounts of E, NE, and other chemicals. Remember the surge of extra energy the body receives when frightened or when exercising? Eventually the extra energy chemicals are also reabsorbed or metabolized, allowing the body to return to normal, to calm down.

"The closest thing I've had to a natural high was the rock climb and I was terrified.... The adrenaline is just pumping through your system and you're just so high off of that your heart is pumping and you sit down. We sat up there about five minutes after the climb and I never felt so good and alone with myself other than when I was using drugs."
18-year-old recovering cocaine abuser

The normal progression of events in regards to physical activity is as follows:

◇ the body demands extra energy;

◇ nerve cells and glands release energy chemicals;

◇ the body transforms chemicals to extra energy;

◇ the person finishes her/his tasks;

◇ most of the extra energy chemicals are reabsorbed.

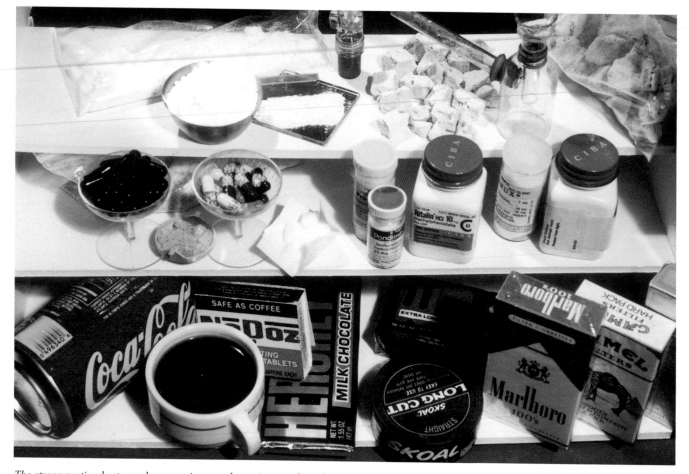

The stronger stimulants, such as cocaine, amphetamines, and amphetamine congeners, are shown on top. The weaker stimulants, like caffeinated drinks and over-the-counter (OTC) medications, are on the lower left with tobacco products on the lower right.

When a person uses strong stimulants, the process is reversed.

◊ Stimulants are ingested, drunk, smoked, injected, or snorted;

◊ the body receives extra energy and the user becomes overly active to use up the extra energy;

◊ with continued use, nerve cells and glands become depleted of energy chemicals;

◊ the body becomes exhausted and demands extra energy;

◊ more stimulants are taken.

"I did it for the adrenaline. I did it to stay awake. I did it 'cause I enjoy life a lot and wanted to get the most out of life. I stayed awake and did it, and did it, and did it."

19-year-old recovering stimulant addict

Stronger stimulants, such as methamphetamine or cocaine, force the release of the energy chemicals and then multiply their effect by keeping the neurotransmitters (E, NE, and dopamine) circulating. It keeps them active either by blocking their reabsorption through reuptake ports on the membrane of the sending neurons and/or by blocking their metabolism when they are released into the synaptic gap. If this process continues, the body is infused with tremendous amounts of extra energy. The energy chemicals are difficult to replace due to depletion of the neurotransmitters stored in the vesicles.

"During the first hours of the coca effect, one cannot sleep but this sleeplessness is in no way distressing. I have tested this effect of coca, which

wards off hunger, sleep, and fatigue and steels one to intellectual effort, some dozen times on myself."

Sigmund Freud (Freud, 1884)

THE CRASH

If strong stimulants are only taken occasionally, the body has time to recover. But if they are taken continuously over a long period of time or in large quantities, the energy and confidence supplies become depleted and the body is left without reserves. It is squeezed dry—exhausted. With stronger stimulants, this crash, its subsequent withdrawal symptoms, and severe depression can last for days, weeks, and in some cases, even months. The severity of the crash depends on the length of use, the strength of the drug, the extent

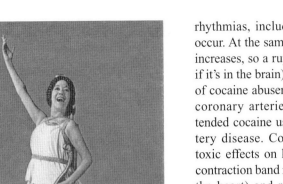

Ritalin®
(methylphenidate)
sparks energy
swiftly

relieves chronic fatigue
and mild depression

Even a born huntress won't quiver with
excitement at the thought of a chase, if
chronic fatigue has her off the track.
When this condition marks your patient
as its quarry, Ritalin can score a therapeutic bull's-eye. You'll find that it gives

In the 1960s, stimulants were actually identified in advertisements as "stimulants." This 1968 ad for Ritalin® listed chronic fatigue, drug-induced lethargy, psychoneuroses (e.g., depression), narcolepsy, senile behavior, and finally hyperactivity disorder as conditions that could be treated with the drug. Since many strong stimulants were heavily regulated or banned in the '70s, methylphenidate (Ritalin®) has been promoted mostly for attention deficit/hyperactivity disorder (AD/HD).

of biochemical disruption, and any pre-existing mental or emotional problems.

"There is only so much you can do and after a while you don't get high anymore, no matter how much more you do. You just need to crash and the depression is terrible: the fatigue, not even being able to walk, not being able to get out of bed, and just being desperate to sleep. The depression lasts up to eight days but it is intensely acute for three or four days in my case."
Recovering 36-year-old female "meth" addict

It is important to remember that the energy and confidence received from stimulants is not a free gift. It is a loan from the rest of the body and must be repaid by giving the body time to recover, to rebuild its supply of stimulatory neurochemicals, and to repair damaged neurons (as much as possible).

CARDIOVASCULAR SIDE EFFECTS

Many stimulants, including nicotine, constrict blood vessels, thus decreasing blood flow to tissues and organs, particularly the skin and extremities. Since blood flow is decreased, tissue repair and healing are slowed. In addition heart rate is increased and, with the stronger stimulants such as cocaine and amphetamines, various heart ar-rhythmias, including tachycardia, can occur. At the same time, blood pressure increases, so a ruptured vessel (a stroke if it's in the brain) is possible. Autopsies of cocaine abusers often reveal clogged coronary arteries indicating that extended cocaine use causes coronary artery disease. Cocaine also has direct toxic effects on heart muscles causing contraction band necrosis (scar tissue on the heart) and resultant heart failure (Karch, 1996).

Polydrug use of a stimulant and a depressant can cause additional, unexpected, and possibly fatal cardiovascular effects. Alcohol and cocaine metabolize to cocaethylene, a potent metabolite that can have more serious effects.

REWARD/PLEASURE CENTER

Cocaine and amphetamines disrupt the reward/pleasure center. Normally this center that exists in all mammals as a survival mechanism gives a surge of pleasure when hunger, thirst, sexual desire, or other need that helps us survive is being been satisfied (Goldstein, 1994). When cocaine or amphetamines are taken, they stimulate this center and signal the brain that hunger is being satisfied although no food is being eaten; that thirst is being satisfied although no liquid is being drunk; and that sexual desire is being satisfied although there has been no sexual activity. This stimulation is perceived as an overall rush and feelings of well-being and pleasure. As the drug is used more and more, the intensity of this rush diminishes but the emotional memories linger on.

NIDA researchers have imaged the limbic system of the brain during cocaine craving using a PET (positron emission tomography) scan. They found that cocaine craving activates this circuitry to an exceptionally high level (Childress, McElgin, Mozley, Reivich, & O'Brien, 1996).

Since the body is fooled into thinking its basic needs have been satisfied, the user can become dehydrated and malnourished. In fact many long-term users of stimulants develop vitamin and

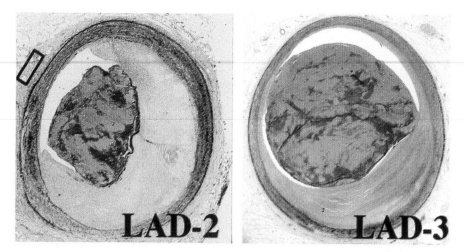

These cross sections of the left anterior descending (LAD) coronary artery are of a 36-year-old long-term IV cocaine user who died from acute myocardial infarction. The thrombus that caused the heart attack can be seen in both cross sections of the lumen (interior) of the LAD. It overlays plaque that has built up over the years, probably due to the cocaine use.

Courtesy of Dr. Rene Virmani, Chairman, Dept. of Cardiovascular Pathology, Armed Forces Institute of Pathology

mineral deficiencies that can damage teeth and cause other health problems.

WEIGHT LOSS

The ability of stimulants to make the body think it has satisfied hunger without eating and thereby cause weight loss is one of the main reasons they are used. Even tobacco can cause a slight appetite loss because of this effect. The fear of gaining weight causes many cocaine, amphetamine, and nicotine users to maintain their habit.

"I was fat from about the age of 8. My doctor put me on amphetamine when I was 16. Unfortunately they made my heart race, so I gave them up. In my senior year I took up smoking and that kept the weight off 'cause when I gave them up 10 years later, I gained about 20 pounds. In college I started drinking coffee to study for exams and that kept my mouth busy doing something instead of eating. Unfortunately I figure I've screwed up my appestat [appetite regulator] or whatever controls appetite 'cause I've kept gain-

ing weight over the years to the tune of 326 pounds."
57-year-old male recovering compulsive overeater

OTHER EMOTIONAL/ MENTAL SIDE EFFECTS

Initially disruption of neurotransmitters by the stronger stimulants tends to increase confidence, create a certain euphoria, and make users feel they can do anything. But as use continues, the balance of dopamine (D), E, NE, and other neurotransmitters transforms these feelings into irritability, talkativeness, restlessness, insomnia, paranoia, aggressiveness, violence, and psychosis. The stronger stimulants cause psychoses and paranoia by increasing the level of dopamine in the central nervous system. The psychosis is hard to distinguish from a real psychosis, including schizophrenia.

"I used to drive around and hear my motorcycle talking to me and I would see faces come out of the trees and I'd see all kinds of crazy stuff. After 10 days of no sleep, it's like living in a dream 'cause I couldn't distinguish

reality from what the drug was doing to me. I was that far gone."
22-year-old "meth" addict living in a therapeutic community

Prolonged or excess use of even milder stimulants, including caffeine, khat, and ephedra can also cause restlessness, talkativeness, insomnia, and irritability.

"It's almost like there's a veneer over the nerves and it takes off that veneer, that coating, and you are just like a live wire. You'll be on a crowded bus and you might go into a rage very spontaneously, without any real cause."
25-year-old "meth" abuser

TOLERANCE & ADDICTION LIABILITY

Because stimulants force the release of extra D (dopamine), E (epinephrine), and NE (norepinephrine), the central nervous system loses some of its ability to synthesize these neurotransmitters. This adds to the rapid development of tolerance, thus causing other physiological changes in the user's neurochemistry, initiating rapid development of physical and psychic dependence. While the physical dependence of extended cocaine and methamphetamine use isn't quite as severe as with heroin, the psychic dependence is as powerful or more powerful and causes severe craving during withdrawal and the subsequent crash. Tolerance and dependence also develop with methamphetamine congeners, caffeine, nicotine, and other milder stimulants. In fact the strongest dependence develops with tobacco. All of these factors lead to the development of habituation, abuse, and addiction with most stimulants.

COCAINE

There is speculation that Robert Louis Stevenson wrote *Dr. Jekyll and Mr. Hyde* under the influence of cocaine that had recently gained public

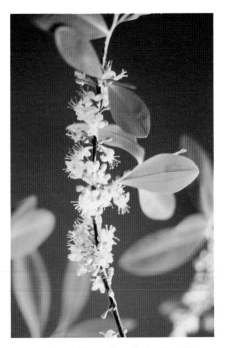

This is the Erythroxylum coca *plant. Two hundred kilograms of coca leaf can be refined to make approximately one kilogram of cocaine.*

Courtesy of the Fitz Hugh Ludlow Memorial Library

attention through the works of a number of scientists, including Sigmund Freud in 1884 (*Über Coca*). The theme of the novel is about the dramatic transformation of Dr. Jekyll when he takes an experimental medication and the consequences of this experimentation. The mania of his alter ego, Mr. Hyde, can be likened to some of the effects of intense use of cocaine, particularly if drug-induced psychosis and paranoia are manifest. This idea of opposites, of ups and downs, of dramatic personality transformations is always present when the effects and side effects of coca and cocaine are examined.

BOTANY, CROP YIELDS, & REFINEMENT

Cocaine is extracted from the coca plant, which grows mainly on the slopes of the Andes Mountains in South America (Colombia, Bolivia, Ecuador, and particularly Peru). Lesser amounts are grown in certain parts of the Amazon Jungle and on the island of

Java in Indonesia. The South American cultivation of the *Erythroxylum coca* and *Erythroxylum novogranatense* plants accounts for 97% of the world's production. The green-yellow shrubs, which grow best at altitudes between 1,500 and 5,000 feet, are 6 to 8 feet tall. The percentage of the alkaloid cocaine that can be refined from the leaves varies from 0.5% to 1.5% by weight. One acre of coca bushes will yield 1.5–2 kilograms of cocaine (Grinspoon & Bakalar, 1985).

◇ The refinement technique is a four- or five-step process depending on the chemicals used (Karch, 1996).

◇ Soak the leaves in lime (or other alkali) and water for three or four days.

◇ Add gasoline, kerosene, or acetone to extract nitrogenous alkaloids.

◇ Discard the waste leaves and add sulfuric or hydrochloric acid to separate the alkaloids from other plant chemicals.

◇ Mix in lime and ammonia to precipitate the basic alkaloids into a crude form of cocaine called "coca paste" ("pasta," "basuco") and then dry it in the sun.

◇ Use a number of chemicals to separate the cocaine hydrochloride from the paste.

Since coca leaves are grown almost exclusively in South America and spoil if transported, the above instructions are useless in other countries.

SMUGGLING & THE STREET TRADE

Because coca leaves are difficult to grow outside of South America and because the extraction process is fairly complex, a highly organized crime cartel developed in order to operate the cocaine trade. Colombian cartels control cultivation and production in the growing countries and much of the street trade in the United States. However, most of the actual smuggling into the United States in recent years has been handled by Mexican gangs, usually by land and sea routes due to increased surveillance of air routes (DEA, 1998).

The United States is responsible for 70% of the world's illegal consumption. Although more than 108 tons of the refined product (cocaine) are seized each year on their way to U.S. markets, an estimated 700 metric tons still get through. The figures for the amount of cocaine produced in Colombia have come under question in 1999 because of larger acreage of the higher yielding *Erythroxylum coca* rather than *Erythroxylum novogranatense* (Lichtblau & Schrader, 1999). Even though the drug use surveys show no great increase in use, authorities think the amount smuggled could be two to three times as much as previously estimated.

◇ At the wholesale level, cocaine prices varied from $10,500 to $36,000 per kilogram of refined cocaine with an average purity of 82%.

◇ From low-level dealers, prices varied from $300 to $2,200 per ounce.

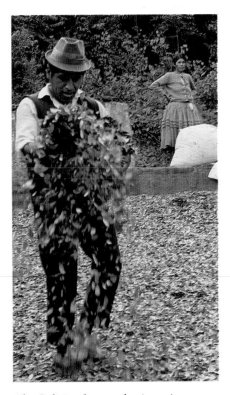

This Bolivian farm worker is sorting coca leaves. It takes 250 kilos of leaves to make 1 kilo of cocaine.

Reprinted, by permission, Alain Labrousse, Observatoire Geopolitique Des Drogues.

◇ At the street level, prices varied from $20 to $200 per gram with an average purity of 57%.

(DEA, 1998)

HISTORY OF USE (*also see History in Chapter 1*)

The effects of cocaine are directly related to the blood levels of the drug. The more cocaine that reaches the brain, the more intense the high, the greater the craving, and the more quickly tolerance, craving, abuse, and addiction occur. Thus when the history of cocaine focuses on the changes in methods of use and the refinement process (the two main factors that control blood cocaine levels), the reasons for the progression from casual coca leaf chewer to dependent "crack" smoker or IV user become clearer.

Chewing the Leaf

Native cultures in South America have used coca leaves for thousands of years for social and religious occasions and to fight off fatigue, lessen hunger, and increase endurance. In particular the Incas in Peru integrated the use of the coca leaf in every part of their lives much as coffee and cigarettes are part of an American's everyday life today. When the Conquistadors conquered the Incan Empire in the sixteenth century, they greatly increased the cultivation and availability of the leaf. They did it for personal profit, to generate government taxes, and to enable the Incans to work at high altitudes digging in the silver mines (Monardes, 1577; Karch, 1997).

The Incas usually chewed the leaf for the juice, adding some lime or ash (from ground shells) to increase absorption by the mucosal tissue in the cheeks and gums. It takes 3–5 minutes for the absorbed coca juice to reach the brain by this route of administration. If the chewer swallows the coca juice, the digestive system breaks down the drug and it takes 30 minutes to reach the brain. A habitual user might chew 12–15 grams of leaves three or four times a day but even so, the maximum amount of cocaine available for absorp-

tion might be just 75 milligrams. The leaves can also be chopped up, mixed with ash, and spooned under the tongue, so the active stimulant alkaloids can be absorbed by the mucosal membranes.

"They take of the leaves of the coca, and they chew them in their mouths, and as they go chewing, they go mingling with it of that powder made of the shells in such sort, that they make it like to a paste, taking less of the powder than of the herb, and of this paste they make certain small balls round, and they put them to dry, and when they will use of them, they take a little ball in their mouth, and they chew them."

Nicolas Monardes, 1577

Even to this day up to 90% of the Indians living in coca-growing regions chew the leaf. In fact in many native homes in Bolivia, visitors are ceremoniously offered pieces of leaves to chew even before refreshments are served. The cocaine blood levels for a coca leaf chewer are about 1/4 of those of smokers and 1/7 of those of IV users (Karch, 1996).

Refinement of Cocaine from Coca

In 1861 Albert Niemann, a graduate student in Gottingen, Germany, isolated cocaine from the other chemicals in the coca leaf. This extraction from the coca leaf produced pure cocaine hydrochloride. Since this extract of the coca leaf was 200 times more powerful by weight than the coca leaf, the stage was set for the widespread use and abuse of cocaine. However, it was 20 years before its use became widespread. This occurred due in part to Karl Koller who discovered the anesthetic properties of the drug and Sigmund Freud who published *Über Coca*. Their writings and other papers promoted the use of the refined cocaine hydrochloride for a variety of ailments including depression, gastric disorders,

asthma, morphine or alcohol addiction. Its use as a local anesthetic or even as an aphrodisiac was also suggested (Guttmacher, 1885). It was the stimulating and mood-enhancing qualities that most interested Freud. However, since cocaine was a new drug that hadn't been studied over time, he made a number of errors of judgment.

"Coca is a far more potent and far less harmful stimulant than alcohol and its widespread utilization is hindered at present only by its high cost.... I have already stressed the fact that there is no state of depression when the effects of coca have worn off."

Sigmund Freud, 1884

Freud's and others' overly optimistic judgments were made using controlled levels of cocaine before dependence and addiction had a chance to develop. When the drug was made more widely available and people had a chance to become chronic users, then the true nature and dangers of refined cocaine became obvious.

Drinking Cocaine

The fact that the newly refined cocaine could be dissolved in water or al-

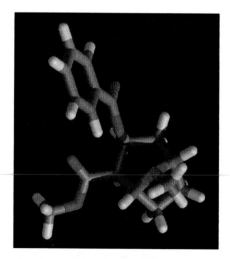

Simulation of the cocaine HCL molecule, $C_{17}H_{21}NO_4$.

Courtesy of the Molecular Imaging Department, University of California Medical Center, San Francisco

cohol made other routes of use possible, namely drinking, injecting, and contact absorption. Beginning in the late 1860s, cocaine wines became popular in France and Italy but it wasn't until a clever manufacturer and salesman, Angelo Mariani, developed Vin Mariani and promoted its use through the first celebrity endorsements (e.g., Thomas Edison, Robert Louis Stevenson, and Pope Leo XIII) that the first cocaine epidemic began. Although the wine contained only a modest amount of cocaine (two glasses of wine contained the equivalent of a line of cocaine), its effect was more than modest because it was used with alcohol (Karch, 1997). It has been found in recent years that alcohol and cocaine form cocaethylene, a metabolite that has stronger and longer-lasting effects than other cocaine metabolites and causes more intense effects than cocaine hydrochloride by itself. It takes 15–30 minutes for the metabolites of cocaine to reach the brain after oral ingestion.

Suddenly in the 1880s and '90s, patent medicines laced with cocaine, opium, morphine, heroin, marijuana, and alcohol became the rage. They were touted as a cure for any ailment including asthma, hay fever, fatigue, and a dozen other illnesses.

Since the drugs induced a high and controlled pain, the perception was that the drugs cured illness rather than just controlling the symptoms. The prolonged use of these and other prescription medications created a large group of dependent users and addicts, the majority being women (Aldrich, 1994).

Injecting Cocaine

The invention of the hypodermic needle in 1857 had a more immediate effect on the use of morphine than on cocaine for two reasons. First, the refinement of morphine from opium occurred 50 years earlier than the refinement of cocaine and second, the use of an opiate painkiller such as morphine had a natural outlet in the Crimean and U.S. Civil Wars and at home as a remedy for dozens of painful illnesses.

Medically the subcutaneous injec-

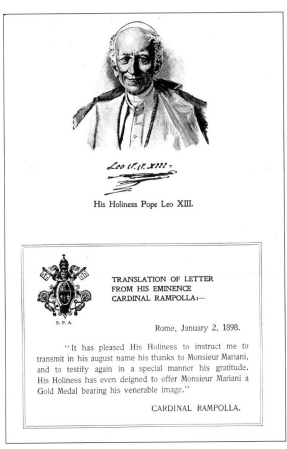

His Holiness Pope Leo XIII.

TRANSLATION OF LETTER FROM HIS EMINENCE CARDINAL RAMPOLLA:—

Rome, January 2, 1898.

"It has pleased His Holiness to instruct me to transmit in his august name his thanks to Monsieur Mariani, and to testify again in a special manner his gratitude. His Holiness has even deigned to offer Monsieur Mariani a Gold Medal bearing his venerable image."

CARDINAL RAMPOLLA.

Angelo Mariani, creator of Vin Mariani, would send free cases of his wine to various celebrities. They, in turn, would send thank you notes and occasionally endorsements that Mariani would then publicize in newspaper advertisements such as this one with Pope Leo XIII. Since the concept of celebrity endorsements was brand new, many well-known people didn't understand what was involved. In addition the abuse potential of cocaine-based products was not understood.
Courtesy of the Fitz Hugh Ludlow Memorial Library

tion of cocaine caused topical anesthesia (for minor surgery) and deadened the pain of skin ulcerations and other diseases. Unfortunately when physicians first began using cocaine medicinally, many were unaware of the overdose potential and a number of deaths occurred.

Injecting cocaine intravenously results in an intense rush within 15–30 seconds and gives the highest blood cocaine level. The rush is more intense than chewing the leaf or drinking and snorting cocaine hydrochloride, so the alteration in brain chemistry and the reward/pleasure center (as well as the satiation center) is more rapid. Since cocaine is rapidly metabolized by the body, IV use means that the rush and subsequent crash will be equally intense.

Snorting Cocaine

The early 1900s gave rise to a popular new form of cocaine use, snorting the chemical into the nostrils. Called

"tooting," "blowing," or "horning," this method gets the drug to the nasal mucosa (not the lungs) and into the brain within three to five minutes. Peak effects take a few more minutes to occur.

"At first, when you put it in your nose, it starts a numbness and you can feel a little drip going down your throat. And then you get hyperactive in 20 minutes. When you smoke it, it's an instantaneous rush."
26-year-old recovering cocaine addict

Snorting cocaine is a self-limiting method of using cocaine. This occurs because cocaine constricts the capillaries that absorb the drug, so the more that is snorted, the slower the absorption. The blood cocaine level is much less than when used intravenously. As the constricting effect of cocaine wears off, the nasal tissues swell causing a runny sniffling nose, characteristic of cocaine snorters. In addition chronic use can kill nasal tissues and in a few cases perforate the nasal septum that divides the nostrils.

Topical Absorption

Besides absorption through mucosa in the nose, gums, and cheeks, cocaine can be absorbed through mucosal tissue in the rectum and the vagina and act as a topical anesthetic. Rectal application is used in parts of the homosexual community (Karch, 1996). Cocaine can also be absorbed through the outer skin but not at levels high enough to cause effects, merely to be detectable in the bloodstream (and cause problems in drug testing). Finally, cocaine makes eye surgery possible because it can be absorbed by the tiny blood vessels in the eye, thereby deadening the eye nerves and constrict blood vessels to slow bleeding. Synthetic topical anesthetics, such as procaine and lidocaine, that mimic the effects of cocaine are used nowadays for eye surgery, dental procedures, and other minor surgeries because they are much less stimulating to the brain. None of the synthetic anesthetics constrict blood vessels and are therefore combined with epinephrine.

Smoking

In 1914 Parke-Davis, a pharmaceutical company, introduced cigarettes that contained refined cocaine in America but the high temperature (195°C or 383°F) needed to convert cocaine hydrochloride to smoke resulted in destruction of many of the psychoactive properties of the drug. Thus chewing, drinking, injecting, and snorting cocaine remained the principal routes of administration until the mid-1970s when street chemists converted cocaine hydrochloride to freebase cocaine. This lowered the vaporization point to 98°C and made the drug smokable. The chemical process also removed the drug's many cuts or diluting agents making it more pure. Unlike the cocaine hydrochloride cigarettes introduced in 1914, freebase cocaine could be smoked without destroying its psychoactive properties. In the early and mid-1980s, an easier method of making freebase cocaine ("crack") was developed setting the stage for another cocaine epidemic.

When absorbed through the lungs, cocaine reaches the brain within only 5–8 seconds compared to the 15–30 seconds it takes when injected through the veins. The smokable cocaine reaches the brain so quickly it causes more dramatic effects before it is swiftly metabolized. This up and down rapid roller coaster effect results in intense craving.

"I prefer snorting because it would never get me that far out there. Freebase would get me out there more quickly and I didn't really like that."
17-year-old male recovering "crack" smoker

This rapid euphoria followed by an intense dysphoria or depression is especially true with smoking coca paste. "Paste" or "pasta," the intermediate product in the refinement of cocaine, can be smoked and was, in fact, the earliest use of freebase cocaine (almost exclusively in South America in the early 1970s). In some studies in Peru where "pasta" smoking is a severe problem, a number of users report perceptual disturbances early on in their history of use indicating that smoking coca paste unbalances brain chemistry more rapidly (Jeri, Sanchez, Del Pozo, & Fernandez, 1992). Unfortunately it contains a number of impurities and toxic chemicals, including kerosene, alkali, and sulfuric acid, so the effect on the lungs can be severe. Further it contains other more powerful brain active alkaloids that are reported to result in a more severe addiction.

PHYSICAL & MENTAL EFFECTS

Medical Use

Cocaine is not only a stimulant, it is also the only naturally occurring topical anesthetic with powerful vasoconstriction effects. It is used in aerosol form to numb the nasal passages when inserting breathing tubes in a patient, to numb the eye or back of the throat during surgery, and to deaden the pain of chronic sores. (This topical anesthetic effect also numbs the nasal passages when the drug is snorted.) Cocaine receptors are also found on the bronchi and smooth muscles of the lungs, so stimulation causes dilation of bronchi. Because of this effect, cocaine has been used to treat asthma.

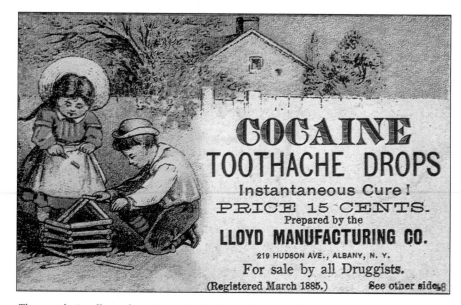

The anesthetic effects of cocaine made the drug a favorite of dentists long before novocaine was synthesized.
Courtesy of the National Library of Medicine, Bethesda

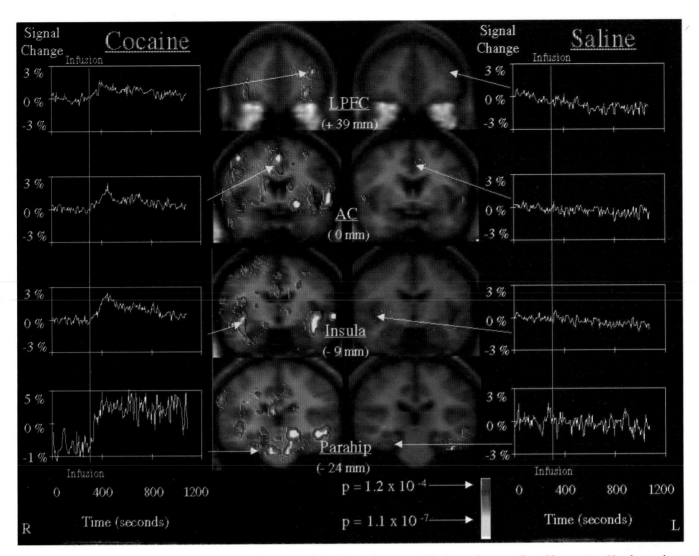

These functional MRI (magnetic resonance imaging) scans on the left show the areas of the brain that are affected by cocaine. Nondrugged brain scans are on the right. The nucleus accumbens/subcallosal cortex (Nac/SCC), amygdala, basal forebrain (BF), and ventral tegmental (VT) areas are highlighted on the left. Notice the stimulation or suppression on the graphs on the left when cocaine is infused.

Courtesy of Hans C. Breiter and the Cell Press

Neurochemistry & the Central Nervous System

Besides topical anesthesia, cocaine's effects (like amphetamines' effects) are the result of its influence on catecholamine neurotransmitters (norepinephrine, epinephrine, and dopamine). Cocaine forces the release of these neurotransmitters and then blocks their reabsorption, so more are available for intense stimulation but they are also more vulnerable to metabolism and eventual depletion. In an experiment with cocaine users, Dr. Nora Volkow at NIDA's Regional Neuroimaging Center

used PET scans to show that cocaine blocked 60% to 77% of the dopamine reuptake sites. At least 47% of the sites had to be blocked for users to feel a drug-induced high (Volkow, Fowler, Wang, et al., 1997). To a lesser extent serotonin and acetylcholine are also affected in a similar fashion.

"I felt real ecstatic, very euphoric. My mind had a great deal of pleasure. I felt like a somebody. I felt like a 'super' person. I could do anything."

32-year-old female recovering cocaine addict

In an experiment at Massachusetts General Hospital, brain scans of 10 cocaine addicts just after injection of the drug showed 90 distinct areas of brain activation, especially the amygdala and nucleus accumbens. Within five to eight minutes of brain activation, all but 13 of the areas became inactive but those 13 are thought to be partly responsible for the intense craving that causes a user to use again and again (Breiter, Gollub, Weisskoss, et al., 1997). Recent studies at Yale, Harvard Medical School, and Northwestern University discovered that a protein called "delta-FosB" sensitized mice to the pleasurable and rewarding effects of cocaine implying that this heightened sensitivity contributes to the intense craving caused by cocaine use (Kelz, Chen, Carlezon, et al., 1999).

Unfortunately the intense stimulation has a price when done frequently. It's like putting 200 volts into a 115-volt light bulb. The bulb burns more brightly but the strain on the filament can eventually burn out the bulb. For example,

◇ catecholamines increase confidence and energy and cause a euphoric rush that seems extremely pleasurable; eventual depletion of the catecholamines causes exhaustion, lethargy, anhedonia (the inability to feel pleasure), and low blood pressure;

◇ acetylcholine increases reflexes, alertness, memory, learning, and aggression but that can turn into muscle tremors, memory lapses, mental confusion, and even hallucinations;

◇ serotonin initially causes elation, raised self-esteem, and increased sexual activity but with excessive use it becomes insomnia, agitation, and severe emotional depression;

◇ dopamine can also overstimulate the brain's fright center causing the paranoia experienced by many stimulant abusers. The fright center is a survival mechanism to warn us of danger but overstimulation causes overreaction. A shadow, sudden movement, or loud voice may seem unbearably threatening.

"A person I know does a shot every 15–20 minutes. He fights sleep. He'll go days without sleeping and he'll collapse. He looks for people hiding under mattresses, behind door hinges, and in books. He asks why you're smiling."
24-year-old recovering intravenous cocaine user

Sexual Effects

Cocaine and amphetamines have similar sexual effects. Cocaine at low doses enhances sexual desire, delays ejaculation, and is considered an aphrodisiac by many users. However with the advent of Viagra®, the initial sexual effects of cocaine have become less desirable. Unfortunately as dosage increases and use becomes chronic, sexual dysfunction, such as the inability to achieve an erection, becomes more common. In addition high-risk sexual behavior and unusual sexual behavior also become more common (Smith & Wesson, 1985).

Aggression, Violence, & Cocaethylene

Disruption of neurotransmitter levels are heavily implicated in the aggression and violence associated with stronger stimulants. When inhibitory functions in the anterior cingulate gyrus and temporal lobes are suppressed; when the emotional triggers in the amygdala are overstimulated; when the fright center in the limbic system is hyperactivated; when the normal function of the temporal lobes are disrupted, then aggression and occasionally violence are often a glance away (Amen, Yantis, Trudeau, et al.,1997).

In a study of domestic violence, researchers found that 67% of the perpetrators had used cocaine the day of the incident and virtually all of those had also used alcohol. Interviews and research seem to indicate that cocaethylene, an active metabolite of cocaine and alcohol when taken together, induces greater agitation, euphoria, and violence than just cocaine alone (Brookhoff, O'Brien, Cook, et al., 1997; Landry, 1992).

Abused mother with kids: "He had me like this [hands on throat] saying 'I'll kill you. I'll kill you.'"

Dr. Brookhoff: "Did the children see it?"

Mother: "Yes, they did. And then he threw the knife in the sink and started laughing and kissed me."

Dr. Brookhoff: "Was he drinking tonight?"

Mother: "Yes."

Dr. Brookhoff: "Does he have an alcohol problem?"

Mother: "Yes."

Dr. Brookhoff: "Does he do any drugs?"

Mother: "Yes."

Doctor. "What drugs does he do?"

Mother: "Well, cocaine."

(Domestic violence case documented on video by Memphis, Tennessee police and Daniel Brookhoff, M.D., Methodist Hospital, Memphis.)

Cocaethylene is produced by the combined presence of alcohol and cocaine in the liver. It reaches the brain as easily as the cocaine and has almost identical effects but is somewhat more toxic. Cocaethylene also seems more likely to induce cardiac conduction abnormalities compared to cocaine and therefore is more likely to induce a heart attack. Since the half-life of cocaethylene is more than three times that of cocaine by itself (2 hours vs. 38 minutes), effects, including high blood pressure, last longer (Karch, 1996; Gold & Miller, 1997). Many cocaine abusers are aware of this extended half-life effect and so "front load" with alcohol to prolong the effects of the more expensive cocaine. However, it is theorized that the extended anxiety and panic attacks that are common with cocaine abusers, even after they quit, could be attributed to the slow elimination of cocaethylene (Randall, 1992).

The paranoia and dysfunctional lifestyle involved with cocaine use engenders excess violence. Autopsies showed that 31% of all homicide victims in New York in the early 1990s had cocaine in their bodies (1,332 out of 4,298 victims). Two-thirds of those who tested positive were 15–34 years of age, 86% were male and 87% were African American or Latino (Tardiff, Marzuk, Leon, et al., 1994).

Cardiovascular Effects

Physiologically it is the cardiovascular system that is most affected by long-term cocaine use. Cocaine affects

Effects of cocaine, besides cardiovascular problems, last beyond detoxification. Memory, manual dexterity, and decision making are disrupted to some extent for up to a month after cessation of use (Bolla, Cadet, & Rothman, 1999).

the circulatory system by direct contact (due to receptors right on the heart and blood vessels) and by its effect on the autonomic nervous system in the brain. The heart rate rises and blood vessels constrict causing a 20–30 unit rise in blood pressure. This means that while more blood is available for central blood vessels to energize muscles and increase blood flow to the heart, less is available for the smaller vessels to heal damaged tissues, aid digestion, and infuse other peripheral systems with sufficient oxygen. This leads to cellular changes including damage to heart muscles, coronary arteries, and other blood vessels.

The more cocaine used and the longer it is used, the greater the damage. The raised blood pressure can also cause a stroke, usually within three hours of use. Chronic cocaine use is similar to chronic stress. The hearts of chronic abusers are often slightly enlarged and coronary arterial blood flow is sluggish. The effects of cocaine can cause atherosclerosis, lesions, and other damage that induces heart dis-

ease. Chronic cocaine use also causes a disorganization in the usual formation of heart muscles resulting in contraction band necrosis on the heart. This makes chronic users more likely to suffer a cocaine-induced heart attack (Karch, 1996).

Neonatal Effects

Smoked, snorted, or injected, cocaine and amphetamines are a particular danger to the fetus of a pregnant woman. When a pregnant woman smokes "crack," within seconds her baby will also be exposed to the drug. Because of the stimulatory effects on the cardiovascular system in particular, the chances of miscarriage, stroke, and sudden infant death syndrome (SIDS) due to increased blood pressure and blood vessel malformations are increased (Gold & Miller, 1997).

"I'd been smoking 'crack' for a couple of years and I had a baby who was born testing positive for 'coke.' Child Protective Services came and placed

her in foster care. It took me two years to get my baby back."
17-year-old recovering "crack" user

In a Toronto inner-city hospital, 12% to 20% of all newborns had been exposed to cocaine (Foreman, Klein, Barks, et al., 1994). Respiratory ailments were more common in those infants. Infants born cocaine affected have been called "jittery babies" because they are agitated, have higher blood pressure, are more irritable, and are sometimes smaller.

Many of the abnormalities in the newborns of drug users have to do more with the lifestyle than the drug itself. For example, amphetamine and cocaine users are generally malnourished, so the fetus suffers from malnutrition. The mothers are more likely to smoke tobacco and to have a venereal or IV drug-induced disease, such as hepatitis and AIDS. A drug-dependent mother is more likely to be indifferent to the daily demands of an infant than a nonuser, so bonding problems, untreated illnesses, and emotional deprivation are more likely.

Despite the severe problems of cocaine toxicity and withdrawal noted in cocaine-exposed fetuses and babies, there is hope. Demonstration projects like those of the Haight-Ashbury Free Clinics' Moving Addicted Mothers Ahead (MAMA) and Ujima House Centers have demonstrated that good prenatal and postnatal care of these infants, along with continued excellent pediatric and parenting resources, results in toddlers who catch up in their emotional and physical development to noncocaine-exposed children by their 8th to 10th birthdays.

Metabolism

Because cocaine is metabolized very quickly by the body, effects disappear faster than with amphetamines and amphetamine congeners. After cocaine has finished working, it is metabolized to ecgonine methyl ester, benzoylecgonine, and if alcohol is present, cocaethylene. The half-life of cocaine is about .5–1.5 hours. This means that half the drug is metabolized to pharmacologically inactive metabolites in that period of time. However, even after the drug has almost disappeared from the blood, effects continue to occur.

The Crash

Since cocaine is metabolized so quickly by the body, the initial euphoria, the feeling of confidence, the sense of omnipotence, the surge of energy, and the satisfied feeling disappear as suddenly as they appeared, so the crash after using cocaine can be particularly depressing. With cocaine this depression can last a few hours, several days, or even weeks.

"I really did want to die and I remember that as being way out of proportion to the actual events of my life although it seemed like my life was over."
Recovering cocaine user

Tolerance

Tolerance to the euphoric effects can develop after the first injection or smoking session. Binge or chronic users have escalated their doses from one-eighth of a gram to three grams per day within only a few days while chasing the initial high or the euphoria. Most cocaine users remember their early experiences with cocaine as the most satisfying (Gold & Herkov, 1998).

Withdrawal, Craving, & Relapse

Contrary to notions held by many researchers until the 1980s, there are true withdrawal symptoms when cocaine use ceases. Although similar to the crash, withdrawal effects can last months, even years, depending on dosage, frequency, length of use, and any pre-existing mental problems. The major symptoms are anhedonia (the lack of ability to feel pleasure), anergia (a total lack of energy), loss of motivation or initiative, emotional depression, and an intense craving for the drug. These symptoms are also common for amphetamine withdrawal. It is these symptoms, particularly craving, that

generally cause the compulsive recovering user to relapse again and again.

◇ The time frame for a typical cycle of compulsive cocaine (or amphetamine) use is as follows:

◇ immediately after a binge, usually lasting several days, the user crashes, sleeps all day long trying to put energy back into the body, and swears off the drug forever;

◇ a few days later the user usually feels much better and may leave or drop out of treatment at this time. This temporary return to normal feelings is called "euthymia";

◇ however, about 1 week to 10 days after quitting, the craving starts to build, the energy level drops, and the user feels very little pleasure from any surroundings, activities, or friends. Emotional depression begins to increase;

◇ so 2–4 weeks after vowing to abstain, users feel the craving and depression build to a fever pitch, and unless they are in intensive treatment, they will usually relapse.

"You know, there's no specific time that I can remember where before I went into relapse that I actually decided to go and use again. That's the cunningness of this thing. The next thing you know, you're just there and you're just doing it. You even ask yourself, 'How the hell did I get into this situation again? What happened?'"
28-year-old female recovering cocaine abuser

Overdose

An overdose of cocaine can be caused by as little as 1/50 of a gram or as much as 1.2 grams. The "caine reaction" is very intense and generally short in duration. Most often it's not fatal. It only feels like impending death. However in 2,000–3,000 U.S. cases every year, death can occur within 40 minutes to 5 hours after exposure. Death usually results from either the initial stimulatory phase of toxicity (seizures, hypertension, stroke, and tachycardia) or the later depression phase terminating in extreme respiratory depression and coma.

"I have seen a friend go through overdose. His skin was gray-green. His eyes rolled back, his heart stopped, and there was a gurgling sound that is right at death; and I had to bring him back and that's enough to put the fear of God in anybody."
Intravenous cocaine user

First-time users, and even those who have used cocaine before, can get an exaggerated reaction, far beyond what might normally occur or beyond what they have experienced in the past. This is partially due to the phenomenon known as "inverse tolerance" or "kindling." As people use cocaine, they get more sensitive to its toxic effects rather than less sensitive as one would expect. One reason for this is that each use of cocaine damages heart muscles causing constriction bands (of scar tissue) that make the user more likely to experience a heart attack on the next use. Heart seizures and death will occasionally occur the morning after heavy use. Research in the mid-1990s indicates that cocaethylene, which lasts in the blood and brain after the cocaine has been metabolized, is responsible for many of the overdoses, particularly if it occurs many hours or even the morning after use (Landry, 1992; Karch, 1997).

Miscellaneous Effects

Formication. A side effect of long-term or high-dose cocaine and amphetamine use is an imbalance to sensory neurons that causes sensations in the skin that feel like hundreds of tiny bugs ("coke bugs," "meth bugs," "snow bugs") are crawling under one's skin. Users on "coke" or "speed" runs have been known to scratch themselves bloody trying to get at the imaginary bugs.

Dental erosions. These frequently occur as a result of either poor dental hygiene, malnutrition, the erosive effects of acidic cocaine that has trickled down from the sinuses to the upper front teeth, and from repetitive and compulsive overbrushing of the teeth while intoxicated.

Seizure. This effect is caused by overdose, stroke, or hemorrhage and occurs in 2% to 10% of regular cocaine users (Karch, 1996). Three times as many women as men have seizures from cocaine overdoses.

Cocaine Psychosis

Real schizophrenia is caused by hereditary imbalances of brain dopamine. Excess dopamine activity, induced by excess cocaine use, can trigger cocaine-induced paranoid psychosis/schizophrenia. Often it is difficult for clinicians to tell the difference between real schizophrenia and cocaine-induced schizophrenia and a drug test is necessary since cocaine abusers are usually not forthcoming about their use. This syndrome was first documented when intensive cocaine experimentation and abuse began during the late 1800s. Also cocaine's effect on the brain may trigger a psychotic break in someone with a genetic potential for schizophrenia.

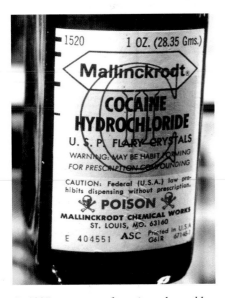

In 1997 one ounce of cocaine, when sold legally in the United States for medicinal purposes, cost about $80. When sold illegally, one ounce of cocaine cost up to $2,000 (DEA, 1998).

Cocaine vs. Amphetamines

Although all the physical and mental effects of cocaine are very similar to the effects of amphetamines, there are differences.

The Price. A heavy cocaine user spends $100 to $300 a day whereas a heavy amphetamine user spends about $50 to $100 a day.

Quality of the Rush or the High. When cocaine or an amphetamine is smoked or injected intravenously, it produces an intense rush followed by a high or euphoria. When either drug is snorted, the intense rush usually doesn't occur, only the euphoria. When an amphetamine or cocaine is drunk, again, there is usually no rush, only the euphoria. Although it is hard to demonstrate experimentally, the majority of users seen at the Haight-Ashbury Clinic claim that the rush and high from cocaine is much greater than that from amphetamine.

Duration of Action. Cocaine's major effects last about 40 minutes; an amphetamine's last 4–6 hours.

Manufacture. Cocaine is plant derived; amphetamines are synthetic.

Methods of Use. Amphetamines are smoked, injected intravenously, snorted, and ingested orally; cocaine is smoked, injected, snorted, applied topically, and occasionally drunk. The most popular ways of doing cocaine are snorting or smoking. Amphetamines are most often snorted or injected.

"Cocaine is more euphoric and not as intense as 'speed.' 'Speed' is very intense and you're going, going, going. The 'coke' is shorter lasting but the cravings are much worse. When I wanted to do 'speed,' it was mainly because I wanted to get things done. I felt 'speed' helped me perform. And the cocaine, I felt like I had absolutely no choice. Cocaine took me down real fast and real hard."
"Crack" cocaine smoker

OTHER PROBLEMS WITH COCAINE USE

Polydrug Use

One of the problems with cocaine is that the stimulation can be so intense that the user needs a downer to take the edge off or to get to sleep. The most common drugs used are alcohol, heroin, or a sedative-hypnotic such as clonazepam, though any downer will do in a pinch. Sometimes the second drug can be more of a problem than the cocaine.

"After the 'coke' would be gone, you'd be all wired up and you couldn't sleep, so I'd always have a little bit of heroin on the side and it'd bring me down. And I wouldn't be all jittery all night and grinding my teeth."
23-year-old recovering cocaine and heroin abuser

Adulteration

Before cocaine reaches the user, usually in powder, flake, or crystalline form, and usually in one-gram size, it is partially adulterated. The street dealer will add an adulterant to lower the purity from 80–90% down to approximately 60% often to pay for his or her own habit or just to make a few extra dollars. Adulteration of cocaine involves dilution with such diverse products as baby laxatives, lactose, vitamin B, aspirin, Mannitol®, sugar, Tetracaine® or Procaine® (topical anesthetics), even flour and talcum powder (Marnell, 1997). When the drug is used intravenously, not only are these diluents put into the bloodstream but so are bacteria and viruses from contaminated needles that can transmit diseases, including hepatitis B and C, blood and heart infections, and AIDS.

COMPULSION

Considering all the problems with cocaine—the expense, the adulteration, the illegality, the possibility of overdose, the physical and psychological dangers—two questions come to mind, "Why do people use cocaine?" and "Why do they use it so compulsively?"

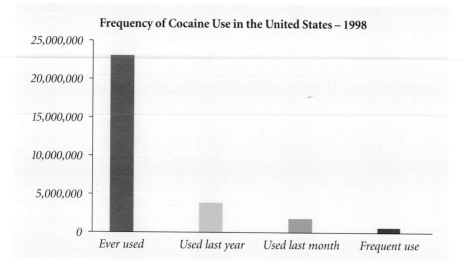

Figure 3-1 •

Of the 23 million Americans who have experimented with cocaine, 3.8 million used it in the past year, 1.7 million used it in the last month, and about 0.6 million used it frequently (51 or more days in the past year). Of these figure, about 1/4 smoke the drug ("crack").

National Household Survey, 1998 (SAMHSA, 1999)

"Most of my friends that I had, they used cocaine before I did and they kind of turned me on to it. We all started getting together and doing it. The sensation at first was like maybe going home and having sex with your old lady."

26-year-old recovering "crack" abuser

Why Do People Start Using Cocaine and Amphetamines?

◇ The drugs mimic pleasurable natural body functions: adrenal energy rush, confidence, euphoria, increased sensitivity, and stimulation of the reward/pleasure center.

◇ It is sometimes easier to get a chemical high instantly than a natural high over a period of time.

◇ People also use these drugs to combat boredom.

◇ People succumb to internal or external peer pressure.

◇ People are curious and the drugs are available.

◇ People use them as a means of alleviating or forgetting personal problems.

◇ Some people use the drugs to escape the effects of the poverty, hopelessness, and filth of their surroundings.

"Well, the first hit of freebase is always the best but you don't ever want to see the last hit. It's like, the more you do, the more you want. . . . I was always broke and I was always trying to find a way to get that high."

26-year-old recovering "crack" abuser

Why Are Cocaine and Amphetamines Used So Compulsively?

◇ Users want to recapture the initial rush (the energy surge and the stimulation of the reward/pleasure (satiation) center, which is extremely intense. Most find that it's hard to reproduce that initial rush but that doesn't stop them from trying.

◇ They want to avoid the crash that is inevitable after the intense high. In many cases a user will shoot up or smoke every 20 minutes, or in some cases, every 10 minutes in a binge episode.

◇ Users want to avoid life's problems such as difficult relationships, lack of confidence, traumatic events, a hated job, or loneliness.

◇ Users respond to the environmental cues that remind them of their drug use. Many seemingly innocuous sensory cues in the environment will trigger memories of smoking, snorting, or shooting and create an overwhelming desire to use again, e.g., seeing white powder, having money in one's pocket, or being in a place where drugs are used.

◇ People use in response to their hereditary predisposition to use. That is, certain people's natural neurotransmitter balance makes them react more intensely to a drug. They are, in essence, presensitized to the drug.

◇ Finally cocaine, in and of itself, changes the neurochemical balance and creates an intense craving that will cause someone to keep shooting, snorting, or smoking until every last microgram is gone, until he or she passes out, or until an overdose occurs.

This final reason for compulsive use of cocaine leads to bingeing, a very common pattern with cocaine. Even cocaine leaf chewing is often done in a binge pattern as noted by Johan von Tschudi, an early explorer of the Amazon Basin. In his 1854 book *Travels in Peru*, he wrote:

"They give themselves up for days together to the passionate enjoyment of the leaves . . . it, however, appears that it is not so much a want of sleep or the absence of food, as the want of coca that puts an end to the lengthened debauch."

(Von Tschudi, 1854)

SMOKABLE COCAINE ("crack," freebase)

"I couldn't bear to be sober. I needed to smoke 'crack' cocaine because smoking

'crack' cocaine takes away all your thoughts. You don't think about reality. You don't think about your bills, 'Oh, I have to pay this tomorrow.' You don't think about yourself. You don't think about nobody around you but 'crack' cocaine."

43-year-old female recovering "crack," heroin, methamphetamine addict

The smokable cocaine epidemic started around 1981, supported at first by after-hours cocaine-snorting clubs, then by freebase parlors, then by "crack houses" (1984), and finally by curbside use and distribution (Hamid, 1992). The words "crack cocaine" didn't appear in the media until 1985, tentatively at first, as if society was trying out a new nickname. By 1986 there seemed to be a "crack" epidemic that crossed all social and economic barriers. By the 1990s the "crack" epidemic had become ingrained in the American psyche as one of the main causes of society's ills: gang violence, AIDS, crime, and addiction. By 1991 the epidemic had begun to wane. By the beginning of the twenty-first century, a small core of "crack" abusers had become entrenched in society, mostly in lower-income groups.

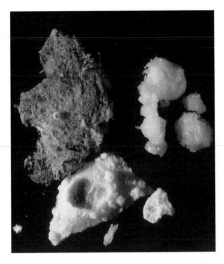

In this collection of "crack" cocaine samples, each "rock" is made in a slightly different manner. The various colors come from the impurities left after heating the mixture.

Some thought that the spread of "crack" to the office, factory, school yard, ghetto, and barrio was generated by media attention. Others thought that the basic properties of smokable cocaine were the cause of the epidemic. Others believed in the natural cycle of any drug epidemic, which seems to last 10–15 years whether it's amphetamine, cocaine, "crack," or heroin. The fact that the use of "crack" continues to be a severe problem despite vastly curtailed media coverage speaks to the addictive nature of smokable cocaine rather than to the influence of the media.

PHARMACOLOGY OF SMOKABLE COCAINE

Attempts to make cocaine smokable go back to the turn of the century but it wasn't until the early '70s when South American cocaine refiners and their workers realized you could smoke cocaine paste, the intermediate step in cocaine refinement, and not destroy its euphoric and stimulating effects. Chemically, cocaine paste is cocaine freebase. The off-white doughy substance contains chemicals such as kerosene, sulfuric acid, and sodium carbonate. It is usually smoked with tobacco or marijuana by the middle- and lower-income classes. When smoked in a marijuana joint, it is called "bazooko" or "basuco." In a study of 158 "pasta" smokers in Lima, Peru, the effects were similar to snorted cocaine but more intense.

"After a few minutes of intense enjoyment, they developed anxiety and vehement wishes to continue smoking, leading to repeated or chain smoking. When they run out of 'paste,' they try to obtain or buy more in a state of compulsive anxiety. The user does not sleep, has no appetite, and his/her only wish is to continue smoking. 'Paste' reaction is so intense that most users, after a few minutes, experience disagreeable sensations (anxiety, compulsions, insomnia, sexual impotency, disquiet, instability, aggressiveness, headaches, and dizziness). Some

patients from the very first puffs experience perceptual disturbances (visual hallucinations)."
(Jeri et al., 1992)

In 1976 in the United States, some clever street chemists found a cleaner way to make cocaine suitable for smoking. The method they developed was called "freebasing" ("basing," "baseballing"). It involves dissolving cocaine hydrochloride in an alkali solution and heating it to create cocaine freebase. After the solution is cooled, ether is added to separate the now fat-soluble freebase from the adulterants in the original cocaine hydrochloride. When the ether/cocaine mixture is separated and evaporated, it leaves behind pure cocaine freebase crystals. Unfortunately the flammability of the ether has caused a number of burn accidents.

Another simpler technique called "cheap basing" or "dirty basing" was developed in the early '80s. It does not remove as many impurities or residues as the freebasing technique, so impurities such as talcum powder and especially baking soda remain. The lumps of smokable cocaine made by this method are usually called "crack" or "fry" because of the crackling sound caused when smoked, or "rock" because the product looks like little rocks.

The converted freebase cocaine, made by either the "basing" method or the "crack" method, has four chemical properties sought by users.

◇ It has a lower melting point than the powdered form (98°C vs. 195°C) so it can be heated easily in a glass pipe and vaporized to form smoke at a lower temperature. Too high a temperature destroys most of the psychoactive properties of the drug.

◇ Since it enters the system directly through the lungs, smokable cocaine reaches the brain faster than when cocaine hydrochloride is snorted.

◇ Freebase cocaine is more fat-soluble than cocaine hydrochloride and so is more readily absorbed by fat cells of the brain, thus causing a more intense reaction.

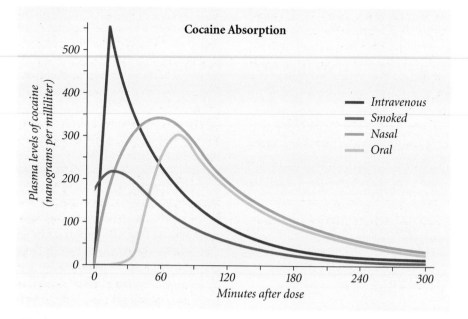

Cocaine Absorption

Plasma levels of cocaine (nanograms per milliliter)

- Intravenous
- Smoked
- Nasal
- Oral

Minutes after dose

Figure 3-2 •

This graph shows the plasma levels of cocaine after equivalent doses were taken through different methods. While smoking gets cocaine to the brain slightly more rapidly than IV use, injection puts a larger amount into the system at one time. When coca leaves are chewed, peak blood plasma levels are about 1/4 to 1/8 of the levels obtained by smoking.

NIDA Research Monograph 99, Research Findings on Smoking of Abused Substances

◊ Users are also able to get a much higher dose of cocaine in their systems at one time because the very large surface area in the lungs (about the size of a football field) can absorb the drug almost instantaneously.

Depending on the way it is synthesized, smokable cocaine has been called "paste," "pasta," freebase, "base," "basay," "crack," "rock," "hubba," "gravel," "Roxanne," "girl," "fry," and "boulya." There is a frequent misperception that "crack" and freebase are different drugs than cocaine. They aren't. They are just different chemical forms of cocaine that make them smokable.

"You get heat energy, heat flashes that go all through your body. You get these pins and needles, depending on the cut, of course."

"Crack" cocaine smoker

EFFECTS & SIDE EFFECTS

The effects of smoking "crack," are almost exactly the same as snorting or injecting cocaine but since smoking cocaine reaches the brain more quickly, the effects and side effects seem more intense. Unfortunately for the "crack" smoker, much of the cocaine is lost to the air; about 50% when smoked in a cigarette and about 75% when smoked in a glass pipe (Siegel, 1992). For this reason much more cocaine has to be smoked than injected. Smoking or using the drug intravenously can produce similar blood levels of cocaine but it is necessary (and easier) to smoke "crack" again and again. All of an injected bolus of cocaine reaches the blood (although some is lost through metabolism before it reaches the brain).

"The feeling that I had on 'crack' cocaine is entirely different than any other drug I have tried. It was that 'crack' cocaine gives you this high where you just seem like there's no worry in the world whereas with heroin and 'speed,' I worried about where my next 'hit' was going to come from."

42-year-old recovering "crack" smoker

Smoking gives a rush, subsequent euphoria, excitation, and arousal that lasts for several minutes. After 5–20 minutes, these feelings are replaced by irritability, dysphoria (general feeling of unease), and anxiety. These feelings lead the user to smoke again. Thus cocaine is almost always used in a binge pattern whether smoked, injected, or even snorted. The user never stops until every last speck is gone.

Acute physical side effects include slurred speech, thirst, coughing, anorexia, dry hands, blurred vision, attention difficulties, and tremors. Chronic use can cause chest pains, sore throat, black or bloody sputum, hypertension, weight loss, insomnia, tremors, and heart damage. Psychological effects of chronic use include cocaine psychosis, paranoia, visual hallucinations, craving, asocial behavior, attention problems, irritability, drug dreams, hyperexcitability, loss of impulse control, auditory hallucinations, lethargy, depression, and social problems (Siegel, 1992).

Some of the more unusual side effects include

◊ **"crack" keratitis** that is abrasions of the eye due to the anesthetic effects of cocaine that make the user unaware of damage caused by rubbing the eye too much;

◊ **"crack" thumb** and **"crack" hands** that are caused by repetitive use of butane lighters to heat up "crack" pipes. A callus builds up on the thumb and the hand has multiple burns;

◊ **"crack" burns** that are superficial burns to the face and hands due to the use of small torches to melt freebase in a short glass pipe. More severe body burns result when the ether explodes during the process.

Respiratory Effects

"I had a lot of coughing after using it and shortness of breath. I didn't really notice it at the time but if I went out to ride my bike or lift weights, I would have a really hard time."

17-year-old male recovering "crack" smoker

Because a user inhales an extremely harsh substance, smoking cocaine can also cause breathing problems, severe chest pains, pneumonia, coughs, fever, and other respiratory complications, including hemorrhage, respiratory failure, and death. "Crack" lung, a relatively new syndrome, describes the pain, breathing problems, and fever that resemble pneumonia (Gold & Miller, 1997). Many "crack" smokers smoke the tar-like black residue in "crack" pipes and overload their lungs with this residue that makes it difficult for the normal clearance mechanisms of the lungs to function, resulting in black or dark brown sputum (Greenbaum, 1993).

Polydrug Abuse

As with snorted and injected cocaine, the intensive use of freebase increases the potential for the abuse of other drugs, especially alcohol, heroin, and sedative-hypnotics. Some smokers combine freebase and marijuana in a combination called "champagne," "caviar," "gremmies," "fry daddies," "cocoa puff," "hubba," or "woolies." In addition users are even mixing PCP with "crack" in a nasty mixture called "space basing," "whack," or "tragic magic." Further there is the addition of freebase cocaine to smokable tar heroin to make a smokable "speedball" called "hot rocks" or "chocolate rocks." Finally, "crack" or cocaine hydrochloride is being used with wine coolers for an oral "speedball" known as "crack coolers." When "crack" is not available, users have switched to shooting and even smoking methamphetamine ("speed"). A mixture of "crank" with "crack" smoked together has also appeared recently and is called "super crank."

Overdose

The most frequent type of overdose that people experience when smoking cocaine is on the mild side: very rapid heartbeat and hyperventilation. However, these reactions are often accompanied by a feeling of impending death. Although most people survive and only get very sweaty and clammy and feel

that they are going to die, several thousand, in fact, are killed by cocaine overdose every year. The deaths result from cardiac arrest, seizure, stroke, respiratory failure, and even severe hyperthermia (extra-high body temperature).

"A friend was freebasing heavily and he started going into convulsions and throwing up blood. It was real awful. I was really scared and I thought he was going to die. Me and my other friend, we just kept freebasing . . . and then when he came out of it, he started freebasing again."
Recovering 16-year-old girl

REASONS FOR THE WIDESPREAD USE OF "CRACK"

Besides the reasons already mentioned for compulsive use of cocaine, such as the search for the first intense rush or avoidance of the downside, there are several other reasons for the compulsive smoking of cocaine. First, smoking does not seem as dangerous as using a contaminated needle. Unfortunately while avoiding needles would remove one source of infection, lowered inhibitions, bartering sex for drugs, and careless high-risk sexual activities lead to higher rates of sexually transmitted diseases, including AIDS and hepatitis B or C. Further, transmission of hepatitis C has been linked to the sharing of the same straw to snort cocaine. Next, smoking a drug is more socially acceptable than injecting it because cigarette, pipe, and cigar smoking are legal and part of our culture.

CONSEQUENCES OF "CRACK" USE

Economic Consequences

The economics of "crack" cocaine have expanded the potential number of users especially among teenagers. The reason is in the packaging. "Crack" is not cheaper than cocaine hydrochloride; it is just sold in smaller units. One gram of cocaine hydrochloride is the standard street sale amount going for

about $60 to $100. Now 1/20 of a gram that has been converted to "crack" or "rock" can be bought for $10 to $20, a manageable sum for teenagers and incidentally about twice the price of cocaine hydrochloride when figured on a per gram basis.

The economics of "crack" cocaine have also created more dealers and these people have a vested interest in keeping users using. Several housing projects in the inner city have become havens for "crack" houses and dealers. A few young dealers are buying new cars and showing off their wealth but the majority of the small-time dealers make just enough to support their own habit or get by. Drug gang homicides are common as local gangs, along with gangs from other countries such as Jamaica, Mexico, and Colombia, control the trade (Dunlop & Johnson, 1992).

"I know it's jive, I know it's negative. I'm trapped in something here. But, I'm used to the money. What else can I do? You gonna send me to McDonalds? After I'm generating this kind of money everyday, I can't go back to McDonalds for $6.50—what is it?—$6.75 an hour today, which is still insulting."
16-year-old "crack" dealer/user

The "crack" trade expanded rapidly in the late 1980s because the dealers used the best sales strategies of a free enterprise system: reduce the price to increase sales; increase the size of the sales force to cover the territory more efficiently; encourage free trade to avoid tariffs and impounding; and create appealing packaging to make the product attractive to a wider segment of the population (Wesson, Smith, & Steffens, 1992).

Social Consequences

"It seems like every time I would hit the pipe, my daughter would say, 'Mommy.' And so I would say, 'Why are you bothering me?' It really made me crazy. I mean, my son, he would

just pick on things and make noise or something just to bother me because he knew that I was doing this."

Recovering "crack" user

Because of the compulsive nature of "crack," addictive "crack" use in the United States had and is still having devastating social ramifications that include the single or even no-parent family, the burned-out grandmother caring for her "crack"-addicted daughter's children, increased rates of abandonment, neglect, and abuse of children, and the formation of an underclass of women who trade sex for "crack." A major impact of "crack" has been a lowering of the price of sex for street prostitutes (Goldstein, Ouellet, & Fendrick, 1992).

"I was selling dope and had three or four thousand dollars a week. I had women coming to me. I never tossed a woman in my life. Those women were coming after me. I mean, you've got to look at both sides of it."

38-year-old male ex-"crack" dealer

"It's two types of women using cocaine. One's a 'tossup' [a woman who trades sex for 'crack']. They're the ones who are down there. They done lost everything they have. They have no self-respect. Me and my sister, we'd work a brother in a minute to get his dope. Once we got his dope— 'Go on, get outta my house.' Me and my sister, we paid our rent, we paid our utilities. We fed our children. We kept clothes on their backs. We kept the house clean. We had not lost our self-esteem. We had not hit rock bottom yet."

24-year-old female recovering "crack" user

In a study of 283 women who exchanged sex for money or "crack," 30% were infected with HIV (Edlin, Irwin, & Faruque, 1994). For many men (particularly in some inner-city African American communities), a major im-

pact on their families and society has occurred because of the high rate of crime associated with "crack" use. There have been high rates of imprisonment, violent deaths, and child abandonment by addicts. In fact about 75% of all inmates in prisons come from single-parent or no-parent homes (Federal Bureau of Prisons, 1997).

Loss

Most drug use is about loss and if one talks to drug users, "crack" cocaine use leads to greater loss than any other drug.

"Well, 'crack' is a drug that is so addictive that it takes your money, your furniture, your home, your car, your clothes.... And then you have to go to places where they feed homeless. And it just takes everything. And when I was on heroin and 'speed,' I had money. I

kept money. I had an apartment. I paid my rent. But the 'crack' cocaine drug was the most awful, the most terrifying drug that I ever experienced."

42-year-old recovering polydrug abuser

✳ AMPHETAMINES ✳

CLASSIFICATION

Amphetamines, known variously as "uppers," "speed," "meth," methamphetamines, "crank," "crystal," "ice," "shabu," and "glass," are a class of powerful synthetic stimulants with effects very similar to cocaine but much longer lasting and cheaper to use. Amphetamines are most often taken orally, injected, or snorted. Recently, smoking methamphetamine has increased in popularity especially with the newer form of methamphetamine, "ice."

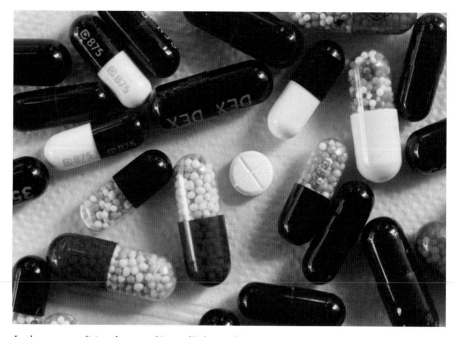

In the past, traditional types of "speed" diverted to street use or manufactured illegally were small tablets of amphetamine or methamphetamine ("crosstops," "whites") originally made in Mexico; Biphetamines® ("black beauties"), a combination of several amphetamine compounds; Dexedrine® ("dexys," "beans"), a dextroamphetamine tablet; Benzedrine® ("bennies"), one of the classic "stay awake" amphetamine pills; and Methadrine® (or Ambar®), a methamphetamine.

Courtesy of the Drug Enforcement Administration Laboratory, San Francisco

There are several different types of amphetamines: amphetamine, methamphetamine, dextroamphetamine, and dextro isomer methamphetamine base. The effects of each type are almost indistinguishable, the major differences being their method of manufacture and their strength.

HISTORY OF USE

Discovery

Amphetamine was synthesized in 1887 in a systematic effort to synthesize ephedrine, a natural extract of the ephedra bush, used for asthma. Interestingly the stimulant qualities and medical applications weren't recognized until the 1930s when Methedrine® (methamphetamine) and Benzedrine® (dextroamphetamine) inhalers were marketed as bronchodilators to help asthmatics breathe. Benzedrine® and Methedrine® were also discovered to be stimulants that could energize the user, counter low blood pressure, reduce the need for sleep, and suppress appetite. The drugs were also used to treat MBD or minimal brain dysfunction, which is what attention deficit/hyperactivity disorder (AD/HD) is called nowadays. The inhalers were sold over the counter until 1959 and prescription Methedrine® wasn't taken off the market until 1968.

Amphetamines were also widely used in pill form during World War II by Allied, German, and Japanese forces to keep pilots alert for extended missions and to keep ground troops awake and somewhat more aggressive in battle. An estimated 200 million Benzedrine® tablets were legally dispensed to U.S. GIs during World War II and another 225 million during the Vietnam conflict between 1966 and 1969 (Miller & Kozel, 1995). Abuse of amphetamines continued in Japan after World War II but the enactment of Japan's Stimulant Drug Program in 1951 brought the problem under control (Fukui, Wada, & Iyo, 1991).

Amphetamines were also used to treat narcolepsy (sleeping sickness), obesity, epilepsy (a subtype), and depression. Concurrently amphetamines came to be abused by students cramming for exams, truckers on long hauls, workers laboring long hours, and soldiers or pilots trying to stay awake for 48 hours straight.

Diet Pills

Pharmaceutical companies in the 1950s and 1960s promoted the hunger-suppressing and mood-elevating qualities of amphetamines. Their advertising led to huge quantities of amphetamines, including Dexedrine® and Dexamyl®, flooding the prescription drug market. Worldwide legal production in 1970 was estimated to be 10 billion tablets (Karch, 1996). In 1970 it is estimated that six percent to eight percent of the American population were using prescription amphetamines mostly for weight loss (Ellinwood, 1973).

"Well, I almost never ate. And when I ate, I ate sugar, colas, cakes, and that was all I ate. I mean, once in a while I'd go to a steak house and treat myself to a fabulous $7.59 steak dinner. I weighed probably 90 pounds and I was anemic and weak but I always felt up and energized because I was always shooting 'speed.'"
38-year-old "speed" user

Street "Speed"

The 1960s were the peak of the "speed" craze that was supplied by both diverted and illegally manufactured amphetamines. The energy for the "Summer of Love," one of the cornerstones of the hippie movement, was fueled by the energy chemicals released by amphetamines as well as by plentiful marijuana and LSD. In a reaction to the "speed" epidemic, the Controlled Substance Act of 1970 classified amphetamines as schedule II drugs and made it hard to buy them legally in the United States. In addition prescription use of the drugs was more tightly regulated. The street market expanded to fill the need, so instead of buying legally manufactured amphetamines that had been diverted, people bought "speed" and "crank" that had been manufactured illegally. The purity rose from an average of 30% in the early '70s to 60% by 1983 (King & Ellinwood, 1997).

"I very seldom ran out in the beginning in the '60s and '70s. It was cheap; people gave it away. It wasn't like using dope. You didn't have to get money together every day."
38-year-old female "speed" user

The most popular form of street "speed" was the "crosstop." Also called "cartwheels" and "white crosses," these were diverted and smuggled into the United States from Mexico. In the early 1970s they cost $5 to $10 per 100 tablets. In the '90s, the price was $1 to $5 per tablet if they could be found. As of 1999 what are most often available are bogus (lookalike) "crosstops" that contain either caffeine or ephedrine instead of amphetamines.

The late 1980s and 1990s saw a resurgence in the availability and abuse of illicit amphetamines, particularly "crank" (methamphetamine sulfate) and "crystal" (methamphetamine hydrochloride—not to be confused with "krystal" which is PCP). Once stymied by the tight control of chemicals needed to produce illegal amphetamines, clever street chemists learned to alter commonly available compounds to produce "speed" products. However, some of the street "meth" was lookalike drugs, including phenylpropanolamine (a decongestant), ephedrine, pseudoephedrine, or simply caffeine tablets disguised to look like amphetamine products.

"Ice"

As the 1990s began, a new, highly potent, and smokable form of methamphetamine, dextro isomer methamphetamine base ("ice," "glass," "batu," or "shabu") had taken center stage, at least in the press. Besides its smokability, greater strength, and longer duration of effects, "ice" had the appeal of a new fad. As with the spread of smokable "crack" cocaine, "ice" was ini-

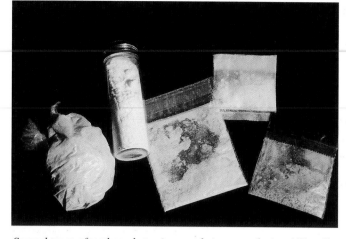

Several types of methamphetamines are being manufactured illegally including "peanut butter meth" on the left.
Courtesy of Lt. Ed Mayer and JACNET, Jackson County, Oregon

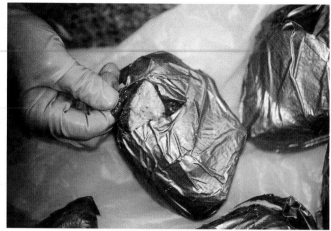

Methamphetamines produced in the United States are smuggled between different states. The "meth" is wrapped in red chili peppers to confuse the smell of drug-sniffing dogs.
Courtesy of Michael Basketti

tially being marketed as a "newer better amphetamine." It cost two to three times as much as "meth" which is surprising because it can be made with a very simple and safe crystallization process.

Surprisingly, perhaps because it is so intense, "ice" did not catch on in the United States as a common drug of abuse except in Hawaii and a few places on the West Coast. However, some Asian countries have a severe "ice" problem. The Philippines was estimated to have 400,000 "shabu" addicts in 1992. The average daily dose was from one to three grams at a cost of $10 to $20 per gram (Wesson, 1992).

Current Use

Licit Use. Amphetamines and methamphetamines are used to treat attention deficit/hyperactivity disorder, narcolepsy, a type of epilepsy, and occasionally for weight control.

Illicit Use. The resurgence in the use of illicit methamphetamines, predominantly "crank" and "crystal meth," occurred during the 1990s. This new "speed" epidemic has been signaled by a dramatic increase in the number of "meth" labs raided by the authorities, particularly in California, Oregon,

Texas, and more recently in the Midwest. While amphetamine use in 1998 was only about 1/2 the peak level of the early 1980s (SAMHSA, 1999), the current growth is troublesome. At a number of treatment centers, many of those coming in for care named "meth" as their primary drug of choice and cause of addiction. An additional worry is that the age of first use has dropped. Some 10–13 year olds are smoking, eating, and snorting "crank." In some high schools "crank," rather than marijuana, is the drug of choice. Some of the reasons for this upsurge are lower prices, increased availability, and current drug fads.

"I started shooting 'speed' and I couldn't keep getting $20 bucks from my mom, you know. I had to either start selling it or start stealing stuff 'cause I had a big habit. So I was stealing cars and I was jacking stereos and I would rip anybody off who gave me money just to get myself high. Incidentally, stealing the car was also a high."
17-year-old recovering IV methamphetamine user

The profile of the typical user is a white male between the ages of 19 and 40. Recently there has been increased

use among women. Historically stimulant epidemics last about 10–15 years and go in waves from one coast of the United States to the other. "Meth" use is sweeping towards the eastern and southern United States. Eventually the intensity of the high and the severity of the side effects of amphetamine abuse become self-limiting and the rapid growth of use levels out.

"Meth" Manufacture

Over the years, much of the street manufacture and dealing of methamphetamines had been taken over by biker gangs (Hell's Angels and Gypsy Jokers) because of the money involved and the partiality of bikers to the drug. But there has been an ever increasing involvement of Mexican gangs in the manufacture and distribution of the drug.

Historically labs made methamphetamines with the P2P method (total synthesis) or by reduction of ephedrine or pseudoephedrine. In raided laboratories, only three percent still used the P_2P method. One of the reasons for the resurgence in the use of methamphetamine is new, somewhat safer, cheaper, and almost odor-free manufacturing techniques (Marnell, 1997). Illicit methamphetamine manufacturing used to be an extremely risky business. The fumes were toxic and explosions could and did occur if the chemicals were handled improperly. Foul odors that emanated from the "cookers" were of great help to law enforcement agencies in locating "meth" labs. Now methamphetamine can even be manufactured on a stove top. The DEA estimates that there are over 300 ways to manufacture methamphetamine (DEA, 1998). It is still risky, particularly for amateurs, but not as risky as before. This increase in the number of street chemists means that it is hard to halt the supply and difficult for users to know what they are getting until they snort it or shoot it into a vein.

Since ephedrine, the principle chemical used in illicit methamphetamine manufacture, is a controlled substance in the United States, it is often smuggled to Mexico from China (where ephedra is extracted from the ephedra bush) or from Germany, where it is synthesized. A small portion is converted to methamphetamine in Mexico but the majority is smuggled into the United States (mainly central and southern California) and then converted to "meth." When ephedrine is not available, pseudoephedrine (found in many OTC cold tablets and medicines) can be used. The other substances used in the manufacture, particularly hydriodic

acid, are also smuggled into the United States from Canada, diverted from legal suppliers, or manufactured illegally.

A record number of 892 "meth" labs were raided in California in 1996 compared to 419 in 1994. The growth of "meth" use and manufacture in the Midwest was emphasized by the 235 labs that were raided just in Missouri. "Meth" cases account for 80% of domestic violence cases and police department drug investigations (DEA, 1998). In 1997 a pound of "meth" bought for $5,000 in California sold for as much as $16,000 in Iowa. Most of the laboratories were small enterprises capable of producing only a pound or so of methamphetamine a day but those run by Mexican gangs (26% of the total and mostly in the West) could cook 10–150 pounds in just two days. The DEA estimates that the Mexican-run labs manufacture 3/4 of the "meth" consumed in the United States. A pound of "meth" wholesales for $4,000 to $20,000, an ounce for $500 to $2,700, and a gram for $40 to $200 (NIDA, 1998).

One other problem with the illegal synthesis of "meth" is the environmental danger of the chemicals used in the process, even with the newer manufacturing methods. Toxins and cancer-causing agents, such as acetone, red

phosphorus, hydrochloric acid, benzene, toluene, sulfuric acid, and lead acetate, are left behind or secretly dumped into streams and landfills. It costs thousands of dollars to clean up each raided laboratory and is dangerous to the health of those doing the cleaning.

EFFECTS

Routes of Administration

Currently, injecting and snorting "meth" are the most popular methods of use although it is also ingested and smoked. Snorting "meth" causes irritation and pain to the nasal mucosa. Intravenous use does put large quantities of the drug directly into the bloodstream and causes a more intense high than snorting or swallowing; however it often causes pain in the blood vessels. Also, with injecting, there is the attendant risk of contaminated needles. Oral ingestion used to be more popular but takes longer to reach the brain and because of the extremely bitter taste of methamphetamines, they are often put into a gelatin capsule or in a piece of paper when taken orally.

"Smoking methamphetamine gives you a good rush. I mean, it's a lot better than snorting it as far as the rush

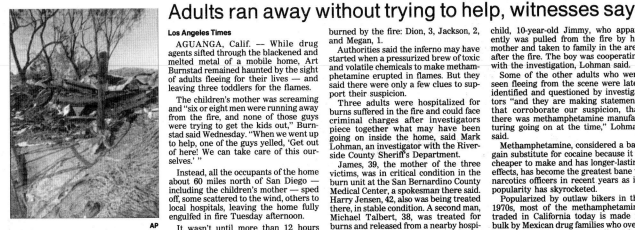

Three toddlers die in meth lab blaze

Adults ran away without trying to help, witnesses say

Los Angeles Times

AGUANGA, Calif. — While drug agents sifted through the blackened and melted metal of a mobile home, Art Burnstad remained haunted by the sight of adults fleeing for their lives — and leaving three toddlers for the flames.

The children's mother was screaming and "six or eight men were running away from the fire, and none of those guys were trying to get the kids out," Burnstad said Wednesday. "When we went up to help, one of the guys yelled, 'Get out of here! We can take care of this ourselves.' "

Instead, all the occupants of the home about 60 miles north of San Diego — including the children's mother — sped off, some scattered to the wind, others to local hospitals, leaving the home fully engulfed in fire Tuesday afternoon.

It wasn't until more than 12 hours later that the bodies of three children were recovered, too burned to recognize. The Riverside County coroner's office tentatively identified them as the chil-

burned by the fire: Dion, 3, Jackson, 2, and Megan, 1.

Authorities said the inferno may have started when a pressurized brew of toxic and volatile chemicals to make methamphetamine erupted in flames. But they said there were only a few clues to support their suspicion.

Three adults were hospitalized for burns suffered in the fire and could face criminal charges after investigators piece together what may have been going on inside the home, said Mark Lohman, an investigator with the Riverside County Sheriff's Department.

James, 39, the mother of the three victims, was in critical condition in the burn unit at the San Bernardino County Medical Center, a spokesman there said. Harry Jensen, 42, also was being treated there, in stable condition. A second man, Michael Talbert, 38, was treated for burns and released from a nearby hospital.

None of the three has been arrested because the investigation is in its earliest stages, Lohman said. He said investiga-

child, 10-year-old Jimmy, who apparently was pulled from the fire by his mother and taken to family in the area after the fire. The boy was cooperating with the investigation, Lohman said.

Some of the other adults who were seen fleeing from the scene were later identified and questioned by investigators "and they are making statements that corroborate our suspicion, that there was methamphetamine manufacturing going on at the time," Lohman said.

Methamphetamine, considered a bargain substitute for cocaine because it is cheaper to make and has longer-lasting effects, has become the greatest bane to narcotics officers in recent years as its popularity has skyrocketed.

Popularized by outlaw bikers in the 1970s, most of the methamphetamine traded in California today is made in bulk by Mexican drug families who oversee teams of cookers who are dispatched to remote locations throughout the state. They confound law enforcement by making large batches of meth, literally over-

AP

DESTROYED — This is all that remains of a mobile home where three children burned to death in

goes. You breathe out and you feel that feeling. It's kind of like shooting but it's different. It's more mellow and it's a shorter high."

Intravenous "meth" user

Because of the dangers in shooting or snorting "meth," some users have taken to smoking "crank," "crystal," or "ice," a potentially more appealing method of use than snorting or injecting. The technique of smoking "crank" or "ice" is similar to smoking freebase cocaine (in a pipe). Smoking gets the drug to the brain faster. No matter how the drug is taken, amphetamines last 4–6 hours compared to only 40 minutes to 1 1/2 hours for cocaine. "Ice," the newest form of methamphetamine, is alleged to last at least 8 hours, some say up to 24 hours, after it is smoked.

Neurochemistry

Amphetamines increase the levels of catecholamines (epinephrine, norepinephrine, and dopamine) in three ways as opposed to cocaine which increases the levels in two ways. Amphetamines and cocaine stimulate the release of catecholamines and they block their reuptake in the sending neuron but only amphetamines block their metabolism. This means that the excess catecholamines exist for a much longer time than cocaine in the synapse, thereby prolonging the effects.

Long-term use of amphetamines causes permanent alterations in the ability of the body to produce these vital neurotransmitters. In animal studies norepinephrine levels were depressed 3–6 months after cessation of use (King & Ellinwood, 1997). Dopamine levels also remained depressed after cessation of use. This means that the user comes to rely on artificial stimulants to keep their dopamine and norepinephrine levels normal, let alone raised. This mechanism is one of the reasons that amphetamines and cocaine generate such compulsive use. The mechanisms will recover somewhat over a long period of time but the imbalance often triggers relapse before that time comes.

In other words **prolonged amphet-**

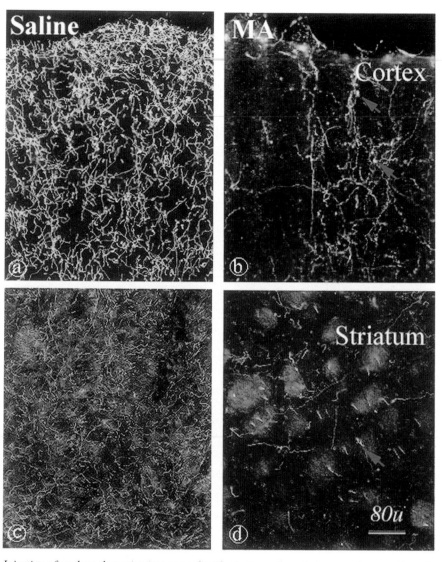

Injection of methamphetamine into normal rat brain tissue (a and c) causes degeneration of serotonin nerve fibers 5-HTT (b and d). Fibers were reduced in a number of regions in the brain, including the frontal and parietal cortices (a and b), hippocampus, striatum (c and d), and thalamus (Zhou & Bledsoe, 1996).

amine use, in and of itself, alters brain chemistry in a way that increases craving. This is also true of cocaine.

In addition to depleting neurotransmitters, researchers in 1996 demonstrated that high-dose methamphetamine use caused definitive degeneration of serotonin fibers in the brain within hours after use (Zhou & Bledsoe, 1996).

Physical Effects

As with cocaine, the initial physiological effects of small to moderate doses of amphetamines include increased heart rate, raised body temperature, rapid respiration, higher blood pressure, extra energy, dilation of bronchial vessels, and appetite suppression.

"I would inject some 'speed' and right after doing it, you get an incredible rush, which some people compare with sexual feelings. And your heart pounds and I've seen people actually pass out from having too much 'speed.' My heart would pound, and I would sweat, and the rush would pass, and then I would just be very high energy."

19-year-old recovering "meth" user.

As with cocaine users, methamphetamine abusers go on binges or "runs," staying up for 3, 4, or even up to 10 days at a time, putting a severe strain on their bodies, particularly the cardiovascular and nervous systems. During these runs, people will try to use their excess energy any way they can—dancing, exercising, cleaning the kitchen at midnight, taking apart a car, or painting the whole house.

"I liked to do little intricate drawings. I would draw for hours; anything small with a lot of detail. I would clean my apartment from top to bottom, even doing my floor with Brillo® pads—my wooden floor—vacuuming my ceiling. If I ran out of stuff to do, I would dump out everything in the vacuum cleaner and vacuum it back up. I didn't like to be outside because I would get paranoid."
38-year-old recovering amphetamine user

Tolerance to amphetamines is pronounced. Whereas 15–30 milligrams per day is the usual prescribed dose, a long-term user might use 5,000 milligrams over a 24–hour period during a "speed run." This means that extended use (or the use of large quantities) will lead to extreme depression and lethargy.

"If I didn't have 'speed,' if I ran out, I would become depressed, very anxiety-ridden. I had suicidal thoughts and I would sleep for long stretches of time 'till I had more 'speed.' And then I would start the whole process over again."
33-year-old recovering "speed" user

Long-term use can cause sleep deprivation, heart and blood vessel toxicity, and severe malnutrition. The blood vessel toxicity can cause extensive damage to cerebral vasculature resulting in multiple aneurysms (the ballooning out of capillary weak spots). With long-term use and hypertensive episodes, the user experiences cerebral hemorrhages (strokes) and arrhyth-

mias, possibly caused by myocardial (heart muscle) lesions (King, 1997). The malnutrition, plus the calcium-leaching effects of amphetamine overuse, often results in bad or rotted teeth. In fact one of the confirming signs of amphetamine abuse is poor dental health.

Finally, if the user has not built up a tolerance, is unusually sensitive, or takes a very large amount, an overdose can occur (convulsions, hyperthermia, stroke, and cardiovascular overexcitation and collapse).

"I shot some 'speed' once and immediately had a seizure. Apparently my heart stopped beating and the person I was with was pounding on my chest. I was real sore and black and blue the next day."
38-year-old methamphetamine user

Mental & Emotional Effects

Amphetamines initially produce a mild to intense euphoria and a feeling of well-being very similar to a cocaine high. But with prolonged use, the unbalanced neurotransmitters (dopamine and norepinephrine) can also induce irritability, paranoia, anxiety, mental confusion, poor judgment, and even hallucinations.

Much like cocaine, amphetamines release neurotransmitters that mimic sexual gratification. Thus they are sometimes used by those who are sexually active and prone toward multiple partners and/or prolonged sexual activity. The drug has also been heavily used in gay populations for sexual endurance. But again, because of the rapid development of tolerance, there is an eventual decrease of sex drive and performance. For many users the rush from shooting or smoking "meth" or "ice" becomes a substitute for sexual activity.

Aggression caused by excessive amphetamine use depends on the dose, the setting, and the preexisting susceptibility to aggression and violence in the user. The increased suspiciousness, paranoia, and overconfidence lead to misinterpretations of others' actions

and hence to violent reactions to perceived threats. Taken to extremes prolonged use can result in violent, suicidal, and even homicidal thoughts. Conversely, in those with hyperactivity disorder, amphetamines can control aggression (King & Ellinwood, 1997).

Excessive amphetamine use can cause amphetamine psychosis, including hallucinations, loss of contact with reality, and pressed speech that is almost indistinguishable from true schizophrenia or paranoid psychosis. It is speculated that the psychosis is caused by excess dopamine activity.

This amphetamine psychosis and listless depression (more common with withdrawal from high-dose intravenous use or heavy smoking of "ice") are usually not permanent although recent research may indicate that the depression may be permanent in some users (Zhou & Bledsoe, 1996).

"I just got so sick of it, you know, just being high for so long. It just messes up your mind. I once stayed up for 23 days with no sleep—not one hour of sleep, not one wink of sleep. When you stay up for that long, you're just like a pile of mush. Your brain's just nothing, you know. You can't even talk. And it just doesn't even feel good. I don't want that feeling anymore."
17-year-old recovering "meth" abuser

Upon cessation of use, the disturbed user will usually return to some semblance of normality after the brain chemistry has been rebalanced, usually within a week. If there was a preexisting mental condition, recovery can take a lot longer. Since extended use can also damage nerve cells, a number of the changes in long-term users, even without pre-existing mental problems, can last a lifetime (Richards, Baggot, Sabol, & Seiden, 1999).

Much of the current interest in "crank," "crystal," and "ice" abuse is concentrated among adolescents and older teenagers, particularly among Asian American and Caucasian American youth. There is also a significant abuse of amphetamines by biker gangs and by gay and lesbian subcultures. Recently there has been an increasing abuse of these drugs in the Hispanic community. One of the reasons for the popularity of the drug is that initially amphetamines induce qualities which we try to teach to young people—alertness, motivation, self-confidence, socialization, excitement, and the ability to work long hours. Unfortunately with drug use, these desirable qualities quickly give way to the opposite effects, including depression, paranoia, and antisocial behavior, among others.

In addition the ability of amphetamines to suppress appetite is one of the main reasons for their current popularity. The projection of an ideal thin body in advertisements helps promote current abuse, much as it did in the '60s and '70s before government regulations limited the legal supply of the drug.

Effects of "Ice"

"Ice" is smokable dextro isomer methamphetamine base. This form of methamphetamine stimulates the brain to a greater degree than the regular methamphetamine but stimulates the heart, blood vessels, and lungs to a lesser degree. The decrease in cardiovascular effects (up to 25% less than that of regular "crank") encourages users to smoke more, resulting in more overdoses and a quicker disruption of neurotransmitters. This disruption means more "tweaking" or severe paranoid, hallucinatory, and hypervigilant thinking, along with greater suicidal depression and addictive use. Detoxification from mental and psychotic symptoms of excessive "ice" use usually takes several days longer than detoxifying from regular methamphetamine abuse.

Right-Handed & Left-Handed Molecules. Manufacturing of "ice" by street chemists represented a significant increase in the sophistication of these illegal laboratories in the United States. "Ice," known pharmacologically as dextro isomer methamphetamine base, is a specific and subtle form of the methamphetamine molecule known to scientists as an optical isomer. When such a molecule is being formed, nature creates mirror images of atomic bonds such that half of the molecules formed are "right-handed" isomers and the other half are "left-handed" isomers (Fig. 3-3).

The amazing feature of this situation is that the two individual isomers often have very different effects on the body. **Dextro** isomer methamphetamine (right-handed) molecule is two to four times stronger in stimulating the brain than the **levo** methamphetamine isomer (left-handed). However, the levo isomer is two to four times stronger in stimulating the heart, blood vessels, and nasal sinuses than the dextro isomer. By the late 1980s street chemists learned that if they used pure left-handed pseudoephedrine to make methamphetamine, it would be trans-

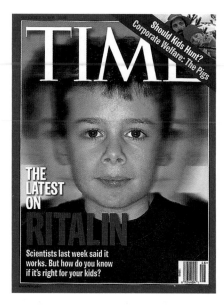

formed to pure right-handed or dextro isomer methamphetamine base which is stronger, lasts longer, and is more smokable than regular "crank" or "crystal meth." It is also less toxic to the cardiovascular system.

AMPHETAMINE CONGENERS

When the prescription use of amphetamines was severely limited because of federal legislation, physicians turned to amphetamine congeners to help treat certain problems that had previously been treated with stronger stimulants. Amphetamine congeners are stimulant drugs that produce many of the same effects as amphetamines but are not as strong. They are also chemically related to amphetamines.

METHYLPHENIDATE (Ritalin® & Attention Deficit/Hyperactivity Disorder [AD/HD])

Methylphenidate (Ritalin®) is one of the most widely used amphetamine congeners. It is prescribed as a mood elevator or as a treatment for narcolepsy, a sleep disorder. However, it is most often prescribed to deal with attention deficit/hyperactivity disorder (AD/HD) (APA, 1994).

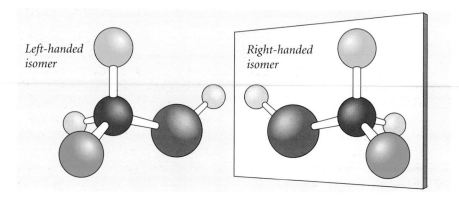

Left-handed isomer

Right-handed isomer

Figure 3-3 •

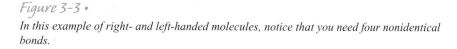

In this example of right- and left-handed molecules, notice that you need four nonidentical bonds.

Diagnosis of AD/HD

This disease is classified under the *International Classification of Diseases (ICD-10)* of the World Health Organization (WHO) into three subtypes: (1) hyperkinetic disorder, (2) disturbance of activity and attention, and (3) hyperkinetic conduct disorder (WHO, 1997, 1998).

In the United States the three subtypes of AD/HD according to the *DSM-IV Diagnostic Manual of the American Psychiatric Association* are: (1) AD/HD, predominantly inattentive type (2) AD/HD, predominantly hyperactive-impulsive type, and (3) AD/HD, combined type.

The person with AD/HD, predominantly inattentive type (attention deficit disorder or ADD),

◊ displays inattention to details that causes careless mistakes in school or at work;

◊ has difficulty sustaining attention at work or play;

◊ doesn't seem to listen when spoken to directly;

◊ doesn't follow through on schoolwork, chores, or duties;

◊ has difficulty organizing tasks or activities;

◊ avoids tasks that require sustained mental effort;

◊ often loses things necessary for tasks or activities;

◊ is often easily distracted by extraneous stimuli;

◊ is often forgetful in daily activities.

The person with predominantly hyperactive-impulsive type (hyperactivity disorder or HD)

◊ often fidgets with hands or feet or squirms in seat;

◊ often leaves seat;

◊ often runs about or climbs excessively in inappropriate situations;

◊ has difficulty playing or engaging in leisure activities quietly;

◊ is often on the go or often acts as if driven;

◊ often talks excessively;

◊ often blurts out answers before questions are completed;

◊ often has difficulty awaiting turn;

◊ often interrupts or intrudes on others.

In diagnosing ADD, HD, or a combination, AD/HD, some symptoms must be present before the age of seven, symptoms should manifest themselves in at least two different settings, there must be evidence of impairment of social functioning, and the symptoms are not better accounted for by other mental disorders (APA, 1994).

"To me, ADD feels like I am always rushing to get something done. I don't allow myself the chance to reflect or think things through. Events keep happening faster and faster and I try to keep up with it. I remember being that way when I was much younger but I wasn't able to look at it with any degree of detachment until now. Other times when I was young, and even now, I'll have one thing I need to do but I go and find 10 things I don't really need to do first, which makes me go faster to get everything done instead of spending the time with the main idea and doing it thoroughly. Taking Ritalin® makes me realize that I have choices I never considered, including not doing things, but it mostly helps me think things through and prioritize."
35-year-old man with AD/HD

Epidemiology

It is estimated that between 2% and 9.5% of all school-age children worldwide have AD/HD. The APA's estimates are 3% to 5% of all school-age children in the United States (APA, 1994). AD/HD is at least three times as prevalent in boys as in girls (Barkley, 1998). Mood changes, social withdrawal, and fear are more common in girls than the aggressiveness and impulsivity found in boys. If one examines children receiving psychiatric treatment, about 40% to 70% of inpatients and 30% to 50% of outpatients could be diagnosed with AD/HD.

The diagnostic tests for AD/HD often rely on diagnostic interview methods but there is still no explicit diagnostic test, so there is controversy about the extent and the severity of this disorder (NIH, 1998). For this reason the use of pharmacotherapy in treatment is still controversial.

Pharmacotherapy for AD/HD

It seems a contradiction but many stimulants in small doses have the ability to focus attention and control hyperactivity. It is theorized that dopamine depletion is one of the main causes for AD/HD and amphetamines or amphetamine congeners force the release of dopamine and prevent its reuptake or metabolism. Amphetamines are also prescribed for this condition as all stimulants, even caffeine, have the ability to focus attention in low doses.

It is estimated that 750,000 to 1,000,000 school children are receiving psychostimulant therapy and the figure is growing. Production of methylphenidate has increased more than 10-fold since 1990 (DEA, 1998). These drugs, such as methylphenidate (Ritalin®), d-amphetamine (Dexedrine®, Adderall®), or pemoline (Cylert®), seem to work in about 75% of AD/HD children. In addition to drug therapy, other adjunctive or separate therapies that are employed include lifestyle changes, education, behavior modification, psychotherapy, and even dietary changes to treat AD/HD.

A recent study by the National Institutes of Health studied the effectiveness of methylphenidate by itself, methylphenidate in conjunction with behavior-management therapy, behavior-management therapy alone, and just standard therapy available in the community. The researchers, working at six separate sites, found that for those with AD/HD alone, methylphenidate by itself was as effective as methylphenidate and therapy and more effective than therapy alone. On the other hand 70% of the children that were studied also had other problems like depression and anxiety. In those cases behavior therapy provided significant benefits especially when used in combination with methylphenidate (Jensen, 1999).

Concerns Regarding AD/HD Pharmacotherapy

In November, 1999 the Colorado Board of Education passed a resolution to discourage teachers from recommending prescription drugs like methylphenidate (Ritalin®) for AD/HD and Luvox® (fluvoxamine maleate), an SSRI antidepressant drug prescribed for obsessive-compulsive disorder.

Methylphenidate is a schedule II drug which means it has addiction liability. Users that get into compulsive use will develop tolerance quickly and increase dosage. Occasionally they will even switch to snorting or injecting the drug to try to recapture the original effects. There are also grave questions about the long-term effects of strong stimulants on children in general and whether this leads to dependence on these kinds of drugs. Concerns include the subjective nature of some AD/HD diagnoses, the confusion with other disorders, or just with the natural exuberance of childhood. The concern in some quarters was strong enough for the military to bar anyone who has used methylphenidate in childhood (after the age of 12) from military service. The military services are exempt from the American Disabilities Act, so they can bar potential enlistees because of AD/HD.

Methylphenidate is occasionally abused and has been diverted to illegal distribution channels, sold on the street, and used as a party drug. A few teenagers even appropriate their younger brother's or sister's supply to party with or to sell. When sold on the streets, methylphenidate tablets (called "pellets") sell for $3 to $10 per tablet.

There is an increased risk of conduct, mood, and anxiety disorders, along with impaired social and cognitive functioning, as the person grows (Biederman et al., 1996). There is an increased risk of alcohol and drug abuse

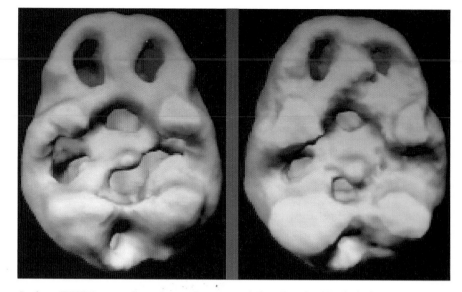

In these SPECT scans of a patient with attention deficit disorder (A), the holes represent areas of the brain that are underactive, especially the area of the prefrontal cortex that controls the executive function (decision making). When Ritalin®, is taken (B), the brain becomes more active because the drug activates neurotransmitters in this region.
Courtesy of the Amen Clinic for Behavioral Medicine, Fairfax, CA (Amen, 1999)

among adults with untreated AD/HD but the reasons for this relationship are hard to pinpoint (Biederman, Wilens, Mick, et al., 1997). Finally, in a group of adolescents in treatment for substance abuse disorders, about half also had diagnosable AD/HD (Horner & Scheibe, 1997). The high occurrence in drug abusers might have several explanations.

◇ It could be an attempt at self-medication.

◇ It could be that AD/HD leads to social alienation and problems with self-esteem, both of which are predictors of problems with alcohol and other drugs.

◇ It could be that the pre-existence of a mental condition makes one more likely to get into compulsive behavior.

◇ It could be that the use of psychoactive stimulants makes one more susceptible to drug use because of neurotransmitter disruption or increased acceptance of the idea of taking drugs to alleviate mental problems.

◇ Finally there could be genetic factors that are common to both

AD/HD and substance abuse disorders. One study found that the chance of an identical twin having the disorder if his brother has the disorder is 11–18 times greater than that of a nontwin sibling (Barkley, 1998). Another study at the University of Oslo found that heritability factors accounted for 80% of the differences between those with the disorder and those without. Other researchers found a strong genetic link between AD/HD and other addictions and impulse-control disorders including heavy alcohol and drug use, compulsive overeating, gambling, and even Tourette's syndrome (Miller & Blum, 1996; Comings, Wu, Chu, et al., 1996; Blum, Braverman, & Cull, et al., 2000).

Nearly half of these children with AD/HD have oppositional defiant disorder, a condition where they overreact to slights, can have outbursts of temper, be stubborn, or act defiant. If left untreated, these can progress to more serious conduct disorders including stealing, vandalism, and arson (NIMH, 1999).

On the positive side, a study at Harvard Medical School showed that boys (6–17 years old) with AD/HD who are treated with stimulants, including Ritalin®, are 84% less likely to abuse drugs and alcohol when they get older compared to those who are not treated (Biederman, Wilens, Mick, et al., 1999).

In the last few years attention has focused on the continued presence of AD/HD in large numbers of adults. Though earlier research had shown a reduction in the continuation of AD/HD symptoms once puberty was reached, the new research indicates the continual need to treat AD/HD patients with drugs like Ritalin® throughout their lives.

DIET PILLS

On September 30, 1999 American Home Products, as the defendant in a class action lawsuit in federal court,

agreed to pay $3.75 billion to $4.8 billion to all people who used two amphetamine congener diet pills, Pondimin® (fenfluramine) and Redux® (dexfenfluramine) and suffered or may suffer heart-valve damage. Prescription records show that approximately 5 million Americans have been prescribed Pondimin® or Redux®. Another amphetamine congener implicated in cases of heart-valve damage is phentermine (Ionamin® and Fastin®). The combination of phentermine and fenfluramine or dexfenfluramine became known as "fen-phen" and like diet pill fads and epidemics going back 50 or 60 years, a severe price was paid for a pharmacological shortcut to weight loss. Though fenfluramine and phentermine had been around 20 years, it wasn't until a 1992 journal article discussed the weight-loss effectiveness of the "fen-phen" combination that the drugs grew in popularity. When dexfenfluramine (Redux®), the right-handed molecular form of fenfluramine, was approved in 1995, the use of these drugs accelerated. It was just two years later that a report by the Mayo Clinic said that its doctors had found 24 cases of heart-valve damage in "fen-phen" users (all women) (Connolly, Crary, McGoon, et al., 1997). Other studies implicating the diet drugs in heart-valve damage soon followed (Khan, Herzog, St. Peter, et al., 1998). In September of 1997 the FDA (Food and Drug Administration) announced the withdrawal of fenfluramine and dexfenfluramine from the market in the United States. In late 1999 three follow up studies of patients who had taken the fen-phen combination or just dexfenfluramine suggested

that the heart-valve problems they suffered were generally not severe, wouldn't worsen over time, and may actually improve after cessation of use (Mayo Clinic, 1999; JACC, 1999; Shively, 1999).

In addition to heart-valve problems, cases of primary pulmonary hypertension (PPH), a potentially fatal cardiopulmonary disease, was found in a number of patients who had used dexfenfluramine. The French government severely restricted its use in 1995 due to PPH. The association of PPH with a diet pill had occurred 30 years earlier when Menocil® (aminorex fumarate), a weight-reducing drug, was withdrawn from European markets.

Other popular amphetamine congeners used as diet pills include phendimetrazine (Preludin®), pemoline (Cylert®), and diethylpropion (Tenuate®, Tepanil®). The stimulation, loss of appetite, and mood elevation caused by them are weaker but similar to the effects of amphetamines with some of the same side effects: excitability, nervousness, and increased blood pressure, heart rate, and respiration. If used to excess, heart irregularities, toxic convulsions, and even stroke, coma, and death can also occur. Despite their widespread use to control appetite and shed weight—there is significant weight loss in the first four to six months—users usually regain and even exceed their starting weights.

In general, diet pills and amphetamines are only recommended for short-term use, so careful monitoring by physicians and review boards is very important. Long-term and high-dose use of diet pills has been associated with the development of abuse and ad-

Diet-drug mix may be deadly, FDA warns

'Fen-phen' linked to heart, lung damage

By Chris Tomlinson
ASSOCIATED PRESS

ROCHESTER, Minn. — A diet-drug combination that is known as "fen-phen" and is taken by millions of Americans may cause serious heart and lung damage, the

Diet drug maker settles for $4.8 billion

By Julie Appleby
USA TODAY

American Home Products agreed Thursday to pay up to $4.8 billion over 16 years to settle claims from consumers who took the weight-loss combo known as "fen-phen."

45 days. If not enough people accept the deal, American could walk away from it.

The proposal includes:

▶ A $1 billion fund for medical tests to check for heart damage for anybody who took the drug and to provide treat-

ment if necessary.

▶ $2.3 billion to pay damages to those who now suffer or later develop moderate to severe heart-valve problems. Payment, based on age and severity of condition, ranges from $500 to $1.4 million.

Those with less severe disease could get more money later if their conditions worsen.

▶ Up to $429 million for plaintiffs' lawyers.

A toll-free number for more information and to register for the settlement is 800-386-2070.

diction even though amphetamine congeners are not as potent as amphetamines.

LOOKALIKES & OVER-THE-COUNTER (OTC) STIMULANTS

LOOKALIKES

The lookalike phenomenon contributed to the abuse of stimulants that began during the 1980s. By taking advantage of the interest in stimulant drugs, a few legitimate manufacturers began to make legal over-the-counter products that looked identical to prescription stimulants. Their various products contained ephedrine and, occasionally, pseudoephedrine (an anti-asthmatic), phenylpropanolamine (a decongestant and a mild appetite suppressant), and caffeine (a stimulant). These were being combined, packaged, and sold as "legal stimulants" in a deliberate attempt to misrepresent the drugs as controlled drugs (Morgan, Wesson, Puder, & Smith, 1987). The same chemicals were also showing up as illicit amphetamine lookalikes, such as street "speed," "cartwheels," and "crank," and as cocaine lookalikes, such as Supercaine®, Supertoot®, and Snow®. The cocaine lookalikes add benzocaine or procaine to mimic the numbing effects of the actual drug.

The problem with the lookalike products is their toxicity when overused, particularly when two or more of the drugs are combined. Also an amphetamine-like drug dependence developed in users who chronically abused the drugs (Tinsley & Wadkins, 1998). The physical problems can be particularly severe since large amounts are required to get a "speed" or cocaine-like high. For these reasons in the early 1980s, the FDA banned the OTC sales of products containing two or more of these ingredients. Since that time the sale of lookalikes persists with individual OTC stimulants being packaged to look like controlled prescription

stimulants. Further some manufacturers have circumvented the combination ban by combining herbs that contain ephedrine, caffeine, or phenylpropanolamine rather than the drugs themselves. (*See Herbal Ecstasy® and Herbal Nexus® in this chapter.*)

OTHER OVER-THE-COUNTER STIMULANTS

Pseudoephedrine and phenylpropanolamine, which have decongestant, mild anorexic, and stimulant effects, are also found in hundreds of allergy and cold medications, often in combination with antihistamines, such as Benadryl®, and in over-the-counter diet pills, like Dexadiet® and Dexatrim®. Individuals who ingest these drugs and drink coffee or other caffeinated beverages often experience anxiety attacks and rapid heartbeats. Caffeine has been sold as an OTC stimulant for years in tablets with trade names such as NoDoz® and Vivarin®.

MISCELLANEOUS PLANT STIMULANTS

Caffeine from the coffee bush and cocaine from the coca bush are often thought of as the principal plant stimulants but worldwide, dozens of plant extracts with stimulant properties have been used for centuries by millions of people, often in the Middle East, Far East, and Africa. These drug-containing plants include the khat bush, betel nuts, the ephedra bush, and the yohimbe tree.

KHAT & METHCATHINONE

Khat ("qat," "shat," "miraa")

In 1992 when the United States sent troops to Somalia, the soldiers were surprised to find a large percentage of the population chewing the leaves, twigs, and shoots of the khat shrub (*Catha edulis*) in order to get amphetamine-like sensations including a mild euphoria and stimulation. In Yemen, another country on the Arabian peninsula, more

than half the population uses khat and it is not unusual for people to spend over 1/3 of their family income on the drug. It is the driving force of the economy in Somalia, Yemen, and other countries in East Africa, southern Arabia, and the Middle East. Such drug usage is not a new development in these countries. In fact references to khat can be found in Arab journals in the thirteenth century. The leaves were used by some physicians as a treatment for depression but mostly it was used in social settings. In gatherings, the stimulatory effects of khat encourage talkativeness. Many homes in some Middle East countries actually have a room dedicated to khat chewing, similar to British homes that have a tearoom or parlor. Khat is used mostly by men in the countries where it is cultivated.

The khat shrub is 10–20 feet tall. Because the main active ingredients lose potency so quickly, the leaves and sprouts are harvested early in the morning, kept moist, and speedily transported to market where they are sold by noon. The fresh leaves and tender stems are chewed and the juice swallowed. Dried leaves and twigs, which are not as potent as the fresh leaves, can be crushed for tea or made into a chewable paste (U.S. Department of Justice, 1992).

The main psychoactive ingredient, cathinone, only has a half-life of approximately 90 minutes, so the leaf must be chewed continuously to sustain a high. Cathinone is a naturally occurring amphetamine-like substance that produces a similar euphoric effect, along with exhilaration, talkativeness, enhanced self-esteem, hyperactivity, wakefulness, aggressiveness, and loss of appetite. Unfortunately side effects include anorexia, tachycardia, hypertension, dependence, chronic insomnia, and gastric disorders (Kalix, 1994). People who use too much khat can become irritable, angry, and often violent. Chronic khat abuse results in symptoms similar to those seen with amphetamine addiction, including physical exhaustion, violence, and suicidal depression upon withdrawal. There are also rare reports of paranoid hallucinations and even overdose deaths. In experiments with monkeys where the animals were allowed to self-administer a drug to see if it was addictive, cathinone was shown to have a powerful reinforcing effect. The binge pattern of use found with cocaine and amphetamines was repeated by the monkeys with cathinone (Goudie & Newton, 1985).

The constant factional battles in Somalia that devastated the country could be partially due to the stimulatory and aggression-inducing effects of khat, along with the struggles to control the money involved in the trade. Worldwide, hundreds of millions of dollars are spent on the drug, even in poor countries. The stimulation and subsequent crash caused by khat has had an economic impact on countries, including reduced work hours, decreased production, income loss, and malnutrition (Giannini, Burge, Shaheen, & Price, 1986). Khat abuse is rare in the United States because of the rapid deterioration of the leaf once it is cut from the branches although recently there was a bust in Monterey County, California for the cultivation and abuse of the khat shrub. Also some street chemists are beginning to develop more stable analogues of cathinone in the United States.

Methcathinone

In the early '90s in the United States, a synthetic version of cathinone called "methcathinone" was synthesized in illegal laboratories, particularly in the Midwest, and sold on the street as a powerful alternative to methamphetamine. It is usually snorted but is also taken orally (mixed in a liquid), intravenously, and smoked in a "crack pipe" or in a cigarette or "joint." Since it is cheap to manufacture, a number of labs have sprung up. By the end of 1994, 34 methcathinone laboratories had been raided in Michigan and recently law enforcement officers have found labs in other Midwest states, including 22 in Indiana and 8 in Wisconsin. Labs have also been found in Washington, Texas, Pennsylvania, and a dozen other states. Like methamphetamine manufacture, ephedrine is

the main raw ingredient for methcathinone synthesis. A gram of the drug sold for $40 to $120 in 1996 compared to methamphetamine which sold for $40 to $200 (DEA, 1998).

Methcathinone (also known as "ephedrone") was originally synthesized by Parke-Davis Pharmaceuticals in 1957 in the United States but rejected for production due to side effects. The formula became widely known in Russia and by the early 1980s, methcathinone manufacture and illicit use was widespread. It has been estimated that 20% of illicit drug abusers in the former Soviet Union use methcathinone (Calkins, Alkan, & Hussain, 1995).

Using methcathinone instead of khat is similar to using cocaine instead of the coca leaf. Methcathinone is more intense than khat, so its addictive properties and side effects can be more intense (and quite similar to those of methamphetamines). Side effects include lack of coordination, labored respiration, and nervousness. PET scans of long-term methcathinone users show lasting reductions in dopamine production that can lead to nervous system and muscular problems, such as Parkinsonism (a dopamine deficiency disease) (Ricaurte et al., 1997).

BETEL NUTS

References to the betel nut (actually seeds of the betel palm, *Areca catechu*) date back more than 21 centuries.

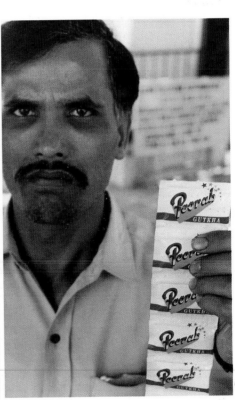

In Mumbai (Bombay) India, betel nut (areca nut) use is widespread. The nut (a) along with the necessary ingredients for use can be bought in thousands of small stalls throughout the city. The nut is chopped and mixed with lime and sweeteners, smeared on a betel leaf, often sprinkled with tobacco (b) and then chewed (c), allowing the active ingredients to be absorbed by the mucosa of the cheek and gums. The residual juice is then spit out. In recent years, a prepackaged product called "gutkha" (d) has become extremely popular. This vendor (who sells tobacco, bidi cigarettes, and gutkha) wouldn't smile for the camera due to his discolored and missing teeth caused by his use of gutkha.

Courtesy of Simone Garlaund

They have been widely used in the Arab world, India, Pakistan, Malaysia, the Philippines, New Guinea, Polynesia, southern China, Taiwan, and some countries in Africa. Marco Polo brought betel nuts back to Europe in 1300. The betel palm is widely cultivated, usually on large plantations, in a number of countries with a tropical climate. Each palm produces about 250 seeds per year.

Today more than 200 million people worldwide use betel nuts not only as a recreational drug but also as a medication. Just in Taiwan 17% of men and 1% of women, an estimated 2 million people, chew the nut on a regular basis. The main active ingredient is arecoline that increases levels of epinephrine and norepinephrine. The effects of these central nervous system stimulants are similar to those of nicotine or strong coffee and include a mild euphoria, excitation, decrease in fatigue, and lowered levels of irritability. Maximum effects occur six to eight minutes after chewing begins. Some users claim that betel chewing lowers tension, reduces appetite, and induces a feeling of well-being (Bibra, 1995). Some users chew from morning until night, others use them only in social situations. Some liken the practice to gum chewing or cola drinking in the West. This drug can also produce psychological dependence.

The betel nut (husk and/or meat) is generally chewed in combination with another plant leaf (peppermint, mustard, etc.) and some slaked lime to make it more palatable. The juice of this mixture stains the teeth and mouth dark red over time. In high doses arecholine can be toxic. Another substance in betel nuts, muscarine, is epidemiologically linked to oesophageal cancer. Up to seven percent of regular users have cancer of the mouth and esophagus. However, the most common danger has to do with tissue damage to mucosal linings of the mouth and esophagus. There is even a prominent and identifiable set of withdrawal symptoms similar to those experienced during withdrawal from other stimulants like caffeine.

In the late 1990s a product called "gutkha" was marketed in India. Gutkha is a sweetened mixture of tobacco, betel nut, and betel leaves. It was sold at price even affordable to children (about 40¢ to 50¢) and packaged to attract their attention. The sales of these products have already reached close to $1 billion due to the habituating nature of these substances. Children as young as 12 have been diagnosed with precancerous lesions in their mouths due to gutkha use when the product had only been available in India for a few years (BDF, 1999).

YOHIMBE

Yohimbine, a bitter spicy extract from the African yohimbe tree (*Corynanthe yohimbe*), can be brewed into a stimulating tea or used as a medicine. It is reported to be a mild aphrodisiac. It seems to increase the activity of the neurotransmitter acetylcholine which results in more penile blood inflow. It also increases blood pressure and heart rate. Yohimbine has been reported to produce a mild euphoria and occasional hallucinations but in larger doses it can be toxic and even cause death by respiratory paralysis (Marnell, 1997). The bark can be bought at some herbal stores, along with a whole series of medicines for "increasing potency" with names like Male Performance®, Yohimbe Power®, Manpower®, and Aphrodyne® (prescription only).

EPHEDRA (ephedrine)

The ephedra bush (*Ephedra equisetina*), found in deserts throughout the world, contains the drug ephedrine. This drug is a mild stimulant that is used medicinally to treat asthma, narcolepsy, other allergies, and low blood pressure. Many use it to make tea; the Mormons brewed it as a substitute for coffee that was forbidden by their religion. Ephedrine, also known as marwath and ma huang, has been mentioned as a stimulant tonic and medication in China for over 5,000 years and is still sold in herbalists' shops today. Ephedrine was isolated and synthesized in 1885 but then was

forgotten for almost 50 years before a scientific paper recommended it for asthma. Its popularity increased dramatically. Up until then epinephrine was the only effective medication used to treat asthma.

Ephedrine has more peripheral effects, such as bronchodilation, and fewer central nervous system effects, such as euphoria, than amphetamines but one of the common side effects of excessive ephedrine use is drug-induced psychosis (Karch, 1996). Extract of ephedrine has been used by athletes for an extra boost but can lead to heart and blood vessel problems. A weightlifter's death in Ohio led to the banning of sales of the extract. Other states have followed suit and banned the sales of all ephedrine-based products. Many lookalike and over-the-counter products that advertise themselves as MDMA, amphetamine substitutes, or other stimulants (e.g., Cloud 9®, Nirvana®) contain ephedrine as the active ingredient.

Natural ephedra and synthetic ephedrine and pseudoephedrine are also the main ingredients in the synthesis of methamphetamine and meth-

FDA Plans Ephedrine Crackdown

Supplements linked to deaths, illnesses

Associated Press

Washington
With at least 17 deaths and 800 illnesses linked to dietary supplements laced with ephedrine, the government said yesterday it will crack down on the pills, tablets and teas that promise to help people lose weight, build muscle and feel more energetic.

The Food and Drug Administration plans to dramatically cut the dose of the herbal stimulant that can be put into any dietary supplement, and to ban the mar-

cathinone and because of the demand for them, a large illegal trade has sprung up.

Herbal Ecstasy® & Herbal Nexus®

In an attempt to cater to some people's desire for abusable stimulants and psychedelics, entrepreneurs have introduced stimulant herbal products. These capsules and tablets combine the herbal form of ephedrine (ephedra), an herbal extract of caffeine (possibly from the kola nut), with other herbs and vitamins and are advertised as Herbal Ecstasy®, Herbal Nexus®, or other catchy names. The use of herbal substances is an attempt to get around the FDA ban on some combinations of these products and to cash in on the current interest in certain psychoactive drugs including MDMA (ecstasy), nexus (CBR), other stimulants, and even marijuana. Some of these herbal products also contain vitamins and are touted as buffers for the toxic effects of the real ecstasy and nexus. Unfortunately the problems, even with herbal ephedra, have caused several states to ban products with any form of ephedra or ephedrine and have provoked a warning from the FDA on the use of any substance containing the drug.

CAFFEINE

Caffeine is the most popular stimulant in the world. It is found in coffee, tea, chocolate, soft drinks, 60 different plants, and hundreds of over-the-counter or prescription medications. It has become ingrained in so many cultures that efforts at any kind of prohibition or reduction of use are doomed to failure. In America there is the morning coffee, the coffee break at work in the morning and afternoon, coffee at meetings and conferences, and even the steaming cup of decaf after dinner to keep the ritual going. As with many psychoactive drugs, the ritual surrounding use of coffee or tea is often as important as the stimulation sought. Some of the rituals include selecting

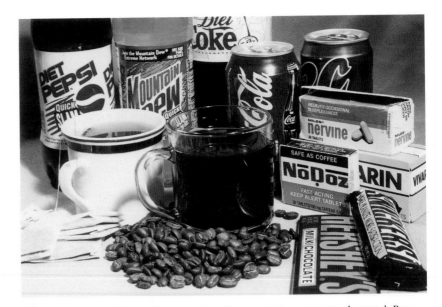

Caffeine concentration in most beverages is only one part in one or two thousand. Pure caffeine extract is a powerful stimulant.

the right coffee, grinding the beans, finding a comfortable or "cool" place to drink, collecting dozens of cups, demitasses, or mugs, reading the newspaper, and finding the right pastry to go with the morning cup.

HISTORY OF USE

Tea is the most widely consumed beverage in the world besides water. In the United States it accounts for 17% of the caffeine consumed (Silverman & Griffiths, 1995). Tea was thought to have been present in China as early as 2700 B.C. but the first written record dates back to A.D. 35. It was used in Japan around A.D. 600 but didn't become an important part of the culture until the fifteenth century. A tea ceremony became an important ritual in Japanese homes and castles. Tea was introduced into Europe around the end of the sixteenth century and immediately became quite popular, particularly in England and subsequently English colonies such as America (Harler, 1984). The Boston Tea Party in 1774, when irate Bostonians threw tea into Boston Harbor to protest a tax on tea, reflected the importance of this psychoactive substance in colonial life. Today the major exporters of tea are India, China, and Sri Lanka while

the major importers are the United Kingdom, the United States, and Pakistan. About 75% of the world's tea is black tea and 22% is green tea.

Coffee was first cultivated in Ethiopia around A.D. 650. Legend says that the stimulant properties of coffee were discovered when Kaldi, an Arab goat herder, noticed the friskiness of his goats when they ate red berries from the coffee bush and tried them himself. Later on, Arabs learned how to prepare a hot drink from the berries rather than just chewing them. Use then spread to Arabia in the thirteenth century and finally to Europe by the fifteenth century. The drink was so stimulating that many cultures banned it as an intoxicating drug. In colonial America it was suggested that the use of tea and coffee led to the use of tobacco, alcohol, opium, and other drugs (Greden & Walters, 1997). Fortunately or unfortunately coffee and tea were also great sources of revenue and the pressure against prohibition was immense both from governments and the general public. The use of caffeinated beverages continued to expand until today, in the United States alone, each coffee drinker consumes about 20 pounds of coffee per year.

Cocoa from the cacao tree was first used in the New World by the Aztecs and Mayan royalty, mostly as an unsweetened drink or as a spice, and brought to Europe by Hernando Cortez in 1528. Widespread use didn't occur until the nineteenth century when the first chocolate bars appeared on the market. There is only a small amount of caffeine in chocolate but the other active ingredient, theobromine, has similar effects.

Caffeinated soft drinks (colas) are carbonated beverages that contain a caffeine-containing extract of the kola nut from the African kola tree (*Cola nitida* or *Cola acuminata*) but mostly caffeine extracted from the process of decaffeinating coffee. The caffeine of the kola nut is released by cracking it into small pieces and then chewing it. The kola nut has been used in some African countries for centuries. The use of the nut for chewing and as a syrup made from powdered kola nut spread to Europe in the mid-1800s. By the late 1800s cola drinks made with carbonated or phosphated liquids, such as Coca Cola®, became popular in the United States (Kuhar, 1995). It is important to note that caffeine is added to other soft drinks and not just colas. Mountain Dew®, orange and even some lemon-lime sodas now contain this drug.

Other plants containing caffeine include guarana, maté (ilex plant), and yoco, found in South America. Guarana is the national drink of Brazil made from the guarana shrub. It has more caffeine than coffee and is made into sweet carbonated beverages. Maté is the most popular caffeine drink in Argentina. It is a tea-like hot drink made from the leaves of a certain holly plant. Maté leaves can be bought in a number of health food stores (Weil & Rosen, 1993). This is not to be confused with Mate de Coca® that contains coca leaves instead of tea leaves.

PHARMACOLOGY

Caffeine is an alkaloid of the chemical class called "xanthines." It is found in more than 60 plant species such as the *Coffea arabica* (coffee), *Thea sinensis* (tea), *Theobroma cacao*

TABLE 3–2 CAFFEINE CONTENT IN VARIOUS SUBSTANCES

Amount of Beverage or Food	Caffeine Content in Milligrams (mg)	
	Average	Range
1 demitasse espresso	200 mg	
1 cup freshly brewed American coffee (6 oz.)	100 mg	90–125 mg
1 cup of instant coffee	75 mg	60–100 mg
1 cup of decaf coffee	3 mg	2–4 mg
1 cup of tea	60 mg	30–100 mg
12 oz. caffeinated soft drink (e.g., Coca Cola®, Mountain Dew®)	45 mg	36–60 mg
Cocoa	25-50 mg	
4 oz. chocolate bar	80 mg	25–100 mg
1 No-Doz® tablet	100 mg	
1 Vivarin® tablet	200 mg	
1 Excedrin® tablet	65 mg	
1 Midol® tablet	32 mg	

(chocolate), or *Cola nitida* (cola drinks). The white, crystalline, bitter-tasting drug was isolated from coffee in 1820. Tea leaves contain a higher percentage of caffeine than coffee but less tea is used for the average cup. Caffeine can be used orally, intravenously, intramuscularly, or rectally, though most consumption is by mouth. The half-life of caffeine in the body is 3–7 hours, so it will take 15–35 hours for 95% of the caffeine to be excreted. School-age children eliminate caffeine twice as fast as adults (Silverman & Griffiths, 1995).

In the United States, per capita consumption of caffeine is 211 milligrams per day, about 2 cups of regular coffee and perhaps a cola; in Sweden, 425 milligrams (85% from coffee); and in the United Kingdom, 445 milligrams (72% from tea). Worldwide, the figure averages about 70 milligrams per day (Silverman, 1995).

◊ About half of all Americans drink 3.3 cups of coffee on any given day and most of that is regular coffee, not the lattes and espressos found in specialty coffees that have exploded in popularity in recent years (Coffee Science Source, 1998).

◊ Twenty percent of adults in the United States consume more than

350 mg of caffeine and 3% consume more than 650 mg.

◊ Caffeinated soft drinks, which are becoming increasingly popular, contain about 30–60 mg of caffeine, approximately half that of regular coffee (COHIS, 1999).

◊ In 1997 Americans consumed about 540 12-oz. cans of soft drinks per person per year at a total yearly cost of $54 billion.

◊ There are about 450 different soft drinks available in the United States of which 65% contain caffeine.

◊ About 16% of the per capita daily consumption of caffeine in the United States is from tea, 16% from soft drinks, while 60% is from coffee (National Soft Drink Association, 1999; COHIS, 1999).

"I start in the morning with a double latte. That's 300–400 milligrams of caffeine. I'll have two Cokes® for lunch, that's another 100 milligrams. Then a couple of cups of regular coffee in the afternoon—another 200 milligrams. That's 700 milligrams minimum. I know plenty of people at work who will have at least 10 cups of coffee besides

the lattes and chocolate bars. They're up to 2,000 milligrams a day. Their tolerance is incredible. They'll drink a cup and fall asleep."

36-year-old caffeinated businessman

PHYSICAL & MENTAL EFFECTS

Medically, caffeine is used in a number of over-the-counter preparations as a decongestant, an analgesic, a stimulant, an appetite suppressant, and for menstrual pain. Nonmedically, caffeine is most widely known and used as a mild stimulant. In low doses (100–200 milligrams) it can increase alertness, dissipate drowsiness or fatigue, and help thinking. Even at doses above 200 milligrams, there can still be increased alertness and performance but, as with any drug, excessive use can cause problems.

At doses of more than 350 milligrams per day (about 5–7 cups of coffee), depending on the susceptibility of the user, anxiety, insomnia, nervousness, gastric irritation, high blood pressure, and flushed face can occur. At doses above 1,000 milligrams, increased heart rate, palpitations, muscle twitching, rambling thoughts, jumbled speech, sleeping difficulties, motor disturbances, ringing in the ears, and even vomiting and convulsions can occur. Caffeine is lethal at about 10 grams (100 cups of coffee).

Consuming 350 milligrams or more of caffeine can lower fertility rates in women and affect fetuses in the womb (e.g., higher blood pressure). A retrospective study at the University of Utah of 2,500 pregnant women found that 6 or more cups of coffee a day almost doubled the risk of miscarriage compared to women who either didn't drink coffee or only drank 1–2 cups a day (Klebanoff, Levine, DeSimonian, et al., 1999). In addition it is thought by a number of researchers that some susceptible women develop benign lumps in their breasts from drinking too much coffee.

Since excessive caffeine use can trigger nervousness, people who are prone to panic attacks should avoid caffeine. A physician or psychiatrist should ask patients who come in with symptoms of anxiety about their caffeine consumption. In fact physicians rarely consider caffeine consumption in their patients with cardiovascular, sleep, gastric, and other problems.

Some researchers also feel that caffeine use makes it harder to lose weight. This difficulty happens because caffeine stimulates the release of insulin. Insulin metabolizes sugar that then reduces the level of sugar in the blood—triggering hunger in the user.

Coronary heart disease, ischemic heart disease, heart attacks, intestinal ulcers, diabetes, and some liver problems have been seen in long-term, high-dose caffeine users, more often in countries with very high per capita caffeine consumption.

TOLERANCE, WITHDRAWAL, & ADDICTION

Tolerance to the effects of caffeine does occur, although there is a wide variation among the ways different people will react to several cups of coffee or tea. Coffee drinkers might eventually need three cups to wake up instead of the usual single cup with lots of cream and sugar. For those with a high tolerance, a cup of coffee can even encourage sleep.

Withdrawal symptoms do occur after cessation of long-term use. These symptoms include headaches, fatigue and lethargy, depression, decreased alertness, sleep problems, and irritability but fortunately most symptoms pass within a few days, although some users say symptoms can last for weeks, even months.

"The headache hits me about five in the afternoon of the day I quit and stays around through the next day. Then I feel tired and my ass drags for the next two weeks. I'll stay off it for a while and then I'll start with half-a-cup and pretty soon I got a pot going all the time plus a couple of six-packs of Diet Coke® in the icebox."

20-year coffee drinker

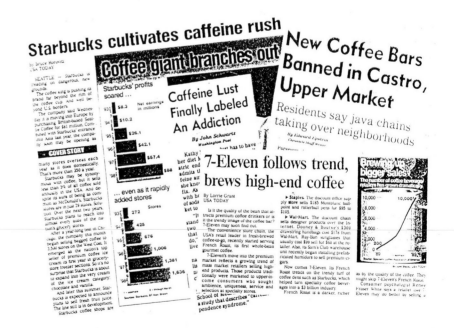

There has been an incredible growth in the number of specialty coffee houses in the United States. Every parking lot seems to have a coffee kiosk and every discount department store and grocery chain store have coffee bars. The number of coffee beverage retailers has grown from 200 in 1989 to more than 10,000 in 1999 and the numbers are accelerating leading to an outcry from neighbors. Starbucks®, the largest of the retailers, had 1,636 stores in 1998 in the United States.

Addiction and dependence can occur with daily intake levels of 500 milligrams (about 5 cups of coffee, 10 cola drinks, or 8 cups of tea), although withdrawal symptoms will occur after cessation of long-term use of 100–200 milligrams per day. Coffee creates a milder dependency than that found with amphetamines and cocaine. It interferes less with daily functioning and is not as expensive as the stronger stimulants. However, two-thirds of those treated for excessive caffeine use (caffeinism) will relapse after treatment back into heavy use.

TOBACCO & NICOTINE

"One of the sounds I remember from growing up in the 1940s and '50s was the sound of my dad's cigarette cough. It started deep in the lungs and ended in an explosion of air. I could tell he was approaching from a block away. I just accepted it as a fact of life. He later became Advertising Director for American Tobacco just when the first Surgeon General's Report on Health and Tobacco was released in 1964. He gave up smoking in 1976 after retiring and died of throat cancer 17 years later, caused by his years of smoking according to his oncologist. Talk about mixed feelings . . . tobacco supported his family then took his life and that of thousands of others."
William Cohen, co-author of Uppers, Downers, All Arounders

Tobacco comes from the leaves and other parts of a plant species belonging to the genus *Nicotiana,* a member of the deadly nightshade family that also includes tomatoes, belladonna, and petunias. There are 64 *Nicotiana* species but most commercial tobacco comes from the milder, broad-leafed *Nicotiana tabacum* plant and a number of its variants. Though tobacco is available in cigarettes, cigars, pipe tobacco, snuff (oral and nasal), and chewing tobacco, cigarettes account for 90% of all tobacco use in America. In a country such as India, chewing tobacco (and chewing the betel nut) is more popular (85% of all adult men). Whether it is smoked, chewed, absorbed through the gums, or even used as an enema, this stimulant ultimately affects many of the same areas of the brain as cocaine and amphetamines though not as intensely.

HISTORY (*also see Chapter 1*)

Native Americans & Tobacco

After several voyages to the New World, Columbus and a number of other French, Portuguese, and Spanish explorers noticed that the Native Americans "drank the smoke" of certain dried leaves and seemed to receive stimulation and sedative effects from the process (O'Brien, Cohen, Evans, & Fine, 1992). The explorers and diplomats introduced tobacco to Europe where it was used for recreation and as a medicine. It was listed as a cure for almost every known disease including ulcerated abscesses, fistulas, and sores. (In this century it is listed as the cause of just as many diseases.) Use spread to Europe, Russia, Japan, Africa, and China in the 1600s and later on to virtually every country in the world. Originally smoking tobacco several times a day in a pipe was the most common form of use but chewing tobacco and using snuff became popular in Europe and America in the eighteenth century because a user didn't have to carry or light a pipe, roll a cigarette, or carry the means to light them. In fact smokeless tobacco remained the preferred method of use until the end of World War I (Benowitz & Fredericks, 1995).

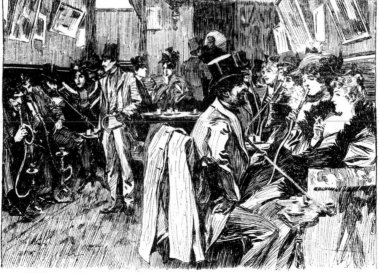

NEW YORK HERALD. SUNDAY. APRIL 28, 1895.

NEW YORK'S NEW SMOKING FAD.

Picturesque Groups and Fighting Talk in the Rooms of the Men from Bagdad.

MANY DAINTY SMOKERS SEEN

A Fashionable Crush Early, and Later Young Men Who Talk Defiance.

GAMBLERS ALSO NUMEROUS.

Turks Have a King of Clubs of Their Own Now and Breathe Slaughter.

A SCENE IN ONE OF THE RECENTLY OPENED TURKISH SMOKING PARLORS.

At the turn of the century, tobacco dens were as notorious as the psychedelic clubs of the 1960s and the "rave" clubs of the '90s.

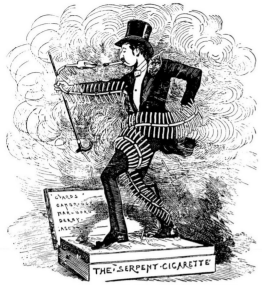

SWELL STRUGGLING WITH THE CIG'RETTE POISONER.

Even back in the late 1800s, the addictive nature of smoking was appreciated. The invention of the cigarette-rolling machine in 1884, along with the development of tobacco strains that weren't as irritating to the throat and lungs, increased cigarette use from 40 a year to 40 a day for many smokers.
Courtesy of the National Library of Medicine, Bethesda

moist snuff—finely chopped tobacco as found in brands such as Copenhagen® and Skoal®—is stuck in the mouth next to the gums where the nicotine is absorbed into the capillaries. With loose-leaf chewing tobacco like Beech Nut® and Red Man®, larger sections of leaf are stuffed into the mouth and chewed to allow the nicotine-laden juice to be absorbed. There were approximately 6 million regular smokeless tobacco users in the United States in 1998 with sales over $1 billion (SAMHSA, 1999). The use of chewing tobacco and snuff is very prevalent in professional and amateur male athletes in America.

Snuff is a fine powder that is most often sniffed into the nose but it is also rubbed on the gums or chewed. Stems and leaves of the tobacco plant are fermented, dried, and then ground into powder. Various scents and flavors are then added to the powder to improve the bitter taste of nicotine. Snuff boxes and use of this form of tobacco were once considered very chic and fashionable throughout the world. Today sniffing snuff is not nearly as popular as smoking or chewing tobacco. This method of use is irritating to mucosal tissues and deadens the sense of smell.

Growth of Cigarette Smoking

The cigarette market expanded greatly because of improved cigarette-manufacturing technology, a milder type of tobacco that allowed for deeper inhalation, lower prices, increased advertising, and more aggressive marketing techniques. World Wars I and II initiated millions of GIs into smoking cigarettes (Slade, 1992). Cigarette companies supplied free or cheap cigarettes to the soldiers in an effort to expand their market. England even stockpiled cigarettes during World War II in case of invasion or an interruption in the supply. Interestingly some of the reasons for the switch to cigarettes were worries about the health risks of smokeless tobacco including the fear that chewing it caused tuberculosis. In the nineteenth and early twentieth centuries, fear of tuberculosis was the equivalent of our present day fear of cancer (O'Brien et al., 1992).

If a user smoked 40 cigarettes a year in the late 1800s, it was not nearly the health problem it is today when the consumption of an average heavy smoker is 30–40 cigarettes a day, or more than 10,000 a year. This new popularity of tobacco not only multiplied the number of smokers, it multiplied the number of dollars made from tobacco. Gross sales of tobacco products

in the United States in 1998 were approximately $46 billion (U.S. Department of Agriculture, 1999). In 1998, 45 million Americans, about 1 in 5, smoked cigarettes regularly (that is more than once a week) (SAMHSA, 1999).

Smokeless Tobacco

The three types of smokeless tobacco, moist snuff, powder snuff, and loose leaf, are still popular. A pinch of

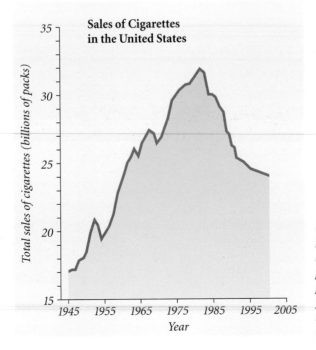

Sales of Cigarettes in the United States

Total sales of cigarettes (billions of packs)

Year

Figure 3-4 •

Sales of cigarettes have climbed from 18 billion packs a year in 1945 to a peak of 32 billion packs a year in 1985. By 2000, U.S. sales had dropped to 24 billion packs.

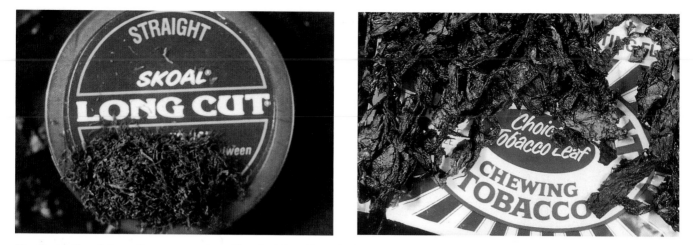

Two forms of smokeless tobacco are moist snuff on the left and loose leaf on the right. More than 120 million pounds of chewing tobacco and snuff were sold in the United States in 1998—20 pounds per user.

PHARMACOLOGY

Tobacco & Cigarettes

When tobacco is burned in a cigarette or cigar, the smoke that is created consists of fine particles and droplets of tar. Tobacco and tobacco smoke contain nicotine and about 4,000 other chemicals, many created by the burning process. About 400 are classified as toxins and 43 are known carcinogens. For example, some of the major by-products in a lit cigarette are tobacco tar, a blackish substance that has direct effects on the respiratory system, and nitrosamines, some of which are carcinogenic (Glantz, 1992).

Nicotine

Nicotine is the most important ingredient in tobacco in terms of cardiovascular and particularly psychoactive effects. The average tobacco leaf (*Nicotiana tabacum*) contains two percent to five percent nicotine. Pure nicotine is colorless, bitter, smelly, and highly poisonous. Mixed in water it is a powerful insecticide. Smoking and inhaling a cigarette delivers nicotine to the brain in five to eight seconds. Chewing tobacco or placing snuff placed on the gums delivers the nicotine in five to eight minutes.

◇ The average cigarette contains 10 milligrams of nicotine but only delivers 1–3 milligrams of that to the lungs when burned and inhaled.

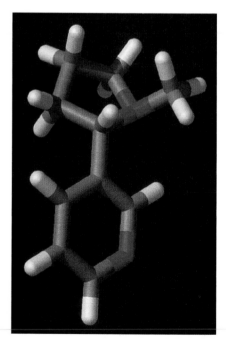

This is a computer simulation of the nicotine molecule, $C_{11}H_{14}N_2$. Nicotine was isolated in 1828 by the German scientists Posselt and Reiman. Besides cigarettes, nicotine is used in insecticides such as Black Leaf 40® that contains 40% nicotine sulfate.

Courtesy of the Molecular Imaging Department, University of California Medical Center, San Francisco

TABLE 3–3   SOME INGREDIENTS FOUND IN CIGARETTE SMOKE

Tobacco Smoke	Common Product	Adverse Health Effects
Cadmium	Artists oil paints	Yellow stains on teeth
Hydrogen cyanide	Gas chamber poison	Breathing difficulty
Vinyl chloride	Garbage bags	Whitening of fingers and pain when cold
Toluene	Embalmer's glue	Inflamed, cracked skin
Benzene	Rubber cement	Drowsiness, dizziness, headaches, nausea
Naphthalene	Paint pigment	Headache, confusion
Arsenic	Rat poison	Pins and needles feeling in hands and feet

Compiled by the California Department of Health Services

About 70 milligrams ingested at one time is fatal. Chain smokers might get up to 6 milligrams in their lungs before rapid distribution and metabolism put a damper on high blood-nicotine levels.

◇ In comparison one chew of tobacco will deliver approximately 4.5 milligrams of nicotine and one pinch of snuff, about 3.6 milligrams.

◇ The actual blood-nicotine level of one cigarette is measured as approximately 25 µg/L or 25 micrograms per liter of blood. The average smoker will maintain a nicotine level of 5–40 µg/L depending on the time of day or night (Schmitz, Schneider, & Jarvik, 1997).

◇ The nicotine in the first cigarette of the day raises the heart rate by an average of 10–20 beats per minute and the blood pressure by 5–10 units.

The effect of nicotine is the main reason for the widespread use of tobacco. Nicotine, a central nervous system stimulant, disrupts the balance of neurotransmitters such as endorphins, epinephrine, dopamine, and particularly acetylcholine. Acetylcholine affects heart rate, blood pressure, memory, learning, reflexes, aggression, sleep, sexual activity, and mental acuity. What nicotine does is mimic acetylcholine by slotting into nicotinic acetylcholine receptor sites, so those cholinergic effects are exaggerated. The release of dopamine makes a smoker feel satisfied and calm, so a cigarette both stimulates and calms.

Scientists have located one of the key proteins in the nicotine receptor that seems to be responsible for the positive reinforcing properties of nicotine. When the scientists developed a strain of mice without the key protein (1 of the 10 proteins that form the nicotinic receptor), the mouse had no desire to self-administer nicotine on a regular basis. Even when injected with nicotine, the level of the calming neurotransmitter dopamine did not increase.

In another experiment PET imaging studies found that smokers had lower levels of the enzymes MAO-A and B (monoamine oxidase A and B) which calm the smoker (Fowler, Volkow, & Wang, et al., 1996).

Nicotine & Craving

Besides the mildly pleasurable effects that smokers receive from tobacco, some of the reasons for continuing to smoke include

◇ the social context, such as drinking and smoking in bars and at a meal;

◇ the ritual aspects of lighting up and smoking;

◇ the perception of smoking as an adult activity;

◇ the desire to manipulate mood;

◇ the desire to be rebellious;

◇ the perception that smoking is sexually attractive.

The two most important reasons that people continue to smoke have to do with weight loss and craving.

Nicotine appears to suppress appetite and increase metabolism. On average, smokers weigh about six to nine pounds less than nonsmokers (Klesges, Meyers, Klesges, & LaVasque, 1989; Schmitz et al., 1997). Since withdrawal from smoking is often accompanied by weight gain, the fear of putting on pounds can keep smokers from quitting or cause relapse when they do quit. A current hypothesis about weight gain is that nicotine raises the metabolic rate to burn more calories and lowers the inherited weight setpoint (Perkins, 1993).

Finally, the most important reason that people continue to smoke is **an intense desire to maintain a certain nicotine level in the blood (and therefore in the brain) in order to avoid withdrawal symptoms.** This need to avoid negative effects by continued use is known as "negative drug reinforcement." In addition the authors believe that the very act of relieving withdrawal symptoms can activate the nucleus accumbens inducing a certain sense of pleasure. This same effect has been postulated for heroin or other opioid withdrawal (Goldstein, 1994).

TOLERANCE, WITHDRAWAL, & ADDICTION

Tolerance

Tolerance to the effects of nicotine develops quite rapidly, even faster than with heroin or cocaine. A few hours of smoking are sufficient for the body to begin adapting to these new toxic chemicals.

"The first time I smoked it was to impress a girl. I got dizzy and high and

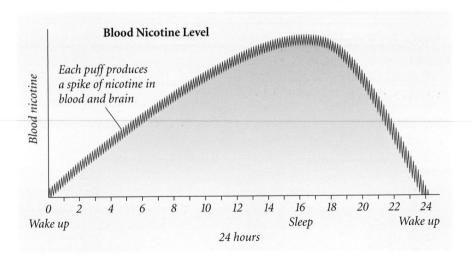

Blood Nicotine Level

Each puff produces a spike of nicotine in blood and brain

Blood nicotine

0 2 4 6 8 10 12 14 16 18 20 22 24
Wake up   Sleep   Wake up

24 hours

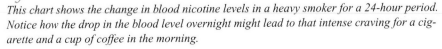

Figure 3-5 •

This chart shows the change in blood nicotine levels in a heavy smoker for a 24-hour period. Notice how the drop in the blood level overnight might lead to that intense craving for a cigarette and a cup of coffee in the morning.

had to sit down. A year later, my 30th cigarette of the day only gave me a mild stimulation and a nagging cough. Now all I have left is the cough, a bunch of smoking rituals, and it costs about three bucks a pack."

Two-pack-a-day smoker

Withdrawal

Withdrawal from a pack- or two-pack-a-day habit after prolonged use can cause headaches, nervousness, fatigue, hunger, severe irritability, poor concentration, sleep disturbances, and intense nicotine craving. It is a true physical dependence that has been built up. One process that occurs is the creation of more acetylcholine receptors particularly the nicotinic receptors (Stein, Pankiewicz, Harsch, et al., 1998). When a person tries to stop using tobacco, the activity of acetylcholine is greatly exaggerated by all these extra receptors, thus making the user restless, irritable, and discontent. Soon the smoker comes to depend on smoking to stay normal, that is, to avoid these withdrawal effects. Also, recent research demonstrated that abrupt withdrawal of nicotine resulted in significant decrease of action in the brain's reward function. This effect lasted for days (Epping-Jordan, Watkins, Koob, & Markou, 1998). The resultant lack of a reward function drives the animal to crave nicotine when its use is discontinued.

The sense of relaxation and well-being that most smokers receive from a cigarette is, in fact, the sensation of the withdrawal symptoms being subdued.

Smokers will try to maintain a constant level of nicotine in the bloodstream and brain. Even when smokers switch to a low tar and nicotine brand, they often increase the number of cigarettes they smoke just to maintain their nicotine target levels. In fact nicotine craving may last a lifetime after withdrawal.

"When I wake up at two or three in the morning, I can't go back to sleep without a cigarette. I just can't. If I try,

I stay awake and fidget. If I smoke, I go back to sleep. I don't know if I have to smoke or just want to."

Two-pack-a-day smoker

Addiction

"I cannot refrain from a few words of protest against the astounding fashion lately introduced from America, a sort of smoke-tippling, which enslaves its victims more completely than any other form of intoxication, old or new. These madmen will swallow and inhale with incredible eagerness, the smoke of a plant they call herba Nicotiana, or tobacco."

German Ambassador to The Hague, c. 1627

The use of tobacco is a pure example of the addictive process. The pleasure received from the direct effects of smoking are not intense as the initial pleasure derived from alcohol, cocaine, or almost any other psychoactive drug. Coughing, dizziness, headache, even nausea are experienced by the novice smoker; the cost of a two-pack-a-day habit can run $3,225 a year at $3.50 a pack; the health problems and premature deaths that result from smoking are too numerous to mention; and yet people continue to smoke. In fact 80% of smokers believe that cigarette smoking causes cancer, yet they still smoke (Harris Poll, 1999).

One of the strongest indications of the addictive potential of tobacco can be seen when you look at the percentage of casual tobacco users who become compulsive users vs. the percentage of casual users of other psychoactive drugs who become compulsive users of those drugs.

◇ Twenty-three million people have tried cocaine. About 600,000 are weekly users, about 2.6%, but only a tiny fraction of cocaine users do it on a daily basis.

◇ Seventy-two million people have tried marijuana but only 6.8 million use it weekly, about 9.4%, and a few percent on a daily basis.

◇ One hundred and seventy-eight million have tried alcohol, yet less than 48 million drink on a weekly basis, about 27%; 20 million drink on a daily basis, about 11%.

◇ One hundred and fifty-two million have smoked cigarettes   60 million of them on a weekly basis (about 40%); 46 million of them on a daily basis (about 30%).

(SAMHSA, 1999)

These figures mean that almost 1/3 of those who ever tried a cigarette became daily habitual users compared with the 11% of alcohol experimenters who become daily abusers. And yet people continue to experiment with cigarettes.

Granted you might say that people want to keep using cigarettes because smoking is really pleasurable and that the choice is theirs. Yet according to one survey, 80% of smokers interviewed say they want to quit and another 10% say they want to limit the amount they smoke. That means that 9 out of 10 smokers are unhappy with their smoking and yet they continue to smoke. Recently the tobacco companies have started to admit that nicotine is indeed addicting.

In many countries the rate of daily use is even higher than in the United States: 50% in China, 40% in England, and 50% in Japan (WHO, 1998). In a British study 90% of teenagers who had smoked just three to four cigarettes at the time of the survey were found to be compulsive smokers years later. This statistic means that even the most casual use of tobacco usually leads to compulsive use. And yet people continue to smoke. Globally 12% of women and 47% of men smoke.

It is worth noting here that nicotine craving is much subtler and less noticeable to the user than the other cravings that occur with drugs like cocaine, heroin, or alcohol. However, the craving is nevertheless extremely powerful and may be associated with what is called a "self-determined nicotine state of consciousness" or "state dependence." **State dependence** means that people will try to achieve a certain mental and physical state which may be neither pleasurable nor objectionable but it is a state with which they are familiar and one that they, and not others, have determined. Many people think that a large part of addiction is created by this desire to be in a familiar physical and mental mood even if it is damaging to the body and mind. In a *USA Today* survey, four out of five smokers and nonsmokers alike believed nicotine is an addictive substance.

Other factors to consider for nicotine addiction are the dramatic decrease in the brain's reward function during withdrawal that causes animals to crave tobacco and eventually relapse (Epping-Jordan et al., 1998). Also recent research indicates that there may be a genetic predisposition to nicotine addiction that makes tobacco use harder to stop for some than for others. The suspect gene is the same reward pathway gene, DRD_2 A_1 allele, implicated in predisposition to alcoholism and other drug addictions (Spitz, 1998).

EPIDEMIOLOGY

One interesting note, in 1994 only 5% of Black high school seniors said they smoked on a daily basis compared to 22% of Whites. In focus groups, children said such things as "Smoking hurts stamina for sports," "Boys don't like girls who smoke," and "We believed the media about the dangers of cigarettes." But a 1997 survey found that the rate for Black teenagers had doubled.

TABLE 3–4   CIGARETTE USE IN THE UNITED STATES—1998

By Age	Ever Used	Used Past Year	Used Past Month
12-17	8 million	5 million	4 million
18-25	19 million	13 million	12 million
26-34	25 million	13 million	11 million
Over 35	100 million	36 million	33 million
Totals	**152 million**	**67 million**	**60 million**

1998 National Household Survey on Drug Abuse (SAMHSA, 1999)

TABLE 3–5   SMOKELESS TOBACCO USE IN THE UNITED STATES—1998

By Sex	Ever Used	Used Past Year	Used Past Month
Male	32 million	9 million	6.1 million
Female	6 million	1 million	0.6 million
Totals	**38 million**	**10 million**	**6.7 million**

National Household Survey on Drug Abuse 1998 (SAMHSA, 1999)

SIDE EFFECTS

Worldwide, in 1997, tobacco caused about 3.5 million premature deaths or 1 out of every 5 premature deaths. This figure will increase to 10 million annually in 20–30 years with 7 million of those deaths in developing countries. The average life span loss to those smokers who die in middle age (before the age of 70) will be 22 years. In China alone about three-quarters of a million smokers (mostly men) die prematurely each year (WHO, 1998).

In the United States, it is estimated that 390,000 smokers will die prematurely in the year 2000 and another 50,000 nonsmokers will die from secondhand smoke. The main reason for the extremely high figures is that often tobacco takes 20, 30, or even 40 years for its most dangerous effects, such as cardiovascular disease, respiratory impairment, and cancer, to become lethal. Most who die from smoking had been smoking more than 20 years, so the immediate warning signs of overdose—heart palpitations, blackouts, hangovers, rages, paranoia, and nausea—common with other psychoactive drugs are missing. Except for the coughing, dizziness, initial nausea, bad breath, green mucous, lower lung capacity, and lowered energy levels, there are no immediate flashing warning signs. Recognizing the warning signs of cocaine, heroin, or alcohol use is a very visceral, very immediate process. Those of tobacco are very subtle and slow. The dangerous side effects weigh directly against the pleasure received. With tobacco, that craving can only be countered by an intellectual appreciation of the long-term dangers. In most cases the crav-

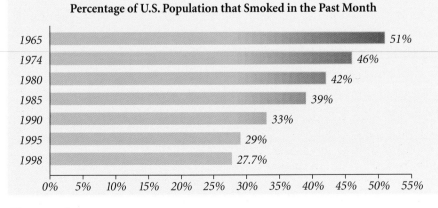

Percentage of U.S. Population that Smoked in the Past Month

1965	51%
1974	46%
1980	42%
1985	39%
1990	33%
1995	29%
1998	27.7%

Figure 3-6 •

Smoking rates in most other countries are higher than in the United States.

National Household Survey on Drug Abuse, 1998

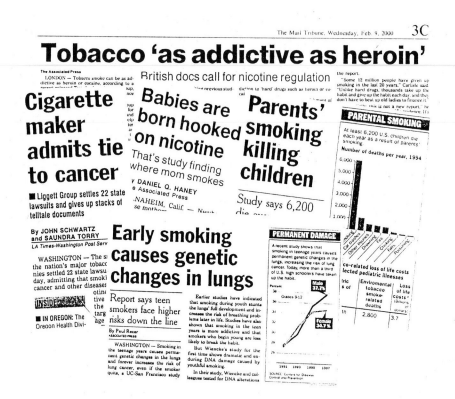

As research continues, the link between smoking and illness becomes overwhelming.

●●●

ing and fear of withdrawal win out over common sense.

Longevity

"I've smoked two packs a day for 36 years and I'm still alive. I'm active and I'm good at my job. In any case I'm not going to live forever, so why should I give up smoking?"

54-year-old smoker

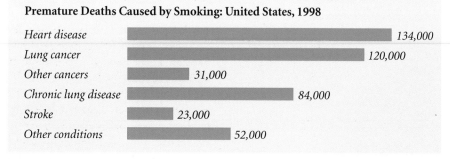

Premature Deaths Caused by Smoking: United States, 1998

Heart disease	134,000
Lung cancer	120,000
Other cancers	31,000
Chronic lung disease	84,000
Stroke	23,000
Other conditions	52,000

Figure 3-7 •

Total estimated premature deaths caused by smoking is 444,000 (CDC, 1999). The average life span of a two-pack-a-day smoker is eight years less than a nonsmoker.

The exceptional 75-year-old smoker who is healthy should not be seen as confirmation that smoking won't shorten life span or impair health. One has to look at the overall statistics. They show that, on average, a two-pack-a-day smoker will live eight years less than someone who doesn't smoke. Almost as important as these premature death statistics is the issue of quality of life. Because of breathing difficulties, poor circulation, and a

dozen other imbalances caused by smoking, a smoker will have more medical complications, be less able to participate in physical activity, and will not be able to live life to the fullest.

Smoking or chewing tobacco affects the body by interacting with the organs and tissues directly or indirectly through the central nervous system.

Cardiovascular Effects

Smoking accelerates the process of plaque formation and hardening of the arteries (atherosclerosis), the major cause of heart attacks, by increasing low-density fats, increasing blood coagulability, and triggering cardiac arrhythmias (irregular beatings of the heart). The inhaled carbon monoxide created by tobacco combustion also accelerates the process of athersclerosis. In addition since nicotine constricts blood vessels, it restricts blood flow and raises blood pressure increasing the risk of a stroke (ruptured blood vessel in the brain). The combination of nicotine and carbon monoxide also increases the risk of angina attacks (heart muscle spasms).

Respiratory Effects

About 85% of men with lung cancer and 75% of women with lung cancer smoke. The most likely culprits are the tars and other products of combustion that are inhaled by the smoker. Cigarette smokers also have a much higher rate of bronchopulmonary disease, such as emphysema, chronic bronchitis, and chronic obstructive pulmonary disease. In addition children who live with smokers have a much higher incidence of asthma, colds, and bronchitis from inhaling secondhand smoke. Finally, environmental pollutants, such as asbestos or volatile chemicals, greatly increase the rates of respiratory illness and cancer in smokers above the rates due to exposure from just smoking alone or breathing dirty air.

Cancer

The increase in lung cancer since the 1930s when the use of cigarettes

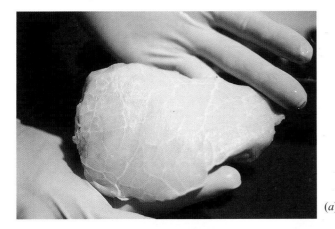

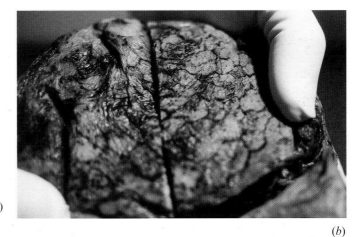

(a)

(b)

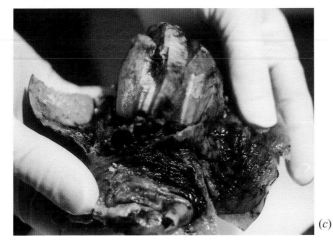

(c)

A normal lung (a) is pink and spongy. It is protected by the ribcage from external damage. Unfortunately smoking deposits tar, other chemicals, and irritants in the alveoli (air sacs) as well as destroying the cilia (fine hairs lining the membranes) that help remove foreign particles. The smoker's lung (b) is blackened by these deposits. Many of the chemicals in tobacco, particularly the tar, cause cancer (c). More than 100,000 people die prematurely from tobacco-induced lung cancer every year.

Courtesy of Leslie Parr

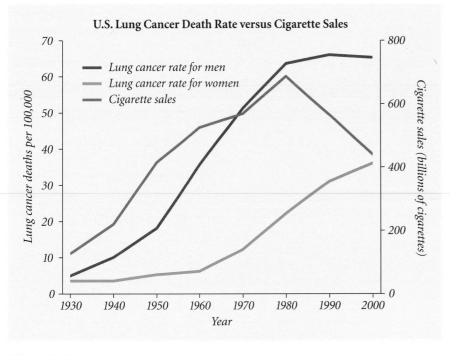

U.S. Lung Cancer Death Rate versus Cigarette Sales

Figure 3-8 •

Since it takes 10–40 years for lung cancer to develop, there is a delay in decreasing rates of lung cancer even though sales among men have declined.

started to accelerate is startling. The rate in men has gone up 15-fold and in women 9-fold. In the graph (Fig. 3-8), we have juxtaposed the per capita smoking rate from 1930 to the present next to the per capita death rate from lung cancer. As the chart shows, in 1988 lung cancer deaths in women surpassed deaths from breast cancer for the first time in history.

Studies at UCLA have shown precancerous alterations in bronchial epithelium occur not only from habitual cigarette smoking but also from habitual smoking of marijuana and/or cocaine (Barsky, Roth, Kleerup, Simmons, & Tashkin, 1998). Pipe and cigar smokers are less likely than cigarette smokers to get lung cancer but more likely than nonsmokers to get not only lung cancer but cancers of the larynx, mouth, and esophagus.

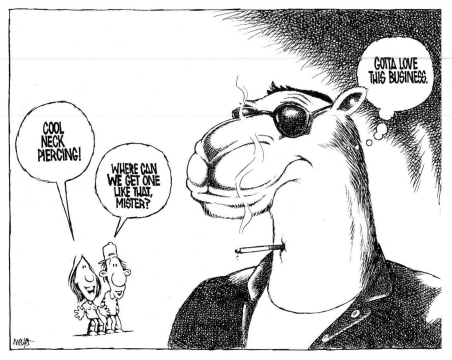

Fetal Effects

The carbon monoxide and nicotine in tobacco smoke reduces the oxygen-carrying capacity of a pregnant mother's blood, so less oxygen gets to the baby, contributing to a lower birth weight and a higher incidence of crib death (sudden infant death syndrome - SIDS). Research indicates that women who smoke heavily during pregnancy are twice as likely to miscarry and have spontaneous abortions as nonsmokers. In one study the offspring of mothers who smoked during pregnancy were four times more likely to have attention deficit/hyperactivity disorder (AD/HD) (Milberger, Biederman, Faraone, & Jones, 1998). There was also an increased risk of early onset conduct disorder and even drug dependence (Weissman, Warner, Wickramaratne, & Kandel, 1999).

Smokeless Tobacco Effects

Tobacco is as addicting in its smokeless form as in its smoked form, even though the nicotine takes 3–5 minutes to affect the central nervous system when chewed or pouched in the cheek compared to the 10 seconds it takes when inhaled from a cigarette. Strangely enough more of the nicotine reaches the bloodstream with smokeless tobacco and the rush is somewhat more intense. The effects of chewing are almost identical to the effects of smoking, including a slight increase in energy, alertness, blood pressure, and heart rate. In the case of tobacco, smoking limits the amount of nicotine that can be put in the body (one milligram from a cigarette) as compared to chewing (four milligrams or more).

The main advantage of smokeless tobacco over cigarettes is the protection it gives the lungs since no smoke is inhaled. Lung cancer rates and other respiratory problems drop dramatically. Unfortunately there are other problems with smokeless tobacco.

"I can't think of a more disgusting habit than chewing tobacco. I broke up with my boyfriend because he was always dripping tobacco juice, spitting, and had those awful brown stains on his clothing. Ugh."
17-year-old high school student

Smokeless tobacco is irritating to the tissues of the mouth and the digestive tract. Many users experience leukoplakia, a thickening, whitening, and hardening of tissues in the mouth. Their gums can become inflamed causing more dental problems, and although the risk of lung cancer is reduced compared to smoking, the risks of oral, pharynx, and esophageal cancers are increased. In addition, since blood vessels are constricted while either chewing or smoking, circulatory problems, the largest health hazard of smoking, are just as grave with smokeless tobacco.

Mental & Emotional Effects

Nicotine can be stimulating, relaxing, or even depressing, often depending on the mood of the smoker. People use it to get going in the morning, to mellow out after a meal, to get ready for bed, to steady their nerves, and even to conclude sex. Some of the emotional effects are related to the settings where tobacco is used: a person might feel more confident holding a cigarette while starting a conversation or talking on the phone to a client. But after continued use, tobacco's effectiveness at calming and relieving anxiety seems more associated with preventing nicotine withdrawal rather than acting as a true sedative. In fact nicotine addicts rarely identify their very first use of tobacco as pleasurable. The vast majority remembers very negative effects from their first exposure: headache, dizziness, nausea, coughing, etc. Yet they continued to use and developed addiction.

BENEFITS FROM QUITTING

A number of beneficial physiologic changes that occur on quitting are the following:

◇ within 36 hours, blood carbon monoxide levels return to normal;

◇ within 48 hours, nerve endings adjust to the absence of nicotine and the senses of smell and taste begin to come back;

◇ within a week, the risk of heart attack drops, breathing improves, and constricted blood vessels begin to relax;

◊ within 2 weeks to 3 months, circulation improves, lung function increases up to 30%, and the complexion looks healthy again;

◊ within 1–9 months, fatigue, coughing, sinus congestion, and shortness of breath decrease and the lungs increase their ability to handle mucus, thereby helping to clean themselves and reduce infection;

◊ within 5 years, the heart disease death rate returns to the rate for nonsmokers;

◊ within 10 years, the lung cancer death rate drops almost to the rate for nonsmokers, precancerous cells are replaced, and the incidence of other cancers decreases;

◊ within 10–15 years, the risk to all major diseases caused by smoking decreases to nearly that of those who have never smoked (WHO, 1998).

(Adapted from Glantz, 1992)

The potential benefits to the lung of quitting may not be so for those who started smoking as a teenager. Recent studies by John Wiencke of UC Medical Center in San Francisco showed that smoking in teenagers caused permanent genetic DNA damage to their lung cells leaving them forever at increased risk to lung cancer even if they quit smoking. Such damage was less likely among smokers who started their use in their 20s (Wiencke, Thurston, Kelsey, Varkonyi, & Wain, 1999).

Mentally there are other beneficial changes:

◊ Initially there is anxiety, anger, difficulty concentrating, increased appetite, and craving due to withdrawal.

◊ After two weeks most of these side effects disappear with the exception of craving and increased appetite.

THE TOBACCO INDUSTRY & TOBACCO ADVERTISING

The Business of Tobacco

Just a handful of companies control the tobacco market in the United States. Philip Morris (Marlboro®, Virginia Slims®, Basic®), R.J. Reynolds/Nabisco® (Winston®, Camel®, Salem®), American Brands (Carlton®, Lucky Strike®, Pall Mall®), British American Tobacco (Kool®), and U.S. Tobacco (Copenhagen®, Skoal®) account for more than 95% of sales ($46 billion in 1998). Over the past 20 years there has also been an aggressive expansion into foreign markets aided by the weakening and dissolution of state-owned and smaller private tobacco companies. Cigarette smoking is growing at a rate of 3% a year in developing countries. The United States consumes about 440 billion cigarettes annually. U.S. exports of cigarettes rose to 250 billion by 1996 but dropped to 151 billion in 1999 (U.S. Department of Agriculture, 1999).

In the 1980s, because of the ever-increasing cost of a pack of cigarettes, many manufacturers came out with generic brands that were cheaper and by 1993 accounted for 25% of U.S. cigarette sales. To win back some of that market, the big manufacturers lowered the prices on name brands.

Bidi cigarettes are made in India but sold in the United States. Their colorful packages seem aimed at children, mainly teenagers. Their nicotine content is 7% to 8% vs. 1% to 2% in American cigarettes. They are sold for $1.50 to $3.50 for a pack of 20 cigarettes.

Advertising

Advertising expenditures by the tobacco industry are over $1 billion a year with another $1.5 billion in giveaways, premiums, promotional allowances to retailers, and other items. Advertising works. As a result of the Joe Camel® advertising campaign, sales of Camels® to teenage smokers from the age of 12–18 more than tripled over a five-year period while the sales to adult Camel® smokers remained the same. The Joe Camel® campaign was finally dropped due to political and social pressure.

However, while the media focused on Joe Camel®, the most popular cigarettes among teenagers have been Marlboro® and Newport®. Among 12th graders in 1998,

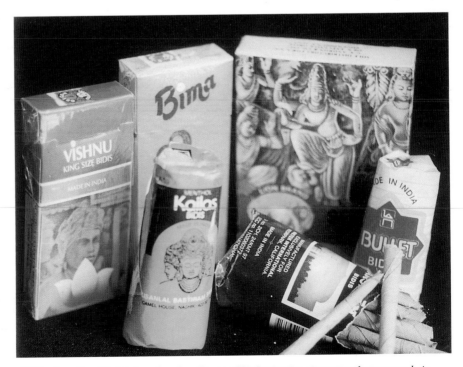

Oddly shaped and brightly colored packages of high-nicotine cigarettes that are made in India are called "bidis."

◇ 65.2 % smoked Marlboro®,

◇ 13.3% smoked Newport®,

◇ 9.6% smoked Camels®.

Ethnically the differences in brand preferences are dramatic.

◇ 58% of White 12th graders and 58% of Hispanic 12th graders preferred Marlboro®,

◇ 8% of Black high school students preferred Newport ®.

(Monitoring the Future, 1999)

Studies have shown that starting to smoke in the teen years is more addictive to the user than starting to smoke during adulthood. Also smokers who begin young are less likely to break the habit than adult onset smokers, making the teen market extremely attractive to cigarette manufacturers (Wiencke et al., 1999).

There is also evidence that because most smokers acquire their habit before the age of 20, tobacco companies have used advertising to appeal to these new young smokers. For example, in a confidential memo, one tobacco company advised its advertising department as follows:

"Thus, an attempt to reach young smokers, starters, should be based, among others, on the following major parameters:

◇ *Present the cigarette as one of a few initiations into the adult world.*

◇ *Present the cigarette as part of the illicit pleasure category of products and activities.*

◇ *In your ads, create a situation taken from the day-to-day life of the young smoker but in an elegant manner have this situation touch on the basic symbols of the growing-up, maturity process.*

◇ *To the best of your ability (considering some legal constraints), relate the cigarette to 'pot,' wine, beer, sex, etc.*

◇ *Don't [their emphasis] communicate health or health-related points."*

Antismoking advertising also works. In Massachusetts, when $70 million was spent in an antitobacco campaign on prime time television, sales of cigarettes dropped 20% compared to a national average drop of 3%.

Regulation

Recognizing that regulations and bad publicity could hurt sales, the U.S. tobacco industry created the Tobacco Merchants' Association and later the Tobacco Institute and the Council for Tobacco Research to lobby against laws they didn't like. They also used these organizations to mute criticism of tobacco and the tobacco industry with their own research, publicity, and information. This strategy is not unusual in business. Most industries have lobbying and public relations groups. What changed, starting in the late 1940s and '50s, was the mounting evidence that tobacco was extremely harmful and extremely addicting, highlighted by the first *Surgeon General's Report to the Nation* in 1967 on the dangers of smok-

Texas tobacco suit settled for $15 billion

By Robert Davis
and Doug Levy
USA TODAY

The tobacco industry will pay Texas about $15 billion in the nation's largest product liability settlement, which will be announced today in Austin.

The deal was finalized Thursday on the eve of a jury trial set to begin today.

Neither side would discuss specifics, but the tobacco industry is believed to have agreed to pay about $15 billion over 25 years to reimburse the state for treating smoking-related illnesses.

Florida's tobacco settlement last summer was $11 billion.

The deal is expected to include millions of dollars for anti-smoking programs and restrictions on advertising. A key theme: cutting sales to kids.

"It is inconceivable that anyone in the state of Texas will have any criticism of" the deal, said Ron Dusek, spokesman for Texas Attorney General Dan Morales; Dusek refused to discuss any aspects of the case.

Texas is the third state to settle its case against the industry, joining Florida and Mississippi.

Texas sued eight tobacco companies and three trade groups in 1996 for $8.6 billion. With damages, the lawsuit grew to $15 billion. The state accused the companies of fraud, controlling nicotine levels to cause addiction and trying to sell to children.

Texas is one of 40 states to sue the tobacco industry. Minnesota is set for trial next week.

The industry is trying to negotiate a "global settlement" in Washington that would trade $368.5 billion for some protec-

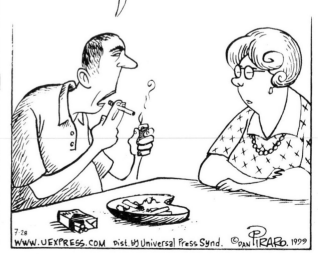

ing. Since that time there has been a continuing battle among the tobacco industry, Congress, smokers, and non-smokers about the legality, availability, and health hazards of smoking.

Laws & Lawsuits

Because of the coughing and tearing caused by secondhand smoke, as well as documented actual health problems, numerous laws have been passed at the state and federal levels prohibiting the use of tobacco products in a variety of spaces and buildings (e.g., sections of restaurants, airplanes, some businesses, federal and state buildings). From indifference to other peoples' habits in the early '80s to a powerful crusade in the '90s, public opinion has changed. Unfortunately tobacco has long been exempt from laws protecting the health of Americans. The principal law that has been superseded is the one that states that no substance that causes cancer may be sold for human consumption. A special statute was voted by Congress exempting tobacco from this law. In 1997 and 1998 tobacco companies gave $220 million in soft-money political contributions (money given to political parties rather than specific candidates)—$138 million to Republicans and $82 million to Democrats (White, 1999). Given the addictive nature of tobacco, some think that such contributions are the equivalent of marijuana or coca growers giving money to politicians to promote drug legalization.

By 1995 the Food and Drug Administration and the Clinton Administration were ready for a full-scale assault on the tobacco industry. The administration said its goal was to cut teenage smoking in half by sharply curtailing "the deadly temptations of tobacco and its skillful marketing" by the industry. The industry said the real aim of the antismoking forces and the new legislation was to outlaw smoking altogether. One of the themes of various tobacco industry campaigns was the right to choose. President Bill Clinton gave the FDA authority to regulate cigarettes because of their nicotine content; that is, because nicotine is addictive, it dam-

ages people's abilities to choose freely whether they want to smoke or not. The FDA declared cigarettes a drug, releasing material and memos from the tobacco industry itself showing that tobacco companies have long believed cigarettes are addictive, mainly because of nicotine. However, the industry countered FDA control in 1999 by claiming that since tobacco was so dangerous to health [sic], the FDA, which was supposed to regulate drugs beneficial to Americans, had no jurisdiction because all they would be able to do by law was outlaw cigarettes. These matters will be in courts for years to come.

The biggest assault on the tobacco industry has come from a number of state governments that are suing the tobacco companies. Some of the suits are for the extra cost of health care due to smoking. Other suits accuse the tobacco industry of manipulating nicotine levels to keep smokers addicted. Brown and Williamson, the nation's 5th largest manufacturer (Chesterfield®, Eve®), settled a lawsuit in 1996 agreeing to pay 5% of its pretax profits or $50 million a year toward programs that help people stop smoking.

$20 Million Awarded In Tobacco Trial in S.F.

▶ **SMOKER**
From Page 1

kowitz, a spokesman for R.J. Reynolds. He said there was no proof that Whiteley relied on statements made by the tobacco companies when she decided to smoke.

Despite the tobacco companies' attempt to "vilify" Whiteley, her lawyer, Madelyn Chaber of San Francisco, said the jury was swayed

To settle two major lawsuits and hopefully forestall further litigation, the major tobacco companies agreed to $40 billion and $206 billion settlements to help pay for the medical costs of tobacco-induced illnesses, to finance smoking prevention campaigns (particularly aimed at teenagers), and to support other state programs. The moneys are to be paid over a period of 25 years.

Secondhand Smoke

Besides the issue of the addictive nature of tobacco and nicotine, a main battle over smoking during the 1990s was over the issue of secondhand smoke (the smoke that is inhaled by nonusers in a room with smokers). It is estimated that one person dies from secondhand smoke (mostly from cardiovascular disease) for every eight smoker deaths. When the issue was first raised in the early 1980s, the evidence was scant but since then the U.S. Surgeon General's Office, the National Research Council, OSHA, and The International Agency for Research on Cancer have concluded that secondhand smoke does cause lung cancer and cardiovascular diseases. Other studies have connected secondhand smoke to other illnesses, including asthma and bronchitis in the children of smokers.

One of the reasons for the danger from secondhand smoke is that the side-stream smoke, mostly from a smoldering cigarette when the user is not inhaling, has higher concentrations of the substances, such as tar, that cause respiratory problems. So while secondhand smoke has small amounts of nicotine, it has 1–40 times the amount of carcinogens found in mainstream (inhaled) smoke.

In 1996 California, Utah, and Vermont, Flagstaff, Arizona, New York City, and Boulder, Colorado had banned smoking in all bars and restaurants despite warnings from the owners that business would drop. The results of a study showed that, in fact, revenues increased in four localities, stayed the same in four localities, and in only one did the rate of increase slow down but not decrease (Glantz & Charlesworth, 1999).

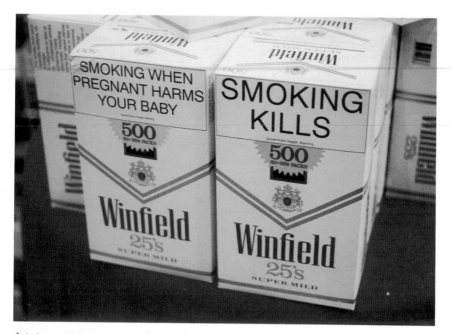

It is interesting to compare the warnings found on American cigarette packages and Australian cigarette packages. The Australians are willing to tell the complete truth about tobacco.

CONCLUSIONS

Stimulants seem like all-American drugs because initially they mimic virtues that are highly prized in our culture: the ability to work hard and stay up late, alertness, confidence, aggression, and mental acuity. Americans want a cup of coffee or a cigarette to wake up; more coffee at work to get going; a cola in the afternoon to carry on; an OTC product or prescription diet pill to hold the appetite down; a snort of methamphetamine to make the work less boring; a daily dose of Ritalin® to hold the kids in line; and a "rock" of "crack" to bring out the party animal. Instant energy, confidence, and gratification are sought.

Compare the use of stimulants to gain energy and confidence to natural methods where energy supplies are replenished through relaxation, sleep, naps, light morning exercise (e.g., tai chi), meditation, good nutrition, and a healthy lifestyle. The natural methods first create the energy supplies and then let them be spent. The chemical methods drain the body of its energy supplies, so it has to shut down to recover. The natural method works time after time. The chemical method causes tolerance and psychological dependence to develop, so the resulting excess use taxes the body's resources and can damage neurochemistry.

Perhaps a new American slogan should be, **"If you want to speed up, slow down."**

CHAPTER SUMMARY

General Classification

1. Uppers are central nervous system stimulants.

2. The seven principal stimulants are cocaine (including "crack"), amphetamines, amphetamine congeners (e.g., Ritalin® and diet pills), lookalike or over-the-counter stimulants, miscellaneous plant stimulants, caffeine, and nicotine.

General Effects

3. By increasing chemical and electrical activity in the central nervous system, stimulants increase energy, raise heart rate, blood pressure, and respiration; they make the user more alert, active, confident, anxious, restless, aggressive, and less hungry.

4. Uppers cause many of their effects by forcing the release of energy chemicals (particularly norepinephrine and epinephrine).

5. Most problems with stimulants occur when the body isn't given time to recover and its energy supply becomes depleted. The user can fall into a severe depression.

6. Cardiovascular side effects can include heart arrhythmias, constricted blood vessels, and heart disease.

7. Another set of problems with the stronger stimulants comes when the stimulated reward/pleasure center does not signal the need for food, drink, or sexual stimulation, resulting in malnutrition, dehydration, or a reduced sex drive.

8. Since stimulants reduce appetite, almost all of them are used to reduce weight, often causing various health problems.

9. Though stimulants initially increase confidence and induce a certain euphoria, excessive use of the stronger stimulants can cause severe neurotransmitter imbalance. A user can become paranoid,

have muscle tremors, become aggressive, and even become psychotic.

10. A major problem with all stimulants is their ability to induce rapid tolerance and ultimately major abuse and addiction problems.

Cocaine

11. Cocaine is noted for the intensity of its stimulation, its high price, and the speed with which it is metabolized in the body. It produces an intense craving and is highly addicting.

12. The coca leaf is chewed and the stimulating juice is absorbed through the stomach in 15–30 minutes. The refined cocaine hydrochloride can be snorted (2–5 minutes), injected (15–30 seconds), or drunk (15–30 minutes). Cocaine freebase ("crack," "rock") is smoked. Smoking is the fastest route to the brain, 7–10 seconds.

13. Cocaine is a topical anesthetic and is used for medical procedures, such as eye surgery, or to desensitize the pain of skin lesions.

14. Cocaine mimics and intensifies natural body functions and highs. The comedown is equally intense, so the user keeps taking the drug to stay up. The brain becomes sensitized to the memory of the pleasurable effects.

15. Cocaine as well as amphetamines initially delay orgasm and so are taken to try and enhance sexual activity but prolonged use eventually causes sexual dysfunction including a decrease in orgasm.

16. Cocaine, especially when used in combination with alcohol, can precipitate violence, often domestic violence.

17. Cocaine can also cause heart damage and damage to the fetus of a pregnant user.

18. Tolerance develops rapidly causing severe psychic dependence.

19. An overdose of cocaine can be the result of as little as 1/50 of a gram or as much as 1.2 grams or more. Most overdose reactions are not fatal but death can come from cardiac arrest, respiratory depression, and seizures.

20. Cocaine is often used in conjunction with other drugs.

21. The compulsion to use cocaine and methamphetamines is often caused by the desire to experience natural body functions such as extra energy, confidence, alertness, and euphoria artificially. The desire to escape mental pain and overcome a sense of hopelessness also makes a person use. People continue using because body chemistry has been changed by the drug, thus creating a compulsion to use.

Smokable Cocaine ("crack," freebase)

22. Freebase cocaine and "crack" are smokable forms of cocaine. "Crack" has more impurities.

23. Smoking freebase cocaine is more intense than snorting cocaine because when smoked in the freebase form, the drug reaches the brain more quickly, can be taken more often, and is more fat-soluble.

24. "Crack" cocaine causes many problems because of the economics of the drug. It is sold in smaller more affordable units but because of its quick metabolism and rapid addiction, its use quickly accelerates to $100–$300-a-day amounts and the profits are large.

Amphetamines

25. Amphetamines are very similar to cocaine, the main difference being that they are synthetic, longer acting, and cheaper to buy.

26. Amphetamines were originally prescribed to fight exhaustion, depression, narcolepsy, asthma, some forms of epilepsy, and obesity but were often taken for their mood-elevating and euphoric properties.

27. Prolonged use of amphetamines can induce paranoia, heart and blood vessel problems, twitches, increased body temperature, dehydration, and malnutrition.

28. Tolerance develops rapidly with amphetamines. Amphetamine and cocaine withdrawal causes physical and emotional depression, extreme irritability, nervousness, anergia, anhedonia, and craving.

Amphetamine Congeners

29. Many diet pills and mood elevators mimic the actions of amphetamines but are not quite as strong.

30. Currently congeners like Ritalin® and Cylert® are used in the treatment of attention deficit/hyperactivity disorders (AD/HD).

31. Diet pills can still cause many of the problems found with amphetamines and can be addicting. The diet pill combination of phentermine and fenfluramine or dexfenfluramine, called "fen-phen," was found to cause heart damage and was taken off the market.

Lookalike & Over-the-Counter (OTC) Stimulants

32. Lookalike drugs were popularized to take advantage of the desire for amphetamines and cocaine. They are composed of over-the-counter stimulants. Heavy use can cause heart and blood vessel problems as well as dependence.

Miscellaneous Plant Stimulants

33. Other plant stimulants, such as khat, betel nut, ephedra, and yohimbe, have been used by hundreds of millions of people, particularly in the Middle East and Africa, since ancient times. They are still used today.

34. A synthetic form of khat, methcathinone, is widely used in Russia and is being made in the United States.

Caffeine

35. Caffeine, particularly coffee, is the most popular stimulant in the world. Besides coffee, caffeine is

found in tea, chocolate (cocoa), caffeinated soft drinks, and a number of over-the-counter products.

36. Tolerance can develop with caffeine. Withdrawal symptoms, such as headaches, depression, sleep problems, and irritability do occur, particularly if consumption is more than five cups a day.

Tobacco & Nicotine

37. Nicotine (tobacco) is the most addicting psychoactive drug. In the United States, at least 46 million people are addicted to cigarettes compared to the 15 million addicted to alcohol.

38. Nicotine addiction causes more deaths than all the other psychoactive drugs combined.

39. One of the main reasons for tobacco's addictive nature, besides the slight stimulation it gives, is the need for the smoker's body to maintain a certain level of nicotine in the blood to avoid severe withdrawal symptoms.

40. Besides shortening a person's life span, tobacco lowers the quality of life.

41. Smokeless tobacco is as addicting and as damaging as tobacco that is smoked.

42. Lawsuits brought by state and federal governments in the United States, as well as individual or class action suits, are being won against the tobacco companies for increasing the addictive nature of their products and for the health damage caused by smoking.

Conclusions

43. Though stimulants initially boost many of the qualities we admire, they have a full share of side effects that cause damage when the substance is over used.

REFERENCES

Aldrich, M. R. (1994). Historical notes on women addicts. *Journal of Psychoactive Drugs, 26* (1), 61–64.

Amen, D. G. (1999). ADD and the Brain. *Amen Clinic for Behavioral Medicine (Online).*

Amen, D. G., Yantis, S., Trudeau, J., Stubblefield, M.S., & Halverstadt, J. S. (1997). Visualizing the firestorms in the brain: An inside look at the clinical and physiological connections between drugs and violence using brain SPECT imaging. *Journal of Psychoactive Drugs, 29*(4), 307–320.

APA (American Psychiatric Association). (1994). *Diagnostic and Statistical Manual of Mental Disorders* (4th ed.). Washington, DC: Author.

Barkley, R. A. (1998). Attention deficit/ hyperactivity disorder. *Scientific American, 9/10/98.*

Barsky, S. H., Roth, M. D., Kleerup, E. C., Simmons, M., & Tashkin, D. P. (1998). Histopathologic and molecular alterations in bronchial epithelium in habitual smokers of marijuana, cocaine, and/or tobacco. *Journal of the National Cancer Institute, 90*(16), 1198–1205.

Benowitz, N. L., & Fredericks, A. (1995). History of tobacco use. *Encyclopedia of Drugs and Alcohol* (Vol. 3, pp. 1032–1036).

Bibra, E. F. (1995). *Plant Intoxicants: Betel and related substances* (Chapter 16, pp.

207–216). Rochester, VT: Healing Arts Press.

Biederman, J., Wilens, T., Mick, E., Spencer, T., & Faraone, S. V. (1999). Pharmacotherapy of Attention-deficit/ Hyperactivity Disorder Reduces Risk for Substance Use Disorder. *Pediatrics, 104*(2).

Biederman, J. et al. (1996). A prospective 4-year follow-up study of attention deficit/hyperactivity and related disorders. *Archives of General Psychiatry, 53*(5), 437–446.

Biederman, J., Wilens, T, Mick, E., et al. (1997). Is AD/HD a risk factor for psychoactive substance use disorders? Findings from a four-year prospective follow-up study. *Journal of the American Academy of Child and Adolescent Psychiatry, 36*(1), 21–30.

Blum, K., Braverman, E. R., Cull, J. G., Holder, J. M., Luck, R., Lubar, J., Miller, D., & Comings, D. E. (2000). "Reward deficiency syndrome" (RDS): A biogenetic model for the diagnosis and treatment of impulsive addictive, and compulsive behaviors. *Journal of Psychoactive Drugs, 32*(1).

Bolla, K., Cadet, J. L., & Rothman, R. (1999). John Hopkins. *Journal of Neuropsychiatry and Clinical Neuroscience.*

Breiter, H., Gollub, R., Weisskoss, R., Kennedy, D., Makris, N, Berke, J., Goodman, J., Kantor, H., Gastfriend, D.,

Riorden, J., Mathew, R., Rosen, B., & Hyman, S. (1997). Acute effects of cocaine on human brain activity and emotion. *Neuron, 19,* 591–611.

BDF. (1999). Gutkha. British Dental Health Foundation on the Internet.

Brookoff, D., O'Brien, K. K., Cook, C. S., Thompson, T. D., & Williams, C. (1997). Characteristics of Participants in Domestic Violence: Assessment at the Scene of Domestic Assault. *JAMA, 277* (17), 1369–1372.

Calkins, R. F. , Alkan, & Hussain. (1995). Methcathinone: The next illicit stimulant epidemic? *Journal of Psychoactive Drugs, 27*(3), 277–285.

CDC (Centers for Disease Control). (1999). Cigarette smoking-related mortality. TIPS, Tobacco Information and Prevention Source. *http://www.cdc.gov/ tobacco/mortali.htm.*

Childress, A. R., McElgin, W., Mozley, D., Reivich, M., & O'Brien, G. (1996). Brain correlates of cue-induced cocaine and opiate craving. *Society for Neuroscience Abstracts 22:365.5.*

Coffee Science Source. (1998). Coffee facts and figures. *http://www.coffeescience. org/factrend.html.*

COHIS. (1999). Caffeine. *http://www.bu. edu/chois/subsabse/caffeine/about.htm# whati.*

Comings, D. E., Wu, S., Chiu, C., et al. (1996). Polygenic inheritance of

Tourette syndrome, stuttering, attention deficit hyperactivity, conduct, and oppositional defiant disorder: The additive and subtractive effect of the three dopaminergic genes-DRD$_2$, D beta H, and DAT$_1$. *American Journal of Medical Genetics, 6*(3), 264–288.

Connolly, H. M., Crary, J. L., McGoon, M. D., et al. (1997). Valvular heart disease associated with fenfluramine-phentermine. *New England Journal of Medicine, 337*(9).

DEA (Drug Enforcement Administration). (1998). *NNICC Report on the Supply of Illicit Drugs to the United States. http://www.usdoj.gov/dea/pubs/intel/nni cc97.htm.*

Dunlop, E., & Johnson, B. D. (1992). The setting for the crack era: Macro forces, micro consequences (1960–1992). *Journal of Psychoactive Drugs, 24*(4), 307–322.

Edlin, B. R., Irwin, K. L., & Faruque, S. (1994). Intersecting epidemics: Crack cocaine use and HIV infection among inner-city young adults. *New England Journal of Medicine, 331*, 1422–1427.

Ellinwood, E. H. (1973). Amphetamine and stimulant drugs. In *Drug use in America: problem in perspective. Second report. Marijuana and Drug Abuse Commission,* 140–157.

Epping-Jordan, M. P., Watkins, S. S., Koob, G. F., & Markou, A. (1998). Dramatic decreases in brain reward function during nicotine withdrawal. *Nature, 393*(6680), 76–79.

Federal Bureau of Prisons. (1997). *http://www.bop.gov.*

Foreman, R., Klein, J., Barks, J., et al. (1994). Prevalence of fetal exposure to cocaine in Toronto, 1990–1991. *Clinical Investment Medicine, 17*(3), 206–211.

Fowler, J. S., Volkow, N. D., Wang, G. J., et al. (1996). Brain monoamine oxidase A inhibition in cigarette smokers. *Proceedings of the National Academy of Sciences, 93,* 14065–14069.

Freud, S. (1884). *Uber Coca.* In R. Byck, (1974). *The Cocaine Papers-Sigmund Freud.* New York: Stonehill.

Fukui, S., Wada, K., & Iyo, M. (1991). History and current use of methamphetamine in Japan. In S. Fukui et al. (Eds.), Cocaine and methamphetamine: Behavioral toxicology, clinical pharmacology and epidemiology. Tokyo: Drug Abuse Prevention Center.

Giannini, A. J., Burge, H., Shaheen, J. M., & Price, W. A. (1986). Khat: Another drug of abuse. *Journal of Psychoactive Drugs, 18*(2), 155–158.

Glantz, S. A. (1992). *Tobacco: Biology & Politics.* Waco, TX: Health Edco.

Glantz, S. A., & Charlesworth, A. (1999). Tourism and hotel revenues before and after passage of smoke-free restaurant ordinances. *JAMA, 281,* 1911–1918.

Gold, M. S., & Miller, N. S. (1997). Cocaine (and crack): Neurobiology. In J. H. Lowinson, P. Ruiz, R. B. Millman, & J. G. Langrod (Eds.), *Substance Abuse: A Comprehensive Textbook* (3rd ed., pp. 181–198). Baltimore: Williams & Wilkins.

Gold, M. S., & Herkov, M. J. (1998). The pharmacology of cocaine, crack and other stimulants. In A. W. Graham & T. K. Schultz, T. K. (Eds.), *Principles of Addiction Medicine* (2nd ed., pp. 137–145). Chevy Chase, MD: American Society of Addiction Medicine, Inc.

Goldstein, A. (1994). *Addiction: From Biology to Drug Policy* (pp. 155–163, 179–180). New York: W.H. Freeman and Company.

Goldstein, P. J., Ouellet, L. J., & Fendrick, M. (1992). From bag brides to skeezers: a historical perspective on sex-for-drugs behavior. *Journal of Psychoactive Drugs, 24*(2), 349–362.

Goudie, A., & Newton, T. (1985). The puzzle of drug-induced taste aversion: Comparative studies with cathinone and amphetamine. *Psychopharmacology, 87,* 328–333.

Greden, J. F., & Walters, A. (1997). Caffeine. In J. H. Lowinson, P. Ruiz, R. B. Millman, & J. G. Langrod (Eds.), *Substance Abuse: A Comprehensive Textbook* (3rd ed.). Baltimore: Williams & Wilkins.

Greenbaum, E. (1993). Blackened bronchoalveolar lavage fluid in crack smokers, a preliminary study. *American Journal of Clinical Pathology, 100,* 481–487.

Grinspoon, L., & Bakalar, J. B. (1985). *Cocaine: A Drug and Its Social Evolution.* New York: Basic Books, Inc.

Guttmacher, H. (1885). New medications and therapeutic techniques. Concerning the different cocaine preparations and their effects. *Vienna Medical Press.* In R. Byck, (1974), *The Cocaine Papers-Sigmund Freud.* New York: Stonehill.

Hamid, A. (1992). The developmental cycle of a drug epidemic: The cocaine smoking epidemic of 1981–1991. *Journal of Psychoactive Drugs, 24*(4), 337–348.

Harris Poll. (1999). *Relapse of compulsive gamblers. USA Today, 1999.*

Harler, C. R. (1984). Tea production. *Ency-*

clopaedia Britannica (Vol. 18, pp. 16–19). Chicago: Encyclopaedia Britannica.

Horner, B. R., & Scheibe, K. E. (1997). Prevalence and implications of attention deficit/hyperactivity disorder among adolescents in treatment for substance abuse. *Journal of the American Academy of Child and Adolescent Psychiatry. 36*(1), 30–36.

JACC. (1999). Fen-phen follow up. *Journal of the American College of Cardiology, 34*(7).

Jensen, P. (1999). Effectiveness of AD/HD therapies. American Medical Association's (NIH study). *Archives of General Psychiatry, Dec. 1999.*

Jeri, F. R., Sanchez, C., Del Pozo, T., & Fernandez, M. (1992). The syndrome of coca paste. *Journal of Psychoactive Drugs, 24*(2). 173–182.

Kahn, M. A., Herzog, C. A., St. Peter, J. V., et al. (1998). The prevalence of cardiac valvular insufficiency assessed by transthoracic echocardiography in obese patients treated with appetite-suppressant drugs. *New England Journal of Medicine, 339*(11).

Kalix, P. (1994). Khat, an Amphetamine-Like Stimulant. *Journal of Psychoactive Drugs, 26*(1), 69–73.

Karch, S. B. (1997). *A Brief History of Cocaine.* Boca Raton, FL: CRC Press.

Karch, S. B. (1996). *The Pathology of Drug Abuse.* Boca Raton, FL: CRC Press.

Kelz, M. B., Chen, J., Carlezon, W. A., et al. (1999). Expression of the transcription factor FosB in the brain controls sensitivity to cocaine. *Nature, 401,* 272–276.

King, G. R. & Ellinwood, E. H. (1997). Amphetamines and other stimulants. In J. H. Lowinson, P. Ruiz, R. B. Millman, & J. G. Langrod (Eds.), *Substance Abuse: A Comprehensive Textbook* (3rd ed.). Baltimore: Williams & Wilkins.

Klebanoff, M. A., Levine, R. J., DeSimonian, R., Clemens, J. D., & Wilkins, D. G. (1999). Maternal serum paraxanthine, a caffeine metabolite, and the risk of spontaneous abortion. *New England Journal of Medicine, 341*(22), 1639–1644.

Klesges, R. C., Meyers, A. W., Klesges, L. M., & LaVasque, M. E. (1989). Smoking, body weight, and their effects on smoking behavior: A comprehensive review of the literature. Psychological Bulletin, 106, 204–230.

Kuhar, M. J. (1995). Cola/Cola Drinks. In J. H. Jaffe (Ed.), *Encyclopedia of Drugs and Alcohol* (Vol. I, pp. 251–252). New

York: MacMillan Library Reference USA, Simon & Schuster MacMillan.

Landry, M. (1992). An overview of cocaethylene. *Journal of Psychoactive Drugs, 24*(3), 273–276.

Lichtblau, E., & Schrader, E. (1999). U.S. fears it badly underestimated cocaine production in Colombia. *Los Angeles Times (12-1-99).*

Marnell, T. (Ed.). (1997). *Drug Identification Bible.* Denver: Drug Identification Bible.

Mayo Clinic. (1999). New fen-phen study finds heart-valve disease may improve after stopping drugs. *Mayo Clinic Proceedings, Dec, 1999. http://www.mayo. edu/comm/mcr/news/news_880.html.*

Milberger, S., Biederman, J., Faraone, S. V., & Jones, J. (1998). Further evidence of an association between maternal smoking during pregnancy and attention deficit hyperactivity disorder: Findings from a high-risk sample of siblings. *Journal of Clinical Child Psychology, 27,* 352–358.

Miller, D., & Blum, K. (1996). Overload: *Attention Deficit Disorder and the Addictive Brain.* Kansas City: Andrews and McMeel.

Miller, M., & Kozel, N. (1995). Am phetamine epidemics. In J. H. Jaffee (Ed.), *Encyclopedia of Drugs and Alcohol* (Vol. I, pp. 110–117). New York: Simon & Schuster MacMillan.

Monardes, N. (1577). *Joyfull Newes Out of the Newe Founde Worlde.* Translated by Frampton, J. Reprinted in 1967. New York, AMS Press, Inc.

Monitoring the Future. (1999). Cigarette brands smoked by American teens. *http://www.umich.edu/~newsinfor/.*

Morgan, J. P., Wesson, D. R., Puder, K. S., & Smith, D. E. (1987). Duplicitous drugs: The history and recent status of lookalike drugs. *Journal of Psychoactive Drugs, 19*(1), 21–31.

National Soft Drink Association. (1999). Soft Drink Facts. *http://www.mariec @nsda.com.*

NIDA (National Institute of Drug Abuse). (1998). Current Trends in drug use worldwide. *NIDA Notes, 13*(2).

NIH (National Institutes of Health). (1998). Diagnosis and treatment of attention deficit hyperactivity disorder: Consensus development conference statement. *http://www.NIH.com.*

NIMH (National Institute of Mental Health). (1999). *Attention Deficit/ Hyperactivity Disorder. NIH Publication No. 96–357.2.*

O'Brien, R., Cohen, S., Evans, G., & Fine, J. (1992). *The Encyclopedia of Drug Abuse* (2nd ed.). New York: Facts on File.

Perkins, K. A. (1993). Weight gain following smoking cessation. *Journal of Consulting Clinical Psychology, 61,* 768–777.

Randall, T. (1992). Cocaine, alcohol mix in body to form even longer lasting, more lethal drugs. *JAMA, 267,* 1043–1044.

Ricaurte, B. et al. (1997). Reductions in brain dopamine and serotonin transporters detected in humans previously exposed to repeated high doses of methcathinone using PET. *Society for Neuroscience Abstracts, 22,* 1915. Also in *NIDA Notes, 11*(5).

Richards, J. B., Baggot, M. J., Sabol, K. E., & Seiden, L. S. (1999). A high-dose methamphetamine regimen results in long-lasting deficits on performance. *Journal of Psychoactive Drugs, 31*(4).

SAMHSA. (1999). *Summary of findings from the 1998 National Household Survey on Drug Abuse.* Rockville, MD: Substance Abuse and Mental Health Services, Office of Applied Studies.

Schmitz, J. M., Schneider, N. G., & Jarvik, M. E. (1997). Nicotine. In J. H. Lowinson, P. Ruiz, R. B. Millman, & J. G. Langrod (Eds.), *Substance Abuse: A Comprehensive Textbook* (3rd ed., pp. 276–290). Baltimore, MD: Williams & Wilkins.

Shively, B. (1999). Fen-phen follow up. *Circulation, Oct, 1999.*

Siegel, R. K. (1992). Cocaine freebase use: A new smoking disorder. *Journal of Psychoactive Drugs, 24*(2), 183–209.

Silverman, K., & Griffiths, R. R. (1995). Coffee. In J. H. Jaffee (Ed.), *Encyclopedia of Drugs and Alcohol* (Vol. I, pp. 250–251).

Silverman, K., & Griffiths, R. R. (1995). Tea. In J. H. Jaffee (Ed.), *Encyclopedia of Drugs and Alcohol* (Vol. III, pp. 1018–1019).

Slade, J. (1992). The tobacco epidemic: Lessons from history. *Journal of Psychoactive Drugs, 24*(2), 99–110.

Smith, D. E., & Wesson, D. R. (1985). *Treating the Cocaine Abuser.* Center City, MN: Hazelden.

Snyder, S. H. (1996). *Drugs and the Brain.* New York: W.H. Freeman and Sons.

Spitz, M. (3-5-98). Gene can help smokers kick the habit. *San Francisco Chronicle,* A4.

Stein, E. A., Pankiewicz, J., Harsch, H. H., et al. (1998). Nicotine-induced limbic cortical activation in the human brain: A functional MRI study. *American Journal of Psychiatry 155*(8), 1009–1015.

Tardiff, K, Marzuk, P. M., Leon, A. C., Hirsch, C. S., Stajic, M., Portera, L., & Hartwell, N. (1994). Homicide in New York City: Cocaine use and firearms. *JAMA 272,* 43–46.

Tinsley, J. A., & Wadkins, D. D. (1998). Over-the-counter stimulants: abuse and addiction. *Mayo Clinic Proceedings, 73*(10), 977–982.

U.S. Department of Agriculture. (1999). Tobacco facts. *U.S. Department of Agriculture's Economic and Statistics System.*

U.S. Department of Justice. (1992). *Khat Factsheet.* Drug Enforcement Administration, Intelligence Division.

Volkow, N.D. Fowler, J. S., Wang, G. J., et al. (1997). Relationship between subjective effects of cocaine and dopamine transporter occupancy. *Nature, 386,* 827–830.

Von Tschudi, J. (1854). Travels in Peru. In S. B. Karch, (1996). *The Pathology of Drug Abuse* (pp. 2–3). Boca Raton, FL: CRC Press.

Weil, A., & Rosen, W. (1993). *From Chocolate to Morphine.* Boston: Houghton Mifflin Company.

Weissman, M. M., Warner, V., Wickramaratne, P. J., & Kandel, D. B. (1999). Maternal smoking during pregnancy and psychopathology in offspring followed to adulthood. *Journal of the American Academy of Child and Adolescent Psychiatry, 38,* 892–899.

Wesson, D. R., Smith, D. E., & Steffens, S. C. (1992). *Crack and ice: Treating smokable stimulant abuse.* Center City, MN: Hazelden.

White, B. (1-11-99). Soft money donations soared despite ongoing investigations. *Washington Post,* A17.

WHO (World Health Organization). (1997). The smoking epidemic: A fire in the Global Village. WHO Press Release: *http://www.who.ch/.*

WHO. (1998). Tobacco epidemic: Health dimensions. WHO Fact Sheet: *http://www.who.ch/.*

Wiencke, J. K., Thurston, S. W., Kelsey, K. T., Varkonyi, A., & Wain, J. C. (1999). *Journal of the National Cancer Institute, 91*(7), 614–619.

Zhou, F. C., & Bledsoe, S. (1996). Methamphetamine causes rapid varicosis, perforation and definitive degeneration of serotonin fibers: An immunocytochemical study of serotonin transporter. *Neuroscience Net, Vol. 1,* Article #00009.

Downers:
Opiates/Opioids &
Sedative-Hypnotics

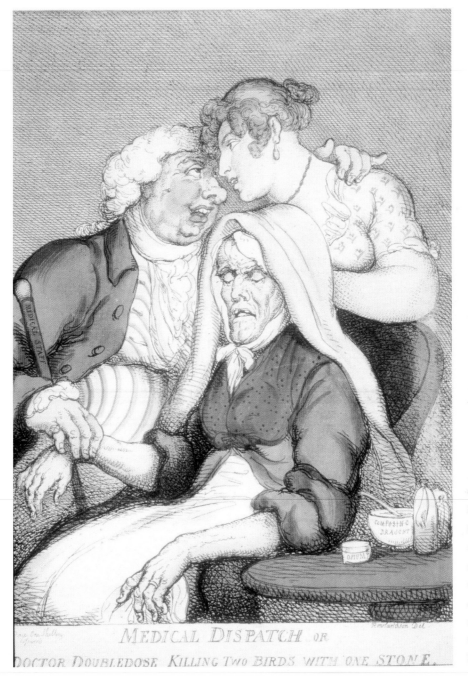

MEDICAL DISPATCH OR
DOCTOR DOUBLEDOSE KILLING TWO BIRDS WITH ONE STONE.

T his nineteenth century illustration satirizes the uncontrolled use of opioids by physicians. Physician-induced opiate (usually morphine) addiction was most common in the late nineteenth and twentieth centuries.

Courtesy of the National Library of Medicine, Bethesda

GENERAL CLASSIFICATION

- **Major Depressants:** The three major downers (depressants) are opiates/opioids, sedative-hypnotics, and alcohol *(see Chapter 5)*.
- **Minor Depressants:** The four minor downers (depressants) are skeletal muscle relaxants, antihistamines, over-the-counter downers, and lookalike downers.

OPIATES/OPIOIDS

- **Classification:** Opiates are natural or semisynthetic derivatives of the opium poppy. Opioids are synthetic derivatives of the opium poppy.
- **History of Use** *(see Chapter 1)*: The efficiency of different routes of administration helps determine the intensity of effects and abuse potential.
- **Effects of Opioids:** Most opioids, such as opium, morphine, and heroin, control pain and possibly induce pleasure. In the process they disrupt the satiation switch. The drugs also suppress coughs and control diarrhea. The opioids' manipulation of naturally occurring neurotransmitters causes the effects.
- **Side Effects of Heroin & Other Opioids:** These drugs create problems because of side effects, increased tolerance, tissue dependence, and severe withdrawal.
- **Additional Problems with Heroin & Other Opioids:** Fetal effects, overdose, drug contamination, dirty needles, high cost, sexually transmitted diseases, abscesses, polydrug use problems, and especially addiction often occur with these drugs.
- **Morphine & Heroin:** Morphine is the standard for pain relief; heroin causes the most social and health problems.
- **Other Opioids:** Codeine, hydrocodone (Vicodin®), methadone, meperidine (Demerol®), and other analgesics (painkillers) are also widely used.

SEDATIVE-HYPNOTICS

- **Classification:** Benzodiazepines, e.g., alprazolam (Xanax®) and diazepam (Valium®), are the most frequently prescribed sedative-hypnotics. Sedatives are calming drugs, whereas hypnotics are sleep-inducing drugs.
- **History:** Calming drugs have always been desired. Sedative-hypnotics have ranged from bromides and chloral hydrate to barbiturates and benzodiazepines.
- **Use, Misuse, Abuse, & Addiction:** Society's attitudes towards sedative-hypnotics swing between avid acceptance and wariness of addictive potential. Misuse and abuse of sedative hypnotics occur due to a variety of reasons.
- **Benzodiazepines:** These sedative-hypnotics were developed as safe alternatives to barbiturates but tolerance, addiction, withdrawal, and overdose still exist. These drugs can impair memory
- **Barbiturates:** Since 1900 more than 2,500 barbiturate compounds were developed (e.g., Seconal®, phenobarbital); they were widely used and abused.
- **Other Sedative-Hypnotics:** These drugs, prescribed for anxiety and other problems, were also abused for their psychic effects. GHB has been abused at "rave" and dance parties.

OTHER PROBLEMS WITH DEPRESSANTS

- **Drug Interactions:** Using two or more downers at one time can lead to overdose. Cross-tolerance and cross-dependence also develop.
- **Misuse & Diversion:** Two hundred million doses of prescription drugs are diverted to illicit channels each year in the United States. Besides diversion, there are problems such as polydrug use, synergism, cross-tolerance, and cross-dependence.
- **Economics:** Americans spent $91 billion on prescription drugs in 1999. Of the $3^{1}/_{2}$ billion prescriptions written, approximately 250 million were for psychoactive drugs, mostly downers. In addition they spent $15–$20 billion each year on over-the-counter medications. Some of the most common are antihistamines, sleep aids, nondepressant analgesics, and anti-inflammatories (PhRMA, 1999).

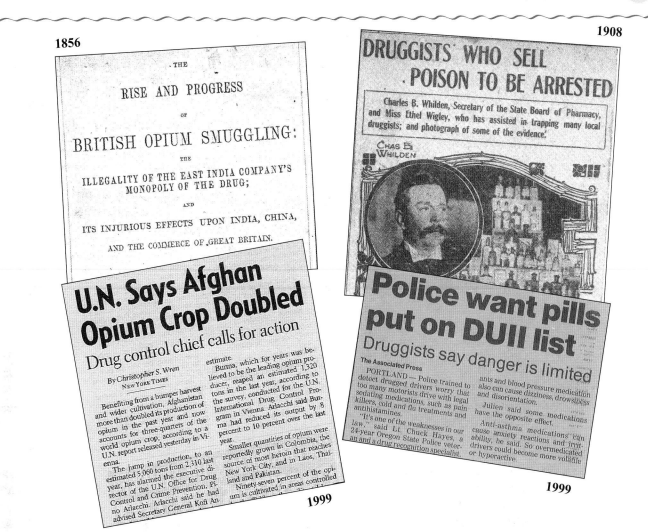

1856

1908

DRUGGISTS WHO SELL POISON TO BE ARRESTED

Charles B. Whilden, Secretary of the State Board of Pharmacy, and Miss Ethel Wigley, who has assisted in trapping many local druggists; and photograph of some of the evidence.

U.N. Says Afghan Opium Crop Doubled

Drug control chief calls for action

By Christopher S. Wren
NEW YORK TIMES

Benefiting from a bumper harvest and wider cultivation, Afghanistan more than doubled its production of opium in the past year and now accounts for three-quarters of the world opium crop, according to a U.N. report released yesterday in Vienna.

The jump in production, to an estimated 5,060 tons from 2,310 last year, has alarmed the executive director of the U.N. Office for Drug Control and Crime Prevention, Pino Arlacchi. Arlacchi said he had advised Secretary General Kofi An-

estimate.

Burma, which for years was believed to be the leading opium producer, reaped an estimated 1,320 tons in the last year, according to the survey, conducted for the U.N. International Drug Control Program in Vienna. Arlacchi said Burma had reduced its output by 8 percent to 10 percent over the last year.

Smaller quantities of opium were reportedly grown in Colombia, the source of most heroin that reaches New York City, and in Laos, Thailand and Pakistan.

Ninety-seven percent of the opium is cultivated in areas controlled

1999

Police want pills put on DUII list

Druggists say danger is limited

The Associated Press

PORTLAND — Police trained to detect drugged drivers worry that too many motorists drive with legal sedating medications, such as pain killers, cold and flu treatments and antihistamines.

"It's one of the weaknesses in our law," said Lt. Chuck Hayes, a 24-year Oregon State Police veteran and a drug recognition specialist.

ants and blood pressure medication also can cause dizziness, drowsiness and disorientation.

Julien said some medications have the opposite effect.

Anti-asthma medications can cause anxiety reactions and irritability, he said. So overmedicated drivers could become more volatile or hyperactive.

1999

GENERAL CLASSIFICATION

"Not only did nothing feel bad, everything felt good; I mean no physical pain; nothing on my mind weighing me down. Everything was just light, fluffy, and warm."
20-year-old male heroin addict

Downers depress the overall functioning of the central nervous system to induce sedation, muscle relaxation, drowsiness, and even coma (if used to excess). They also often cause disinhibition of impulses and emotions. Unlike uppers that release and enhance the body's natural stimulatory neurochemicals, depressants produce their effects through a wide range of biochemical processes at different

sites in the brain and spinal cord as well as in other tissues and organs outside the central nervous system.

Some depressants mimic the actions of the body's natural sedating or inhibiting neurotransmitters (e.g., endorphins, enkephalins, GABA) whereas others directly suppress the stimulation centers of the brain. Still others work in ways scientists haven't yet fully understood. Because of these variations, the depressants are grouped into a number of subclasses based on their chemistry, medical use, and legal classification.

The three major classes of depressants are opiates/opioids, sedative-hypnotics, and alcohol. The four minor classes of depressants are skeletal muscle relaxants, antihistamines, over-

the-counter sedatives, and lookalike sedatives.

MAJOR DEPRESSANTS

OPIATES/OPIOIDS

Opiates and opioids, such as morphine, codeine, hydrocodone (Vicodin®), oxycodone (Percodan®), methadone, propoxyphene (Darvon®), and even heroin, were developed for the treatment of acute pain, diarrhea, coughs, and a number of other illnesses. Most illicit users take these drugs to experience euphoric effects, to avoid emotional and physical pain, and to suppress withdrawal symptoms.

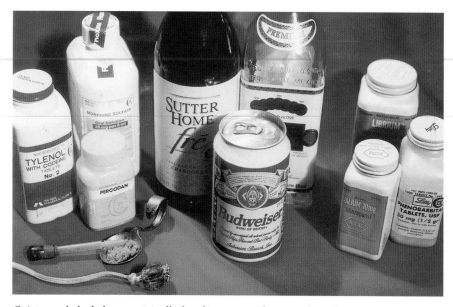

Opiates and alcohol were originally found in nature, whereas sedative-hypnotics were created in laboratories.

SEDATIVE-HYPNOTICS

Sedative-hypnotics, also referred to as solid alcohol, represent a wide range of synthetic chemical substances developed to treat nervousness and insomnia. The first, barbituric acid, was created in 1864 by Dr. Adolph Von Bayer. Other barbiturates followed (phenobarbital, Seconal®) until more than 2,500 had been created. Bromides, paraldehyde, and chloral hydrate were also widely used until the late 1940s and occasionally until the '80s. Chloral hydrate is still used. Since 1950 dozens of different sedative-hypnotics, such as Miltown® (meprobamate), Doriden®, Quaalude®, Mandrax® (banned), Rohypnol®(banned), and especially benzodiazepines, e.g., Valium® and Xanax®, have been created. All have toxic side effects and can cause tissue dependence. Benzodiazepines are the most widely used prescription drugs although antidepressants such as Prozac® have taken over a substantial share of the market.

ALCOHOL (*see Chapter 5*)

Alcohol, the natural by-product of fermented plant sugars or starches, is the oldest psychoactive drug in the world. It has been widely used over the centuries for social, cultural, and religious occasions. It is used for a number of medical remedies, from sterilizing wounds to lessening the risk of heart attacks. Because of its overall depressant effect, this liquid sedative has been used to reduce stress and lower inhibitions. Abuse also makes alcohol the world's most destructive drug in terms of health consequences, such as cirrhosis of the liver, mental deterioration, ulcers, and impotence. Social consequences of alcohol abuse include violence, crime, absenteeism, marital problems, and automobile accidents. In the United States alone it is estimated that 48 million Americans drink at least once a week while anywhere from 12–14 million are active problem drinkers and alcoholics, depending on one's definition of alcohol abuse and addiction (SAMHSA, 1999).

MINOR DEPRESSANTS

SKELETAL MUSCLE RELAXANTS

Centrally acting skeletal muscle relaxants include carisoprodol (Soma®), chlorzoxazone (Parafon Forte®), cy-clobenzaprine (Flexeril®), and metha-carbamol (Robaxin®). They are synthetically developed central nervous system depressants aimed at areas of the brain responsible for muscle coordination and activity. They are used to treat muscle spasms and pain. Whereas the current abuse of these products is rare, their overall depressant effects on all parts of the central nervous system produce reactions similar to those caused by other abused depressants. Recently carisoprodol has been abused.

ANTIHISTAMINES

Antihistamines, found in hundreds of prescription and over-the-counter cold and allergy medicines, including Benadryl®, Actifed®, and Tylenol P.M. Extra®, are synthetic drugs that were developed during the 1930s and 1940s for treatment of allergic reactions, ulcers, shock, rashes, motion sickness, and even symptoms of Parkinson's Disease (PDR, 1999). In addition to blocking the release of histamine, these drugs cross the blood-brain barrier to induce the common and oftentimes potent side effect of depression of the central nervous system resulting in drowsiness. Even antihistamines are occasionally abused for their depressant effects.

OVER-THE-COUNTER DOWNERS

Over-the-counter depressants, such as Nytol®, Sleep-Eze®, and Sominex®, are sold legally in stores without the need for a prescription. Depressants that were used in the 1880s became marketed as sleep aids or sedatives in the twentieth century. Scopolamine in low doses, antihistamines, bromide derivatives, and even alcohol constitute the active sedating components in many of these products. As with other downer drugs, these products are occasionally abused for their sedating effects.

LOOKALIKE DOWNERS

Lookalike sedatives were advertised along with lookalike stimulants in the early 1980s. The great commercial success of the lookalike stimulants encouraged shady drug manufacturers to sell products that looked like prescription downers. These companies took legally available antihistamines and packaged them in tablets and capsules so they resembled restricted depressants, such as Quaalude®, Valium®, and Seconal®. As with the other antihistamines, lookalike sedatives cause drowsiness as a side effect, thereby mimicking some of the effects of more potent downers. They are rarely found nowadays except in magazine ads for legal downers.

OPIATES/OPIOIDS

Opiates/opioids, some of the oldest and best documented groups of drugs, have been the source of continual and occasionally explosive worldwide problems, e.g., nineteenth century Opium Wars in China, the rise of drug crime cartels, drug gangs in Mexico, and the spread of AIDS and hepatitis C from infected needles. Heroin receives the most publicity but other opiates/opioids, including hydrocodone, codeine, meperidine (Demerol®), and fentanyl, also create problems and can be used compulsively.

In the 1970s the discovery of the body's own natural opiate painkillers, endorphins and enkephalins, significantly changed our understanding of opiates/opioids as well as the whole field of addictionology, biochemical research, and pain management (Goldstein, 1994).

CLASSIFICATION

OPIUM, OPIATES, & OPIOIDS

Opium is processed from the milky fluid of the unripe seed pod of the opium poppy plant (*Papaver somniferum*). It is also extracted from the entire plant (called "poppy straw"). There are other poppy plants but only the *Papaver somniferum,* which is one to five feet tall, produces opium. There are over 25 known alkaloids in opium but the two most prevalent, called "opiates," are morphine (10–20% of the milky fluid) and codeine (0.7–2.5%) (Karch, 1996; Marnell, 1997). Although a small amount of opium is used to make antidiarrheal preparations, e.g., tincture of opium and paregoric, virtually all the opium coming into this country is refined into morphine, codeine, and thebaine. The main reason for the decline in the popularity of opium is the availability of semisynthetic and synthetic prescription opioids.

◇ Semisynthetic opiates, e.g., heroin, hydrocodone (Vicodin®), oxycodone (Percodan®), or hydromorphone (Dilaudid®), are made from the three opium alkaloids.

◇ Fully synthetic opiate-like drugs include meperidine (Demerol®), methadone, and propoxyphene (Darvon®).

◇ Finally, there are synthetic opioid antagonists (naloxone and naltrexone) that block the effects of opiates and opioids.

HISTORY OF USE (see Chapter 1)

The ancient Sumerians, Egyptians, and Chinese recorded the paradoxical nature of opium in their medical texts, listing it as a cure for all illnesses, a pleasurable substance, and a poison. Socrates, when he was ordered to commit suicide, drank from a cup that contained not only hemlock but also opium. Ironically, modern day euthanasia or assisted-suicide formulas often include morphine or other opioids. Greek writings told of the gods' use of opium for mystical or mythical purposes—Greek heroes, such as

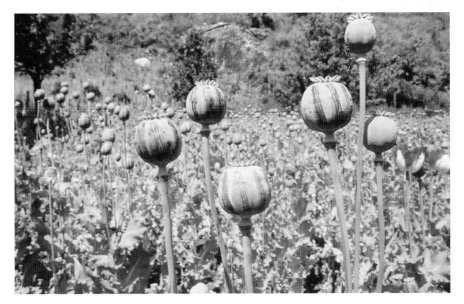

An illegal opium poppy field on the northern border of Thailand shows the flowers and the unripe seed pods that contain the raw opium. The pod is scored on the sides allowing the resinous white substance to ooze out of the incisions. The air dries it to a gummy dark brown and the next morning it is scraped off, pressed into balls, and collected. Most of it is sold to a processor who transforms it to morphine. It can then be shipped or smuggled as morphine or it can be further transformed to heroin.
Courtesy of George Skaggard

TABLE 4–1 OPIATES/OPIOIDS

Generic Drug Name	Trade Names	Street Names
OPIATES (Opium Poppy Extracts)		
Opium (schedule II)	Pantopon®, Laudanum®	"O," op, poppy
Diluted opium, (schedule III)	Paregoric®	
Morphine (schedule II)	Infumorph®, Kadian®, Roxanol®	Murphy, morph, "M," Miss Emma
Codeine (schedule III)	Empirin® w/codeine,	Number 4s (1 grain),
(usually w/aspirin	Tylenol® w/codeine	Number 3s (1/2 grain)
or Tylenol®)	Doriden® w/codeine	Loads, sets, 4s & doors
Thebaine (schedule II)	None	None
SEMISYNTHETIC OPIATES		
Diacetylmorphine (schedule I)	Heroin	Smack, junk, tar (chiva, puro, goma, puta, chapa pote), Mexican brown, China white, Harry, skag, shit, Rufus, Perze, "H," horse, dava, boy
Hydrocodone (schedule III)	Vicodin®, Hycodan®, Lortab®, Lorcet®, Zydone®, Norco®	
Hydromorphone (schedule II)	Dilaudid®	Dillies, drugstore heroin
Oxycodone (schedule II)	Percodan®, Tylox®	Percs
SYNTHETIC OPIATES (Opioids)		
Methadone (schedule II)	Dolophine®	Juice
Propoxyphene (schedule IV)	Darvon®, Darvocet-N®, Wygesic®	Pink ladies, pumpkin seeds
Meperidine (schedule II)	Demerol®, Mepergan®	
Fentanyl (schedule II)	Sublimaze®	Street derivatives are misrepresented as China white
Pentazocine (schedule IV)	Talwin®	Part of Ts and blues
Levorphanol (schedule II)	Levo-Dromoran®	
Levo-alpha-acetylmethadol (schedule II) (long-acting methadone)	LAAM®	Lam
Buprenorphine (schedule V)	Buprenex®	
Oxymorphone (schedule II)	Numorphan®	
Butorphanol (schedule IV)	Stadol®	
OPIOID ANTAGONISTS		
Naloxone	Narcan®	
Naltrexone	Revia®	

Jason, used opium to sedate monsters and other creatures. Hippocrates, the Father of Medicine, prescribed it for sleep, internal ills, and epidemics (Hoffman, 1990; Latimer & Goldberg, 1981).

Over the centuries, experimentation with different methods of use, development of new refinements of the drug, and synthesis of molecules, which act like the natural opiates, have slowly increased not only the benefits of these substances but also their potential for abuse.

ORAL INGESTION

Opium, from the Greek word *opòs* meaning juice or sap, was originally chewed, eaten, or blended in various liquids and drunk. Though the drug was used extensively to induce drowsiness, reduce pain, and control diarrhea, the abuse potential of opium was relatively low because it had a bitter taste, the concentration of active ingredients was low, and the supplies were limited. When taken orally the drug must go

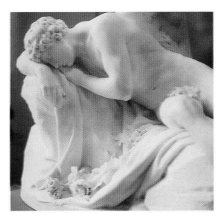

Morpheus, the son of Hypnos, the Greek god of sleep, is shown with opium poppy flowers strewn at his feet. The word morphine comes from Morpheus.
Sculpture by Jean Antoine Houdon, Louvre Museum, Paris. Courtesy of Simone Garlaund

through the entire digestive system before it enters the bloodstream and makes its way to the brain 20 or 30 minutes later. Although the addictive potential of opium was recognized, it was felt that the benefits far outweighed any dangers.

The use of opium in medications and potions continued through the Middle Ages and into the Renaissance (in the early 1500s) when it was popularized by the Swiss alchemist Paracelsus who concocted a tincture of opium called "laudanum" (powdered opium in alcohol) that he prescribed for dysentery, pain, diarrhea, and coughs (O'Brien, Cohen, Evans, & Fine, 1992). Over the next three centuries, other opium mixtures were developed, especially paregoric (opium in alcohol plus camphor), for the treatment of diarrhea. Paregoric is still available as a prescription drug.

SMOKING

The introduction of the pipe from North America to Europe and Asia, particularly China, via Portuguese traders in the sixteenth century set the stage for the widespread nonmedical use of opium. Smoking puts more of the active ingredients of the drug into the bloodstream by way of the lungs; it

also does it quickly. The drug begins to reach the brain in as few as six to eight seconds. The higher concentration of the opiate produces a strong sense of euphoria, relaxation, and well-being, thereby encouraging abuse.

Although opium smoking was initially limited to the middle and upper classes in China (because of the high cost of the drug), it became such a large problem that it was banned in 1729. Unfortunately the opium trade had become so lucrative, especially in China, that it was impossible to shut it off. In the early 1800s when prohibition was again tried, the powerful trading companies of the West and Japan, e.g., the East India Company of England, along with their governments, forced the Chinese government to continue the trade (Latimer, 1981). As a result of the Opium Wars, Hong Kong was ceded to the British.

As the supplies became more plentiful, use increased. Opium smoking was introduced to the United States by some of the 70,000 Chinese workers who were brought over to build the railroads and mine gold, copper, and mercury. The biased and bigoted reaction to these Asian immigrants resulted in headlines that screamed "yellow fiends" and "seducers of white women" and resulted in a spate of prohibitory laws that focused on opium smoking. This was somewhat surprising since the majority of opiate addicts at that time were white women who used large quantities of prescribed and over-the-counter opium and morphine-based medications. Surveys in the 1880s showed that between 56% and 71% of opium addicts were women (Hoffman, 1990). One of the current methods of smoking is to heat some heroin on tin foil and inhale the fumes through a straw. This method is called "chasing the dragon."

REFINEMENT OF MORPHINE, CODEINE, & HEROIN

In 1805 the German pharmacist Frederich Serturner refined morphine from opium and found it to be 10

times stronger and therefore a much better pain reliever but its greater strength promoted more compulsive use. The refinement of morphine benefited wounded soldiers in war, especially the Crimean War and the U.S. Civil War. Unfortunately it also increased the potential for opiate addiction or morphinism.

In 1832 codeine, the other major component of opium, was isolated. It got its name from the Greek word *kodeia,* which means poppyhead. Since it was only 1/5 the strength of morphine, it was often used in cough syrups and patent medicines.

In 1874 the British chemist C.R. Alder Wright refined heroin from morphine. He chemically altered morphine to produce diacetylmorphine (heroin) in an attempt to find a more effective painkiller that didn't have addictive properties. This powerful opiate stayed on the shelf until 1898 when an employee of Bayer and Company® thought it should be promoted for coughs, chest pain, tuberculosis, and pneumonia (Trebach, 1981). Unfortunately since heroin crossed the blood-brain barrier much more rapidly than morphine, the rush and subsequent euphoria came on more quickly and was more intense (although Bayer® chemists mistakenly claimed it caused less respiratory depression than codeine) (Karch, 1996). The new drug created a subculture of compulsive heroin users in the twentieth century. It was estimated that there were between 250,000 and 1,000,000 opium, morphine, and heroin abusers in the United States shortly after the turn of the century.

IV USE

Another major development of the nineteenth century regarding opiates was the development of the hypodermic needle in 1853. Intravenous use can inject high concentrations of the drug directly into the bloodstream through the veins. It takes 15–30 seconds for an injected opiate or opioid to affect the central nervous system. If the drug is injected just under the skin

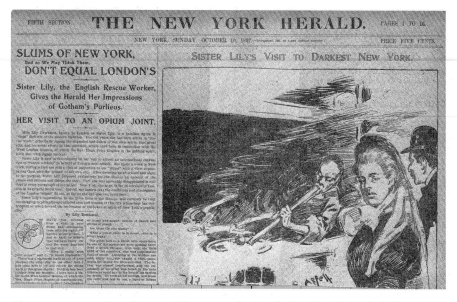

This is a representation of a turn of the century "opium den" in New York (which does not exist today). Newspapers periodically ran stories that demonized Chinese opium dens.
Courtesy of the National Library of Medicine, Bethesda

the habit of sniffing or snorting heroin (also called insufflation and intranasal use). It takes five to eight minutes for the drug to enter the nasal capillaries and reach the central nervous system. From the turn of the century until the 1920s, heroin addicts were split evenly between "sniffers" and "shooters" (Karch, 1996). Since more of the drug is needed when snorted to get the same high as when injected, low prices of heroin encourage insufflation, especially for those who are afraid of the needle. This route was popular with heroin-using GIs in Vietnam because of the easy availability and high purity of the drug. Approximately half of all heroin addicts entering treatment began their heroin use by insufflation (Casriel, Rockwell, & Stepherson, 1988).

or in a muscle ("skin popping" or "muscling"), the effects are delayed by 5–8 minutes. Until the development of the hypodermic needle, oral use of morphine and smoking of opium induced a certain euphoria and relief from physical and emotional pain, but with the large amount of drug that could be injected at one time, an intense rush also occurred. The intensity of the rush made compulsive drug-seeking behavior more likely.

PATENT MEDICINES

During the mid- to late-1800s, opiates became so popular that hundreds of tonics and medications, such as Mrs. Winslow's Soothing Syrup, or McMunn's Elixir of Opium, came on the market to treat everything from tired blood to coughs, diarrhea, and toothaches (Armstrong & Armstrong, 1991). Just before the turn of the century, the use of opioids for nervousness and pleasure (recreational use) by the middle and upper classes also came into vogue. Whether it was a reaction to the strict Victorian mores and behaviors of the time or simply an exciting experimentation, the number of opium parlors and the use of opium increased.

Women addicts outnumbered male users in the late 1800s and early 1900s when opium, morphine, and heroin were still readily available and physicians were not fully aware of the addictive potential of drugs. Iatrogenic (physician-induced) addiction was a common problem. In fact four to eight times as many prescriptions with opioids were written back then. IV morphine was prescribed for anything from anemia, asthma, and cholera to nervous dyspepsia, insanity, neuralgia, and vomiting. Some of the more famous female opiate users and addicts were the writers Elizabeth Barrett Browning, George Sand, Charlotte Bronte, and Louisa May Alcott; the pioneering social worker Jane Addams; and the well-known actress Sarah Bernhardt (Aldrich, 1994).

"I arrived on the stage in a semiconscious state, yet delighted with the applause I received."
Sara Bernhardt, 1890 (Palmer & Horowitz, 1982)

SNIFFING & SNORTING

In addition to drinking, eating, smoking, and injecting opiates, new immigrants from Europe introduced

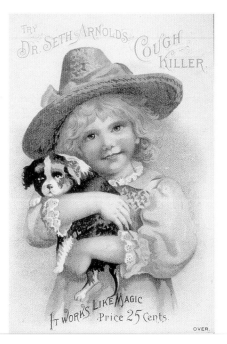

Many patent medicines and cure-alls contained opium as the main active ingredient. Although the ingredients were not advertised, opium, codeine, and morphine were used in many cough syrups, such as Dr. Seth Arnold's Cough Killer, Mrs. Winslow's Soothing Syrup, and opium-based laudanum became popular.
Courtesy of the National Library of Medicine, Bethesda

"You know you're in more pain because when you snort it; it takes a lot to go through your system. When you shoot it, you get it right away. So when you get sick from snorting it, it's just like someone tearing your guts out."

58-year-old male in recovery with a 35-year habit

Many "sniffers" never graduate to injecting heroin and take a perverse pride in their method of use. On the other hand, many IV users look down on "sniffers." "Sniffers" seem to use with other "sniffers" much as IV users "shoot up" with other IV users.

TWENTIETH CENTURY

Rising concern over the perceived problems caused by use and abuse of opium, morphine, and especially heroin spurred various governments to action. Casual nonmedical use of opiates was declared illegal at the beginning of the twentieth century by the international community through The Hague Resolutions and by the United States through The Pure Food and Drug Act in 1906 and The Harrison Narcotics Act in 1914. In 1924 production of heroin in the United States was prohibited. The gradual proliferation of laws also increased the jail population. Commitments to federal prisons for violations of the narcotics law rose from 63 in 1915 to 2,529 in 1928 (about 1/3 of all federal prisoners) (Musto, 1973).

In the first two decades of the twentieth century, opioid addiction was considered a medical problem and was treated by physicians. Alcoholism was considered more debilitating and certainly more expensive than opioid addiction and a number of treatment centers were opened.

The availability or prohibition of different opioids shifted methods of use. When the importation of smokable opium was banned in 1909, it produced a shift to heroin because opium prices rose drastically while heroin remained less expensive (Zule, Vogtsberger, & Desmond, 1997).

Because these restrictions limited supply and made opium and heroin valu-

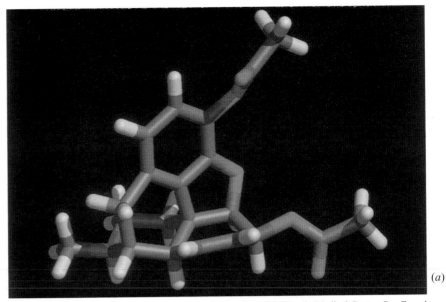

(a)

Courtesy of the Molecular Imaging Department, University of California Medical Center, San Francisco

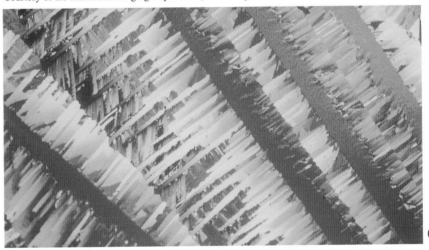

(b)

Courtesy of Michael W. Davidson, © Institute of Molecular Biophysics, Florida State University, Tallahasse, FL

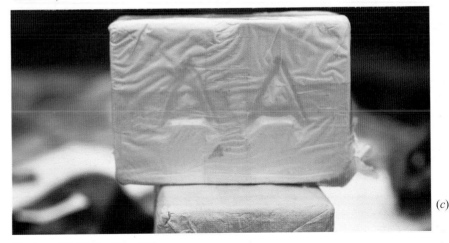

(c)

Courtesy of the Michael Skaggard

There are a number of ways drugs can be viewed: (a) as a computer simulation of the heroin molecule, which is designated as diacetyl morphine, (b) as a microphotograph of the heroin crystal, (c) as a block of processed heroin weighing one kilogram.

able commodities, growing, processing, and distributing opiates/opioids, especially heroin, became major sources of revenue for criminal organizations worldwide. These groups include the Chinese Triads, the Mafia and the French Connection, Mexican narcoficantes, African traffickers, the Russian Mafia, and most recently the Colombian Cartel.

In addition diversion of legal prescription opiates/opioids, such as hydrocodone, cough syrups, and oxycodone, through theft, bogus purchases from phony or even legitimate companies, and forged prescriptions has created an illegal market of pills and injectables.

"I went to different physicians. I would rip off prescription pads and since I worked in the medical field, writing my own prescriptions was no problem except that I committed a felony every time I did it, which was once a week. I never got caught but I always lived in mortal fear that they would get me."
Recovering Darvon® (propoxyphene) user

Currently an estimated 1.7 million Americans use prescription opiates/opioids illicitly every month compared to 130,000 to 800,000 heroin abusers. (The estimates of heroin users vary radically. For example, New York City alone is estimated to have 200,000 heroin addicts.) Approximately 2.4 million Americans have tried heroin (SAMHSA, 1999). In 1996 there were approximately equal numbers of injectors and snorters with a much smaller percentage of smokers (NIDA, 1996). Recently, snorting and smoking heroin have increased in popularity in the United States due to an influx of heroin from Colombia and Mexico as well as Southeast and Southwest Asia. Large percentages of "sniffers" and smokers are more likely to be found in the eastern half of the United States (NIDA, 1998). Some of the "snorters" mix it with water and snort it out of a Visine® spray bottle.

(*NOTE*: **For the rest of this chapter, we will use the generic term OPIOID to denote both natural and** semi-synthetic **OPIATES and synthetic OPIOIDS.**)

EFFECTS OF OPIOIDS

Medically, physicians most often prescribe opioids to deaden pain, control coughing, and stop diarrhea. Nonmedically, users self-prescribe opioids to get a rush, to induce euphoria, to drown out emotional pain, or to try to feel normal by preventing withdrawal symptoms. But to truly comprehend opioids, it is important to understand how pain and pleasure are connected to the nervous system.

PAIN

Pain, such as the pain of burned skin or a broken bone, is a warning signal that tells us whether we are being damaged physically. It sends a message to the spinal cord and on to the brainstem and medial portion of the thalamus in our brain, which in turn tells the body to protect itself from further damage (Jaffee, Knapp, & Ciraulo, 1997). The pain message is transmitted from nerve cell to nerve cell by a neurotransmitter called substance "P."

If the pain is too intense, the body tries to protect itself by softening the pain signals. It reduces pain by flooding the brain and spinal cord with endorphins. These endorphins attach themselves to opioid mu and kappa receptor sites on the membranes of sending nerve cells in the pain pathway, telling them not to send substance "P" (Fig. 4-1).

However, many signals still get through. If the pain remains unbear-

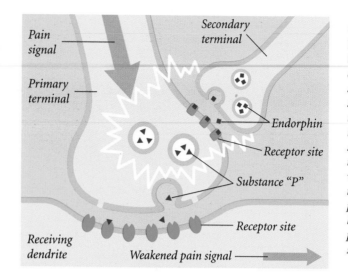

Figure 4-1 •

Natural Pain Suppression. *This diagram of a synapse shows that when pain signals are being transmitted through the nervous system, a secondary terminal releases endorphins, which then slot into receptor sites on the primary terminal and limit the release of the pain neurotransmitter, substance "P."*

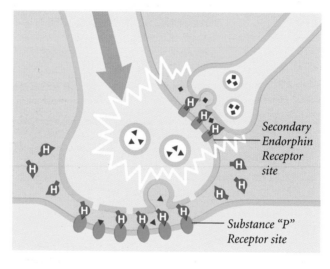

Figure 4-2 •

Artificial Pain Suppression. *Heroin (or any opioid) slots into the secondary endorphin receptor sites limiting the release of substance "P." It also blocks most of the substance "P" that gets through by slotting into the primary substance "P" receptor sites on the receiving dendrite of the next neuron.*

able, opioid medications can be used to relieve the agony. These drugs are effective because they act like the body's endogenous endorphins and enkephalins. Opioid medications not only limit the release of substance "P," they also help block what little does get through to the receiving neuron (Fig. 4-2).

The effects of the various opioids are similar to each other. The differences have to do with how long the drug lasts, how strong it is per gram, and how toxic it is to the body. For example, heroin, codeine, and Darvon® will relieve pain from four to six hours but the heroin will have much stronger effects. Because heroin is relatively short acting, an addict might use it as many as four times a day. The pain-killing effects of fentanyl, on the other hand, will barely last an hour but it is strong enough to be used as an anesthetic during surgery. Pain control is not only limited to physical pain.

"When you are loaded on heroin, you can watch your best friend get hit by a car, all your friends could be dying, your dog could come down with rabies, and you could get AIDS, herpes, and cancer all at once and you don't care. You're separated from it and blocked off from your emotions."
18-year-old female heroin addict.

Decreased anxiety, a sense of serenity, drowsiness, and a deadening of unwanted emotions are often experienced by opioid users. This is due to the drug's inhibiting effect on the locus coeruleus on top of the brainstem and its influence on the dopinergic reward pathway. Experiments have shown that severe stress alone can activate endorphins to mitigate emotional pain (Goldstein, 1994). In fact in one animal experiment, the greater the stress, the more the use of morphine to relieve the stress was remembered, thus imprinting the concept that emotional upset can be relieved by drugs (Will, Watkins, & Maier, 1998). This negative reinforcement uses many of the same brain

mechanisms that cause positive reinforcement of drug-seeking behavior.

PLEASURE

The other major effect of opioids involves endorphins, dopamine, and the mesolimbic dopaminergic reward pathway or the reward/pleasure center, which includes the nucleus accumbens. As described in Chapter 2, this system, through a variety of mechanisms, positively reinforces an action that is good for the body's survival. The normal activation of this system gives a surge of pleasure that encourages repetition of the action, e.g., encourages the person to drink when thirsty, eat when hungry, have intercourse when sexually aroused. It then senses satiation and turns this mechanism off. If the reward/pleasure center is not being activated by dopamine on a regular basis or if it is dysfunctional, a person will not feel good, will not feel rewarded, and will not feel pleasure. Instead there will be a feeling of emptiness and depression. Recent animal research suggests that, in addition to giving a surge of positive reinforcement, dopamine release in this pathway helps the brain remember (unconsciously) what was done, so it can be done again in the future (Wickelgran, 1997).

"The last shot is never good enough. You're always looking for a certain shot. You're looking for the same shot you had when you first did the drug, which you'll never get again."
22-year-old recovering heroin addict

Searching for a high or relief from pain, which can feel like a high, some people try opioids because these drugs artificially activate this reward pathway. Opioids activate this pathway by

◇ slotting into the receptor sites meant for endorphins/enkephalins;

◇ inhibiting the action of GABA resulting in increased activation of the reward pathway (Nutt, 1998);

◇ glutumate receptor activation that enhances responsiveness of dopa-

mine neurons resulting in activation of the reward pathway (Carlezon Boundy, Haile, et al., 1997);

◇ increasing the number of glutamate receptors (GluR1) on dopamine releasing neurons (Carlezon et al., 1997);

◇ reducing the number of dopamine receptors (down regulation) that cause the release of more dopamine to activate the pathway.

Of the various opioids, heroin has the strongest effect on the reward pathway.

"I didn't have to deal with anything while I was on heroin. I didn't have to process information. My whole life was geared to just one thing, getting that next fix of heroin. You stop processing life. You stop processing thought."
49-year-old parolee in a therapeutic treatment community

SATIATION

When the natural (endogenous) endorphins and enkephalins relieve pain or give a surge of pleasure (positive reinforcement), various cells in the brain monitor the action and when the need is filled, the signal goes out, "mission accomplished," "that's enough," "you can stop now." Powerful psychoactive drugs, including heroin, can disrupt this cutoff switch in a variety of ways and reinforce the desire to continue the behavior. As mentioned in Chapter 2, the on-off switch can be stuck in the on position; it can be ignored because the pleasure is still desired; or it can disrupt communication with the new brain. Genetically some people are more susceptible to disruption of the switch. In others, excessive drug use is the more powerful factor. Whatever the genetic susceptibility, the more frequently this circuit is overloaded by heroin or other powerful opioids, the greater the malfunction of the satiation switch (Hyman, 1998).

RECEPTOR SITES

There are actually multiple natural opioid receptor sites for the body's own opioids (endorphins, enkephalins, and dynorphins). The main receptors are mu, delta, kappa, and possibly sigma. They are found in the brain, the spinal cord, the digestive track, various organs, and a dozen other sites. Opioid drugs (exogenous opioids) slot into these same receptor sites but cause more intense reactions than the body's own (endogenous) opioids. Also the stronger the opioid drug (e.g., heroin vs. codeine), the greater the effects. But each opioid drug has a unique affinity for each site. At one synapse the drug might act like an agonist and trigger effects; at another it might act as an antagonist, blocking changes; at a third, it might work as a combination agonist and antagonist. For example:

◇ mu receptors trigger the reward/pleasure center, block pain transmission, and depress the autonomic nervous system, including respiration, blood pressure, endocrine release, pupil contraction, and the gastrointestinal tract;

◇ kappa receptors seem to induce dysphoria rather than euphoria as well as mediate pain at the spinal cord level (Jaffe et al., 1997; Simon, 1997; Gold, 1998).

So one drug, such as fentanyl, will affect pain more than heroin that might have a greater influence on the rush and euphoria.

COUGH SUPPRESSION & DIARRHEA CONTROL

Besides pain control, opioids are used to suppress coughs and control diarrhea. They suppress coughs by controlling activation of the cough center in the brainstem that signals the body to cough when the breathing tract is stimulated. Currently, codeine- and hydrocodone-based cough medications are still widely prescribed.

Diarrhea is also controlled because opioids affect areas in the brainstem that inhibit gastric secretions and depress intestinal muscles. Constipation can be a severe problem in surgical patients or those with intractable pain who use opioids over a long period.

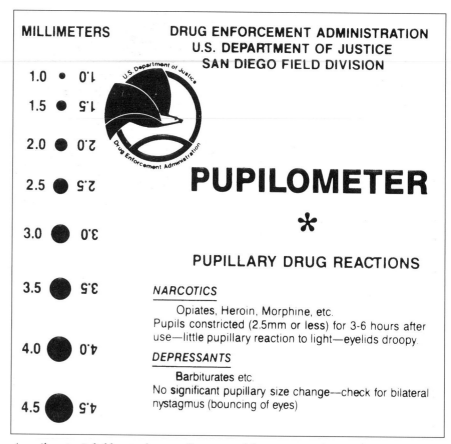

A pupilometer is held up to the eyes of a suspected drug user in order to compare the size of pupils against normal standards. Since opioids contract pupils, pupil size is a strong indicator of drug use. (Cocaine and methamphetamines can dilate pupils.)

SIDE EFFECTS OF HEROIN & OTHER OPIOIDS

PHYSICAL EFFECTS

Opioids affect almost every part of the body: heart, lungs, brain, eyes, voice box, muscles, cough and nausea centers, reproductive system, digestive system, excretory system, and the immune system. Some of the major side effects are

◇ insensitivity to warning pain signals, which is a desired effect but can keep a user from treating a damaging ailment such as abscesses;

◇ lowered blood pressure;

◇ lowered pulse and respiration rate;

◇ confusion.

Some of the other side effects of the stronger opioids are mild but quite identifiable in the heavier user, particularly with heroin:

◇ eyelids droop and the head nods forward;

◇ speech becomes slurred and slowed;

◇ the walking gait and coordination are slowed;

◇ pupils become pinpoint and do not react to light;

◇ skin dries out and itching increases.

Other effects are less visible:

◇ suppression of the cough center in the brain can hinder clearance of phlegm in those users with respiratory ailments such as emphysema and tuberculosis;

◇ opioids also trigger the nausea center; some heroin addicts know a batch of heroin is good if it makes them vomit.

"It hit from the feet going up to the head. I was yelling at him to take the needle out and I was on the toilet seat. I mean, I hugged that toilet bowl for hours, vomiting."
21-year-old heroin user

And finally

◇ though opioids are used to stop diarrhea, they cause chronic constipation;

◇ opioids affect the hormonal system; a woman's period is delayed and a man produces less testosterone while sexual desire is dulled, often to the point of indifference.

"When I'm on heroin, I can't have an orgasm. It's just one of those things. I can have sex for hours and it starts to get painful. Heroin makes my whole body numb; I don't want to move around and I don't want to have sex when I'm high. When you're not high, it is all right but when you are high, it's shitty."
24-year-old dealer/heroin addict

TOLERANCE, TISSUE DEPENDENCE, & WITHDRAWAL

The desire for relief from pain and the experiencing of pleasure (the rush, mood elevation, and/or euphoria), combined with tolerance, tissue dependence, and withdrawal, are the main reasons for the addictive nature of opioids.

"After a while they [#4 codeine tablets] didn't really have any effect on me and the pain was taking over with the drug, so I started taking more codeine. And I took more, and more, and finally, I was going through like two bottles of codeine a week."
Recovering codeine abuser

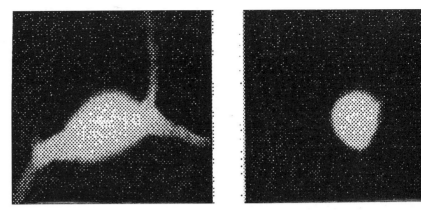

Figure 4-3 •
The dopamine-producing neuron on the left is from the ventral tegmental area of a rat that was not exposed to morphine. Chronic administration of morphine caused the shrunken neuron on the right. The researchers were able to prevent the shrinkage by administering naltrexone, an opioid antagonist that blocks the effects of morphine or by administering BDNF (brain-derived neurotropic factor) or GDNF (glial-derived neurotropic factor).
Courtesy of Eric J. Nestler, Yale University

Tolerance

Tolerance occurs when the body tries to neutralize the heroin (or any other psychoactive drug) by a variety of methods. It may

◇ speed up the metabolism, particularly in the liver;

◇ desensitize the nerve cells to the drug's effects;

◇ excrete the drug more rapidly out of the body through urine, feces, and sweat;

◇ alter the brain and body chemistry to compensate for the effects of the drug.

The body's adjustment requires the user to increase dosage if the same effects are desired. Since tolerance occurs rapidly with opioids, such as morphine, users might need 10 times as much drug in as short a period as 10 days (Jaffe, 1990).

"Since the first day I started using heroin, I was using it every day. I thought it was a joke that people wouldn't get addicted the first time but I went ahead and did it anyway. After about two weeks of use, I ran out of money and I found out how bad I could get sick. I wish I wasn't sick

any of the time but it's kind of like a requirement. Once you're a junkie, you've got to be sick."
27-year-old female heroin addict.

There is almost no limit to the development of opioid tolerance. After a year of opioid use, a terminal cancer patient was using 5 fentanyl patches, 20 Demerol® tablets, and continuous morphine suppositories. This limitless tolerance compares to a drug such as nicotine where 3 packs a day are usually the upper limit (Goldstein, 1994).

Tissue Dependence

The adaptation of the body to the effects of a drug will often permanently alter brain chemistry. An animal study by Dr. Eric Nestler and colleagues at Yale University showed that chronic administration of morphine to rats actually reduced the size of dopamine-producing cells (in the ventral tegmental area) by 1/4 (Fig. 4-3) (Nestler & Aghajanian, 1997). This means that when chronic morphine (or heroin) use is stopped, the body has less ability to produce its own dopamine and therefore less ability to feel elated or even normal. This depletion intensifies the desire to use the drug again.

"It gets to the point where you're not getting high anymore. You're just existing and using to get well everyday."

22-year-old female heroin abuser

This and many other changes in body chemistry result in physical dependence since the body relies on the drug to stay normal. Chronic opioid drug use also decreases the firing rate of cells in the brain's locus coeruleus. Researchers also found that animals that were allowed to become physically dependent, then were withdrawn from the drug, and then readministered the drug, would become physically dependent more rapidly. The same pattern is true for humans, explaining why each relapse leads to more rapid addiction.

Tolerance and physical dependence can extend to other opioids. That is, if users build a tolerance and a physical dependence to heroin, they will also have a tissue dependence and tolerance to morphine, codeine, and other opioids.

"My tolerance to Demerol®, morphine, and things like that was tremendous. I had to have tons of the stuff. I went to have a local surgery and they were like, 'Okay, how's that?' and I was like, 'Is this just a test or what?'"

35-year-old recovering opioid addict

This cross-dependence is the basis for methadone maintenance treatment where one opioid is substituted for another less damaging one. However, tolerance and physical dependence appear to be receptor specific, so a drug, such as heroin, that works at the mu receptors will not create as much of a tolerance as a drug that works at kappa receptors (Jaffe et al., 1997). This is known as "**select tolerance**." For example, if a user takes codeine regularly, he/she will develop a tolerance to the nauseating side effect quicker than to the pain-killing effect.

Withdrawal

Withdrawal occurs when tissue dependence has developed and the per-

TABLE 4–2   OPIOID WITHDRAWAL SYMPTOMS

Bone, joint, and muscular pain	Insomnia
Anxiety	Sweating
Runny nose	Diarrhea
Rapid pulse and tachycardia	High blood pressure
Coughing	Dilated pupils
Hyper-reflexes and muscle cramps	Yawning
Anorexia	Chills and goose bumps
Teary eyes	Vomiting
Fever	Stomach cramps

son suddenly stops using. The body has changed enough to trigger this rebounding effect as it tries to return (too quickly) to normal.

"You get deep deep muscle and bone pains. There's no way to get comfortable and you fluctuate between being chilly and sweating a lot. You can either be constipated or have diarrhea. You're in total body agony that nothing relieves. It's real uncomfortable. I have actually, and this is not a figure of speech, I have been going through withdrawal where I wished I was dead."

35-year-old recovering heroin user

In general, short-acting opioids, like heroin, morphine, and Dilaudid®, result in more severe withdrawal symptoms that begin within 8–12 hours after cessation of chronic use, reach peak intensity within 48 hours, and then subside over a period of 5–7 days. Long-acting opioids, like methadone, will delay the symptoms from 36–48 hours, reach peak intensity in 4–6 days, and persist for 14 days or more (Jaffe et al., 1997). Other opioids, such as codeine, Percodan®, and Darvon®, have withdrawal phenomena somewhere between those two extremes. One reason the hyperactivity of withdrawal occurs is the sudden release of excess norepinephrine that has been produced but not released during use of the opioid because the

drug inhibits the neural release of these neurotransmitters in the locus coeruleus (Gold, 1998).

It is important to remember that although opioid and particularly heroin withdrawal feels like an incredibly bad case of the flu, it is almost never life threatening as is withdrawal from alcohol or sedative-hypnotics. Unfortunately since opioid withdrawal symptoms can be painful and seem so frightening or create so much anxiety, particularly for heroin addicts, the fear of withdrawal becomes a greater trigger for continued use than even the desire to repeat the rush.

"I would rather die a hundred times over of a horrible, burning, flesh-eating death than to be dope sick. Dope sickness is when you get cramps from your toes to your inner thighs and it just totally encircles your legs and you can't walk."

19-year-old polydrug abuser with major depression

ADDITIONAL PROBLEMS WITH HEROIN & OTHER OPIOIDS

NEONATAL EFFECTS

Most opioids, especially heroin and morphine (and its metabolites), quickly cross the placental barrier between the fetus and the mother, thereby sending large doses of the drug to the developing infant. Pregnant users have a greater risk of miscarriage, placental separation, premature labor, breech birth, stillbirth, and seizures. When a baby is born to an addicted mother, the child is also addicted and since babies are much smaller than adults, the tissue dependence and withdrawal symptoms are more severe. These symptoms can last five to eight weeks and unlike adults, babies in withdrawal can die.

OVERDOSE

"I've OD'd six to eight times and luckily I came back. I've been really dead you know, like out for five minutes, not breathing, no heartbeat or anything and I've come back. So I know what my limit is and I know not to push it."
22-year-old heroin addict.

Overdose occurs when so much of the drug enters the brain that the nervous system shuts down. Blood pressure drops, the heart beats too weakly to circulate blood, and lungs labor and fill with fluid. Severe respiratory depression is the major cause of death with heroin overdose. The person passes out and, unless quickly revived, will slip into a coma and die. It is estimated that 3,000–4,000 people die from heroin overdoses each year (NIDA, 1998). There were about 70,000 emergency room visits for heroin in 1998 compared to 142,000 for cocaine. These figures have more than doubled in the past 10 years (DAWN, 2000).

"You know, people who do heroin aren't worried about dying because like if three people die from a new batch of heroin, everybody wants to know where they are getting that heroin, so they can go get some because it's the best and they figure they will just do a little less."
41-year-old recovering heroin addict

Heroin overdose can be counteracted by a shot of an opioid antagonist,

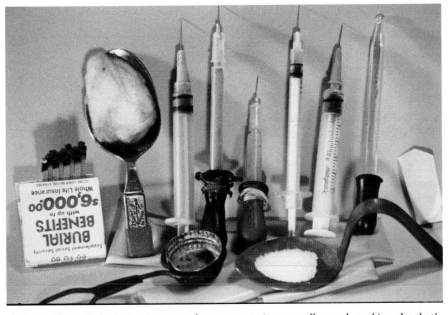

Addicts will use diabetics' syringes, eyedroppers, veterinary needles, and anything else that's handy to inject their heroin or other opioid.

naltrexone, to block and reverse the life-threatening effects of too much drug. This also obliterates the high and if the overdose victim is an addict, will cause severe withdrawal effects.

DIRTY & SHARED NEEDLES

The most dangerous problem with opioids, the one that causes the most illness and death, is dirty or shared needles, along with contaminated drugs. Needles are used because they put a large amount of the drug into the bloodstream at one time. Unfortunately users can also unknowingly inject adulterants, such as powdered milk and procaine, or dangerous bacteria and viruses, including hepatitis B and C, endocarditis, malaria, syphilis, flesh-eating bacteria, gas gangrene, and the HIV virus that causes AIDS.

Hepatitis C & HIV

Various studies have shown that 50% to 90% of all needle-using heroin addicts carry hepatitis C. Even those with less than one year of IV drug use had a positive rate of 71.4%. Once infected, 20% to 40% will develop liver disease and 4% to 16% will develop

liver cancer (Payte & Zweben, 1998). Since the hepatitis C virus (HCV) was identified in 1988 and a test devised for it, the number of cases of HCV caused by transfusion has dropped dramatically but IV drug use transmission remains high and they have created a well of infection to be spread to their partners or co-users.

"The person that introduced me to the needle at home guaranteed me it had never been used by anybody. And after I used, I looked at the needle and realized that it was not a new needle. And I was high and I didn't care and after that, I didn't care as much either."
29-year-old recovering heroin addict who has been infected with HIV

The transmission of HIV by IV drug use is also substantial. More than half of IV drug users carry the HIV virus although the percentages vary radically from city to city. In San Francisco 4.3% of IV drug users are HIV positive while in New York the figure is as high as 80% because of the greater sharing of needles. It is estimated that

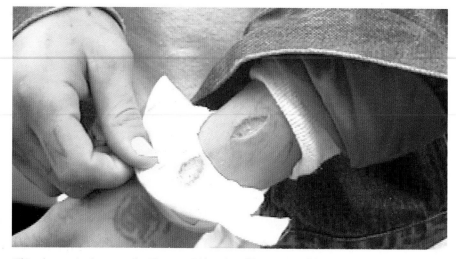

This abscess in the arm of a 25-year-old heroin addict occurred because of infectious organisms that were transmitted by contaminated needles or drugs. Abscesses are more common in opioid abusers than stimulant abusers, even though stimulant abusers shoot up more often.

◊ 26% of all U.S. AIDS cases (173,693 of 679,739) were transmitted to an IV drug user by a contaminated needle;

◊ 10.5% (69,886) were transmitted to heterosexual or homosexual partners of IV drug users through sexual relations (CDC, 1999).

Internationally the figures are worse. In Burma, for example, the World Health Organization estimated that between 74% to 91% of the country's IV heroin addicts are HIV positive.

Excess needle use continually traumatizes the blood vessels, often causing them to collapse. This is why injection drug users are forced to switch to locations other than the cubital fossa opposite the elbow. Injection sites include the wrist, between the toes, in the neck, or even in the dorsal vein of the penis.

Abscesses & Other Infections

Abscesses and ulcerations caused by soft tissue infections are common in IV drug users since most heroin abusers will shoot up four to six times a day, often with a contaminated needle. The most common infectious organisms are *staphylococcus aureus* and *beta-hemolytic streptococci* (Orangio,

Pitlick, & Latta, 1984). If the infection is too deep or too far along, often part of the flesh has to be cut away. In addition adulterants such as cotton can lodge in the skin. Other signs of IV drug use are lesions or "tracks," which are scars on the skin often caused by constant inflammation at the injection site and hyperpigmentation.

"This is my first abscess here and, well, you can see the 'tracks' where I use. This thing used to be like a big old hole, like that. And they'd have to scrape it in there and they'd put gauze in there. It's really no funny matter."
40-year-old recovering heroin addict

One of the worst infections is necrotizing fasciitis, an infection that destroys fascia and subcutaneous tissue but is not immediately visible on the surface. Bacteria like *clostridium perfinges* and variant strains of *streptococcus* and *staphylococcus* are known to cause this condition which has been known as infection by flesh-eating bacteria.

Endocarditis, an infection of heart valves, is found more often in IV drug users. Research points to a variety of organisms (including those involved in abscesses) that are dislodged from the injection site and lodge in heart valves.

Cotton fever is another illness found more frequently in IV drug users. It is caused by endotoxins (which thrive in cotton) being injected into the system. The term cotton fever is also used by addicts to describe any short-term bacterial infection resulting in the symptoms of fever, chills, tremors, aches, and pains.

Dilution & Adulteration

The purity of heroin has increased almost 10–fold since 1987 (DEA, 1998).

"The first 'China white' I got . . . looked like a 20 hitter. I know that if I was shooting up, then I probably would have OD'd. A 20 hitter means that you could take 1 gram and throw 19 grams of cut on it and it'd still be good, still get you off."
36-year-old recovering heroin addict

One of the reasons an overdose occurs is that street drugs can vary radically in purity. Street heroin varies from 0% to 99% pure, so if a user is expecting 3% heroin and gets 30%, the results could be fatal. Dilution of an expensive item like heroin with a cheap substitute, e.g., powered milk, starch, sugar (dextrose, lactose), baby laxative (Mannitol®), aspirin, Ajax®, quinine, caffeine, or talcum powder, is extremely common. Because of increased production and a proliferation of street chemists, it is also much easier to come across synthetic high-potency opioids. The average heroin purity for retail-level heroin according to the DEA in 1996 was 36% compared to 3% to 4% purity just 10 years before. Part of the reason is the influx of very pure Southeast Asian and South American heroin (DEA, 1998).

Cost

Contrary to popular belief promoted by television and movies that show heroin addicts as derelicts, criminals, and people who have a mental illness, a majority of heroin users (73%) are gainfully employed (ONDCP, 2000). However, because of the buildup of tolerance and the high cost of heroin, a great many users must turn to illegal methods to pay for their habits. The cost of a heroin habit can range from $60 to $200 a day depending on the level of use.

"I had two other friends and one was blackmailing a pharmacist. We'd get outdated drugs they were supposed to throw away. We'd pick them up in the alley and we'd get gallons and gallons of cough syrup and any other narcotics pills."
38-year-old male recovering heroin addict

Additional costs to society result from the treatment of infections, HIV, and other illnesses contracted through intravenous heroin use.

The overwhelming need to support an opioid habit makes antisocial behaviors, such as robbery, prostitution, dealing drugs, and eventual involvement with the legal system, almost inevitable. It is estimated that 60% of the cost of supporting a habit is gotten through consensual crime, including prostitution and drug dealing, and supplemented by welfare payments and occasional work. Most of the remaining 40% comes from shoplifting and burglary.

"When we were really strung out, we were spending $150 to $200 a day to feel normal. It's one thing to spend that kind of money and get loaded but when you're spending that kind of money to just function as a human being, it's irritating."
32-year-old recovering heroin addict

POLYDRUG USE

Multiple Drug Use

A heroin user might start with heroin in the morning to stop withdrawal symptoms and calm down. Later he might drink some alcohol or take some "speed" to get energetic and in the evening might use marijuana to relax.

Mixing

Opioids are often used at the same time with other drugs. A common opioid combination is cocaine or amphetamine with morphine or heroin. This combination, called a "speedball," can enhance the painkilling and euphoric effects of both drugs (Karch, 1996). Many methadone users use clonazepam (Klonopin®) to enhance their maintenance dose because the combination feels somewhat like a heroin high. Recently, because of the drop in street heroin prices and the rise in marijuana prices, some dealers are spiking poor quality marijuana with heroin to give it an extra kick and sell it as high quality pot. Unfortunately opioids can have additive and synergistic effects when used with marijuana or most other depressant drugs, such as alcohol and benzodiazepines. These combinations increase the potential for respiratory depression, lethargy, possible overdose, and even death.

"I'd be waiting and waiting and during the time that I was waiting, I'd be getting drunk. By the time I got around to doing my shot, I was already drunk. I'd hit up and boom, I'd be on the floor."
36-year-old male heroin user in treatment

Morphing

Since the depression from heroin can be so great, abusers might use an upper to change their mood. They then might get so wired from the cocaine or methamphetamine that they will use alcohol or heroin again to come down. At night they might be dragging around so much they'll use another stimulant.

Cycling

A number of heroin addicts will go off their drug for several weeks and switch to a cheaper high to give the body a chance to lower its tolerance and tissue dependence, often in an attempt to reduce the cost of their addiction. They might switch to alcohol, benzodiazepines, or marijuana in the interim and then cycle on and off heroin for the next few months.

Sequentialing

Someone might use heroin for several years and then switch to alcohol because they can't stand the IV drug user's lifestyle. After a few years of alcohol and a bloated liver, they might then switch to marijuana only to switch back to heroin once again a few years later.

"I used to do three lines of cocaine in each nose while dancing. And then some guy that I met in the club introduced me to heroin. So I started using heroin for like three years and then I started 'speedballing' which is speed and heroin mixed. And then I did everything else while working at the club. I smoked marijuana, I did acid, I popped diet pills, and I drank."
38-year-old recovering addict

These polydrug patterns from mixing to sequentialing are encountered with other abused drugs and are not just seen in opioid abusers.

FROM EXPERIMENTATION TO ADDICTION

Experimentation with alcohol, marijuana, and tobacco used to begin much earlier than experimentation with heroin but that gap has closed dramatically. In 1994 the average age of first heroin use was about 21 years old. In 1997 that figure had dropped to 17.6 years of age (NIDA, 1998). Generally it takes an average of a year of sporadic use for someone to develop a daily habit, although some users with a predisposition to opioid addiction might jump to daily use within 15 days.

"I'd wake up in the morning and before I'd go to work (when I was working), I'd have to do a hit of dope just to function. I'd have to do a hit of dope just to get out of bed. I'd have to do a hit of dope to go to the bathroom. It wasn't a matter of getting high

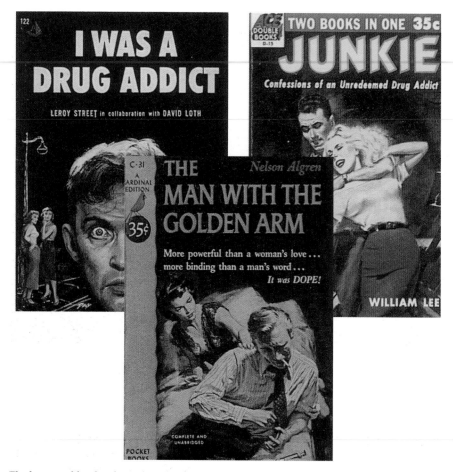

The heroin addict has been the subject of numerous pulp fiction novels and hundreds of motion pictures. However, the attitude of the public towards the "dope fiend" has changed since the 1950s when many of these novels were written.

anymore; it was a matter of getting functional."
Recovering 38-year-old male heroin abuser

In addition the user has to get something from the drug besides just relief from withdrawal symptoms to want to keep returning to the drug. That something could be the rush, a numbing of the emotions, or temporary relief from pain. Unfortunately for many users, the onset of tolerance, tissue dependence, and addiction, negates many of the benefits that were originally sought. In other cases the drug works too well.

"After a while you're not just killing your pain; you start to kill your feelings, any feelings you might have

regardless of whether you're having pain. It's not the pain that you're killing. It's never really the pain. It's the feelings that you have."
36-year-old recovering heroin abuser

If an opioid user has passed from experimentation to abuse or addiction, treatment becomes a physiological as well as a psychological process. Physically the addict has to be detoxified from the heroin or other opioid, often with the use of medications such as Darvon® (a milder opioid than heroin), methadone (a long-lasting opioid), LAAM® (a very long-lasting opioid), and buprenorphine (a powerful opiate agonist at low doses and an antagonist at high doses). Psychologically the addict has to learn a new way of living.

The Vietnam Experience

The road from experimentation to addiction can be better understood by looking at the use of heroin in Vietnam by U.S. soldiers from 1967 to the end of the war in 1973. Lee N. Robins (a psychiatrist at Harvard) and others tested several groups of GIs, first while still stationed in Vietnam and then after they had been returned to the United States. Almost half the GIs had experimented with opium or heroin. Twenty percent had been addicted at one time and reported withdrawal symptoms. Since heroin was so readily available, experimentation was easy, even for those who were too young to drink. So the usual progression from alcohol, cigarettes, and marijuana to heroin or cocaine was reversed. According to Robins, the most startling part of the study was that only 5% of those who had become addicted in Vietnam relapsed within 10 months after they returned to the United States and only 12% relapsed even briefly within 3 years. Most of the returning GIs didn't even go through treatment (Robins, 1994). This seems to suggest that even though tissue dependence caused by use of drugs can be powerful, other factors including preexisting sensitivity determined by heredity and environment have at least an equal or possibly greater influence.

MORPHINE & HEROIN

MORPHINE & PAIN CONTROL

Morphine

In 1805 morphine was the first alkaloid to be isolated but it wasn't fully synthesized until 1952. It remains the standard by which effective pain relief is measured. Morphine is processed from opium into white crystal hypodermic tablets, capsules, suppositories, oral solutions, and injectable solutions. This analgesic may be drunk, eaten, absorbed under the tongue, absorbed rectally by suppository, or injected into a vein, a muscle, or under the skin. Different routes of administration have

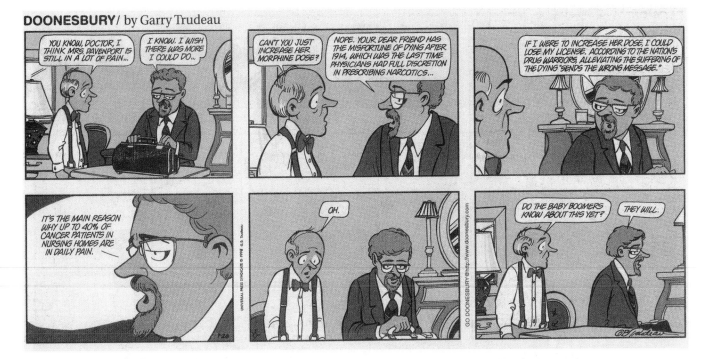

DOONSBURY © 1998, G. B. Trudeau. Reprinted, by permission, UNIVERSAL PRESS SYNDICATE. All rights reserved.

different effects. For example, three to six times more morphine must be taken orally to achieve the same effects as taking a smaller amount intravenously.

The liver is the principal site of metabolism and along with other tissues converts the morphine into metabolites that more readily cross the blood-brain barrier. Some of the morphine is excreted quickly in the urine. The metabolites such as morphine-3-glucuronide are possibly more potent than morphine (Karch, 1996). Morphine remains in measurable amounts in the plasma for four to six hours and can be detectable in the urine for several days.

Therapeutic Pain Control

When morphine or any other opioid is used in a hospital or by prescription for pain control, one of the fears and concerns of doctor and patient alike is the possible development of tissue dependence and addiction. A second concern is that the opioid will mask clues to cancer or other serious disease. Finally the physician is concerned that the patient is faking symptoms (malingering) in order to get drugs to supply their addiction (purposive withdrawal). These three concerns might keep some physicians from prescribing sufficient pain medications even when appropriate. In fact iatrogenic addiction (physician-induced addiction) is very rare but iatrogenic relapse or manipulation to obtain opioids may be very frequent.

"I had been masking the pain for so long that I didn't know how much pain I had or didn't have and when I didn't really have pain, per say, that was pathological. I couldn't deal with the slightest little thing."
37-year-old recovering prescription opioid addict

Since some level of tissue adaptation occurs with even the initial dose of an opioid, some care does need to be taken in prescribing. Part of the problem is the confusion between physical dependence and addiction. **Physical dependence**, as described above, is a physical adaptation of the body to a drug that will result in withdrawal symptoms when the drug is stopped. Since the severity of the withdrawal symptom is directly related to length of use and amount taken, most short-term use of pain medications will result in only mild withdrawal symptoms. Other factors, such as hereditary and environmental susceptibility, have to come into play. It is important for the physician to learn about risk factors such as

◇ physical health (e.g., kidney and liver function),

◇ drug abuse, medical drug use, and mental health history.

In addition the physician has to

◇ develop a working diagnosis and treatment plan;

◇ discuss risks vs. benefits and compliance with the patient;

◇ keep up-to-date on recent trials of medications or consult with someone familiar with the drug;

◇ get constant feedback from the patient as to effects, efficacy, and side effects;

◇ be willing to modify type of medication and dosages;

◇ keep accurate records concerning effects and patient reaction (adapted from Verhaag & Ikeda, 1991).

HEROIN—A WORLD VIEW

Since the 1930s heroin has captured more headlines than any other opioid. There are 5–10 million serious heroin users worldwide while a dozen countries are battling the growth, use, and exportation of heroin on their own soil. Since 1992 there has been a steady increase in heroin use worldwide but especially in the United States, due mostly to increased supplies and decreased cost. Even with the increase in supplies, the United States still consumes only three percent (10–15 metric tons) of the world's heroin supply. Since 1986 worldwide production of illicit opium, the raw ingredient to make heroin, has more than doubled according to the DEA and the International Narcotics Control Board.

The area of Southeast Asia known as the Golden Triangle (Myanmar [Burma], Northern Thailand, and Laos) is the largest producer and exporter of illegal opium and heroin. It is also one of the largest users. Thailand and Burma have 1/2 million addicts each. Golden Triangle heroin, known on the street as "China white" in its exportable form, can be up to 99% pure. Attempts to control or limit the growing and refining operations in the Golden Triangle are difficult and dangerous. The following is a description of some of the jungle refining operations by an international narcotics agent.

"The Golden Triangle is an area of constant motion as far as the narcotics trade is concerned. From year to year, the different insurgent groups are continually forming new alliances and dissolving old ones based on economics of the narcotic trade rather than the ideologies of the different groups. The groups have their own armies, often containing 3,000 to 7,000 men. Golden Triangle opium is grown in Burma,

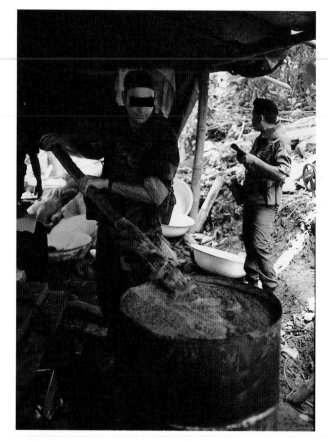

A narcotics agent and Thai soldier stand at an illegal opium jungle laboratory in Thailand that has just been raided. The 55-gallon barrel is filled with cooked opium, ready to be transformed into 20 kilograms of morphine and then into an equal weight of heroin. A small jungle laboratory such as this can process 60 kilograms of number four heroin (very pure) every four days.
Courtesy of George Skaggard

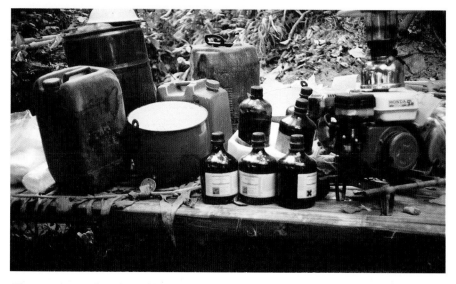

The various jars, barrels, and bags contain the chemicals needed to process opium to morphine to heroin. They contain ether, hydrochloric acid, acetic anhydride or AA, lime, ammonium chloride, charcoal, and sodium carbonate.
Courtesy of George Skaggard

Laos, and Thailand by ethnic hill tribes. Ethnic Chinese in the area contract the opium growing by providing the tribes with seeds and cash.

The Chinese middlemen collect the opium on a cash basis from the growers and refine it into the world's purest heroin in nearby jungle refin-

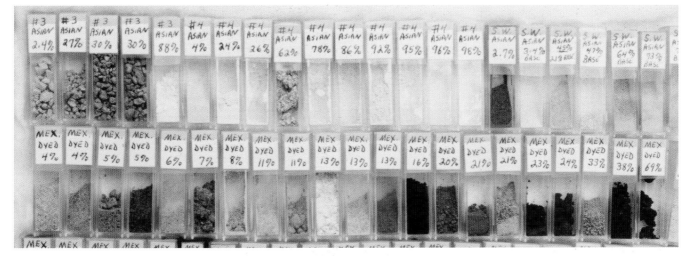

These are just a few samples of heroin seized by the Drug Enforcement Administration. Note that many highly diluted samples are dyed to make them appear a purer form of the drug.

Courtesy of Robert Sager, former lab chief, Drug Enforcement Administration

• •

eries. The refineries are of two types: those run by large organized insurgent groups or small independently syndicated groups. Large laboratories, usually found on the Burmese side of the border, make 200 kilograms of heroin at a time. There are about 200 of these large laboratories. The smaller laboratories on the Thai side of the border refine about 60 kilograms at a time. Those were the only ones we could raid because of political considerations. The work force of the larger labs includes 10 guards and 20 lab technicians. Security is usually provided by ex-military insurgents armed with M-16 rifles, machine guns, and grenade launchers.

Both groups' refineries are typically located in rough jungle-covered ravines near small streams. The refining equipment is easily portable and mostly primitive; enameled pots, 55-gallon drums, and wood-fueled stoves. The chemists, usually ethnic Chinese, follow a process handed down from chemist to chemist. Traditionally,

precursor chemicals used in the manufacture of heroin are transported through Thailand from sources in Malaysia, Singapore, Western Europe, Japan, and Bangkok. Extraction of morphine from opium takes from 1-2 days and heroin synthesis requires an additional 12—14 hours.

After processing, the heroin is stored in the jungle until it is marketed in nearby Thai border towns to buyers from various countries. Then utilizing Thailand's efficient transportation and banking systems, the heroin retraces the precursor chemicals' route. Initially the drugs are hauled by pack-mule or horse caravans carrying up to 3,000 kilograms at a time. The heroin finally arrives in Malaysia, Singapore, or Hong Kong where it is smuggled to the rest of the world's markets, including the United States.

International narcotics agent working in the Golden Triangle

Southwest Asian heroin from Afghanistan and Pakistan (known as

the "Golden Crescent") is the other major source. Myanmar and Afghanistan supply 92% of the world's production. Other Southeast Asian types of heroin include Indian, Cambodian, and Malaysian or Sri Lankan pink heroin (usually around 50% pure). India is the largest legal grower of opium but it is highly regulated and the vast majority of the crop is used for medical purposes (NIDA, 1998).

There has been a major increase in the production and abuse of heroin in Southwest Asia. From Afghanistan, Iran, Pakistan, Turkey, and Lebanon comes a product that is known as "Persian brown" or "Perze," which can be more than 90% pure. Several of these countries that grow opium now also have exploding addict populations. For example, there are an estimated 1.9 million opioid users in Pakistan.

"Persian heroin is simply raw processed morphine. The process to take raw morphine and turn it into white is a very expensive and lengthy chemical process which takes experts, so dealers are just giving you less quality for ridiculous prices."

28-year-old recovering male heroin smoker

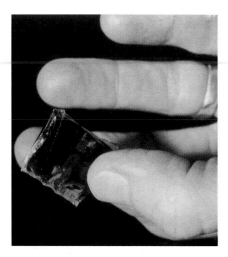

A small sample of Mexican "tar" heroin, the most common type of heroin sold in the United States, is packed in a little plastic bag.

Courtesy of JACNET, Jackson County, Oregon

Since the 1940s Mexico has been a major supplier of heroin to the United States. In the 1980s a relatively new form of Mexican heroin, known as "tar" or "black tar," took over much of the market on the West Coast, although it is still only five percent of heroin seizures. Perhaps the United States/ Mexico border is more porous than other routes. "Tar" heroin is extremely potent, 40% to 80% pure, but also has more plant impurities than the Asian refinement of the drug. A small chunk (black or brown) the size of a match head, which is enough for two to five doses, costs about $20 to $25. "Tar" heroin, also called "chapapote," "puta," "goma," "chiva," and "puro," is unique in that it's sold as a gummy pasty substance rather than the usual powder form. "Tar" dissolves easily in water and is also more likely to be smoked than other types of heroin. In 1995 an ounce of heroin on the East Coast of the United States, at the low-level dealer level, was as high as $8,000, while on the West Coast, an ounce could go for $3,000 (DEA, 1998).

"I came from the Midwest where we mostly get 'China white' and that to me is a whole lot cleaner than 'tar.' I'd

never seen an abscess or anything like that. People on the West Coast have abscesses all the time because here it is 'black tar.' The stuff I see when I break it down, there's so much crap in it. It's like, 'yuck,' I can't believe I put that 'shit' in my veins but I do it anyway."
27-year-old female heroin addict

In addition several countries have major refining facilities or act as major transshipment points for heroin. These transshipment countries include the Netherlands, Canada, Italy, France, and Nigeria (the latter also produces its own heroin). Also many ex-Soviet Republics and satellites (e.g., Albania, Armenia, Uzbekistan, Kazakhstan, and Turkmenistan) are involved in production and transshipment of heroin.

Although some homegrown opium exists in the United States, most heroin is imported. A few criminal organizations still control most of the trade and have adapted to changing times. For example, with the return of Hong Kong to the People's Republic of China in 1997, many of the triads (Chinese criminal organizations) based in Hong Kong decided that their headquarters would be wiped out if they

stayed. In response they increased their presence in other countries and tried to expand their markets and the number of users. This expansion has also led to a large increase in Asian gangs' involvement with heroin trafficking in the United States.

The Asian gangs and the Mafia have also increased the importation of cheaper smokable heroin to encourage many young users to try it in order to create a new market. This is what happened with cocaine when the availability of smokable "crack" cocaine expanded the number of cocaine users. At the present time injection is the preferred means of abusing heroin in the West, although in most Asian and Middle Eastern countries, it is smoked. Occasionally it is snorted.

"If anybody has the delusion that smoking's all that much different than shooting heroin, they're in for a big surprise. It's just as easy to get addicted smoking heroin as it is shooting heroin."
34-year-old heroin smoker

Alarmingly in the early 1990s, a number of Colombian cocaine cartels

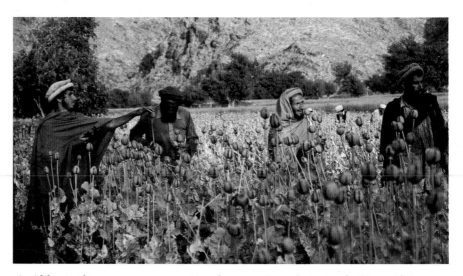

An Afghani militia man scrapes raw opium from an opium poppy capsule. Many militias around the world fund their military operations with money from growing and trafficking drugs.

Reprinted, by permission, Alain Labrousse, Observatoire Geopolitique Des Drogues.

diversified and started to grow and distribute opium poppies (in addition to their fields of coca shrubs) in an effort to cash in on the growing heroin market. Their existing cocaine distribution channels enabled them to expand rapidly. By the end of the 1990s, Colombian heroin was involved in the majority of drug busts (although the amounts were relatively small) (DEA, 1998). They also sold purer and cheaper heroin to compete with the Mafia and the Asian gangs.

OTHER OPIOIDS

CODEINE

"For me, codeine is just weak heroin. It doesn't do much for me. Codeine just stops the pain and stops your nose from running. It just gets you able to function enough in order to go get you some heroin."

42-year-old male recovering heroin user

Codeine is extracted directly from opium or refined from morphine. It is about 1/5 as strong as morphine and is generally used for the relief of moderate pain. The most common drugs mixed with codeine are aspirin or acetaminophen because of synergistic analgesia (the drugs compliment each other's strength). Codeine is also commonly used to control severe coughs (Robitussin AC®, Cheracol®). It is a schedule V drug in cough syrups and is even sold over the counter in some states. It is a schedule II or schedule III (if mixed with other drugs) prescription drug when used for analgesia. Codeine used to be the most widely prescribed and abused prescription opioid in the United States and other countries but hydrocodone (Vicodin®) has taken over that dubious honor. Some addicts drink large amounts of cough syrup to relieve heroin withdrawal or just to get slightly loaded. One of the problems with codeine, as with many opioids, is that it triggers nausea. One of the reasons many

physicians prescribe hydrocodone for moderate pain is because it seems to cause less nausea. The half-life of codeine is about 3 hours and the drug will be detectable in the blood for up to 24 hours and in the urine for up to 2 or 3 days.

HYDROCODONE (Vicodin®, Hycodan®, Tussend®, Norco®)

More than 50 million prescriptions were written for hydrocodone (Vicodin®) in 1998 (American Druggist, 1999). This most widely prescribed semisynthetic opioid has many of the same actions as codeine but produces less nausea. Four times as many prescriptions for hydrocodone for analgesia were written as compared to codeine. It is also used in cough preparations, called "antitussives", e.g., Hycomin Syrup®. A number of people who were prescribed hydrocodone for pain became dependent on this schedule III ophioid. As with other opioids, respiratory depression and masking of illness can be dangerous especially when other depressants, including alcohol, different opioids, analgesics, and antianxiety agents, are used at the same time. About 337 deaths are reported each year due to hydrocodone overdose, although more occur when used with other depressants (DAWN, 1997). Seventeen out of 20 DEA field divisions mentioned hydrocodone abuse as a problem. In frequency of mentions, oxycodone (Percodan®) was next, then codeine, and finally hydromorphone (Dilaudid®) (DEA, 1999).

"I injured myself and I was on hydrocodone, you know. It's kind of a super painkiller and it felt good. I'd

take one, next hour and a half I'd be real sleepy and lightheaded... be dizzy. It's like being drunk. I developed a small addiction to it, you know. It was an easy escape; pop a pill, drink some water. Drown my fears away, drown the pain away... feel good for a while."

24-year-old weightlifter

METHADONE (Dolophine®)

Methadone is only one of two legally authorized opioids used to treat heroin addiction through a program known as methadone maintenance (*see Chapter 9*). Under this harm reduction program started in New York in 1965, methadone is used as a legally dispensed substitute for heroin. The addict comes into the clinic every day to receive a dose. On a few occasions (e.g., when the methadone user has to go out of town) a take-home dose is given for the following day or two. Methadone is usually mixed with fruit juice or in tablets for take-home doses. There are approximately 115,000 heroin addicts involved in methadone treatment in more than 900 methadone treatment programs nationwide. Methadone is also used to detoxify a heroin abuser who has become physically dependent.

Because this long-acting synthetic opioid reduces drug craving and blocks withdrawal symptoms for 24–72 hours, it diminishes the craving for heroin, which has a shorter duration of action, causes more intense highs and lows, and is illegal. The disappearance of the intense need to use heroin again and again and come up

---

with increasing amounts of money has led to a dramatic decrease in crime among those in methadone maintenance. Like any opioid, methadone also has painkilling and depressant effects that can be used in clinical situations. The analgesic effects only last 4–6 hours.

Like heroin, methadone is addicting and must be monitored closely to prevent diversion into illegal channels. Despite heavy regulation of methadone clinics and tight controls of the supply, methadone is still sold on the street, abused, and responsible for a number of overdoses every year. Addicts will combine methadone with other drugs, such as clonazepam (Klonopin®), clonidine (Catapres®), carisoprodol (Soma®), and alprazolam (Xanax®), in order to intensify the high and make it resemble the feeling they get from heroin.

Recently there have been proposals, research, and trials by the U.S. Department of Health and Human Services among others to make methadone treatment more convenient and bring it into the mainstream of health care. Rather than have recovering addicts get their methadone only from methadone clinics, the drug would also be available through certified physicians and nonmethadone drug clinics. There is also a proposal to move methadone treatment out from the scrutiny of the FDA to the oversight of SAMHSA (Substance Abuse and Mental Health Services Administration) which would decrease the amount of regulations that cover its use.

HYDROMORPHONE (Dilaudid®)

Hydromorphone, a short-acting semisynthetic opioid, can be taken orally or injected. Hydromorphone is refined from morphine, a process that makes it 7–10 times more potent on a gram-for-gram basis than morphine and shorter-acting opioids. Hydromorphone is used as an alternative to morphine for the treatment of moderate to severe pain. Since it is more potent, it has a higher abuse potential than morphine. Illegally diverted Dilaudid® is becoming increasingly attractive to cocaine users for the drug combination known as a "speedball," (hydromorphone and cocaine or methamphetamine). A 4-milligram tablet of Dilaudid® sold on the street varies from $30 to $70 (DEA, 1998). Though it is quite potent, just a few deaths from overdose are reported each year.

OXYCODONE (Percodan®)

This semisynthetic derivative of codeine is used for the relief of moderate to severe pain. Oxycodone is most often taken orally, often in combination with aspirin or acetaminophen. By this route it usually takes about 30 minutes before the effects appear and these effects last from 4–6 hours. Its pain-relieving effect is much stronger than codeine but weaker than that of morphine or Dilaudid®.

MEPERIDINE (Demerol®, Pethidine®)

A synthetic phenylpiperidine derivative, this short-acting opioid is one of the most widely used analgesics for moderate to severe pain, though it is only 1/6 the strength of morphine. It is most often injected, though it can be taken orally. This drug can be neurotoxic in large doses. Demerol® affects the brain in such a way that it causes as much sedation and euphoria than morphine but less constipation and cough suppression. Since it is eliminated by the kidneys, patients with impaired kidneys should avoid the drug. Though less potent by weight than morphine, it is often the opioid most often abused by medical professionals.

PENTAZOCINE (Talwin NX®)

Talwin NX®, prescribed for chronic or acute pain, comes in tablets or as an injectable liquid. It has about half the potency of morphine and acts as a weak opioid antagonist as well as an opioid agonist. This drug used to be frequently combined and injected with an antihistamine drug ("Ts and blues") for the heroin-like high. Increased vigilance and reformulation of Talwin® (including the addition of naloxone, a more powerful opioid antagonist) by its manufacturer have almost stopped these problems, although some abusers still abuse Talwin NX® orally by itself. There are no emergency room reports of pentazocine overdoses perhaps because of its reformulation. However it still retains an abuse potential and is therefore classified as a controlled drug.

PROPOXYPHENE (Darvon®, Darvocet®, Propacet®, Wygesic®)

Used for the relief of mild to moderate pain, Darvon® is often prescribed by dentists. More than 20 million prescriptions were written for propoxyphene in 1998 (American Druggist, 1999). It is taken orally for moderate pain with the effects lasting four to six hours. Propoxyphene is occasionally used as an alternative to methadone maintenance and for heroin detoxification, especially for younger addicts, because it has only 1/2 to 2/3 the potency of codeine. The older the user, the slower the metabolism, so the drug is more potent. Misuse of this drug makes someone susceptible to overdose or addiction. Four percent of opioid fatalities in 1994 (351 cases) involved propoxyphene (often in combination with alcohol).

"After seven years of doing Darvon®, I started having withdrawals after three to four hours from the last pill that I had taken, so I was addicted to my watch. Then it got to where it was like two hours, so I needed like 14 or 16 Darvons® to get through the day."
Recovering 43-year-old female Darvon® abuser

Although it has abuse potential, Darvon® and especially Darvon-N® (a naptholate salt) continues to be used successfully in the detoxification of heroin addicts.

FENTANYL (Sublimaze®)

Fentanyl is the most powerful of the opioids (50–100 times as strong as morphine on a weight-for-weight basis). It is used intravenously during and after surgery for severe pain. Structurally this synthetic phenylpiperidine derivative is related to meperidine (Demerol®). It is also available in a skin patch to give steady pain relief for patients with intractable pain. A fentanyl lollipop was introduced in 1994 to be used by children for postoperative pain. Unfortunately fentanyl is popular with some surgical assistants and anesthesiologists due to its availability and strength.

DESIGNER HEROIN

There are street versions of fentanyl (alpha, 3-methyl) and meperidine (MPPP) manufactured in illegal laboratories. They are extremely potent and can cause drug overdoses and even damage to the nervous system. Sold as "China white," these drugs bear witness to a growing sophistication of street chemists who now can bypass the traditional smuggling and trafficking routes of heroin. Since these designer drugs are made without controls on purity or dosage, they represent a tremendous health threat to the opioid-abusing community. There have been numerous outbreaks of overdose deaths due to ultrapotent fentanyl being sold as normal-potency heroin.

"When I first got out here on the West Coast, I found out that it ['China white'] wasn't white dope at all. It was fentanyl and it wasn't even pharmaceutical fentanyl. It was bathtub fentanyl and people were dying on it."
Dealer/heroin user

If improperly made, street Demerol® (MPPP) can contain a chemical, MPTP, which destroys the brain cells that control voluntary muscular movement and rapidly cause the degenerative nerve condition known as "Parkinson's Disease." This degeneration causes a condition known as the "frozen addict," when the addict loses the ability to make any physical movements for the rest of his or her life.

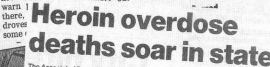

LAAM® (l-alpha acetyl methadol)

LAAM® is another opioid that is used for heroin replacement therapy similar to methadone maintenance. It prevents withdrawal symptoms and lasts for about 2–3 days compared to methadone's duration of action of 24–72 hours. This reduces visits to the clinic for the drug to every other day or 3 days a week. It also reduces the need for take-home doses, thereby reducing the potential of street trade with the drug. The half-life of LAAM® is 48 hours and the half-life of active LAAM® metabolites is 96 hours. Though the drug was developed in the late 1940s as a possible substitute for morphine, the slow onset and long duration of toxic action made it unsuitable for pain management (Rawson, Hasson, Huber, et al., 1998). It has been studied since the mid-1960s as a treatment for opioid-dependent individuals but it wasn't until 1993 that the U.S. Food and Drug Administration made LAAM® available for clinical use. The main detriment to the use of LAAM®, according to a survey of LAAM® clinics, seems to be the complicated paperwork and regulatory hurdles involved with use along with staff attitude towards the drug (Rawson, 1998).

The drug itself seems to work as well as methadone. In 1999 a proposal was made to move the monitoring of LAAM® as well as methadone out of the FDA and into SAMHSA in an effort to decrease the bureaucratic paperwork associated with their use. LAAM® has now been given approval to be the second opioid agonist drug (after methadone) to be legally used in the treatment of opioid addiction.

NALOXONE, NALTREXONE (Narcan®, Revia®)

Naloxone and naltrexone are opioid antagonists. They block the effects of endogenous as well as exogenous opioids. Naloxone is effective in treating heroin or opioid drug overdose. When a heroin overdose victim is injected with the drug, opioid effects are immediately reversed and the person snaps back to consciousness in a matter of seconds. When the drug wears off, the patient can fall back into a coma because the heroin is still in the system. Often naloxone needs to be repeated until the heroin is completely metabolized by the body.

"I just remember finding a vein finally and then waking up with a plastic

tube in my nose, getting hit in the chest by a paramedic. Then everything went from black to light and they're standing over me and I was really pissed off at them for killing my buzz. And they're like, 'We just saved your life,' and I said, 'Maybe I didn't want you to. You just wasted $20.' But after a while, I thought about it and I know I could have died.'"

20-year-old male heroin addict in recovery

Naltrexone (Revia®) is used to prevent relapse and help to break the cycle of addiction for opioids. Taking naltrexone daily effectively blocks the effects of heroin and any other opioid. Naltrexone is also being used to reduce craving for alcohol and cocaine to support detoxification and abstinence. A time-release version of naltrexone (Naltrel®) is being developed that would only need to be injected once a month. Naltrexone is legally approved to treat heroin addiction.

BUPRENORPHINE (Buprenex®)

Buprenorphine is a powerful opioid agonist at low doses and an opiate antagonist at high doses. In low doses it is used as an analgesic alternative to morphine. It is being used experimentally as an alternative to methadone for detoxification and induction of methadone maintenance because it is more attractive to addicts and limits the supplementary use of heroin or other opiates and opioids by addicts.

CLONIDINE (Catapres®)

This nonopioid is often used to diminish the opioid withdrawal symptoms such as nausea, anxiety, and diarrhea. Since it acts on norepinephrine receptors to control their overactivity, one of the main causes of severe withdrawal symptoms, it shortens withdrawal time from almost a month down to a couple of weeks in some cases.

SEDATIVE-HYPNOTICS

CLASSIFICATION

More than 57 million prescriptions were written for sedative-hypnotics (mostly benzodiazepines) in 1998 in the United States (PhARM, 1999). Use in other countries is also widespread. These drugs are usually prescribed to control anxiety, to control the symptoms of anxiety or panic attacks, to induce sleep, to relax skeletal muscles, to control hypertension, to diminish severe alcohol or heroin withdrawal symptoms, and to prevent seizures. Many more prescriptions used to be written for sedative-hypnotics in the '60s, '70s, and '80s, particularly benzodiazepines, but the use of psychiatric medications for emotional depression, e.g., tricyclic antidepressants and the newer antidepressants, e.g., Prozac® and Zoloft®, have taken over a significant part of sedative-hypnotics' share of the market. At least 88 million prescriptions were written in 1998 for psychiatric medications.

Almost all sedative-hypnotics are available as pills, capsules, or tablets though some, such as diazepam (Valium®) and lorazepam (Ativan®), are

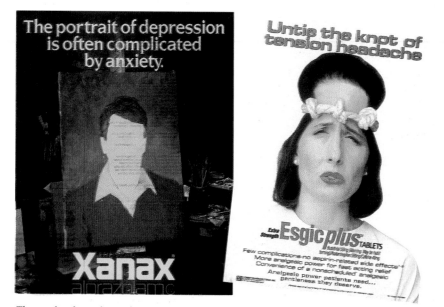

The market for sedative-hypnotics is in the billions of dollars. Advertising used to be directed at those with prescriptive authority but recently prescription drug advertisements in print and on television have directed their message at the consumer so they will "suggest" a certain drug to their doctor.

used intravenously for more immediate effects in seizure and panic attacks. The two main groups of sedative-hypnotics are benzodiazepines and barbiturates. There are also a number of other non-benzodiazepine/nonbarbiturate sedative-hypnotics

The effects of sedative-hypnotics are generally similar to the effects of alcohol (e.g., lowered inhibitions, physical depression, sedation, muscular relaxation) and like alcohol, sedative-hypnotic drugs can cause memory loss, tolerance, tissue dependence, withdrawal symptoms, and addiction. The obvious basic difference between the two depressants is their potency; on a gram-by-gram basis, sedative-hypnotics are much more potent than alcohol.

Sedatives, such as alprazolam (Xanax®), diazepam (Valium®), and meprobamate (Miltown®), are calming drugs, also called "minor tranquilizers." Some benzodiazepines, for example, act on the neurotransmitter GABA (gama amino butyric acid), serotonin, and dopamine to help control anxiety and restlessness. Sedatives are also capable of causing muscular relaxation, body heat loss, lowered inhibitions, reduced intensity of physical sensations, and reduced muscular coordination in speech, movement, and manual dexterity. They are also used to help with alcohol or heroin detoxification and to control seizures.

Hypnotics, such as short-acting barbiturates and benzodiazepines, work on the brainstem, inducing sleep along with depression of most body functions, including breathing and muscular coordination. Some sedatives are used as hypnotics and some hypnotics are used as sedatives, so it is sometimes difficult to separate the two functions.

HISTORY

Calming and sleep-inducing drugs have been around for millennia. The ones used in ancient cultures were natural plant-derived substances (especially opium) that were discovered through natural experimentation. In the last hundred years, with the increasing sophistication of chemical processes, many of the sedative-hypnotics have been developed in the laboratory.

At the turn of the century, bromides, paraldehyde, and chloral hydrate were commonly used. Though chemically they were quite different, they all depressed the central nervous system.

◇ **Bromides,** used as sedatives or anticonvulsants, were first introduced

TABLE 4–3   SEDATIVE-HYPNOTICS

Name	Trade Name	Street Name
BENZODIAZEPINES		
Alprazolam	Xanax®	
Chlordiazepoxide	Librium® Libritabs®	Libs
Clonazepam	Klonopin®	
Clorazepate	Tranxene®	
Diazepam	Valium®	Vals
Estazolam	Pro-Som®	
Flunitrazepam (banned in U.S.)	Rohypnol®	Ruffies, roofies, roachies
Flurazepam	Dalmane®	
Halazepam	Paxipam®	
Lorazepam	Ativan®	
Oxazepam	Serax®	
Prazepam	Centrax®	
Quazepam	Doral®	
Temazepam	Restoril®	
Triazolam	Halcion®	
BARBITURATES		
Amobarbital	Amytal®	Blue heaven
Aprobarbital	Alurate®	
Butabarbital	Barbased®, Butisol®	
Butalbital	Esgic®, Fiorinal®	
Hexobarbital	Sombulex®	
Mephobarbital	Mebaral®	
Methohexital	Brevital®	
Pentobarbital	Nembutal®	Yellows, yellow jackets, nebbies
Phenobarbital	Luminal®	Phenos
Secobarbital	Seconal®	Reds, red devils, F-40s
Equal parts secobarbitol & amylbarbital	Tuinal®	Rainbows, tuies, double trouble
Talbutal	Lotusate®	
Thiamylal sodium	Surital®	
Thiopental sodium	Pentothal®	
NONBENZODIAZEPINE, NONBARBITURATE SEDATIVE-HYPNOTICS		
Bromides		
Chloral hydrate	Noctec®, Somnos®	Jelly beans, Mickeys, knockout drops
Ethchlorvynol	Placidyl®	Green weenies
GHB (gammahydroxybutyrate)		Grievous bodily harm, liquid E, fantasy, Georgia home boy
GBL (gamma butyl lactone)	Blue Nitro®, Revivarant®, Insom-X®, Revivarant G®, Gamma G®, GH Revitalizer®, Remforce®	
Glutethimide (obsolete)	Doriden®	Goofballs, goofers
Glutethimide & codeine	Doriden® & codeine	Loads, sets, setups, hits, C & C
Meprobamate	Equinil®, Miltown®, Meprotabs®, Deprol®	Mother's little helper
Methaprylon	Noludar®	Noodlelars
Methaqualone (only illegal forms)	Quaalude®, Soper®, Somnafac®, Parest® Optimil®, Paraldehyde	Ludes, sopes, soapers, Qs
Zolpidem	Ambien®	

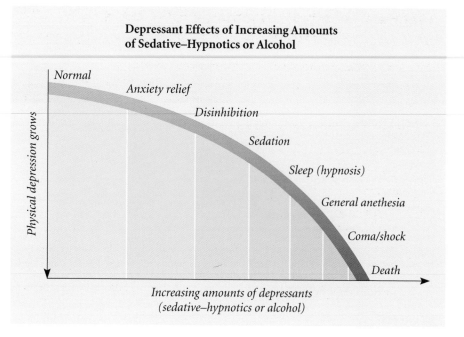

Depressant Effects of Increasing Amounts of Sedative–Hypnotics or Alcohol

Normal

Anxiety relief

Disinhibition

Sedation

Sleep (hypnosis)

General anethesia

Coma/shock

Death

Physical depression grows

Increasing amounts of depressants (sedative–hypnotics or alcohol)

Figure 4-4 •

As this chart shows, the different strengths of sedative-hypnotics can be used simply to calm or to anesthetize for surgery. When users self-medicate with sedative-hypnotics and/or alcohol, they often lose track of where they will end up on the scale.

in the 1850s and often sold over the counter but they had a long half-life and so prolonged or non-supervised use could build up toxic doses in the body.

◇ **Chloral hydrate** was used both as a sedative and as a hypnotic. It is still occasionally used to this day because the margin of safety is better than barbiturates for sleep problems.

◇ **Paraldehyde** was used to control the symptoms of alcohol withdrawal. Despite its offensive odor and tendency to become addictive, it is still occasionally used to treat alcoholics (Hollister, 1983).

◇ **Barbiturates** were first developed at the end of the nineteenth century and slowly grew in popularity; they peaked in the 1930s and 1940s. Phenobarbital, secobarbital, and pentobarbital were among the hundreds of compounds synthesized from barbituric acid. Appreciation of the toxic potential of barbiturates due to a low therapeutic index, low degree of selectivity,

along with a high dependence and addictive potential, instilled an apprehension of use and encouraged researchers to look for new classes of sedative-hypnotics.

◇ **Meprobamate (Miltown®)** was developed in the late '40s and '50s. This long-acting sedative replaced many long-acting barbiturates, including phenobarbital. Its popularity peaked from 1955 to 1961 when benzodiazepines took center stage.

◇ **Glutethimide (Doriden®)** was tried but it seemed to have many of the disadvantages of barbiturates without too many advantages. It was also weaker than phenobarbital and subject to abuse when it was used in combination with codeine ("loads," "sets," and "setups") in order to potentiate the effects of both drugs. It is no longer manufactured in the United States.

◇ **Benzodiazepines** were discovered in 1957 at Roche Laboratories in a deliberate search for a safer class of sedative-hypnotics. When

Librium® (chlordiazepoxide) and Valium® (diazepam) were synthesized and marketed in 1960 and 1963 respectively, they quickly became immensely popular because they were less toxic than barbiturates, meprobamate, and glutethimide, although many of the sites of action in the central nervous system were similar to those of the barbiturates. Over the years more than 3,000 compounds were developed although only a couple of dozen were marketed and released (Sternbach, 1983). To this day benzodiazepines dominate the market for sedative-hypnotics. Although they are less toxic than other sedatives, benzodiazepines are very addictive and have a dangerous withdrawal reaction.

USE, MISUSE, ABUSE, & ADDICTION

In the twentieth century, society's attitude towards the use of psychiatric medications has swung like a pendulum. The free use of barbiturates in the '30s and '40s along with the vision of a drug-controlled society as written about in Aldous Huxley's *Brave New World* led to the search for nonaddictive alternatives. But the widespread use of Miltown® in the '50s, which eventually led to an attitude of "better living through chemistry" in the '60s, seemed to fulfill Huxley's fears. Benzodiazepines were hailed as miracle drugs and prescribed in huge amounts (100 million prescriptions per year in the United States by 1975) and again, fear of becoming a drug-dependent society came to the fore. As a result a kind of guerrilla warfare has occurred which pits some of those in the medical and treatment communities who want to have the freedom to prescribe benzodiazepines as they see fit against the others who feel that overuse of prescription drugs needs to be brought under control. Even within some drug companies, there is a conflict between the research/development departments that want to develop drugs with very targeted effects and marketing departments that would like to have their drugs approved for as many conditions as possible and used for extended periods of time.

When used properly, sedative-hypnotics can be useful therapeutic adjuncts to treating a variety of psychological and physical conditions. When misused they can cause undesirable side effects, dependence, abuse, addiction, and even suicides.

"I stopped marijuana and hallucinogens 12 years ago and then told myself that I was not using drugs 'cause I was using prescription drugs. I stopped after a while . . . after a 4-year period."
38-year-old female recovering polydrug abuser

Sedative-hypnotic (as well as opioid) misuse can occur through several mechanisms:

◊ when patients overuse the drugs prescribed by the physician;

◊ when patients use them in combination with other psychoactive drugs to potentiate or counteract effects;

◊ when they borrow the drug from a friend to self-medicate;

◊ when they divert the drug from legal sources through forged prescriptions, buying on the black market, or stealing to get high or medicate emotional pain.

"I would go over and visit people and the first thing, within five minutes, I would go to the bathroom, go over into the medicine cabinet and flush the toilet so no one in the other room would hear me. I'd trash the medicine cabinet and if I didn't find anything there, I'd go through the drawers."
43-year-old recovering prescription drug user

Over the years, in popular and scientific literature and movies, sedative-hypnotics have been associated with both accidental and intentional drug

TABLE 4–4 MENTIONS OF DRUG PROBLEMS IN EMERGENCY ROOMS - 1999

In many cases, more than one drug is found in incoming patients.

Drugs	% of total drug mentions (more than 100% due to polydrug use)
1. Alcohol in combination with other drugs	34%
2. Cocaine	30%
3. Heroin/morphine, codeine, or other opioids	20%
4. Marijuana	15%
5. Benzodiazepines (Xanax®, Valium®, Ativan®, Klonopin®)	11%
6. Acetaminophen, aspirin, ibuprofen	11%
7. Antidepressants (Trazodone®, Elavil®, Prozac®)	7%
8. Methamphetamine/amphetamine	4%
9. Antihistamine	1%
10. OTC sleeping aids	1%

(DAWN, 2000)

overdoses. Many movies use the image of an empty vial of prescription drugs to indicate a suicide attempt or the need for stomach pumps.

In the *Annual Emergency Room Data Survey,* physicians list which drugs cause medical problems severe enough to make people seek medical attention. The above list shows which drugs are reported most often. Overall, there are more than a 1/2 million visits to emergency rooms for drug problems such as overdose, dependence, withdrawal syndrome, and drug interactions.

Studies of sedative-hypnotic drug misuse and overdose conducted by the National Institute of Drug Abuse (NIDA) reveal some factors that contribute to abuse or overdose with these drugs.

◊ Since sedatives impair memory, awareness, and judgment, individuals fail to realize or forget how many sedatives they have ingested to help them get to sleep or to relieve stress. Rather than waiting long enough for the full dosage of the drug to affect them, they continue to take more of the drug and accidentally reach a toxic state.

This effect has been called "drug automatism."

◊ Ignorance of additive and synergistic effects resulting from combining these drugs with alcohol or other sedatives is widespread.

◊ Selective tolerance to some effects of the drug but not to its toxic effects results in a narrowing window of safety where the amount needed to produce a high comes closer to the lethal dose of the drug.

◊ Adolescent attitudes of invulnerability promote risk-taking behavior in respect to the amount of drug ingested.

BENZODIAZEPINES

Benzodiazepines are the most widely used sedative-hypnotics in the United States. This class of drugs was developed in the late 1940s and 1950s as an alternative to barbiturates. Since benzodiazepines have a fairly safe therapeutic index, many health care professionals initially overlooked their peculiarities, e.g., the length of time

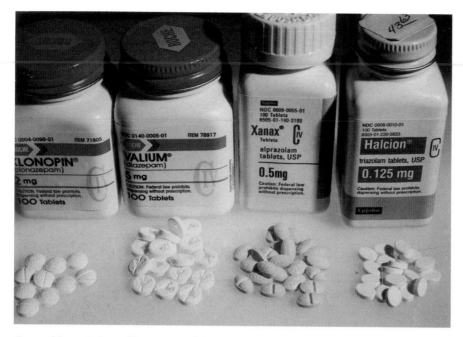

Some of the main benzodiazepines include alprazolam (Xanax®), diazepam (Valium®), clonazepam (Klonopin®), and triazolam (Halcion®).

they last in body tissues, their ability to induce tissue dependence at low levels of use, and the severity of withdrawal from the drug. For these reasons almost all recommendations for benzodiazepine use today emphasize it should be used short term and for specific conditions, not as a long-term medication, such as an antidepressant or blood pressure drug.

"They began to treat my headaches with Valium® because Valium® was 'the wonder drug.' You can't overdose on Valium®. No way you can kill yourself. They were wrong about it."

45-year-old recovering benzodiazepine abuser

MEDICAL USE OF BENZODIAZEPINES

Medically benzodiazepines are used to

◇ manage anxiety disorders;

◇ provide short-term treatment for the symptoms of anxiety and panic disorders;

◇ control anxiety and apprehension in surgical patients and to diminish recall of the procedure;

◇ treat sleep problems;

◇ control skeletal muscular spasms;

◇ elevate the seizure threshhold (anticonvulsant) and control seizures;

◇ control acute alcohol withdrawal symptoms, e.g., severe agitation, tremors, impending acute delirium tremens, and hallucinosis.

"The enclosed space of the MRI x-ray they were going to slip me into really triggered one of my claustrophobic panic attacks, so we couldn't finish. I was yelling, 'get me outta here' along with some nasty threats to do them bodily harm. The next time, they gave me some Valium® and though I still felt nervous, it did calm me enough so I could have the scan done. It seemed like a dream."

50-year-old female without any drug problem

NONMEDICAL USE OF BENZODIAZEPINES

Since the desirable emotional and physical effects of benzodiazepines are very similar to alcohol, they are sometimes used for the same reasons

a person drinks. A double-blind study on nondrug addicts compared the effects of low-dose diazepam injections and alcohol injections. The subjects found the highs from each of the drugs to be extremely similar, however higher-dose diazepam produced more physical impairment (Schuckit, Greenblatt, Gold, & Irwin, 1991).

Benzodiazepines alone can be abused but they are most often abused in conjunction with other drugs. "Speed" and cocaine users often take a benzodiazepine to come down from excess stimulation. Heroin addicts frequently take a benzodiazepine when they can't get their drug of choice and alcoholics use them to prevent life-threatening withdrawal symptoms, such as convulsions. For example, depending on the study, 20% to 40% of alcoholics and 25% to 50% of heroin- or methadone-maintained addicts use benzodiazepines (Miller & Gold, 1990). In another study at a treatment center, 10% of polydrug clients abused benzodiazepines. They were more likely to be older than 30 years, white, well-educated, and female (Malcolm, 1993). Almost 100% of benzodiazepine addicts report dependence on or addiction to other drugs (Busto, Sellers, Naranjo, et al., 1986).

"If I threw down 10 Valium®, I didn't really feel that much. It wasn't like taking Nembutal® or other barbiturates where you get a real rush. I would have to take an awful lot to feel anything. It relieved certain anxieties; it alleviated depression. You tell the doctor, 'I'm depressed.' 'Okay, take some Valium®.'"

38-year-old recovering female benzodiazepine abuser

NEUROCHEMISTRY & GABA

Benzodiazepines have been shown to exert their sedative effects in the brain by potentiating (magnifying) a naturally occurring neurotransmitter, called GABA (gamma amino butyric acid), in the cerebellum, cerebral cortex, and limbic system (Potokar & Nutt, 1994). GABA is recognized as the most important inhibitory neurotransmitter, so when a drug, like alprazolam (Xanax®), greatly increases the actions of GABA, it increases the inhibition of anxiety-producing thoughts and over-stimulating neural messages. Other sedating neurotransmitters, such as serotonin and dopamine, are also potentiated.

Most benzodiazepines, e.g., prazepam, are prodrugs. This means that the liver converts a certain percentage of a drug, like diazepam (Valium®), to a metabolite (e.g., nordiazepam). The metabolites can be as active or even more active than the original drug itself. The metabolite of diazepam can be further converted to temazepam and oxazepam (Jenkins & Cone, 1998). (These last two active metabolites are also manufactured separately by pharmaceutical companies as Restoril® and Serax®.) The metabolites along with the original drug are very fat-soluble (lipophilic) and so stay in the body for a long time.

Specific benzodiazepines have been developed to treat specific conditions. For example, short-term alprazolam (Xanax®) is used for immediate relief of the symptoms of generalized anxiety disorder and panic disorder; triazolam (Halcion®) is used for short-term (7–10 days) treatment of insomnia; diazepam (Valium®) is used to gain relief from skeletal muscle spasms caused by inflammation of the muscles or joints or to control seizures, such as those that occur during severe alcohol or barbiturate withdrawal; intravenous Valium® is used as a sedative just before surgery.

TOLERANCE, TISSUE DEPENDENCE, & WITHDRAWAL

Tolerance

Tolerance to benzodiazepines develops as the liver becomes more efficient in processing the drug. However, age-dependent tolerance also occurs with these drugs, meaning that a younger person can tolerate much more of these benzodiazepines than someone older. The effect of a dose on a 50-year-old first-time user can be 5

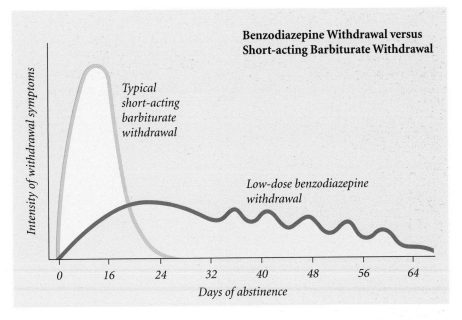

Figure 4-5 •
The delay in the occurrence of withdrawal symptoms can be dangerous to benzodiazepine abusers who stop using abruptly.

or 10 times stronger than the same dose on a 20 year old.

"I started taking Valium® when I went out to parties 'cuz I found that it gives me . . . it was the same as drinking. But liquor gave me headaches, which I was trying to prevent. So I forget when, exactly, it started controlling me. I started taking, oh, 10 a day, or 5 at a time. Then pretty soon, I'd pop 10 at a time."
Recovering benzodiazepine abuser

Tissue Dependence

Physical addiction to the benzodiazepine can develop if the patient takes 10–20 times the normal dose daily for a couple of months or longer, or takes a normal dose for a year or more. Since many benzodiazepines are slowly deactivated by the body over a period of several days, even low-dose use can lead to addiction when these drugs are taken daily over a number of years. In addition the pleasant mental effects and hypnotizing aspects of the drugs (reinforcement) can result in a mental or psychological dependence.

Withdrawal

After high-dose continuous use for about one to three months or lower-dose use for at least one to two years, withdrawal symptoms can be severe. Withdrawal symptoms can be

◇ recurrence of the symptoms that were being treated with the benzodiazepine,

◇ rebound or magnification of the symptoms that were being treated,

◇ pseudowithdrawal where the user exaggerates the recurrence of symptoms,

◇ true withdrawal in a patient who has become physically dependent, often caused by low GABA and excess epinephrine and norepinephrine.

The drug is long lasting, so with true withdrawal the onset of symptoms is delayed—about 1 day for short-acting and up to 5 days for long-acting benzodiazepines. The symptoms can last 7–20 days for short-acting and up to 28 days for long-acting benzodiazepines (Eickelberg & Mayo-Smith, 1998).

Since many of the symptoms of

TABLE 4–5   PLASMA HALF-LIFE OF BENZODIAZEPINES

This table shows the length of time various benzodiazepines remain in the body and continue to affect the user.

Chemical (Trade) Name	Half-Life
Very long acting	
Halazepam (Paxipam®)	30–200 hours
Prazepam (Centrax®)	30–200 hours
Flurazepam (Dalmane®)	90–200 hours
Intermediate acting	
Clonazepam (Klonopin®)	18–50 hours
Chlordiazepoxide (Librium®)	7–46 hours
Diazepam (Valium®)	14–90 hours
Short acting	
Alprazolam (Xanax®)	6–20 hours
Temazepam (Restoril®)	5–20 hours
Oxazepam (Serax®)	6–24 hours
Lorazepam (Ativan®)	9–22 hours
Very short acting	
Triazolam (Halcion®)	2–6 hours

true withdrawal are similar to the symptoms of an anxiety or depressive disorder, it can be hard to judge the level of dependence. First a craving for the drug occurs to avoid the withdrawal symptoms, followed by tremor, muscle twitches, nausea and vomiting, anxiety, restlessness, yawning, tachycardia, cramping, hypertension, inability to focus, sleep disturbances, and dizziness. Some people even experience a temporary loss of vision, hearing, or smell and other sensory hypersensitivity while in withdrawal; occasionally they have hallucinations (Miller, 1990; Eickelberg, 1998). The symptoms continue and peak in the first through third weeks. These symptoms occasionally include multiple seizures and convulsions which can be fatal.

"I stopped taking them and on the third day, I remember I was sweating. I changed the sheets on the bed. I took a shower. I was fairly relaxed and I went into a convulsion. I don't remember what happened. All I can remember is waking up and all my front teeth

were knocked out. I ended up going through about 80 convulsions."
Recovering Valium® abuser

The persistence of benzodiazepines (Table 4-5) in the body from low or regular doses taken over a long period of time results not only in prolonged withdrawal symptoms but in symptoms that erratically come and go in cycles separated by 2–10 days. These symptoms are sometimes bizarre, sometimes life threatening, and all are complicated by the cyclical nature of the severity. Short-acting barbiturates, on the other hand, follow a fairly predictable course where the symptoms come and then go and do not return. Called the "**protracted withdrawal syndrome**," the symptoms of benzodiazepine withdrawal may persist for several months after the drug has been terminated.

BENZODIAZEPINE OVERDOSE

The reason actual overdoses and suicides have decreased with the in-

creased use of benzodiazepines and decreased use of barbiturates is that the benzodiazepines have a much greater therapeutic index, the lethal dose of a drug divided by its therapeutic effective dose. The therapeutic index of barbiturates is 10 to 1 while the therapeutic index of benzodiazepines is 700 to 1. With barbiturates it means that 10 times a therapeutic dose in an individual who has not developed tolerance can be fatal. For benzodiazepines, 700 times the therapeutic dose can be fatal. However, this margin of safety is diminished when benzodiazepines are taken in combination with alcohol. In addition to alcohol, the sedative-hypnotics have additive and synergistic effects with other depressant drugs, including other benzodiazepines, phenothiazines, MAO inhibitors, barbiturates, opioids, and other antidepressants (PDR, 1999).

Symptoms of overdose include drowsiness, loss of consciousness, depressed breathing, coma, and death if left untreated, however, it might take 50 or 100 pills to cause a serious overdose. Yet street versions of the drug, often misrepresented and sold as Quaaludes®, are so strong that only 5 or 10 pills can cause severe reactions.

MEMORY IMPAIRMENT, ROHYPNOL®, & DATE RAPE

Benzodiazepines impair the ability to learn new information. They disrupt the transfer of information from short- to long-term memory (Juergens & Cowley, 1998; American Psychiatric Association, 1990). The amnestic effect of benzodiazepines (medically known as "retrograde amnesia" and commonly called a "drug black out" or "brown out") helps patients forget traumatic surgical and other medical procedures. This effect has unfortunately been used by a few sexual predators to cause a victim to forget they were sexually assaulted.

The drug most associated with date rape is the benzodiazepine called Rohypnol® (flunitrazepam). Rohypnol®, like other benzodiazepines, also causes relaxation and sedation. Rohypnol® or another very short-acting benzodiazepine is slipped into an alcoholic beverage and when drunk incapacitates the person, lowers inhibitions, and disrupts the memory. This illicit use began in Europe in the 1970s but didn't start appearing in the United States until the 1990s. Flunitrazepam is 10 times more potent, by weight, than Valium® and is short acting (2–3 hours) although it has a long half-life (15–35 hours) and so frequent use will cause a build-up of the drug in the body's tissues. When taken with alcohol, the safety margin is greatly reduced. It used to be possible to fill a Rohypnol® prescription in Mexico and then bring it into the United States but in 1996 the Food and Drug Administration banned all imports of the drug, even for personal use. Special laws adding 20 more years to the sentence of anyone convicted of using Rohypnol®, GHB, or any drug to assault someone or commit violence, was enacted in 1996 (*see GHB in this chapter*).

BARBITURATES

Though barbituric acid was first synthesized in 1863, it remained a medical curiosity until 1903 when it was synthesized to barbital (Veronal®). The chemical modification made it possible for the drug to enter the nervous system and induce sedation. It was originally believed to be free of the addictive propensities of opiates and opioids. Phenobarbital came next in 1913 and since then, about 50 of the 2,000 other barbiturates that have been released have been marketed. By the time there had been extensive clinical experience with the drugs, dangers such as overdose, severe withdrawal symptoms, dependence, and addiction had become apparent (Lukas, 1995). Since the peak of their use in the '40s and '50s and their abuse in the '50s, '60s, and '70s, their licit and illicit use has declined dramatically.

EFFECTS

◊ The long-acting barbiturates, such as phenobarbital, last 12–24 hours

TABLE 4–6   CLASSIFICATION OF BARBITURATES

Long acting	phenobarbital (Luminal®), mephobarbital (Mebaral®)
Intermediate acting	amobarbital (Amytal®), aprobarbital (Alurate®), butabarbital (Butisol®), talbutal (Lotusate®)
Short acting	butalbital, hexobarbital (Sombulex®), pentobarbital (Nembutol®), secobarbital (Seconal®)
Ultra short acting	methohexital (Brevital®), thiamylal (Surital®), thiopental (Pentothal®)

and are used mostly as daytime sedatives or to control epileptic seizures.

◊ The intermediate-acting barbiturates, such as butabarbital, are used as sedatives and last 6–12 hours.

◊ The short-acting compounds, including butalbital and in the past, Seconal® ("reds") and Nembutal® ("yellows"), last 3–6 hours and are used to induce sleep. They can cause pleasant feelings along with the sedation (at least initially), so they are more likely to be abused.

◊ The very short-acting barbiturates, such as Pentothal®, are used mostly for anesthesia and can cause immediate unconsciousness. The high potency of these barbiturates makes them extremely dangerous if abused.

As with benzodiazepines, barbiturates affect GABA therefore acting as a brake on inhibitions, anxiety, and restlessness. Because they can induce a feeling of disinhibitory euphoria, barbiturates seem to have a stimulatory effect but the drugs eventually become sedating. To even a greater extent than with benzodiazepines, the effects of barbiturates are very similar to the effects of alcohol. Excessive or long-term use can lead to changes in personality and emotional state, such as mood swings, depression, irritability, and boisterous behavior (Lukas, 1995).

The effects of barbiturates often depend on the mood of the user and the setting where taken. An agitated

barbiturate user might become combative, whereas a tired barbiturate user in a quiet setting might go to sleep.

"I'd take Seconals® and they made me feel great. I wouldn't hesitate to say anything; I'd just talk and talk, and sometimes I'd want to fight. It made me very rowdy. But I thought I was on top of the world. I thought I was great. And now when I see other people when they take it, they look like idiots. I guess that's what I was, you know, an idiot."
Recovering barbiturate user

TOLERANCE, TISSUE DEPENDENCE, & WITHDRAWAL

Tolerance to barbiturates develops in a variety of ways. The most dramatic tolerance, **dispositional tolerance** (metabolic tolerance), results from the physiologic conversion of liver cells to more efficient cells which metabolize or destroy barbiturates more quickly. The other process, **pharmocodynamic tolerance,** causes the nerve cells and tissues that are directly affected by the drug to become less sensitive.

Tissue dependence to barbiturates occurs when 8–10 times the normal dose is taken daily for 30 days or more.

Within 6–8 hours after using short-acting barbiturates, users will begin to experience withdrawal symptoms, such as anxiety, agitation, loss of appetite, nausea, vomiting, increased heart rate, excessive sweating, abdominal cramps, and tremulousness. The symptoms tend to peak on the second or third day. The more intense the use, the more severe the symptoms. Withdrawal symptoms resulting from heavy tissue dependence are very dangerous and can result in convulsions within 12 hours to 1 week from the last dose.

"I'd go into a state of complete unconsciousness and I'd wake up in the hospital with IVs in me. They'd try to straighten me out and they would let me go from the hospital and then I'd do the same thing."

32-year-old male recovering barbiturate user

OTHER SEDATIVE-HYPNOTICS

GHB (gammahydroxybutyrate)

GHB is a rapidly acting, strong, central nervous system depressant. GHB, a metabolite of GABA, an inhibitory neurotransmitter but now synthetically produced, was used as a sleep inducer in the 1960s and 1970s. By the 1990s, this white powder, which is taken orally, had also become popular among bodybuilders because it changed the ratio of muscle to fat and was thought to increase the levels of growth hormone in the body. It also induced an effect similar to methaqualone, alcohol, or even heroin intoxication—euphoria and sedation—and so in recent years it became popular in "rave" clubs along with other club drugs like LSD, "ecstasy," and Rohypnol®. It has been called "liquid ecstasy," "scoop," "Georgia home boy," "easy lay," or "grievous bodily harm" (NIDA, 1999).

The side effects are increased dreaming, lack of coordination, nausea, respiratory distress, and occasionally seizures. Like any sedative, it can be dangerous when used with other depressants including alcohol. The drug was initially available in health food stores or by mail order and described

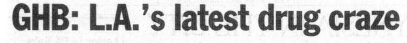

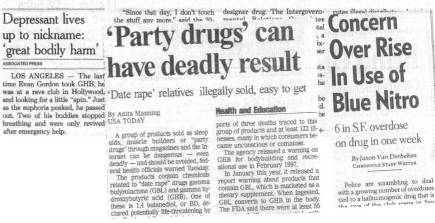

as a nutrient rather than a sedative. By the 1990s the FDA decided there were enough health risks to take it off the market. Street chemists have since rushed to fill the void.

GHB is usually dissolved in water or alcohol by the capful or teaspoonful or as a premixed solution. A dose costs $5 to $10. The effects last three to six hours. With one gram there is a feeling of relaxation. With two grams the relaxation increases while heart rate and respiration fall. Balance, coordination, and circulation are disrupted. With two to four grams, coordination and speech become impaired. A deep sleep similar to a coma can occur with side effects including nausea, vomiting, depression, delusions, hallucinations, possibly seizures, amnesia, and coma with a greatly reduced heart rate. It can be addicting (ONDCP, 1998).

Because of the amnestic effects of GHB, it has been used by sexual predators to lower the inhibitions and defenses of women. Its use spurred the passage of the Drug-Induced Rape Prevention and Punishment Act of 1996, which increased federal penalties for use of any controlled substance to aid in sexual assault or violence.

GBL (gamma butyl lactone)

Increased legal scrutiny of GHB has resulted in the abuse of GBL in 1999. GBL is a prodrug (or active metabolite of GHB). It is also an in-

gredient in liquid paint stripper and available through chemical suppliers in the United States. It was quickly formulated into a mint-flavored elixir for the "rave" club scene. These elixirs, sold under the trade names of Blue Nitro®, Revivarant®, Revivarant G®, Gamma G®, GH Revitalizer®, Remforce®, and Insom-X®, were responsible for up to 75 toxic reactions by early 1999. Some abusers have even drunk diluted paint stripper or even "huffed" the hardware store products containing GBL. Many states are now urging the FDA to take regulatory action against GBL.

METHAQUALONE (Quaalude®, Mandrax®)

Although widely used at one time as a sleep aid, the heavy abuse of Quaalude® led to the withdrawal of this product from the legitimate market. This change led to a tremendous increase in the illicit production of Quaalude®, known as bootleg "ludes," which look identical to the original prescription drug. The active chemical in Quaalude®, methaqualone, is manufactured by street chemists or smuggled in from Europe, South Africa, or Colombia. In Europe and other countries, Mandrax® (methaqualone and an antihistamine) had great popularity in the 1970s and 1980s. The antihistamine exaggerated the effect of the methaqualone. Today South Africa still has many Mandrax® abusers. However there is no guarantee that the street versions of these drugs contain actual methaqualone and even when they do, the dosage may vary dramatically making an overdose more likely. The reasons for the popularity of methaqualone are its overall sedative effect and the prolonged period of mild euphoria caused by suppression of inhibitions. This disinhibitory effect is similar to that caused by alcohol.

ZOLPIDEM (Ambien®)

This short-acting hypnotic with a 2.5 hour half-life has a lower risk of addiction than most benzodiazepines, so it is prescribed for some sleep disorders. Excess use can cause nausea, diarrhea, headaches, dizziness, and drowsiness the following day. As with benzodiazepines, zolpidem can cause memory, performance, and learning impairment. By itself zolpidem rarely causes overdose deaths except in combination with other depressants.

ETHCHLOVYNOL (Placidyl®)

Called "green weenies" on the street, Placidyl® is one of the older sedative-hypnotics. It is still a controlled prescription drug and is subject to limited abuse. Placidyl® is about the equivalent of Doriden® in potency, with similar toxic and addictive effects but is shorter acting.

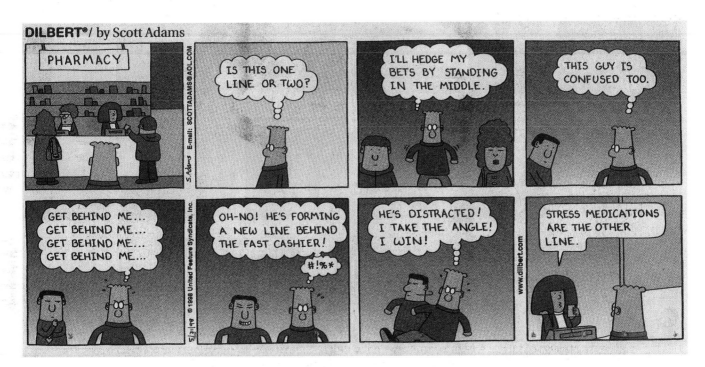

OTHER PROBLEMS WITH DEPRESSANTS

DRUG INTERACTIONS

SYNERGISM

If more than one depressant drug is used, the poly-drug combination can cause a much greater reaction than simply the sum of the effects. One of the reasons for this synergistic effect lies in the chemistry of the liver.

For example, if alcohol and Valium® (diazepam) are taken together, the liver becomes busy metabolizing the alcohol, so the sedative-hypnotic passes through the body at full strength. Alcohol also dissolves the Valium® more readily than stomach fluids, allowing more Valium® to be absorbed rapidly into the body. Valium® exerts its depressant effects on parts of the brain different from those affected by alcohol. Thus, when combined, alcohol and Valium® cause more problems than if they were taken at different times. Exaggerated respiratory depression is the biggest danger with the use of alcohol and another depressant. That combination also causes more blackouts (a period of amnesia or loss of memory while intoxicated).

"I took my little medication with me one night, drinking in the bar. I played some pool and that's all I remember.

This was on a Sunday. When I woke up, it was Wednesday."
Recovering polydrug abuser

The synergistic effect causes 4,000 deaths a year. In addition almost 50,000 people are treated in emergency rooms because of adverse reactions to multiple drug use.

CROSS-TOLERANCE & CROSS-DEPENDENCE

Cross-tolerance is the development of tolerance to other drugs by the continued exposure and development of tolerance to another drug. For example, a barbiturate addict who develops a tolerance to a high dose of Seconal® is also tolerant to and can withstand high doses of Nembutal®, phenobarbital, anesthetics, opiates, alcohol, Valium®, and even blood-thinner medication. One explanation of cross-tolerance is that many drugs are metabolized or broken down by the same body enzymes. As one continues to take barbiturates, the liver creates more enzymes to rid the body of these toxins. The unusually high levels of these enzymes result in tolerance to all barbiturates as well as other drugs also metabolized by those same enzymes.

Cross-dependence occurs when an individual becomes addicted or tissue dependent on one drug, resulting in biochemical and cellular changes that support an addiction to other drugs. A heroin addict, for example, has altered body chemistry such that he or she is also likely to be addicted to another opiate/opioid, e.g., hydrocodone, oxycodone, meperedine, morphine, codeine, methadone, or propoxyphene (Darvon®). As in this example, cross-dependence most often occurs with different drugs in the same chemical family. A diazepam (Valium®) addict is also tissue dependent on alprazolam, lorazepam, and other benzodiazepines. A heavy butalbital user is also tissue dependent for phenobarbital. Cross-dependence has also been documented to some extent with

opiates/opioids and alcohol; cocaine and alcohol; and benzodiazepines and alcohol.

MISUSE & DIVERSION

"His wife had a stash of pills that was just marvelous, you know; 500 sleepers, uppers and downers and everything; you name it. I couldn't wait to be invited to dinner because I'd get, you know, I'd just fill up."
43-year-old female recovering sedative-hypnotic addict

As a class, sedative-hypnotic drugs and prescription opioids are frequently misused and diverted to abuse from legitimate prescribing practices. Unfortunately, unscrupulous, addicted, or out-of-date medical professionals also participate in unethical, criminal, or inappropriate prescribing practices.

One pattern of illicit use with sedatives and/or opioids results when a patient is treated for multiple medical complaints by many different physicians and each prescribes a different sedative or opioid that is then dispensed by different pharmacies. For example, Dalmane® will be prescribed for sleep; Serax® for anxiety; Xanax® for depression; Valium® for muscle spasms; and Librax® for stomach problems. Each prescription, in and of itself, may be at a nonaddictive level but all these prescriptions combined result in a tissue-dependent dose of benzodiazepines.

"This one doctor, he gave me Nembutal®, Darvon®, a little phenobarbital, Valium®, and Compazine®. I would call the drugstore and get those five drugs, all at one time. And they'd be delivered to my house, free of charge. My medical insurance is paying for them. I mean, luxury, right there."
Recovering 43-year-old sedative-hypnotic abuser

Because of their widespread use for a variety of medical indications, sedative-hypnotics and opioids are also subject to forged prescriptions or prescription manipulations (photocopying or changing dosage or number of refills) that provide an abuser with enough drugs for diversion to illicit street sales or to feed an addiction. To combat this problem, many states have added triplicate prescriptions for benzodiazepines and other stringent mechanisms to prevent diversion, much as they have done for opioids. Many physicians and psychiatrists see triplicate prescriptions for benzodiazepines as an intrusion in their practice of medicine.

"I couldn't just deal with one pharmacist taking 40 pills a day because they would turn you in to the FDA. They'd turn you in and the doctor would get in trouble, so I had to get several drugstores working for me."
43-year-old recovering sedative-hypnotic abuser

Another form of diversion is smuggling drugs that are legal outside the United States. Recently flunitra-

A13

Prescription Drug Smuggling On the Rise

Illegal injections linked to cross-border Tijuana imports

LOS ANGELES TIMES

LOS ANGELES — Major shipments of Mexican prescription drugs are being smuggled into Southern California from Tijuana, fueling greater sales through illegal back-room clinics and storefronts, state and federal officials say.

The pervasive black-market sales, mainly by Latino merchants, has emboldened shop owners not only to sell pharmaceuticals to immigrant customers but to take a more dangerous new step: Some merchants are giving injections and practicing medicine on customers.

Police in the Orange County city of Tustin are investigating whether the illegal practice contributed to the death last week of 18-month-old Selene Segura Rios. The girl died two hours after receiving what her parents were told was a penicillin injection in the back room of a toy store.

She was the second Latino child in the last 10 months to die after receiving injections from unlicensed practitioners in Orange County.

"Stores selling illegal prescription drugs of all kinds are a pervasive problem in the Hispanic community," said Howard Ratzky, supervising drug investigator for the state Department of Food and Drug. "It's very hard to stop, and nobody knows how many stores out there are engaging in this."

Ratzky said the issue has gone beyond "the trend of an unlicensed store selling prescription drugs." Some stores, he said, "have begun offering medical treatment by people identifying themselves as physicians." A U.S. Customs agent in San Diego also noted a growing number of cases where people who sell the

▶ TIJUANA: Page A17 Col. 5

zepam (Rohypnol®), a drug that is not sold in the United States, has been illegally making its way into dance and "rave" clubs and into the drug-using community.

Misuse and diversion aren't the only ways that bad reactions and physical problems can occur due to prescription drugs. A study led by Dr. Bruce Pomeranz at the University of Toronto estimated that each year between 76,000 and 137,000 Americans die and an additional 1.6–2.6 million are injured due to bad reactions from legally prescribed prescription drugs and over-the-counter medication. The figures do not include drug abuse or prescribing errors. While some disagree with the magnitude of the numbers, they agree that the problem is very real and unfortunately common.

Some of the actions that could help control prescription drug abuse as described by Peter Lurie and Philip R. Lee at the University of California Medical Center in San Francisco are

◊ better education of physicians regarding pharmacotherapy and the effects of drugs;

◊ better education and research regarding pain control and the use of opioids;

◊ more accurate information regarding drugs rather than just inserts or overdone PDR information;

◊ limited interaction between drug company detailers (salesman);

◊ increased role for the pharmacist in identifying drug interactions and inappropriate prescribing;

◊ more careful prescribing in hospitals and nursing homes;

◊ greater patient participation in deciding which drug to use;

◊ more attention to patient feedback to judge effectiveness of drugs;

◊ more testing in geriatric populations to make sure prescribed drugs are not debilitating;

◊ limited prescribing of certain powerful drugs to specialists;

◊ limited prescribing of psychoactive drugs (e.g., duplicate and triplicate prescriptions for scheduled drugs);

◊ less drug advertising in medical journals; more peer scrutiny of prescribing practices of fellow physicians.

(Adapted from Lurie & Lee, 1991.)

ECONOMICS

In 1999 Americans spent about $91 billion or nine percent of their total medical expenditures of $1 trillion dollars on prescription medications. This was about 1/3 of the world's total expenditures for prescription drugs (PhRMA, 1999). It was also three times the amount spent just 10 years ago (Fig. 4-6). Americans also spent about $15 billion on over-the-counter drugs such as aspirin, laxatives, sunscreens, and vitamins. At the current rates of growth, both figures will double over the next 10–15 years.

In contrast to the $106 billion spent on prescription and over-the-counter drugs, about

◊ $50–60 billion were spent on illegal drugs,

◊ $75 billion on tobacco, and

◊ $140 billion on alcohol (ONDCP, 1999; PhRMA, 1999).

Legal psychoactive drugs, including psychiatric medications, account for approximately 10% to 12% of prescriptions written in the United States. The other prescriptions include cardiovascular medications, antibiotics, menopause medications, hormones, birth-control pills, ulcer medications, diabetes-control medications, antihistamines, thyroid drugs, and bronchodilators.

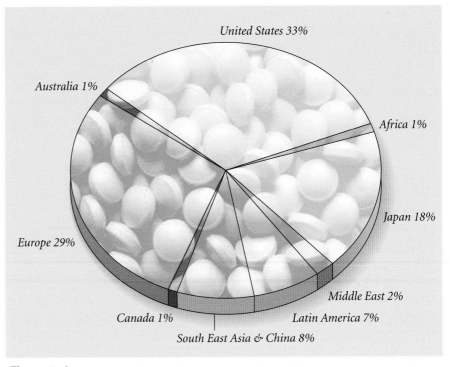

Figure 4-6 •
World Prescription Drug Market, 1996. Source: IMS Health, 1998.

TABLE 4–7 TOP-SELLING PRESCRIPTION DRUGS IN THE UNITED STATES

CLASS OF MEDICATION	# OF PRESCRIPTIONS
(based on the 200 top-selling prescriptions filled at 35,000 community pharmacies in 1998)	
Cardiovascular medications	
antihypertensives	159,558,000
beta blockers	54,921,000
anticholesterol	62,114,000
heart regulators	35,133,000
diuretics	51,850,000
miscellaneous cardiovascular	19,961,000
Total	**383,537,000**
Antibiotics (amoxicillin, cephalexin, penicillin, tetracycline)	**207,009,000**
Pain medications	
opioids (e.g., hydrocodone, propoxyphene, codeine)	93,627,000
NSAIDS and corticosteroids	83,466,000
skeletal muscle relaxants	13,343,000
Total	**190,436,000**
Psychiatric medications	
antidepressants (Prozac®, Zoloft®, tricyclics)	88,246,000
anxiolytics (benzodiazepines such as Xanax®)	57,482,000
antipsychotics (Risperdol®)	3,874,000
Total	**149,602,000**
Menopause/hormone therapy (Premarin®, Norvasc®)	**98,765,000**
Ulcer/stomach medications (Prilosec®, Zantac®)	**68,614,000**
Diabetes medications (Glucophage®, Humulin®, Rezulin®)	**60,715,000**
Oral contraceptives	**52,299,000**
Antihistamines (Claritin®, Zytec®, Allegra®, Promethazine®)	**51,008,000**
Thyroid medications (Synthroid®)	**48,456,000**
Bronchodilators (Albuterol®)	**39,405,000**
Anticonvulsants (Dilantin®)	**18,415,000**
Electrolytes (potassium chloride)	**16,180,000**
Antifungals (Lotrisone®)	**11,605,000**
Miscellaneous (for osteoporosis, impotence, expectorant, gout, iron supplement, antismoking, migraine, AD/HD)	**44,500,500**
TOTAL U.S. PRESCRIPTIONS	**3,545,572,000**

Adapted from: Scott-Levin Associates. (American Druggist, 1999)

CHAPTER SUMMARY

GENERAL CLASSIFICATION

1. Downers are central nervous system depressants.

2. The three major depressants are opiates/opioids, sedative-hypnotics, and alcohol.

3. The four minor depressants are skeletal muscle relaxants, antihistamines, over-the-counter sedatives, and lookalike sedatives.

OPIATES/OPIOIDS

Classification

4. Opiates (from the opium poppy) and opioids (synthetic versions of opiates) were developed for the treatment of acute pain, to control diarrhea, and to suppress coughs.

5. Opiates include opium, morphine, codeine, heroin, hydrocodone, hydromorphone (Dilaudid®), and oxycodone (Percodan®). Opioids include methadone, propoxyphene (Darvon®), meperidine (Demerol®), and fentanyl.

History of Use

6. The change in routes of administration (from ingestion to smoking to snorting to injection) along with refinement and synthesis of stronger opioids (from opium to morphine to heroin to fentanyl), have increased the effectiveness as well as the addiction liability of opioids.

7. Opium and morphine were very popular in patent medicines, in prescription medicines, and as social/recreational drugs.

Effects of Opioids

8. Opiates/opioids mimic the body's own natural painkillers, endorphins and enkephalins. These analgesic drugs block the transmission of pain messages to the brain by substance "P."

9. Opiates/opioids can also cause euphoria by stimulating the reward/pleasure center. The satiation switch can be disrupted by opioids. The drugs also control diarrhea and suppress the cough mechanism.

Side Effects of Heroin & Other Opioids

10. Opioids mask pain signals, depress heart rate, slow respiration rate, depress muscular coordination, increase nausea, induce pinpoint pupils, cause itching, and cause mental confusion.

11. A physical tolerance to opioids develops rapidly, increasing the speed with which the body becomes physically dependent on the drug.

12. Withdrawal from opioids is like an extreme case of the flu. People do not usually die from opiate/opioid withdrawal, although they can die from overdose.

Additional Problems with Heroin & Other Opioids

13. Opioids cross the placental barrier and affect fetuses. Babies can be born addicted to opioids and can die from opioid withdrawal.

14. Overdose kills 3,000–4,000 heroin users each year, mostly through extreme respiratory depression.

15. Contaminated needles transmit hepatitis C and HIV in increasing numbers. Injecting heroin also causes abscess (skin infections). Endocarditis, cotton fever, and flesh-eating disease also occur.

16. Adulteration of drugs, the high cost of an addiction (up to $200 a day), and the dangers of polydrug use add to the dangers of use.

17. The age of first use of heroin has decreased dramatically over the past five years (from 21 down to 17.6 years old). The progression

from experimentation to physical dependence can occur in a month or two. Addiction depends more on other factors such as genetics and early environment. Most returning Vietnam veterans who had developed physical dependence while in Vietnam did not continue use showing that addiction is much more than just physical (tissue) dependence.

Morphine & Heroin

18. Morphine, the standard for severe pain relief, can be taken by mouth, by injection, or by suppository. The therapeutic use of opioids for pain is subject to much controversy. Some doctors underprescribe due to fear of patient addiction.

19. "China white" heroin from Asia, Mexican "tar" heroin, and recently Colombian white heroin are the most widely used in the United States.

20. Heroin can be injected, smoked, or snorted. All three methods of use are very addicting.

Other Opioids

21. Codeine, which is refined directly from opium, used to be the most widely used and abused prescription opioid.

22. Hydrocodone, a synthetic version of codeine, has become the most widely used and abused prescription opioid.

23. Methadone is a longer-lasting opioid that heroin addicts use to avoid withdrawal and the addicting highs caused by heroin use. A number of synthetic and semisynthetic opioids, such as hydromorphone (Dilaudid®), oxycodone (Percodan®), meperidine (Demerol®), propoxyphene (Darvon®), and fentanyl, have made their way to the illicit market. Highly potent syn-

thetic heroin designer drugs (fentanyl and Demerol® derivatives) have appeared on the street, thus increasing the danger of overdose.

24. Other drugs used to treat opiate/opioid addiction are LAAM®, a long-acting opioid, naloxone and naltrexone (opioid antagonists), buprenorphine, propoxyphene (Darvon®) and clonidine.

SEDATIVE-HYPNOTICS

Classification

25. The two main groups of sedative-hypnotics are barbiturates and benzodiazepines.

26. Sedatives (minor tranquilizers) are calming drugs used mostly to treat anxiety. Hypnotics are mainly used to induce sleep.

History

27. Early civilizations used opioids as calming drugs but over the last 150 years, sedative-hypnotics have included bromides, chloral hydrate, paraldehyde, barbiturates, Miltown®, and benzodiazepines

Use, Misuse, Abuse, & Addiction

28. Societal acceptance of sedative-hypnotics has varied from decade to decade from avid acceptance to fear of overuse. They are usually prescribed to control anxiety, induce sleep, relax muscles, and act as mild tranquilizers but many physicians are afraid of physical dependence and addiction.

29. Withdrawal from sedative-hypnotics after extended use is dangerous. Overdosing and severe withdrawal symptoms are more strongly associated with barbiturates rather than with benzodiazepines.

30. Overdose is commonly accepted as the main danger of sedative-hypnotics, particularly when used with other depressants such as alcohol.

Benzodiazepines

31. Benzodiazepines include alprazolam (Xanax®), diazepam (Valium®), clonazepam (Klonopin®), temazepam (Restoril®), and lorazepam (Ativan®).

32. Benzodiazepines are usually used medically to manage anxiety, treat sleep problems, control muscular spasms and seizures, and subdue the symptoms of alcohol withdrawal. They are used nonmedically to calm down, induce a mild euphoria, and lower inhibitions.

33. Benzodiazepines work on the inhibitory transmitter GABA as well as serotonin and dopamine.

34. Benzodiazepines can stay in the body for days, even weeks. After tolerance and tissue dependence have developed, withdrawal symptoms can occur many days after ceasing use.

35. The memory loss caused by benzodiazepines especially Rohypnol® is sometimes used to take sexual advantage of a woman.

Barbiturates

36. More than 2,000 barbiturates have been developed over the last 100 years.

37. Barbiturates include Seconal® ("reds"), Nembutal® ("yellows"), and phenobarbital.

38. These drugs are mostly used to control seizures, induce sleep, and lessen anxiety but benzodiazepines and other psychiatric drugs have replaced their use over the past 40 years.

Other Sedative-Hypnotics

39. GHB, a strong depressant, has become popular in the party scene. Effects include sedation and euphoria. GBL is also used in the same way as GHB.

40. Nonbarbiturate sedative-hypnotics include street methaqualone (Quaalude®), meprobamate (Miltown®, Equanil®), and ethchlovynol (Placidyl®).

41. Methaqualone (Quaalude®) is only available from illicit sources. The drug causes an overall sedation, mild euphoria, and suppression of inhibitions.

OTHER PROBLEMS WITH DEPRESSANTS

Drug Interactions

42. Alcohol and sedative-hypnotics used together can be especially life threatening. They cause a synergistic (exaggerated) effect that can suppress respiration and heart functions.

43. Cross-tolerance and cross-dependence occur within the sedative-hypnotic class of drugs, within the opioid class of drugs, and to a lesser extent among sedative-hypnotics, opioids, and alcohol.

Misuse & Diversion

44. Hundreds of millions of doses and prescriptions of sedative-hypnotics and prescription opioids are diverted to illicit channels each year.

Economics

45. Over $91 billion dollars are spent by Americans on prescription drugs. Of the 3½ billion prescriptions written each year, 250 million were for psychoactive drugs, particularly opioids, sedative-hypnotics, skeletal muscle relaxants, and nondepressant psychiatric drugs (antidepressants).

REFERENCES

Aldrich, M. R. (1994). Historical notes on women addicts. *Journal of Psychoactive Drugs, 26*(1), 61–64.

American Druggist. (1999). The top 200 drugs. *American Druggist, 216*(2).

American Psychiatric Association. (1990). *Task Force Report on Benzodiazepines.* Washington, DC: American Psychiatric Association Press.

Armstrong, D., & Armstrong, E.M. (1991). *The Great American Medicine Show.* New York: Prentice Hall.

Busto, U., Sellers, E. M., Naranjo, C. A., et al. (1986). Withdrawal reaction after long-term therapeutic use of benzodiazepines. *The New England Journal of Medicine, 315,* 854–859.

Carlezon, W. A. Jr., Boundy, V. A., Haile, C. N., Lane, S. B., Kalb, R. G., Neve, R. L., & Nestler, E. J. (1997). Sensitization to morphine induced by mediated gene transfer. *Science, 277*(5327), 812–814.

Casriel, C., Rockwell, R., & Stepherson, B. (1988). Heroin sniffers: Between two worlds. *Journal of Psychoactive Drugs, 20*(4).

DAWN (Drug Abuse Warning Network). (2000). *Mid-Year 1999 Preliminary Emergency Department Data from the Drug Abuse Warning Network.* Rockville: SAMHSA.

DAWN. (1999). *Drug Abuse Warning Network Annual Medical Examiner Data 1998.* Rockville: SAMHSA.

DEA (Drug Enforcement Administration). (1999). *Heroin. DEA Publications. www.usdoj.gov/dea/pubs/abuse/chap2/narcotic/heroin.htm.*

DEA. (1998). Colombian heroin a major threat. 62% seized in the United States originates in South America. DEA Press Release. *http://www.usdoj.gov.dea/pubs/pressrel/pr960903.htm.*

Eickelberg, S. J., & Mayo-Smith, M. F. (1998). Management of sedative-hypnotic intoxication and withdrawal. In A. W. Graham & T. K. Schultz (Eds.), *Principles of Addiction Medicine* (2nd ed., pp. 441–456). Chevy Chase, MD: American Society of Addiction Medicine.

Gold, M. S. (1998). The pharmacology of opioids. In A. W. Graham & T. K. Schultz (Eds.), *Principles of Addiction Medicine* (2nd ed.). Chevy Chase, MD: American Society of Addiction Medicine.

Gold, M. S. (1990). Benzodiazepines: Tolerance, dependence, abuse, and addiction. *Journal of Psychoactive Drugs, 22*(1), 23–34.

Goldstein, A. (1994). *Addiction: From Biology to Drug Policy.* New York: W. H. Freeman and Company.

Hoffman, J. P. (1990). The historical shift in the perception of opiates: From medicine to social medicine. *Journal of Psychoactive Drugs, 22*(1), 53–62.

Hollister, L. E. (1983). The pre-benzodiazepine era. *Journal of Psychoactive Drugs, 15*(1–2), 9–13.

Hyman, S. (1998). An Interview with Steven Hyman, M. D. In *Moyers on Addiction. PBS Online.*

Jaffe, J. H., Knapp, C. M., & Ciraulo, D. A. (1997). Opiates: Clinical aspects. In J. H. Lowinson, P. Ruiz, R. B. Millman, & J. G. Langrod (Eds.), *Substance Abuse: A Comprehensive Textbook* (2nd ed., pp.51–84). Baltimore: Williams & Wilkins.

Jaffe, J. H. (1990). Drug addiction and drug abuse. In: A. G. Gilman, T. W. Rall, A. S. Nies, & P. Taylor, (Eds.), *Goodman and Gilman's the Pharmacological Basis of Therapeutics* (8th ed., pp. 522–573). New York: Pergammon Press.

Jenkins, A. J., & Cone, E. J. (1998). Pharmacokinetics: Drug absorption, distribution, and elimination. In S. B. Karch (Ed.), *Drug Abuse Handbook* (pp. 181–184). Boca Raton, FL: CRC Press.

Juergens, S. M., & Cowley, D. R. (1998). The pharmacology of sedative-hypnotics. In A. W. Graham & T. K. Schultz (Eds.), *Principles of Addiction Medicine* (2nd ed., pp. 117–130). Chevy Chase, MD: American Society of Addiction Medicine.

Karch, S. B. (1996). *The Pathology of Drug Abuse* (pp. 281–406). Boca Raton, FL: CRC Press.

Latimer, D., & Goldberg, J. (1981). *Flowers in the Blood: The Story of Opium.* New York: Franklin Watts.

Lukas, S. E. (1995). Barbiturates. In J. H. Jaffe (Ed.), *Encyclopedia of Drugs and Alcohol* (Vol. I, pp. 141–146). New York: Simon & Schuster Macmillan.

Lurie, P., & Lee, P. R. (1991). Fifteen solutions to the problems of prescription drug abuse. *Journal of Psychoactive Drugs, 23*(4), 349–357.

Marnell, T. (Ed.). (1997). *Drug Identification Bible.* Denver: Drug Identification Bible.

Miller, N. S., & Gold, M. S. (1990). Benzodiazepines: Tolerance, dependence, abuse, and addiction. *Journal of Psychoactive Drugs, 22*(1).

Nestler, E. J. & Aghajanian, G. K. (1997). Molecular and Cellular Basis of Addiction. *Science, 278,* 58–63.

NIDA (National Institute of Drug Abuse). (1999). Rohypnol and GHB. *NIDA Infofax.http://www.nida.nih.gov/Infofax/RohypnolGHB.html.*

NIDA. (1996). Research Report: Heroin Abuse & Addiction. *http://www.nida.nih.gov/ResearchReports/Heroin/Heroin.html.*

NIDA. (1998) Current trends in drug use worldwide. *NIDA Notes, 13*(2).

Nutt, D. J. (1998). The Neurochemistry of Addiction. In A. W. Graham & T. K. Schultz (Eds.), *Principles of Addiction Medicine* (2nd ed.). Chevy Chase, MD: American Society of Addiction Medicine, Inc.

O'Brien, R., Cohen, S., Evans, G., & Fine, J. (1992). *The Encyclopedia of Drug Abuse.* New York: Facts on File.

Observatoire Geopolitique des Drogues. (1996). *The Geopolitics of Drugs.* Boston: Northeastern University Press.

ONDCP (Ofice of National Drug Control Policy). (2000). *National Drug Control Strategy: 2000 Annual Report.* Bethesda: National Drug Clearinghouse.

ONDCP. (1999). *National Drug Control Strategy: 1999 Annual Report.* Bethesda: National Drug Clearinghouse.

ONDCP. (1998). Gamma hydroxyburyrate (GHB). *Office of National Drug Control Policy Fact Sheet. http://www.whitehousedrugpolicy.gov.*

Orangio, G. L., Pitlick, S., & Latta, P. (1984). Soft tissue infections in parenteral drug abusers. *Annals of Surgery, 199,* 97–100.

Palmer, C., & Horowitz, M. (Eds). (1982). *Shaman Woman, Mainline Lady: Women's Writings on the Drug Experience.* New York: Quill.

Payte, J. T. (1997). Methadone maintenance treatment: The first thirty years. *Journal of Psychoactive Drugs, 29*(2).

Payte, J. T., & Zweben, J. E. (1998). Opioid maintenance therapies. In A. W. Graham, & T. K. Schultz (Eds.), *Principles of Addiction Medicine* (2nd ed., pp. 557–570). Chevy Chase, MD: American Society of Addiction Medicine, Inc.

PDR. (2000). *Physicians' Desk Reference* (53rd ed.). Montvale, NJ: Medical Economics Company.

PhRMA. (1999). Industry Profile, 1998. *PhRMA (Pharmaceutical Research and Manufacturers of America Publications). http://www.phrma.org/publications/industry/profile98.*

Potokar, J., & Nutt, D. J. (1994). Anxiolytic potential of benzodiazepine receptor partial agonists. *CNS Drugs, 1*, 305–315.

Rawson, R. A., Hasson, A. L., Huber, A. M., McCann, M. J., & Ling, W. (1998). A 3-year progress report on the implementation of LAAM in the United States. *Addiction, 93*(4), 533–540.

Robins, L. N. (1994). Lessons from the Vietnam Heroin Experience. *The Harvard Mental Health Letter. http://www.mentalhealth.com/mag1/p5h-sbo3.htm.*

SAMHSA (Substance Abuse and Mental Health Services Administration). (1999). *Preliminary Results from the 1998 National Household Survey on Drug Abuse.* Rockville: SAMHSA.

Schuckit, M. A., Greenblatt, D., Gold, E., & Irwin, M. (1991). Reactions to ethanol and diazepam in healthy young men. *Journal Study of Alcohol, 52*(2), 180–187.

Simon, E. J. (1997). Opiates: Neurobiology. In J. H. Lowinson, P. Ruiz, R. B. Millman, & J. G. Langrod (Eds.), *Substance Abuse: A Comprehensive Textbook* (2nd ed., pp. 148–156). Baltimore: Williams & Wilkins.

Sklair-Tavron, L., Shi, W. X., Lane, S. B., Harris, H. W., Bunny, B. S., & Nestler, E. J. (1996). Chronic morphine induces visible changes in the morphology of mesolimbic dopamine neurons. *Proceedings of the National Academy of Sciences, 93*, 11202–11207.

Sternbach, L. H. (1983). The benzodiazepine story. *Journal of Psychoactive Drugs, 15*(1–2), 15–17.

Trebach, A. (1981). *The Heroin Solution.* New Haven, CT: Yale University Press.

Verhaag, D. A., & Ikeda, R. M. (1991). Prescribing for chronic pain. *Journal of Psychoactive Drugs, 23*(4).

Will, M. J., Watkins, L. R., & Maier, S. F. (1998). Uncontrollable stress potentiates morphine's rewarding properties. *Pharmacology, Biochemistry, and Behavior, 60*(3), 655–664.

Zule, W. A., Vogtsberger, K. N., & Desmond, D. P. (1997). The intravenous injection of illicit drugs and needle sharing: An historical perspective. *Journal of Psychoactive Drugs, 29*(2).

Downers:
Alcohol

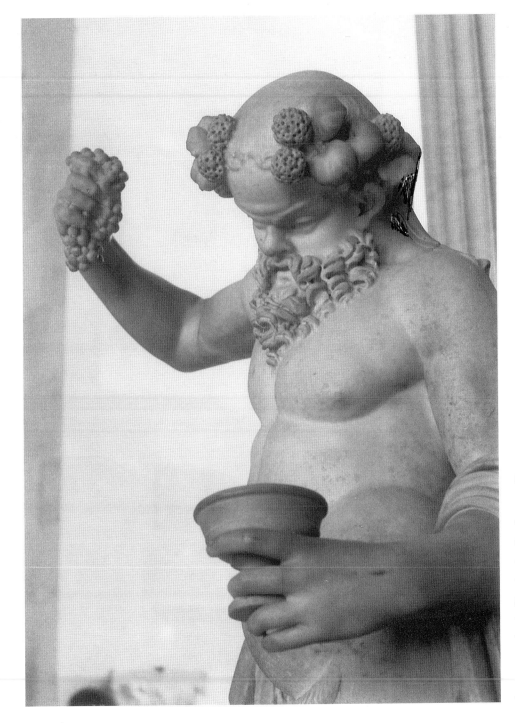

B acchus, also called
"Dionysus," was the ancient
Greek god of wine and
ecstasy. The worship of
Dionysus flourished for a
long time in Asia Minor by
followers called "Bacchants."
Lodges of Bacchus were
suppressed throughout Italy
in 186 B.C.

*Louvre Museum, Paris. Courtesy of
Simone Garlaund*

- **Overview**
  - ◇ **Statistics:** Alcohol is the oldest and most widely used psychoactive drug and is legal in most countries. About 113 million Americans drank alcohol last month and 12–14 million Americans have a drinking problem.
  - ◇ **History (*also see Chapter 1*):** Grain was cultivated for bread and alcohol about 10,000 years ago. Mead (fermented honey), beer (fermented barley), wine (fermented grapes and fruit), and finally distilled spirits (usually made from grain) were discovered by succeeding generations.
  - ◇ **The Legal Drug:** Throughout history, societies have wavered between prohibition, temperance, and unrestricted drinking in their laws and morals regarding alcoholic beverages.
- **Alcoholic Beverages:** Alcohol is fermented from the sugar or other carbohydrates found in grapes and other fruits, vegetables, or grains. Ethyl alcohol (ethanol) is the main psychoactive component in all alcoholic beverages. Beer made from grain is about 5% alcohol, wine made from grapes and other fruits is about 12% alcohol, and distilled liquor made from grains or wines is about 40% alcohol.
- **Absorption, Distribution, & Metabolism:** Though alcohol is absorbed by the body at different rates depending on weight, gender, age, and a dozen other factors, it is metabolized at a steady rate, mostly by the liver, and subsequently excreted through urine, sweat, and breath. The higher the blood alcohol concentration (BAC), the more severe the effects. A BAC of .08 to .10 signifies legal intoxication in the United States.
- **Desired Effects, Side Effects, & Health Consequences:** For alcohol, as with other drugs, use ranges from abstinence, experimentation, and social/recreational use, to habitual use, abuse, and addiction (alcoholism).
  - ◇ **Low- to Moderate-Dose Episodes:** If a person is not at risk (at risk means pregnant, in recovery from addiction, or affected by mental or physical health problems), there are some health benefits from light to moderate alcohol use. In general, sedation, muscle relaxation, and lowered inhibitions accompany low-dose use. The neurotransmitter GABA is most affected by alcohol.
  - ◇ **High-Dose Episodes:** A range of effects occurs, from decreased alertness and exaggerated emotions, up to shock, coma, and death. Effects are directly related to the amount, frequency, and duration of use. They also depend on the tolerance to alcohol developed by the user. Blackouts are common.
  - ◇ **Chronic High-Dose Use:** Excessive chronic drinking causes tolerance and tissue dependence. Withdrawal symptoms can occur upon cessation of drinking. This type of use does major damage to the brain, liver, stomach, and other body organs.
- **Addiction (alcoholism)**
  - ◇ **Classification:** Historically there have been many attempts to classify alcoholism, especially as a disease. Alcohol addiction is caused by a combination of heredity, environment, and drinking alcohol or using psychoactive drugs.
  - ◇ **Long-Term Effects of Addiction (alcoholism):** Depending on a drinker's habits and susceptibility, organ damage, particularly liver damage, cardiovascular problems, nutritional deficits, and polydrug use interactions can occur. Alcohol addiction also impairs important life processes, e.g., relationships, job, self-worth, and even spiritual beliefs.
  - ◇ **Polydrug Abuse:** Alcohol is often abused in connection with other drugs, thus aggravating the problem.
- **Other Problems:** Self-medication for mental problems is common. There are a wide variety of diseases and traumas caused directly or indirectly by alcohol that can kill. Alcohol is also the leading cause of birth defects including fetal alcohol syndrome (FAS). One hundred and thirty thousand deaths from alcohol-related accidents, health problems, suicide, and violence, as well as 25% of hospital visits are due to alcohol.
- **Epidemiology:** Heredity, environment, gender, age, social status, ethnic group, and culture help determine the level of alcohol use (from experimentation to addiction) in an individual.
- **Assessment:** Tests such as the Addiction Severity Index or the Michigan Alcoholism Screening Test are used to determine levels of use, abuse, and addiction.
- **Conclusions:** Since alcoholism can take anywhere from 3 months to 30 years to develop, it is important for drinkers to assess their susceptibility to compulsive use and their present level of use.

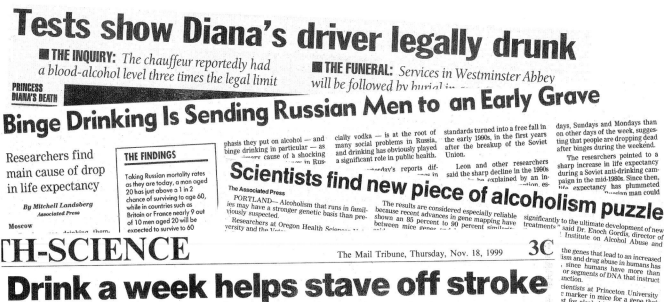

Tests show Diana's driver legally drunk

■ **THE INQUIRY:** *The chauffeur reportedly had a blood-alcohol level three times the legal limit*

■ **THE FUNERAL:** *Services in Westminster Abbey will be followed by burial in*

PRINCESS DIANA'S DEATH

Binge Drinking Is Sending Russian Men to an Early Grave

Researchers find main cause of drop in life expectancy

By Mitchell Landsberg
Associated Press

Moscow

THE FINDINGS

Taking Russian mortality rates as they are today, a man aged 20 has just above a 1 in 2 chance of surviving to age 60, while in countries such as Britain or France nearly 9 out of 10 men aged 20 will be expected to survive to 60

phasis they put on alcohol — and binge drinking in particular — as ... cause of a shocking ... in Rus-

cially vodka — is at the root of many social problems in Russia, and drinking has obviously played a significant role in public health.

...erday's reports dif-

standards turned into a free fall in the early 1990s, in the first years after the breakup of the Soviet Union.

Leon and other researchers said the sharp decline in the 1990s ... he explained by an in-

days, Sundays and Mondays than on other days of the week, suggesting that people are dropping dead after binges during the weekend.

The researchers pointed to a sharp increase in life expectancy during a Soviet anti-drinking campaign in the mid-1980s. Since then, life expectancy has plummeted ...ssian man could

Scientists find new piece of alcoholism puzzle

The Associated Press

PORTLAND— Alcoholism that runs in families may have a stronger genetic basis than previously suspected.

Researchers at Oregon Health Sciences University and the Vete...

The results are considered especially reliable because recent advances in gene mapping have shown an 85 percent to 90 percent similarit... ...

significantly to the ultimate development of new treatments," said Dr. Enoch Gordis, director of Institute on Alcohol Abuse and

the genes that lead to an increased ...ism and drug abuse in humans has , since humans have more than or segments of DNA that instruct ...nction.

...cientists at Princeton University ...c marker in mice for a gene that ...st for alcohol in mice.

...J study is the first to demonstrate ...for physical dependence on alco-...a tendency to drink.

...s sponsored by the National In-...ol Abuse and Alcoholism.

TH-SCIENCE

The Mail Tribune, Thursday, Nov. 18, 1999   3C

Drink a week helps stave off stroke

The Associated Press

As little as a single glass of wine or beer per week can significantly reduce a man's risk of a stroke, according to the biggest study ever to examine the link.

The study found that light to moderate ...

But until now, the evidence of an effect on strokes has been less convincing.

The American Heart Association estimates that 600,000 people in the United States suffer a stroke each year. It is the third leading cause of death in this country, and the leading cause of serious long-term disability.

one a day reduces the risk, and the lesser amount was about as good as the higher one.

There were not enough heavy drinkers in the study to look at the effects of more than one a day, but the heart association warns that drinking to excess can raise blood pressure and, in fact, lead to a stroke.

light to moderately.

"Absolutely it has benefits, but it also has harm," said study co-author Julie E. Buring, an epidemiologist at Harvard-affiliated Brigham and Women's Hospital in Boston. She and other researchers warned of liver damage, the dangers of drunken driving and the

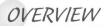

OVERVIEW

STATISTICS

In the last 15 years in Asia

◇ India's alcohol consumption has risen by 171%;

◇ Indonesia's alcohol consumption has risen 500%.

Last month in Europe

◇ only 1 in 10 men and 1 in 5 women abstained from alcoholic beverages;

◇ the lowest rate of abstinence in the European Union was Denmark—2.1% for men and 6.1% for women;

◇ the highest rate of abstinence was Ireland—24.5% for men and 36.3% for women.

Last month in the United States

◇ about 113 million Americans (41% of the population) had at least a can of beer, a glass of wine, or a cocktail; 10–12 million of this group are considered heavy drinkers;

◇ about 3/4 of the 6 million college students had a drink and 1/2 of those were heavy drinkers.

In the last two weeks in the United States

◇ about 16% of 8th grade students had five or more drinks at one sitting (1999);

◇ about 31% of high school seniors had five or more drinks at one sitting (1999).

Yesterday

◇ about $220 million were spent at bars, restaurants, and liquor stores for those drinks;

◇ champagne toasts were made to 7,000 brides and grooms.

Also yesterday in the United States, unfortunately

◇ from 25% to 30% of all U. S. hospital admissions were due to direct or indirect medical complications from alcohol;

◇ about 1/2 the murder victims and 1/2 the murderers drank alcohol;

◇ more than 1/2 of the 300 rapes that occurred involved alcohol;

◇ alcohol was a factor in 40% of all violent crimes;

◇ about 20,000 crimes that occurred involved alcohol or other drugs.

And yesterday, in Europe

◇ between 4.5 million and 7.7 million European children woke up in a house with parents who were problem drinkers;

◇ almost 30% of French men and 11% of French women drank excessively (over 28 drinks per week for men and 14 drinks per week for women).

And worldwide last year

◇ over 2 million people died due to alcohol;

◇ approximately 10% of all diseases and injuries were directly due to alcohol.

(SAMHSA, 1998; NCADI, 1999; Eurocare, 1999; NIAAA, 1999; Justice Department, 1998; Bureau of Alcohol, Tobacco, and Firearms, 1998; University of Michigan, 1999)

HISTORY (*also see Chapter 1*)

Alcohol is the oldest known and most widely used psychoactive drug in the world. It has presumably been present since airborne yeast spores started fermenting plant sugars into alcohol about 1½ billion years ago.

The mists of prehistory cloak our ancient ancestors' discovery of alcohol. Perhaps it was first found by accident when a bunch of grapes or a basket of plums was left standing in a warm place, allowing the fruit sugar to ferment into alcohol (O'Brien & Chafetz, 1991). Perhaps some wild fermented honey was found, diluted with water, and sampled. The drink would later be called "mead" (Waugh, 1968). Early people enjoyed the taste, the mood-altering effects, or both. Curiosity was followed by experimentation and it was discovered that the starch in potatoes, rice, corn, fruit, and grains could also be fermented into alcohol. Further experimentation found the value of alcohol as a solvent for medicines and as a medicine or tonic in and of itself.

Eventually the desire to have ready access to the pleasurable effects as well as the health benefits of beer and wine led humans to search out the raw ingredients with which to manufacture alcoholic beverages and produce them systematically. In fact some historians believe that the first civilized settlements were created to ensure a regular supply of grapes for wine, grain and hops for beer, and poppies for opium-based narcotic drugs (Keller, 1984).

We know that ancient societies were using alcohol around 8000 B.C., about the same time that agriculture developed. Archeologists have found a recipe for beer, along with alcohol residues in clay pots, in Mesopotamia and Iran dating from 5400–3500 B.C. (Goodwin & Gabrielli, 1997). Except for some Moslem countries, the use of alcohol is documented in all civilized societies throughout history, in myths, religions, rituals, stories, hieroglyphs, sacred writings, songs, or in commercial records written on papyrus scrolls or clay tablets. The Babylonian *Epic of Gilgamesh* says wine grapes were given to the earth as a memorial to fallen gods. The *Bible* contains more than 150 references to wine (O'Brien, 1991).

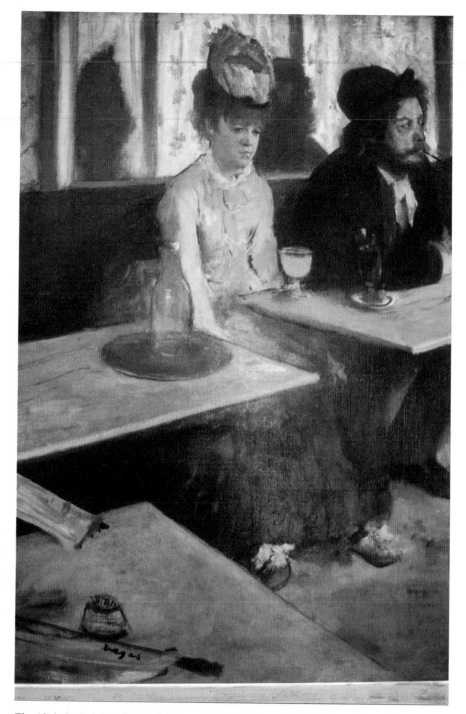

The Absinthe Drinkers *by Edgar Degas, 1876. Absinthe, a distilled liquor that is 68% alcohol, was first produced commercially in 1797. It proved so powerful and dangerous due to a toxin in the wormwood that could cause delerium and death that it was banned in France in 1915 and subsequently by many other countries. Many dissolute artists overindulged in absinthe during the nineteenth century. Currently it is making somewhat of a comeback in the United States and some European countries.*
Musée D'Orsay. Courtesy of Simone Garlaund

THE LEGAL DRUG

Historically the acceptability of alcohol has been intertwined with cultural, social, and financial imperatives. Whether it is used as a reward for pyramid workers, as a solvent for opium in the cure-all known as "laudanum," as a sacrament for Jewish or Christian religious ceremonies, as a substitute for contaminated water supplies, or as the focus of the Anti-Saloon League, alcohol has been the object of desire or of vilification depending on moral attitude, availability, social acceptability, and the politics of the prevailing government. Because beer, wine, and liquor are so widely available and legal in most societies (except Muslim countries) and because they are promoted by custom and advertising, many people do not think of alcohol as a drug.

Almost every country has had periods in their history where alcohol use was restricted or banned completely. Those prohibitions were usually rescinded (Langton, 1995).

◊ The *Chinese Canon of History,* written about 650 B.C., recognized that complete prohibition was almost impossible because men loved their beer (Keller, 1984).

◊ Many Buddhist sects in India prohibited alcohol starting in 500 B.C. and continuing to the present day.

◊ Alcohol was prohibited in ancient Persia by the ruling Islamic culture because of widespread health problems such as malnutrition caused by excess consumption; overindulgence was common in the upper classes.

◊ When alcohol was distilled around A.D. 800, the medicinal qualities of the drug were reemphasized because the increased concentration led to more intense physiological and psychological effects.

◊ In sub-Saharan Africa, the idea of banning alcohol was usually avoided because home-brewed beers had great nutritional value.

◊ In the Middle Ages in Europe, drinking was tolerated by all classes although pubs and drinking establishments were sometimes thought to be places where sedition or heresy could arise, so the more

notorious establishments were closed down (Heath, 1995). Drunkenness was often reserved for festive or religious occasions.

◊ The *Gin Epidemic* in England in the 1700s emphasized that unrestricted use often led to abuse and addiction because of the desirability and nature of the drug. The unrestricted sales of gin (20 million gallons per year in England alone) and the resulting problems of public inebriation, illness, and death, subsequently led to severe restrictions on its manufacture and increased taxes on gin just a few decades after its use was promoted by the British government (O'Brien, 1991).

◊ Official prohibition of alcohol by the government of the United States lasted for 13 years starting in 1919 but pressure by those who wanted to drink, including the Wet Party, led to the repeal of Prohibition.

◊ The industrial revolution that freed people from the land and expanded leisure time also led to the increased recreational use of alcohol

beverages. Globally alcoholism and problem drinking are always more prevalent in developed countries than in the developing countries (WHO, 1999).

Contemporary society's view of the heavy drinker is more forgiving than its view of even an occasional cocaine, heroin, or LSD user. The contradictions surrounding alcohol's accepted place in society and the disfavor in which most other psychoactive drugs are held are not lost on the younger generation.

"Alcohol is heavily social, so one of the problems that I have with prohibition attitudes is that society drinks as much as we do. And because it is legal, I feel I am still part of society even when drunk, whereas with illicit drugs like marijuana, I feel I am stepping outside of what is acceptable."
19-year-old college freshman

Although it is legal and widely available, alcohol is nonetheless a powerful psychoactive drug and is classi-

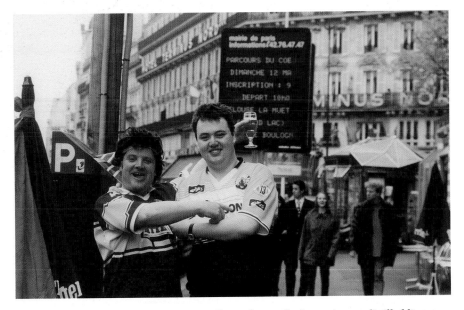

Alcohol is a legal drug in most countries. The preference for beer, wine, or distilled liquors depends on the country's culture, on the availability of certain kinds of beverages, and on the specific occasion. These soccer fans are consoling themselves after their team's defeat. It is of interest to note that they would be in the same place, doing the same drinking to celebrate a victory rather than a loss.
Courtesy of Simone Garlaund

fied as a central nervous system depressant. In small doses it relaxes, sedates, and reduces inhibitions. In moderate doses, even over long periods of time, it continues to relax, sedate, and lower inhibitions in nonsusceptible people. It is however a toxin and in large enough doses can kill a drinker through acute alcohol poisoning—a person often passes out before drinking enough to die.

"I took my 16-year-old brother to a college victory party with my teammates. Three hours later my friend told me my brother had passed out. We called 911 and they told me at the emergency room they had never seen someone with that high a blood alcohol concentration who had still lived. He had been drinking straight vodka from a paper cup."

22-year-old college senior

ALCOHOLIC BEVERAGES

THE CHEMISTRY OF ALCOHOL

There are hundreds of different alcohols. Some are made naturally through fermentation while most that are used industrially are synthesized. Some of the more familiar alcohols include

◇ ethyl alcohol (ethanol, grain alcohol), the main psychoactive component in all alcoholic beverages;

◇ methyl alcohol (methanol or wood alcohol), a toxic industrial solvent;

◇ isopropyl alcohol (propanol or rubbing alcohol), used in shaving lotion, shellac, antifreeze, antiseptics, and lacquer;

◇ butyl alcohol (butanol), used in many industrial processes (O'Brien, 1991).

Ethyl alcohol, often called "grain alcohol," is the least toxic of the alcohols. Few people drink pure ethyl alcohol because it is too strong and fiery

tasting. By convention any beverage with an alcohol content greater than 2% is considered an alcoholic beverage.

In addition to ethyl alcohol, alcoholic beverages also include trace amounts of other alcohols, such as amyl, butyl, and propyl alcohol, that result from the production process and storage (e.g., in wooden barrels). These organic alcohols plus other components produced during fermentation are called "congeners." They contribute to the distinctive taste and aroma of alcoholic beverages. Beer and vodka have a relatively low concentration of congeners; aged whiskies and brandy have a relatively high concentration (Lichine, 1990). It is thought that congeners may contribute to the severity of hangovers and other toxic problems of drinking, though it is clear that the main culprit is ethyl alcohol.

Alcohol occurs in nature when airborne yeast feeds on the sugars in honey and any watery mishmash of overripe fruit, berries, vegetables, or grain. It then excretes ethyl alcohol and carbon dioxide. Elephants, bears, and deer as well as birds and insects have been observed in a state of intoxication, exhibiting unsteady and erratic behavior after eating fermented mixtures.

TYPES OF ALCOHOLIC BEVERAGES

The principle categories of alcoholic beverages are beer, wine, and distilled spirits. When fruits ferment, the product is wine. When grains ferment, beer is produced. Spirits with different concentrations of alcohol can be distilled from fermented barley (whiskey), wine, or various other beverages. Each

country seems to have its national or local drinks; Mexican pulque, made from cactus; Russian kvass, made from cereal or bread; Asian kumiss, made from mare's milk; and even California garlic wine. The actual consumption of beer vs. wine, vs. distilled alcohol depends very much on the culture of that country. For example, Germans drink six times as much beer per capita as they do wine; the French drink twice as much wine as the Italians (Eurocare, 1999).

Beer

Beer brewing and bread making were probably started about the same time in the Neolithic era, about 8000 B.C. The raw ingredients were produced the same way, in cultivated fields. Some of the first written records concerning beer were found in Mesopotamian culture dating back to about 3000–4000 B.C. The Mesopotamians taught the Greeks how to brew beer and Europe learned from the Greeks.

Beer is produced by first allowing cereal grains, usually barley, to sprout in a tub of water where an enzyme called "amylase" is released. After the barley malt is crushed, the amylase helps convert the starches to sugar. This crushed malt is boiled into a liquid mash. It is then filtered, mixed with some hops (an aromatic herb first used around A.D. 1000–1500) and yeast, and allowed to ferment. Beer includes ale, stout, porter, malt liquor, and bock beer. The difference among beers has to do mainly with the type of grain used, the fermentation time, and whether they are top-fermenting beers (those that rise in the vat) or bottom-fermenting beers. The top-fermenting beers are more flavorful

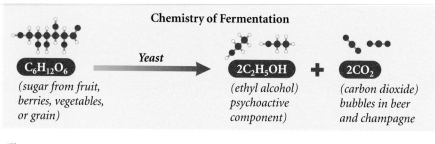

Chemistry of Fermentation

$C_6H_{12}O_6$
(sugar from fruit, berries, vegetables, or grain)

Yeast

$2C_2H_5OH$
(ethyl alcohol) psychoactive component)

$+$

$2CO_2$
(carbon dioxide) bubbles in beer and champagne

Figure 5-1 •

Yeast feeds on sugar and excretes alcohol and carbon dioxide.

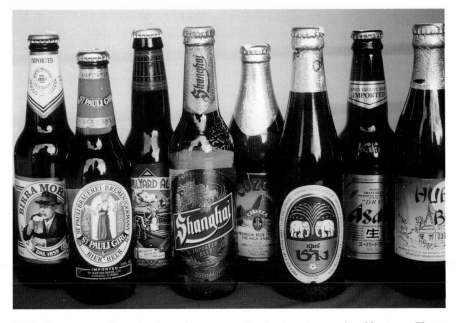

Virtually every country makes beer either as a national enterprise or a local business. These beers and ales come from Thailand, Vietnam, Peru, Germany, Italy, Japan, China, and Colorado.

ese saké rice wine). One species of grape, *Vitas vinifera,* which comes in more than 5,000 types, is used almost exclusively to make most of the grape wine in the world. It was probably the same species that was used 6,000 years ago in the Middle East (Amerine, 1985). Grapes with a high sugar content are preferred because it's the sugar that ferments into alcohol. A disease-resistant hybrid of *Vitas vinifera,* grafted onto several American species, was heavily planted worldwide, particularly in temperate climates found in France, Italy, California, New York, Argentina, and Spain. Wine had a short shelf life until the 1860s when Louis Pasteur showed that heating it would halt microbial activity and keep the wine from turning into vinegar (pasteurization).

Grapes are crushed to extract their juices. Either the grapes contain their own yeast or yeast is added and fermentation begins. The kind of wine produced depends on the variety of grape used, the quality of the soil, the ripeness of the grapes, the climate and weather, and the balance between acidity and sugar. The color and flavor of a particular wine further depend on how long the fermenting liquid is in contact with the grape skins. Red wines are left in contact with skins longer, thus increasing the amount of tannin in the wine. (Some people are allergic to red wines

and include ales, stouts, porters, and wheat beers. The bottom-fermenting beers include the most popular pale lager beers, e.g., Budweiser®, Coors® (Lukas, 1995). Traditional home-brewed beers are dark and full of sediment, minerals, vitamins, (especially B vitamins), and amino acids, and thus have appreciable food value, unlike modern beers that are highly filtered.

The alcohol content of most lager beers is 4% to 5%; ales are 5% to 6%, ice beers have 5% to 7%, malt liquors have 6% to 9%, while light beers are only 3.4% to 4.2% alcohol.

Wine

In some early cultures, beer was the alcoholic beverage of the common people and wine was the drink of the priests and nobles, possibly because vineyards were more difficult to establish and cultivate. In Egypt however, pharoahs did have beer entombed with them in their pyramids to sustain them on their journeys and to offer a gift to the gods. Ancient Greek and Roman cultures seem to have preferred wine; the ruling class kept the best supplies for themselves (Heath, 1995). They also

cultivated vineyards in many of their colonies. After the fall of the Roman Empire, many monasteries in Germany, France, Austria, and Italy carried on the cultivation of grapes and even hybridized new species.

Wines are usually made from grapes, though some are made from berries, other fruits (peach wine, plum wine), and even starchy grains (Japan-

TABLE 5–1   PRODUCTION & CONSUMPTION OF BEER & WINE IN EUROPE & THE UNITED STATES—1996

	Beer Production in Hectoliters	Beer Consumption in Liters per Capita	Wine Consumption in Liters per Capita
Germany	114,800	131.7	22
Denmark	9,591	117.6	28
Luxembourg	481	109.0	58
England	59,139	103.6	13
United States	200,000	95.0	20
Spain	24,879	64.7	30
France	19,493	39.6	60
Italy	11,455	103.6	59

The United States produces the most beer but Germany, Denmark, Luxembourg, and England have a higher per capita consumption (Eurocare, 1999).

One hectoliter = 26.4 gallons   one liter = .2642 gallons

because of their high tannin and histamine content.) White wines typically are aged from 6–12 months and red, from 2–4 years. Once bottled, wines continue to age and to improve in taste.

European wines contain from 8% to 12% alcohol, whereas U.S. wines have a 12% to 14% alcohol content. Wines with higher than 14% alcohol content are called "fortified wines" because they have had pure alcohol or brandy added during or after fermentation. Their final alcohol content is 17% to 21%. Wine coolers that are usually diluted with juice contain an average of 6% alcohol (Matthews, 1995).

Distilled Spirits (liquor)

The alcoholic content of naturally fermented wine is limited to about 14% by volume. At higher levels the concentration of alcohol becomes too toxic and kills off the fermenting yeast, thus halting the conversion of sugar into alcohol. In areas outside of Asia, drinks with greater than 14% alcohol weren't available until about A.D. 800 when the Arabs discovered distillation. This eventually led to the production of distilled spirits such as brandies, whiskies, vodka, and gin.

Brandy is distilled from wine, rum from sugar cane or molasses, vodka from potatoes, whiskey and gin from grains. Distilled spirits can be produced from many other plants including figs and dates in the Middle East or the agave plants in Mexico from which mescal or tequila is made.

One of the results of the invention of distilled beverages is that it became much easier to get drunk. Alcoholism rose in Europe after the introduction of spirits, i.e., the London Gin Epidemic. Similarly alcoholism became a major social problem in the early United States with the manufacture of increasing amounts of corn whiskey that was easier and more profitable to transport and market than bushels of corn. Grains and other sugar-producing commodities could be reduced in volume into more potent and higher-priced commodities that could be easily transported by wagon or in the holds of ships.

ABSORPTION, DISTRIBUTION, & METABOLISM

ABSORPTION & DISTRIBUTION

When someone drinks an alcoholic beverage, it is slightly diluted by digestive juices in the mouth and stomach. Because alcohol is readily soluble in water and doesn't need to be digested, it immediately begins to be absorbed and distributed. Absorption of alcohol into the bloodstream takes place at various sites along the gastrointestinal tract, including the stomach, the small intestines, and the colon. It enters the capillaries through passive diffusion.

Though most drugs must be passed into the intestine for absorption, alcohol is one of the few that is partially absorbed through the stomach. In men about 20% of the alcohol is absorbed

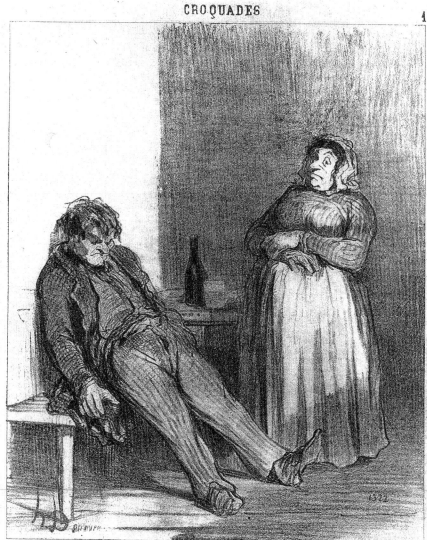

CROQUADES

— Ma femme, t'as tort de me blâmer… comme l'a dit un fameux philosophe… y n'y a que de boire du vin sans soif qui distingue l'homme du reste des animaux

The caption of the sketch by Henri Daumier says, "My wife, you are wrong to blame me . . . as a famous philosopher has said, 'It's only drinking wine when you're not thirsty that distinguishes man from the rest of the animals.'"

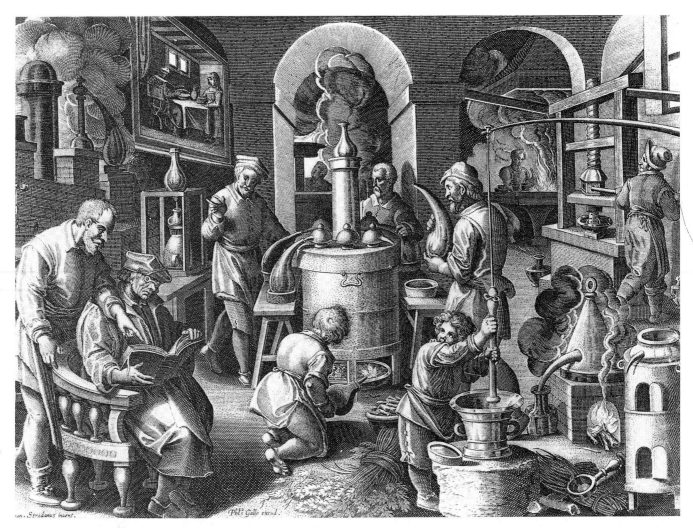

Distillatio by Philip Galle. Distillation in this sixteenth century Dutch laboratory supplies alcohol for making medicines and for drinking. In distillation a liquid is boiled and the vapors are drawn off, cooled, and condensed into a liquid. A clear, colorless, almost 100% pure grain alcohol distillate can be created using this process.

Courtesy of the National Library of Medicine, Bethesda

by the stomach wall while in women there is almost no absorption by the stomach. Given the same body weight, women and men differ in their processing of alcohol. Women have higher blood alcohol concentrations than men do from the same amount of alcohol. A woman who weighs the same as a man and drinks the same number of drinks as a man absorbs about 30% more alcohol and feels its psychoactive effects faster and more intensely (NIAAA, 1990).

This difference between women's and men's reaction to alcohol results from three possible explanations.

◊ Women have a lower percentage of body water than men of comparable size, so there is less water to dilute the alcohol in women resulting in higher alcohol concentrations in the blood.

◊ Women have less active alcohol dehydrogenase enzyme in the stomach to break down alcohol, so less alcohol is metabolized before getting into the blood, also resulting in higher concentrations.

◊ Finally, changes in gonadal hormone levels during menstruation affect the rate of alcohol metabolism, again resulting in higher blood concentrations at different points in the cycle (NIAAA, 1990).

Thus chronic alcohol use causes greater physical damage to women than to men—female alcoholics have death rates 50% to 100% higher than male alcoholics (NIAAA, 1990).

The alcohol that isn't absorbed in the stomach passes into the small intestines where it is absorbed into the bloodstream and partially metabolized by the liver and then quickly distributed throughout the body. Since alcohol molecules are small, water-soluble, lipid-soluble, and move easily through capillary walls by passive diffusion, they can enter any organ or tissue and in the case of pregnancy, can even cross the placental barrier into the fetal circulatory system (O'Brien, 1991). Once alcohol reaches

TABLE 5–2 APPROXIMATE PERCENTAGE OF ALCOHOL IN CERTAIN BEVERAGES (BY VOLUME)

WINE

Unfortified, natural: red, white, rosé	12–14%
Fortified, dessert: sherry, port, muscatel	17–21%
Champagne	12%
Vermouth	18%
Wine cooler	6%

BEER

Regular beer	4–5%
Light beer	3–7%
Malt liquor	6–9%
Ale	5–6%
Ice beer	5–7%
Low-alcohol beer	1.5%
Nonalcoholic beers (Odoul's®, Sharpe's®)	0.5%

LIQUORS & WHISKEYS

Bourbon, whiskey, scotch, vodka, gin, brandy, rum	40–50%
Tequila, cognac, Drambui®	40%
Amaretto®, Kahlua®	26%
Everclear®	95%

(Note: To calculate the proof of a product, double the alcohol content: e.g., 40% alcohol = 80 proof, 100% alcohol = 200 proof.)

the brain and passes through the blood-brain barrier, psychoactive effects gradually begin to occur.

The highest levels of blood alcohol concentration occur 30–90 minutes after alcohol is drunk. How quickly the effects are felt is determined by the rate of absorption. Absorption is influenced by an individual's weight, body chemistry, and factors such as emotional state (e.g., fear, stress, fatigue, or anger), state of health, body fat, food taken with the alcohol, and even the outside temperature. Women absorb more alcohol during the premenstrual period than at other times.

Other factors that speed absorption and cause a faster high in both men and women are

◊ increasing either the amount drunk or the drinking rate;

◊ drinking on an empty stomach;

◊ using high alcohol concentrations in drinks, up to a maximum of 40–50%;

◊ drinking carbonated drinks, such as champagne, sparkling wines, soft drinks, and tonic mixers;

◊ warming the alcohol (e.g., hot toddies, hot saké).

Factors that slow absorption and cause a slower high are

◊ eating before or while drinking (especially meat, milk, cheese, and fatty foods);

◊ diluting drinks with ice, water, or fruit juice that lower the amount of alcohol available for absorption.
(Jones & Pounder, 1998; Longenecker, 1994).

METABOLISM

Because the body treats alcohol as a toxin or poison, elimination begins as soon as it is ingested. Approximately 2% to 10% of the alcohol is eliminated directly without being metabolized; a small amount is exhaled via the lungs while additional amounts are excreted through sweat, saliva, and urine. The re-maining 90% to 98% of alcohol is neutralized through metabolism (mainly oxidation) by the liver and then by excretion through the kidneys and lungs (Jones, 1998).

Alcohol is metabolized in the liver, first by alcohol dehydrogenase (ADH) into acetaldehyde, which is very toxic to the body and especially the liver, and then by acetaldehyde dehydrogenase (ALDH) into acetic acid that is finally oxidized into carbon dioxide (CO_2) and water (H_2O) (Fig. 5-2). The varying availability and efficiency of ADH and ALDH, due in part to hereditary capabilities, accounts for some of the variation in people's reaction to alcohol (Bosron, Ehrig, & Li, 1993).

◊ As mentioned earlier, women have less ADH in the stomach than men, so they are less able to metabolize alcohol, thus they will have a higher

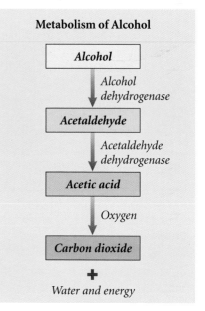

Metabolism of Alcohol

Figure 5-2 •

Metabolism is accomplished in several stages involving oxidation. First the enzyme alcohol dehydrogenase (ADH), found in the stomach and the liver, acts on the ethyl alcohol (C_2H_5OH) to form acetaldehyde (CH_3CHO), a highly toxic substance. Acetaldehyde is then quickly acted on by a second enzyme, acetaldehyde dehydrogenase (ALDH), that oxidizes it into acetic acid (CH_3COOH). Acetic acid is then further oxidized to carbon dioxide (CO_2) and water (H_2O).

BAC than men for an equal amount of ingested alcohol (NIAAA, 1990).

◇ About half of all Japanese, along with some other Asian populations (e.g., Chinese), are born with a more efficient ADH called "atypical ADH" and a less efficient form of ALDH known as "KM ALDH1," thus when they drink even small amounts of alcohol, the toxic acetaldehyde builds up (up to 10 times the normal amount) and causes a flushing reaction due to vasodilation. Tachycardia and headaches also occur. At higher doses, edema (water retention), hypotension, and vomiting occur (Goedde, Harada, & Agarwal, 1979, 1983; Teng, 1981; Woodward, 1998). Though Asians have a higher rate of abstention and lower rate of alcoholism, Asian-Americans' rate of alcoholism is higher, showing that environmental and cultural influences can overcome biological propensities (Lee, 1987).

◇ Although there is no confirming research, it is suspected that the high rate of alcoholism and the high rate of cirrhosis of the liver in Native Americans is due to disruptions in the ALDH and ADH systems as well as a tradition of binge drinking patterns.

◇ Some speculate that if a person has the wrong ALDH, then the normal benefits of light to moderate drinking are not present, therefore the main benefit sought in drinking is getting high—not relaxing, not whetting one's appetite, not becoming more social—only getting high, which takes large amounts of alcohol. The health risks of such a binge pattern are much greater.

Besides ALDH irregularities, drugs such as aspirin also inhibit metabolism of alcohol and lead to higher blood alcohol concentration in both men and women.

In many countries, alcoholic beverages are used primarily as a source of nutrition while in others they are used primarily for their mind-altering effects. Alcohol is a very concentrated energy source, almost as much as pure fat but they are empty calories, i.e., high caloric content with no real food value. On average, alcoholics get half their energy intake from alcohol and, as a result, are much more susceptible to malnutrition, particularly thiamine, folate, and other vitamin B deficiencies. This is in addition to digestive upsets and pancreatic problems. Disruption of liver function also leads to disrupted digestive patterns (Lieber, 1998).

"We get drunk and we have fun. We have a good time. That's what we're about. And I'm healthy. I'm in better shape than any of you guys . . . well maybe not on the inside. My stomach's kind of messed up a little bit. I can't drink liquor that good. I did take blood tests. I get my results on Friday . . . I forgot."

25-year-old male alcohol abuser

Blood Alcohol Concentration (BAC)

Though absorption of alcohol is quite variable, metabolism occurs at a defined continuous rate. About one ounce of pure alcohol is eliminated from the body every 3 hours. Thus we can usually predict the amount of alcohol that will be circulating through the body and brain and how long it will take that amount to be metabolized by the liver and eliminated via urination, sweating, and breathing. However, each person's actual reaction and level of impairment can vary widely, depending on drinking history, behavioral tolerance, and a dozen other factors. It takes about 15–20 minutes for alcohol to reach the brain via the blood and cause impairment but more time for it to enter the urine. It takes 30–40 minutes after ingestion to reach maximum blood alcohol concentration (NIAAA, 1997).

This blood alcohol concentration table (Table 5-3) measures the concen-

TABLE 5–3 APPROXIMATE BLOOD ALCOHOL CONCENTRATION FOR DIFFERENT BODY WEIGHTS

No. of Drinks	1	2	3	4	5	6	7	8	9	10
Male										
100 lbs.	.043	.087	.130	.174	.217	.261	.304	.348	.391	.435
125 lbs.	.034	.069	.103	.139	.173	.209	.242	.287	.312	.346
150 lbs.	.029	.058	.087	.116	.145	.174	.203	.232	.261	.290
175 lbs.	.025	.050	.075	.100	.125	.150	.175	.200	.225	.250
200 lbs.	.022	.043	.065	.087	.108	.130	.152	.174	.195	.217
225 lbs.	.019	.039	.058	.078	.097	.117	.136	.156	.175	.195
250 lbs.	.017	.035	.052	.070	.087	.105	.122	.139	.156	.173
Female										
100 lbs.	.050	.101	.152	.203	.253	.304	.355	.406	.456	.507
125 lbs.	.040	.080	.120	.162	.202	.244	.282	.324	.364	.404
150 lbs.	.034	.068	.101	.135	.169	.203	.237	.271	.304	.338
175 lbs.	.029	.058	.087	.117	.146	.175	.204	.233	.262	.292
200 lbs.	.026	.050	.076	.101	.126	.152	.177	.203	.227	.253

If a person drinks over a period of time, the alcohol is metabolized at a rate of .015 per hour. Use the following table to factor in the time since the first drink.

TIMETABLE FACTORS

Hours since first drink	1	2	3	4	5
Subtract from BAC	.015	.030	.045	.060	.075

Drink Equivalency

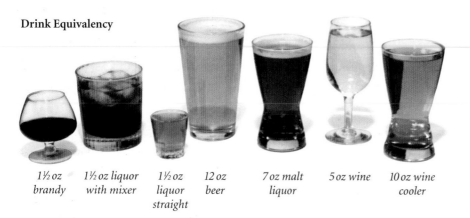

1½ oz brandy   1½ oz liquor with mixer   1½ oz liquor straight   12 oz beer   7 oz malt liquor   5 oz wine   10 oz wine cooler

Figure 5-3 •

One drink is defined as: 1½ oz. brandy, 1½ oz. liquor w/wo mixer, 12 oz. lager beer, 7 oz. malt liquor, 5 oz. wine, 10 oz. wine cooler.

tration of alcohol in a drinker's blood. In most states, legal intoxication is .08 or .10. Some think it should be .05 for safety. In general alcohol is metabolized at the rate of 1/4 oz. to 1/3 oz. per hour. The unit of measurement for BAC is weight by volume, e.g., milligrams per deciliter, but can be expressed as a percentage, e.g., .10% alcohol by volume (Bailey, 1995).

For example, if a 200 lb. male has five drinks in two hours, his blood alcohol would be .108 minus the timetable factor of .030, so his BAC would be about .078 and he would be legally sober enough to drive in many states. If his 200 lb. female companion has five drinks in two hours, her blood alcohol level would be .126 minus the timetable factor of .030, so her BAC would be .096 and not only would she be quite a bit more intoxicated than her companion even though they weighed the same and drank the same amount over the same period of time but she would also be legally drunk in many states.

DESIRED EFFECTS, SIDE EFFECTS, & HEALTH CONSEQUENCES

LEVELS OF USE

The effects of any drug depend on the dosage. The same substance can be a poison, a powerful prescription medicine, or an over-the-counter mild medication depending on the dose and frequency of use. Alcohol is no exception; it can be used in low, moderate, or high doses and it can be used infrequently or often. As with other psychoactive drugs, there are escalating patterns of use.

Abstention (no use)

"My brother experimented with Puerto Rican rum on New Year's Eve when he was 15. He threw up on me on the way to the toilet. That took care of his drinking for five years and mine forever."

54-year-old nondrinker

Experimentation (use for curiosity with no subsequent drug-seeking behavior)

"The first time I tried beer . . . well when you're a little boy, your dad says, 'Go get me a beer.' You pop it open for him and they let you take a sip every once in a while as long as mom's not looking. It tasted good. When you're 10 or 12, you don't really know what alcohol is, you just experience it every once in a while."

33-year-old drinker

Social/Recreational Use (sporadic infrequent drug seeking with no established pattern)

"We know which dorm has the drinkers, so when we feel like a bit of a party and a few drinks, that's where we go. They're more serious about their drinking; they like '40s [40 oz. malt liquor bottles or cans] but I can take it with a grain of salt."

20-year-old college sophomore

Habituation (established pattern of use with no major negative consequences)

"I think the pleasure left. The maintenance thing was . . . now I didn't know how to live any other way. This was the only way I knew how to have fun. This was the only way I knew how to feel better. But it didn't work and it took me awhile to realize that it had become a habit."

36-year-old recovering alcoholic

Abuse (continued use despite negative consequences)

"I always got Bs, and then my grades dropped down to Ds, and then I started failing my classes, and I skipped school, and I got suspended all the time for that when I got caught. I'd skip school and I'd go get high or we'd just skip it because we were always high and we thought it was boring."

15-year-old high school dropout in treatment

Addiction (compulsion to use, inability to stop use, major life dysfunction with continued use)

"I would have the shakes, just really sick. I mean my body could not take alcohol at all. I would be sick in the morning like for days . . . and hard to go to work and hard to take care of my children, hard to do my daily chores. It took me a long

time to get well in the morning until I realized there was a magical cure. I could start drinking bloody Mary's or something that wouldn't upset my stomach and I would be all right again. But then what would happen was once I started I couldn't stop, so I was back on the merry-go-round again."

33-year-old recovering alcoholic

LOW- TO MODERATE-DOSE EPISODES

There are no conclusive studies that drinking small amounts of alcohol, even over an extended period, has negative health consequences for men, nor are there conclusive indications that infrequent mild intoxication episodes have no lasting adverse health consequences for most male drinkers. While this statement may be physiologically correct, alcohol's disinhibiting effect at low doses can result in automobile crashes and legal problems, along with unwanted pregnancies and sexually transmitted diseases, including HIV/AIDS, from high-risk sexual activity. This not withstanding, studies have shown that drinking two drinks of alcohol, especially two glasses of wine or less each day, has some positive health benefits for men including decreased coronary artery disease (NIAAA, 1999). The situation for women, except in relationship to heart benefits, is quite the opposite. Several studies demonstrate that even low levels of drinking in women with a certain genetic susceptibility can result in major health consequences such as an increase in breast cancer (Thun, Peto, Lopez, et al., 1997; Zhang, Schatzkin, Kreger, et al., 1998). Further, studies demonstrate that women who drink are at higher risk to develop liver cirrhosis, pregnancy problems, and even AIDS when they drink moderate amounts of alcohol (NIAAA, 1997; Maher, 1997).

In addition low-level alcohol use is generally not safe for people who

◊   are pregnant;

◊   have certain preexisting physical or mental health problems that are aggravated by alcohol;

◊   are allergic to alcohol, nitrosamines, or other congeners and additives;

◊   have a high genetic/environmental susceptibility to addiction;

◊   have had a history of abuse and addiction problems with alcohol or other drugs in the past.

Sometimes it is difficult to define moderate drinking because each person has a different definition. We will define moderate drinking as drinking that doesn't cause problems for the drinker or for those around him or her (Alcohol Alert, 1992). However, drinkers begin to have pathological consequences to alcohol when they have more than two drinks per day in men and zero to one drink per day in women. Severe effects and long-term health and social consequences usually result from high-dose use episodes and frequent high-dose or chronic use.

Low- to Moderate-Dose Use: Physical Effects

Therapeutic Uses. Alcohol is used as a solvent for other medications since it is water- and lipid-soluble. It is used as a topical disinfectant. Isopropyl alcohol is used as a body rub to reduce fever since it evaporates so quickly. Ethanol has been used as a pain reliever for certain nerve-related pain; systemically it is used to treat methanol and ethylene glycol poisoning; it is occasionally used to prevent premature labor (Woodward, 1998).

Desired Effects. Some people who drink alcoholic beverages think that they taste good, quench the thirst, and relax one's muscle tension. Consumed in low doses before meals, alcoholic beverages activate gastric juices, improve stomach motility, and stimulate the appetite. They produce a feeling of warmth since vessels dilate and blood flow to subcutaneous tissues increases (Woodward, 1998). Alcohol has a slight dehydrating effect on the body, so when people add caffeinated beverages (which act as diuretics) to their drinking, they can overheat on a hot day.

Light to moderate use of alcohol

(up to one drink a day for women and two drinks a day for men) has been shown to reduce the incidence of heart disease (Boffetta & Garfinkel, 1990). Whether the cause is the increase in high-density lipoproteins, particularly HDL_3, a different interaction with lipoproteins, or simply the decrease in tension that a drink can induce, light to moderate use reduces plaque formation. The doses must be low enough not to cause liver damage, induce other adverse health effects, or trigger heavier drinking. Of course any beneficial effects may also be obtained through exercise, low-fat diets, stress-reduction techniques, and an aspirin a day. (On autopsy many "winos" have clean blood vessels and badly damaged livers, hearts, and brains.) *The American Heart Association Guidelines on Alcohol Consumption* says that one to two drinks per day for men and one drink per day for women seems to lower the health risk but because of the dangers involved if the drinking increases, any recommendation concerning alcohol should be in consultation with a physician (AHA, 1996).

Researchers at Columbia University found in a study of 677 stroke victims that those who have one or two drinks a day have a lower risk of strokes because alcohol keeps blood platelets from clumping (Sacco, Elkind, Boden-Albala, et al., 1999). But again since heavy drinking actually increases the risk of stroke, and even moderate drinking has unwanted side effects, and since no benefit is shown in recommending moderate drinking to abstainers, using alcohol as a stroke-preventive measure should only be done in consultation with a physician.

Sleep. Alcohol is often used by people to get to sleep particularly if anxiety is causing insomnia. In fact alcohol does decrease the time it takes to fall asleep but it also seems to disturb the second half of the sleep period especially if consumed within an hour of bedtime (Landolt et al., 1996; Vitiello, 1997). Drinking also seems to have an effect on obstructive-sleep apnea, a disorder where the upper breathing passage (pharynx) narrows or closes during sleep causing the person to come awake, often a number of times during a sleep period, thus leading to fatigue. Those with alcoholism have an increased risk of sleep apnea and those with the condition seem to aggravate their disease by drinking (Miller, et al., 1988; Dawson, Bigby, Poceta, & Mitler, 1993).

Low- to Moderate-Dose Use: Psychological Effects

The effects of alcohol, particularly the physical effects (as with most psychoactive drugs), are dependent on the amount and frequency taken. The mental and emotional effects are also conditioned by the setting in which the drug is used along with the mood and general psychological makeup of the user (Peele, 1995). In general, alcohol affects people psychologically by lowering inhibitions, increasing self-confidence, and promoting sociability. It calms, relaxes, sedates, and reduces tension. But for someone who is already lonely, depressed, suicidal, or angry, the depressant and disinhibiting effects of alcohol can deepen these emotions, so for some drinkers that means sociability and talkativeness and for others, verbal or physical aggressiveness and even violence.

"I started out drinking when I was about 15 out of peer pressure but it made me forget about everything. It felt like a whole new way of life. I was happy; I was gregarious; I was outgoing . . . more extroverted . . . I guess I love dancing and I thought I was Ginger Rogers in that I thought I could do anything."
42-year-old recovering alcoholic

Disinhibition & GABA. The blocking of inhibitions is caused by alcohol's action on the higher centers of the brain's cortex, particularly that part of the brain that controls reasoning and judgment. Alcohol first affects the cortex and then it acts on the lower centers of the limbic system that rule mood and emotion.

Alcohol's psychological effects stem from the drug's interaction with the brain's neurotransmitters, particularly met-enkephalin (which can reduce pain), serotonin (scarcity causes depression and excess causes anxiety), dopamine (which can give a surge of pleasure), and particularly gamma amino butyric acid (GABA). GABA is the major inhibitory neurotransmitter in the brain, so by activating the inhibiting effects of GABA, alcohol lowers inhibitions and slows down all of the brain processes (Valenzuela & Harris, 1997).

"The pleasure then that I liked was just getting high, just feeling like other people feel. Like I don't know if you call this, 'feeling human.' I guess so 'cause you're high and you fit in with everyone else."
36-year-old recovering polydrug abuser

Other neurotransmitters affected by alcohol are endorphins, corticotropin, and acetylcholine.

Low- to Moderate-Dose Use: Sexual Effects

More than any other psychoactive drug, alcohol has insinuated itself in the lore, culture, and mythology of sexual and romantic behavior: a beer "kegger" party to look for a date, a rum and coke before sex, or champagne to celebrate an anniversary. Almost half of a group of 90,000 college students at a number of two and four-year institutions believed that alcohol facilitates sexual opportunities (Presley et al., 1997). Whether it does so because of actual psychological and physiological changes or because of expectations that it will is still open to question.

"It's no mystery why guys in college fraternities, many of whom don't have all that much money, still come up with plenty of money to have outrageous amounts of alcohol and let any woman in for free. The whole point is they're setting up an environment whereby people are going to get more

drunk. Women's inhibitions and a guy's inhibitions are going to get lowered."
23-year-old college counselor

The acceptability of using alcohol extends to high school students. A survey done for the U.S. Surgeon General found that 18% of females and 39% of males say it is acceptable for a boy to force sex if the girl is stoned or drunk (Surgeon General, 1992).

"It doesn't matter if alcohol was involved in the situation. He raped me. It doesn't matter. There's more attention paid to the fact that there was alcohol involved than the fact that a woman was assaulted . . . and that her life changed and that all of these things happened as a result of that. Alcohol's involved in almost every social situation but it doesn't mean that we recognize it or validate it."
22-year-old female college senior

Alcohol's physical effects on sexual functioning are closely related to blood alcohol levels. In low doses alcohol usually increases desire in males and females, usually heightening the intensity of orgasm in females and slightly decreasing erectile ability and delaying ejaculation in males (Blume, 1997; Wilson & Lawson, 1976). Alcohol dilates peripheral blood vessels making it difficult to maintain an erection.

HIGH-DOSE EPISODES

High-Dose Use: Physical Effects of Intoxication

Intoxication is a combination of both psychological mood, expectation, and past drinking experience as well as the physiological changes caused by elevated blood alcohol levels. In most states a person is legally intoxicated when the BAC reaches .10. However, the effects of legal intoxication can be partially masked by experienced drinkers. Experiments have indicated that there is a so-called expectancy effect, such that someone who has not consumed alcoholic beverages but thinks he or she has can exhibit signs of intoxication.

Binge drinking is defined as consuming five or more drinks in a row at one sitting for males and four or more in a row for girls. About 43% of college students say they are binge drinkers while 23% say they binge frequently (Wechsler, Lee, Kuo, & Lee, 2000). In the general population by comparison, only 15.6% binge while 5.9% admit to heavy use (heavy drinking is defined as five or more drinks in one sitting at least five times a month). As with college students, any person who binge drinks is more likely to have hangovers, experience injuries, damage property, and have trouble with authorities (Presely et al., 1997).

However after enough drinks are consumed, expectation, setting, and the mood of the drinker cease to have a strong influence and the depressant effects of the alcohol take over (depending on the tolerance of the drinker). As more alcohol is drunk, blood pressure is lowered, motor reflexes are slowed, digestion and absorption of nutrients becomes poor, body heat is lost as blood vessels dilate, and sexual performance is diminished. In fact every system in the body is strongly affected. Slurred speech, staggering, loss of balance, and mental confusion are all signs of an increased state of intoxication.

High-Dose Use: Alcohol Poisoning (overdose)

If truly large amounts of alcohol are drunk too quickly, severe alcohol poisoning occurs and depression of the various systems can lead to unconsciousness (passing out), coma, and death. Some clinicians use a BAC level of .40 as the threshold for alcohol poisoning.

However, even blood alcohol concentration levels of .02 or greater can result in severely depressed respiration and vomiting while semiconscious. The vomit can be aspirated or swallowed, blocking air passages to the lung, resulting in asphyxiation and death. This can also cause infections in the lungs.

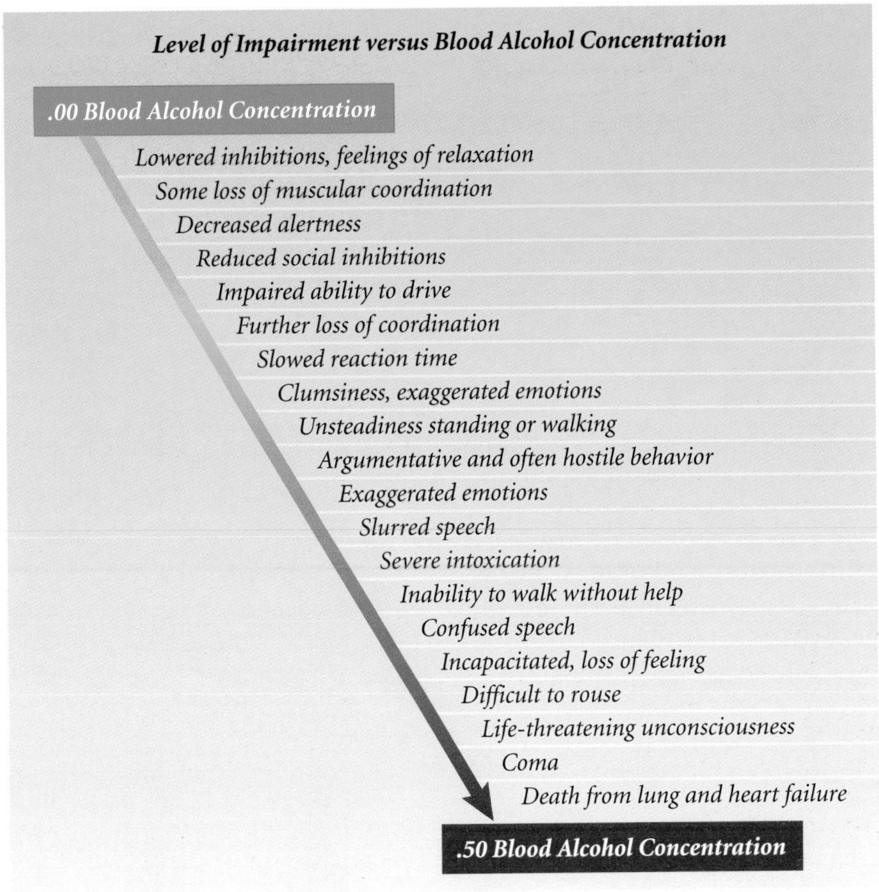

Level of Impairment versus Blood Alcohol Concentration

.00 Blood Alcohol Concentration

Lowered inhibitions, feelings of relaxation
Some loss of muscular coordination
Decreased alertness
Reduced social inhibitions
Impaired ability to drive
Further loss of coordination
Slowed reaction time
Clumsiness, exaggerated emotions
Unsteadiness standing or walking
Argumentative and often hostile behavior
Exaggerated emotions
Slurred speech
Severe intoxication
Inability to walk without help
Confused speech
Incapacitated, loss of feeling
Difficult to rouse
Life-threatening unconsciousness
Coma
Death from lung and heart failure

.50 Blood Alcohol Concentration

Figure 5-4 •

As consumption increases, the amount of alcohol absorbed increases and therefore the effects increase but at different rates depending on the physical and mental makeup of the drinker.

High-Dose Use: Mental & Emotional Effects

"I remember being beat up physically and being emotionally abused and drinking a gallon of wine and feeling like I just wanted to be out of it. And for me, that was the way to deal with the pain. I think women tend to do those things; either they'll take drugs with the perpetrator to have some kind of relationship or after they've been beat up, use alcohol or drugs as a way of not to deal with the pain."

43-year-old ex-wife of abuser

Alcohol depresses other functions of the central and peripheral nervous systems. Initial relaxation and lowered inhibitions at low doses often become mental confusion, mood swings, loss of judgment, and emotional turbulence at higher doses. At a BAC of .05, the thinking and judgment of a drinker become impaired. At a BAC concentration of .10, the level designating legal intoxication in many states, a drinker may demonstrate slurred speech and beyond that level, progressive mental confusion and loss of emotional control. Heavy alcohol consumption before sleep, as with light to moderate consumption, may also interfere with the REM (rapid eye movement) or dreaming sleep essential to feeling fully rested. Chronic alcoholics may suffer from fatigue during the day and insomnia at night, as well as nightmares, bed wetting, and snoring.

High-Dose Use: Blackouts

Some alcoholics suffer blackouts during heavy drinking bouts. During blackouts, a person is awake and conscious and seems to be acting normally but afterwards cannot recall anything that was said or done. Sometimes even a small amount of alcohol may trigger a blackout. Blackouts, which are caused by an alcohol-induced electrochemical disruption of the brain, are often early indications of alcoholism. They are different from passing out or loss of consciousness during a drinking episode since any drinker can pass out from too much alcohol. A drinker can also have a brownout, which is a partial recall of events. A possible indicator of this phenomena and therefore a marker for alcoholism is the reduced amplitude of an electroencephalograph (EEG) event-related potential (ERP) brain wave called the "P3 or P300 wave." This wave demonstrates cognition, decision-making, and processing of short-term memory. This reduced ERP is found in alcoholics and their young sons but not in social drinkers (Begleiter, 1980; Blum, Brauerman, Cull, et al., 2000).

"With alcohol I was out of control because I would drink to the point where I didn't know what I was doing, which made it easier for the man to do whatever he wanted and my not realizing it until the next day or the next morning when I woke up and looked over and didn't have any recollection of what had happened."
32-year-old recovering female binge drinker

High-Dose Use: Hangover

Hangover, a withdrawal syndrome, is the body's response to excessive amounts of alcohol. The effects of a hangover can be most severe many hours after alcohol has been completely eliminated from the system. Typical effects include nausea, vomiting, headache, thirst, dizziness, mood disturbances, abbreviated sleep, sensitivity to light and noise, dry cottony mouth, inability to concentrate, and a general depressed feeling. Some research shows that those with a high susceptibility to alcoholism suffer more severe hangovers and often continue drinking to find relief (NIAAA, 1998). Those with a genetic risk for alcoholism experience more acute withdrawal symptoms and more severe hangovers (Span & Earleywine, 1999).

The causes of hangover are not clearly understood. Additives (congeners) in alcoholic beverages are thought to be partly responsible although even pure alcohol can cause hangovers. Irritation of the stomach lining by alcohol may contribute to intestinal disorders. Low blood sugar, dehydration, and tissue degradation may also play their parts. Symptoms vary according to individuals but it is evident that the greater the quantity of alcohol consumed, the more severe the aftereffects (Swift & Davison, 1998).

High-Dose Use: Sobering Up

A person can control the amount of alcohol in the blood by controlling the amount drunk and the rate at which it is drunk. But the elimination of alcohol from the system is a constant. As mentioned, the body metabolizes alcohol at the rate of 1/4 oz. to 1/3 oz. per hour. Until the alcohol has been eliminated and until hormones, enzymes, body fluids, and bodily systems come into equilibrium, hangover symptoms will persist. An analgesic may lessen the headache pain while fruit juice can help hydrate the body and correct low blood sugar but neither coffee, nor exercise, nor a cold shower cures a hangover. Feeling better comes only with rest and sufficient recovery time.

CHRONIC HIGH-DOSE USE

Chronic High-Dose Use: Tolerance & Tissue Dependence

The effect of alcohol on different drinkers varies widely due to the varying rates at which tolerance develops. Dispositional (metabolic) tolerance, pharmacodynamic tolerance, behavioral tolerance, and acute tolerance are four ways the body tries to adapt to the effects of alcohol and protect itself. The result of tolerance is that the chronic drinker is able to handle larger and larger amounts of alcohol. It also increases the body's dependence on alcohol to stay in physiological balance (tissue dependence).

"Well I started drinking one beer and then I went on to two. A week later I went on to a six-pack, and then through the years I went on to two six-packs and then I ended up drinking tequila. I used to drink a fifth of tequila two years after I got addicted to the alcohol. So I drank tequila most of the day and I used to numb myself."
38-year-old recovering female alcoholic

Dispositional (metabolic) tolerance means the body changes the way it metabolizes alcohol. As a person drinks over a period of time, the liver adapts to create more enzymes to process the alcohol and its metabolite acetylaldehyde (Tabakoff, 1992; Lieber, 1991). This accelerated process eliminates alcohol more quickly from the body. It also accelerates the elimination of other prescription drugs lessening their effectiveness. In addition since liver cells are also being destroyed by drinking and by the natural aging process, the liver eventually becomes less able to handle the alcohol. A heavy drinker who could handle a fifth of whiskey at the age of 30 can become totally incapacitated by half a pint of wine at the age of 50. This process is called "**reverse tolerance.**"

"In the very beginning I got sick, which was a signal. But I thought that happened to everybody. As time went on I learned to develop a tolerance for it and I could drink an awful lot. But then eventually that reversed and it didn't take very much for me to get drunk and out of control and I had blackouts and things like that."
37-year-old recovering alcoholic

Pharmacodynamic tolerance means brain neurons and other cells become more resistant to the effects of alcohol by increasing the number of re-

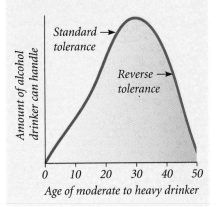

How Aging and Heavy Drinking Affect Liver's Ability to Handle Alcohol

Figure 5-5 •

This graph shows the decrease in liver capacity to process alcohol as a person ages. As the liver is taxed and poisoned by the alcohol, its capacity is diminished to the point where an older chronic drinker can get tipsy on just one drink.

ceptor sites needed to produce an effect or by creating other cellular changes that make tissues less responsive to alcohol. When GABA receptors are activated by ethanol, they change over time to become less sensitive not only to ethanol but to GABA, benzodiazepines, and other GABA agonists as well (Valenzuela & Harris, 1997).

Behavioral tolerance means drinkers learn how to "handle their liquor" by modifying their behavior or by trying to act in such a way that they hope others won't notice they are inebriated. If they practice acting normally while under the influence, they learn behavioral tolerance more quickly (Vogel-Sprott, Rawana, & Webster, 1984).

Acute tolerance also develops to high-dose alcohol use. This rapid tolerance starts to develop with the first use of alcohol, or in animal experiments, with the first injection of alcohol. It is the body's method of providing instant protection to the poisonous effects of ethanol.

Tolerance does not develop equally to all the effects of alcohol, so while a person may learn how to walk steadily with a .14 BAC, they might have trouble performing a task that requires manual dexterity.

Chronic High-Dose Use: Withdrawal

As mentioned a hangover can be a mild withdrawal syndrome after a heavy drinking episode but with alcoholics, withdrawal can be more serious, peaking within 24–36 hours after cessation of chronic-high dose use. Symptoms can include

◊ rapid pulse or sweating,

◊ hand tremors,

◊ insomnia,

◊ nausea or vomiting,

◊ transient visual, tactile, or auditory hallucinations and illusions,

◊ psychomotor agitation,

◊ anxiety,

◊ and in 10% to 33% of the cases depending on the group studied, grand mal seizures.

(APA, 1994)

"I would be more afraid of quitting alcohol than heroin, 'cause with drinking, you go into convulsions and you are really sick. I thought I was going to die from the pain in my stomach—the throwing up, the sweating, and the diarrhea. You don't have any energy and you know if you just took a drink you'd feel better.

And with heroin you get some muscle cramps and you throw up and you get a little diarrhea but you're not going to get convulsions. You're not going to die. You can die from kicking alcohol."

35-year-old female recovering alcohol/heroin abuser

In less than five percent of serious cases of alcohol withdrawal, **delirium tremens,** called "**DTs**," occurs. DTs usually begins 6–48 hours after the last drink in a period of long heavy drinking and can last for 3–10 days, although some cases have been reported to last up to 50 days (Mayo-Smith, 1998). The dramatic symptoms can include trembling over the whole body or grand mal seizures, severe auditory, visual, and tactile hallucinations, disorientation, insomnia, and delirium. The DTs is a serious condition requiring hospitalization. Untreated the mortality rate ranges from 10% to 20%.

Since the main symptoms of severe withdrawal can combine with medical complications, such as malnutrition, pneumonia, depressed respiration, liver problems, or physical damage, medical care for an alcohol abuser or alcoholic needs to be a consideration in any course of treatment.

GABA & Withdrawal. Alcohol at first increases the effectiveness of GABA at its receptor sites, thus preventing the actions of the brain's energy chemicals norepinephrine (NE) and epinephrine (E). This decrease in NE/E makes the person drowsy and depresses other body functions. Over time the brain compensates by creating an excess of NE/E and even more GABA. During withdrawal the rebound excess of NE/E causes anxiety, increased psychomotor activity, tachycardia, hypertension, and occasionally seizures. Normally the GABA would control these effects, however with prolonged use the receptor sites of GABA become less sensitive (tolerant) and therefore less able to control the hyperactivity (Blum & Payne, 1991).

Current research also explores the role of serotonin in the alcohol withdrawal process. A 30% reduction in the availability of brainstem serotonin transporters was found in chronic alcoholics, which correlate with their self-reported ratings of depression and anxiety during withdrawal. In animal studies reduced serotonin has been associated with impaired impulse control and increased alcohol consumption (Heinz, Ragan, Jones, et al., 1998).

Kindling. With many long-term heavy drinkers, a process called "kindling" occurs. What happens is that repeated bouts of drinking and withdrawal actually intensifies subsequent withdrawal symptoms and can cause seizures. The theory is that the repeated presence of alcohol actually alters brain chemistry, impairing the body's natural defenses against damage from alcohol (Becker, 1998).

ADDICTION (alcoholism)

For about 10% to 12% of the 140 million adults in the United States who drink, the use of alcohol has developed into addiction. The incidence of alcoholism in men is approximately two to three times greater than in women (14% of male drinkers vs. 6% of female drinkers). In addition onset of alcoholism usually occurs at a younger age in men than in women (SAMHSA, 1998). In terms of consumption 20% of drinkers consume 80% of all alcohol (Greenfield & Rogers, 1999).

CLASSIFICATION

Early Classifications

Over the years there have been many attempts to classify different types of alcoholism. The purpose of classification is to develop a framework by which an illness or condition can be studied systematically rather than relying strictly on experience. According to scientific literature from the nineteenth and early twentieth centuries, researchers developed 39 classifications of alcoholics, e. g., acute, periodic, and chronic oenomania; habitual inebriety; continuous and explosive inebriate; and dipsomaniac among others.

E. M. Jellinek

In 1941 psychiatrist Karl Bowman and biometrist E. M. Jellinek presented an integration of 24 classifications of alcoholism that had appeared over the years in scientific literature. They integrated the 24 classifications into four types:

1. Primary or true alcoholics; immediate liking for alcohol and rapid development of an uncontrollable need

2. Steady endogenous symptomatic drinkers; alcoholism is secondary to a major psychiatric disorder

3. Intermittent endogenous symptomatic drinkers; periodic binge drinking, again often with a psychiatric disorder

4. Stammtisch drinkers; drinkers in whom alcoholism is precipitated by outside causes, often start as social drinkers.

Twenty years later in 1960, Jellinek in his landmark book *The Disease Concept of Alcoholism* proposed five types of alcoholism: alpha, beta, gamma, delta, and epsilon. Gamma and delta alcoholics were considered true alcoholics (Jellinek, 1961).

◇ **Gamma alcoholics:** mainly they have a high psychological vulnerability but also a high physiological vulnerability; they develop tissue tolerance quickly; they lose control quickly; and their progression to uncontrolled use is marked.

◇ **Delta alcoholics:** mainly they have strong sociocultural and economic influences, along with a high physiological vulnerability; they also acquire tissue dependence rapidly and it's hard for them to abstain; their progression to alcoholism is much slower than gamma alcoholism.

(Babor, 1995; Jellinek, 1961)

Modern Classifications

As valuable as Jellinek's classification was, the scientific basis for alcoholism wasn't as clear cut as with other illnesses and conditions. Four developments starting in the 1950s led to a deeper understanding of alcoholism.

◇ First was the discovery of the nucleus accumbens, an area of the brain that gives a surge of pleasure and a desire to repeat the action when stimulated by electricity or by psychoactive drugs (Olds & Milner, 1954; Olds, 1956).

◇ Next was the discovery of endogenous neurotransmitters, starting in the '70s, which showed that drugs worked by influencing existing neurological pathways and receptor sites in the central nervous system including the reward pathway that researcher James Olds and others had hinted at in the '50s and '60s (Goldstein, 1994).

◇ In the 1980s and '90s, genetic research tools developed insights into genetic influences on addiction; in 1990 the first gene that seemed to have an influence on vulnerability to alcoholism was discovered (Noble, Blum, Montgomery, & Sheridan, 1991; Blum, Braverman, Cull, et al., 2000).

◇ In the '90s, imaging techniques visualized the actual reaction of the brain to drugs.

These developments took classification of alcoholism and addiction away from empirical classification to a more measurable and visible basis.

Type I & Type II Alcoholics. Based on an extensive study of Swedish adoptees and their biological or adoptive parents, type I alcoholism (also called "milieu-limited") is defined as a later onset syndrome that can affect both men and women. It requires the presence of a genetic and environmental predisposition; it can be moderate or severe; and takes years of drinking to trigger it (much like Jellenek's delta alcoholic). Type II alcoholism (also called "male-limited") mostly affects sons of male alcoholics, is moderately severe, is primarily genetic, and is only mildly influenced by environmental factors (Cloninger et al., 1996; Bohman, Sigvardson, & Cloniger, 1981).

Type A & Type B Alcoholics. T. F. Babor and his colleagues introduced the A/B typologies in 1992. They are similar to Cloninger's type I/II typologies. Type A, like type I, is a later onset of alcoholism, less family history of alcoholism, and less severe dependence. Type B, like type II, refers to a more severe alcoholism with an earlier onset, more impulsive behavior and conduct problems or disorders, more co-occurring mental disorders, and more severe dependence (Babor, Dolinsky, Meyer, et al., 1992).

The Disease Concept of Alcoholism

Much of the current research in the treatment of alcoholism is based on the disease concept. However, the idea of alcoholism as a disease goes back thousands of years but only recently has the concept become widely accepted. Both the World Health Organization and the American Medical Association view alcoholism as a specific disease entity (O'Brien, 1991). In 1992 a medical panel from the American Society of Addiction Medicine and the National Council on Alcoholism and Drug Dependence defined alcoholism as follows:

> **"Alcoholism is a primary chronic disease with genetic, psychosocial, and environmental factors influencing its development and manifestation. The disease is often progressive and fatal. It is characterized by impaired control over drinking, preoccupation with the drug (alcohol), use of alcohol despite adverse consequences, and distortions in thinking, most notably denial. Each of these symptoms may be continuous or periodic."**

(Morse, Flavin, et al., 1992)

"I don't consider myself an alcoholic. I have five drinks a day—and that's an average. It's always three and sometimes it's a lot more but it's never interfered with my work. I haven't been to the doctor for 15 years. But since it's never interfered with my work, I see nothing wrong with sitting down and having a drink."
Avowed habitual drinker

Heredity, Environment, & Psychoactive Drugs

Instead of focusing on typologies, it is useful to look at addiction and alcoholism as a continuum of severity that depends, to varying degrees, on genetic predisposition, environmental influences due to the family, workplace, school, or community, and from the action of psychoactive drugs themselves, which can alter the body's neurochemistry and instill craving (*see Chapter 2*).

Family studies, twin studies, animal studies, and adoption studies are showing stronger and stronger **genetic influences** particularly in severe alcoholism (Nutt, 1998; Anthenelli & Schuckit, 1998; Knop, Goodwin, Teasdale, et al., 1984; Blum et al., 1996; Li, Lumeng, McBride & Chao, 1986; Goodwin, 1997). A recent twin study that assessed alcohol-related disorders among 3,516 twins in Virginia concluded that the genetic influence was 48% to 58% of the various influences, a rate much higher than postulated in the past (Prescott & Kendler, 1999). It is theorized that several genes have an influence on one's susceptibility to alcoholism and other drug addictions. A person could have one, several, or all of the genes that make a person susceptible to addiction not just a single gene such as the dopamine D_2 allele receptor gene that governs the number of dopamine receptor sites in the reward pathway of the brain that signals euphoria (Blum et al., 2000). Other markers for a strong genetic influence are a tendency to have blackouts, a greater initial tolerance to alcohol, an impaired decision-making area of the brain, a major shift in personality, an impaired ability to learn from mistakes, and retrograde amnesia.

I'm an adult child of an alcoholic. I came from a long history in my family of alcoholism—my father, my mother, all of his brothers. My father died of alcoholism. So I think growing up in that environment was very depressing and so I think I was depressed for a long time and didn't know it.
43-year-old recovering alcoholic

For other people, the **environmental factors** are the overwhelming influences: child abuse, poverty, poor nutrition, alcohol and other drug-abusing friends and relations, and extreme stress.

"When I was younger I was always surrounded by alcohol and drugs. My mom was an alcoholic, my sister used, and so did my two stepbrothers and

stepsister. My stepdad also used to grow [marijuana]. So I was kind of around it a lot."
19-year-old recovering alcoholic

And for some the physiological effects of **alcohol and other drugs** change neurochemistry and are most important.

"After a while it got to the point where I didn't care what it tasted like. You just wanted that buzz to keep going. The brain was craving alcohol. It was the hard liquor and the higher volume of alcohol involved with it, I think. To this day I still like the taste of Jack Daniels and I watch myself real close."
Recovering 32-year-old alcoholic

In the end what is important varies with the point of view of the person involved. To a researcher or scientist, classification and a systematic view of the science of alcoholism is important. To a psychiatrist, counselor, or social worker, the causes and chemistry of addiction are important because they lead to strategies to counteract craving and lack of control. To the problem drinker or alcoholic, any help, knowledge, or methods that will keep them sober and lessen the craving are important. To all involved, understanding the harm that chronic use can cause is important.

LONG-TERM EFFECTS OF ADDICTION (alcoholism)

Most psychoactive drugs affect a single type of receptor or neurotransmitter, i.e., anandamide receptor for marijuana; endorphin receptor for heroin; or norepinephrine, epinephrine, and dopamine neurotransmitters for cocaine. Alcohol on the other hand interacts with receptors, neurotransmitters, cell membranes, intracellular signaling enzymes, and even genes. Therefore the effect of long-term alcohol abuse on neurochemistry and cellular function is wide-ranging and profound (NIAAA/Congress, 1997).

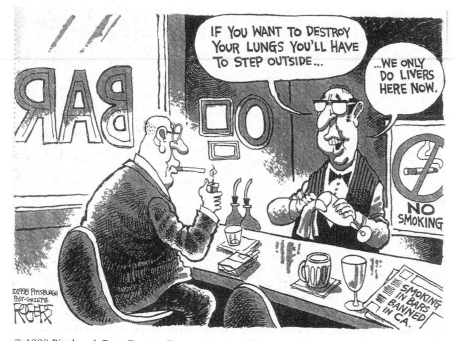

Liver Disease

Since 80% of the alcohol drunk passes through the liver and must be metabolized, high-dose and chronic drinking inevitably affect this crucial organ. In the United States approximately 10% to 35% of heavy drinkers develop alcoholic hepatitis while 10% to 20% develop cirrhosis (NIAAA, 1993).

Alcoholic hepatitis causes inflammation of the liver, areas of fibrosis, necrosis, and damaged membranes. It can take months or years of heavy drinking to develop this condition, which is manifested by jaundice, liver enlargement, tenderness, and pain. It is a serious condition that can only be arrested by abstinence from alcohol but even then the scarring of the liver and collateral damage remains (Moddrey, 1988).

Cirrhosis, the most advanced form of liver disease caused by drinking, is the leading cause of death among alcoholics. Approximately 10,000 to 24,000 Americans die each year from cirrhosis due to alcohol consumption (DeBakey, Stinson, Grant, & Dufour, 1996). When alcohol kills liver cells, the tissues do not regenerate, they scar. The damaging effects of alcohol occur not only because

alcohol itself is toxic but because the metabolic process produces metabolites, such as free radicals and acetaldehyde, that are even more toxic than alcohol itself (Kurose, Higuchi, Kato, Miura, &

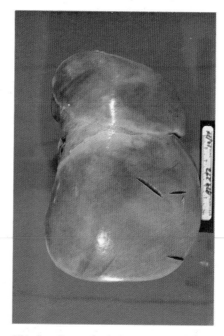

This fatty liver of a drinker is caused by accumulation of fatty acids. When drinking stops, the fat deposits usually disappear.
Courtesy of Boris Ruebner, M.D.

Ishii, 1996). Cirrhosis, like alcoholic hepatitis, is not amenable to treatment although abstinence can often arrest the progression of the disease.

In addition accumulation of fatty acids in the liver, a condition called **"fatty liver,"** can begin to occur after just a few days of heavy drinking. Abstention will eliminate much of the accumulated fat. When the liver becomes damaged due to cirrhosis, fatty liver, or hepatitis, its ability to metabolize alcohol decreases, thus allowing the alcohol to travel to other organs in its original toxic form. Even persistent moderate drinking can then begin to damage the liver.

"I would have taken better care of my body if I knew I would live this long."
Mickey Mantle

Digestive System

While lower doses of alcohol can aid digestion, moderate to higher doses stimulate the production of stomach acid and delay the emptying time of the stomach. Excessive amounts can cause acid stomach, diarrhea, and peptic ulcers.

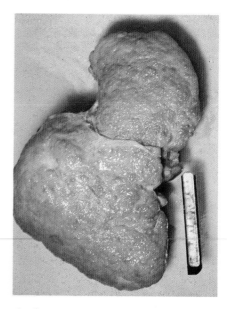

Cirrhosis of the liver takes 10 or more years of steady drinking. The toxic effects of alcohol cause scar tissue to replace healthy tissue. This condition remains permanent, even when drinking stops.
Courtesy of Boris Ruebner, M.D.

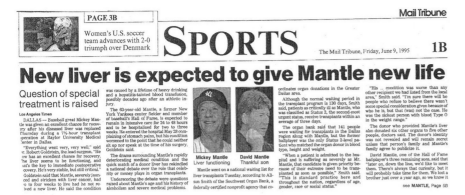

SPORTS

The Mail Tribune, Friday, June 9, 1995   **1B**

New liver is expected to give Mantle new life

Question of special treatment is raised

Los Angeles Times

DALLAS — Baseball great Mickey Mantle was given an excellent chance for recovery after his diseased liver was replaced Thursday during a 7½-hour transplant operation at Baylor University Medical Center in Dallas.

"Everything went very, very well," said Dr. Robert Goldstein, the lead surgeon. "He now has an excellent chance for recovery. The liver seems to be functioning, and that's the key to immediate postoperative recovery. He's very stable, but still critical."

Goldstein said that Mantle, severely jaundiced and stricken with liver cancer, had two to four weeks to live had he not received a new liver. He said the condition

was caused by a lifetime of heavy drinking and a hepatitis-tainted blood transfusion, possibly decades ago after an athletic injury.

The 63-year-old Mantle, a former New York Yankees center fielder and member of baseball's Hall of Fame, is expected to remain in intensive care for 24 to 48 hours and to be hospitalized for two to three weeks. He entered the hospital May 28 complaining of stomach pains, but his condition worsened to the point that he could neither sit up nor speak at the time of his surgery, Goldstein said.

The drama surrounding Mantle's rapidly deteriorating medical condition and the quick match of a donor liver has rekindled a national debate over the role that celebrity or money plays in organ transplants.

Underscoring the debate were questions raised about Mantle's age and his history of alcoholism and severe medical problems.

Mickey Mantle
Liver functioning

David Mantle
Thankful son

Mantle went on a national waiting list for liver transplants Tuesday, according to Allison Smith of the Southwest Organ Bank, a federally certified nonprofit agency that co-

ordinates organ donations in the Greater Dallas area.

Although the normal waiting period in the transplant program is 130 days, Smith said, patients as critically ill as Mantle, who was classified as Status 2, the second-most urgent status, receive transplants within an average of three days.

The organ bank said that 141 people were waiting for transplants in the Dallas region along with Mantle, but the former ballplayer was the only Status 2-level patient who matched the organ donor in blood type, height and weight.

"When a patient is admitted to the hospital and is suffering as severely as Mr. Mantle, that candidate is given priority because of their extreme need to be transplanted as soon as possible," Smith said. "This is standard practice here and throughout the nation, regardless of age, gender, race or social status."

"His ... condition was worse than any other recipient we had listed from the local area," Smith said. "I'm sure there will be people who refuse to believe there wasn't some special consideration given because of who he is, but that (was) not the case. He was the sickest person with blood Type O in the weight range."

The donor who provided Mantle's liver also donated six other organs to five other people, doctors said. The donor's identity was not revealed and will remain secret unless that person's family and Mantle's family agree to publicize it.

David Mantle, one of the Hall of Fame ballplayer's three remaining sons, said that "later on, down the line, we'd like to meet them. There's always that curiosity, but it will probably take time for them. We lost a brother just over a year ago, so we know it

see MANTLE, Page 5B

Mickey Mantle's liver failed because of heavy drinking and cancer. He had a liver transplant but the cancer had spread throughout his body. He died in 1995.

Gastritis (stomach inflammation) is common among heavy drinkers as are inflammation and irritation of the esophagus, pancreas (pancreatitis), and small intestine. Serious disorders including ulcers, stomach hemorrhage, and gastrointestinal bleeding are also linked to heavy drinking (Lieber, 1998). Damage to the liver also causes problems with digestion and proper metabolism.

Alcohol contains calories (about 140 in a 12-oz. beer) but almost no vitamins, minerals, or proteins. Heavy drinkers receive energy but little nutritional value from their drinking. As a result alcoholics may suffer from primary malnutrition, including vitamin B$_1$ deficiency leading to beriberi, heart disease, peripheral nerve degeneration, pellagra, scurvy, and anemia (caused by iron deficiency). In addition because heavy drinking irritates and inflames the stomach and intestines, alcoholics may suffer from secondary malnutrition (especially from distilled alcohol drinks) as a result of faulty digestion and absorption of nutrients, even if they eat a well-balanced diet.

Cardiovascular Disease

Though light drinking is associated with lowered risk of heart disease and stroke, chronic heavy drinking is related to a variety of heart diseases including hypertension (high blood pressure) and cardiac arrhythmias (abnormal irregular heart rhythms) (Klatsky, 1988). Heavy drinking increases

the risk of hypertension by a factor of two or three. Cardiomyopathy, an enlarged, flabby, and inefficient heart, is found in heavy chronic drinkers since acetylaldehyde damages heart muscles. One form of irregular heart rhythm is called "holiday heart syndrome" because it appears in patients from Sundays through Tuesdays or around holidays after a large amount of alcohol has been consumed. Heavy drinking in-

creases the risk of stroke and other intracranial bleeding within 24 hours of a drinking binge (Geller, 1997). The exact mechanism for many of the cardiovascular problems is not definitely known but the connection is clear.

Nervous System

Alcohol limits the brain's ability to use glucose and oxygen, thus killing brain cells as well as inhibiting message transmission. Low to moderate use does not seem to cause permanent functional loss whereas chronic high-dose use causes direct damage to nerve cells. Malnutrition can also injure brain cells and disrupt brain chemistry.

Both physical brain damage and impaired mental abilities have been linked to advanced alcoholism. Brain atrophy (loss of brain tissue) has been documented in 50% to 100% of alcoholics (Parsons, 1977). Breathing and heart-rate irregularities caused by damage to the brain's autonomic nervous system have also been traced to brain atrophy. **Dementia** (deterioration of intellectual ability, faulty memory, dis-

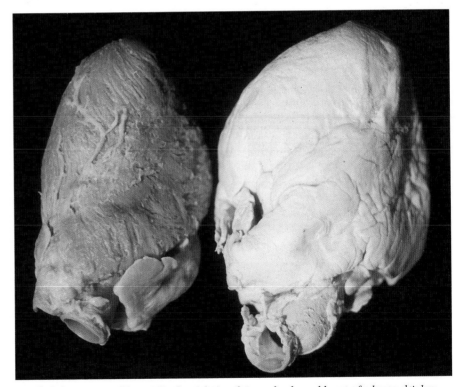

On the left is a normal heart. On the right is a fatty and enlarged heart of a heavy drinker.
Courtesy of Leslie Parr

orientation, and diminished problem-solving ability) is a further consequence of prolonged heavy drinking.

One of the more serious diseases due to brain damage caused by chronic alcoholism and thiamine (vitamin B_1) deficiency is Wernicke's encephalopathy whose symptoms include delirium, visual problems, imbalance, and muscle tremors. The other serious condition that involves thiamine deficiency is Korsakoff's syndrome; its symptoms include disorientation, memory failure, and repetition of false memories (Goodwin, 1997).

Hippocrates wrote about the association between alcohol and seizures/epilepsy more than 2,000 years ago. The prevalence of epilepsy is up to 10 times greater in those with alcoholism (Devantag, Mandich, Zaiotti, & Toffolo, 1983). While the seizures could be caused by head trauma due to drunkenness or other causes, the direct damage to neurological systems as well as the neurological storm caused by withdrawal are strongly implicated.

Reproductive System

Female. While light drinking lowers inhibitions, prolonged use decreases desire and the intensity of orgasm. In one study of chronic female alcoholics, 36% said they had orgasms less than 5% of the time. Chronic alcohol abuse can inhibit ovulation, decrease the gonadal mass, delay menstruation, and cause sexual dysfunction (Blume, 1997). Heavy drinking also raises the chances of infertility and spontaneous abortion.

Male. Again, low to moderate levels of alcohol can lower inhibitions and enhance the psychological aspects of sexual activity but the depressant effects soon take over. Chronic use causes effects beyond a temporary inability to perform. Long-term alcohol abuse impairs gonadal functions and causes a decrease in testosterone (male hormone) levels. Decreased testosterone causes an increase in estrogen (a female hormone) that can lead to male breast enlargement, testicular atrophy, low sperm count, loss of body hair, and

loss of sexual desire. About 8% of alcoholics are impotent and only half can recover sexual function during sobriety. When returning to sexual activity, a recovering alcoholic may experience excessive anxiety; dysfunction can be intensified by one or two bad performances. Also alcohol may lead to increased risk-taking behavior, especially unprotected sex that leads to an increased potential for HIV and other sexually transmitted diseases.

Cancer

Breast Cancer. Although the association between drinking and breast cancer is clear, there is contradictory evidence concerning the association between drinking small amounts of alcohol and the incidence of breast cancer (*see discussion earlier in this chapter under low- to moderate-dose episodes*). A study of 1,200 women with breast cancer showed an association between moderate alcohol use and breast cancer—even amounts as low as one drink a day increased the risk by 50%. In fact 25% of all breast cancer is associated with even brief use of alcohol (Bowlin, 1997). However, another study said that moderate to heavy drinking was more likely to cause breast cancer (Ellison, 1999).

Other Cancers. The risk of mouth, throat, and esophageal cancer are 6 times greater for heavy alcohol users, 7 times greater for smokers, and an astonishing 38 times greater for those who smoke and drink alcohol (Blot, 1992).

Other Systemic Problems

Musculoskeletal System. Alcohol leeches minerals from the body causing a 5- to 10-fold greater risk of a fracture of the femur, the wrist, vertebrae, and the ribs. The unbalancing of electrolytes by chronic or acute use, along with direct toxic effects, can cause myopathy (painful swollen muscles).

Dermatologic Complications. The reddish complexion of chronic al-

coholics is caused by rosacea, psoriasis, eczema, and facial edema, all of which are potentiated by the toxic effects of alcohol. Skin problems also arise from nutritional deficiencies.

Immune System. Excessive drinking has been linked to infectious diseases such as respiratory infections, tuberculosis, pneumonia, and cancer. Heavy drinking may disrupt white blood cells and in other ways weaken the immune system, resulting in greater susceptibility to infections.

Other Susceptibilities. Alcohol can cause a host of other problems.

◇ Alcohol may be a contributing cause for diabetes.

◇ Chronic drinking can cause atrophied muscle fibers, resulting in flabby muscles.

◇ It can also cause weight loss, more so for alcoholic women than alcoholic men, due to damage to the digestive system.

POLYDRUG ABUSE

Most illicit drug users drink alcohol. The reasons vary.

◇ Stacking: Alcohol taken before using cocaine will prolong and intensify the "coke's" effects by creating the metabolite cocaethylene, which also seems to trigger greater violence.

◇ Morphing: Drinking alcohol to come down off a three-day speed run.

◇ Multiple drug use: Taking speed to wake up, drinking at noon to relax, smoking a joint in the afternoon, and then taking alcohol to get to sleep.

◇ Replacement: Drinking alcohol to get loaded if the desired shot of heroin or sedative-hypnotic capsule is unavailable.

◇ Mixing: Drinking alcohol and shooting cocaine to get a "speedball" effect.

◇ Sequentialing: Switching from alcohol to another addiction when the effects of the alcohol have become too damaging; most addicts have sequenced through several addictions.

◇ Cycling: Binge drink for a week, and then only smoke marijuana for a week, and then back to the alcohol.

"I used downers just to come down off the alcohol because I was so shaky. And then I would try using amphetamines just to lift me up so I wouldn't drink so much. But what I would do was stay awake longer and drink more, so that didn't work."
43-year-old recovering polydrug abuser

Polydrug abuse has become so common that treatment centers have had to learn how to treat simultaneous addictions. Although the emotional roots of addiction are similar no matter what drug is used, the physiological and psychological changes that each drug causes, particularly during withdrawal, often have to be treated differently. For example, if a client of the Haight-Ashbury Detox Clinic has a serious alcohol and benzodiazepine problem, the Clinic has to be extremely careful detoxifying the client. That is because Librium®, a benzodiazepine sedative-hypnotic, is one of the drugs used to control the symptoms of delirium tremens caused by alcohol withdrawal.

There is a strong association between smoking and drinking. Approximately 70% of alcoholics are heavy smokers (more than one pack a day) compared to 10% of the general population. The converse is not as dramatic: smokers are only 1.3 times as likely as the general population to drink alcohol compared to nonsmokers. There is also a strong link between early use of tobacco and alcohol. Adolescents who smoke are three times more likely to begin using alcohol while smokers are 10 times more likely to become alcoholics than are nonsmokers (Shiffman & Balabanis, 1995).

OTHER PROBLEMS

SELF-MEDICATION & MENTAL PROBLEMS

Often alcohol is drunk because the person has an existing mental problem such as major depression, schizophrenia, bipolar illness (manic-depression), or panic disorder. The person uses alcohol to try to control the symptoms or to avoid asking for psychiatric help.

"I would pick up some beer to put me out of it. I didn't like the effect that regular psychiatric drugs, such as antidepressants, had on my brain and I'd rather just put myself out with the booze."
Patient with major depression and an alcohol problem

Sometimes alcohol is used for other reasons—to overcome boredom or control restlessness. Unfortunately what happens is that the attempt to self-medicate by drinking can take on a life of its own and create a new set of problems or aggravate an existing one. For example, a person may use alcohol to escape depression although chronic alcohol abuse may actually contribute to depression (Miller, Klamen, Hoffman, & Flaherty, 1995). A study of adults with panic disorder showed that the subjects reported significantly less anxiety and fewer panic attacks when drinking. The use of alcohol to control the symptoms resulted in a higher rate of alcohol use disorders among those with panic disorder (Kushner, Mackenzie, Fiszdon, et al., 1996).

"The problems did get worse when I was drinking. That was one reason that I never figured out I was a manic-depressive. I figured I was depressed because I was drunk all the time."
Alcoholic with manic-depression

Alcoholics are

◇ 21 times more likely to have an antisocial personality disorder,

◇ 3.9 times more likely to have a drug abuse disorder,

◇ 6.2 times more likely to have manic depressive disorder,

◇ 4 times more likely to have schizophrenia.

(Helzer & Pryzbeck, 1988)

The majority of alcoholics who come into treatment are initially diagnosed as suffering from depression. In addition about 1/3 of alcoholics suffer an anxiety disorder.

"The alcohol, that came later on. It intensified my depression and intensified everything. I already felt bad about

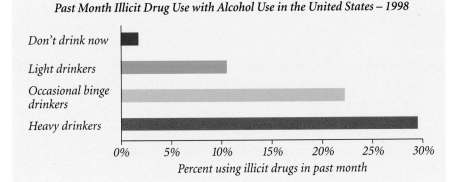

Past Month Illicit Drug Use with Alcohol Use in the United States – 1998

Figure 5-6 •
This chart shows that excessive drinking is associated with the use of other illicit drugs. Whether it's the association with other people who drink and use drugs, the lowering of inhibitions that makes other drug use acceptable, or the desire for stronger and stronger experiences, the association is quite clear.

TABLE 5–4   SOME ALCOHOL-RELATED CAUSES OF DEATH

Diseases (directly caused by alcohol)	Diseases (indirectly caused by alcohol)	Injuries/adverse effects (indirectly caused by alcohol)
Alcoholic psychoses	Tuberculosis	Boating accidents
Alcoholism	Cancer of the lips, mouth, and pharynx	Motor vehicle, bicycle, other road accidents
Alcohol abuse	Cancer of the larynx, esophagus, stomach, and liver	Airplane accidents
Nerve degeneration		Falls
Heart disease	Diabetes	Fire accidents
Alcoholic gastritis	Hypertension	Drownings
Fatty liver	Stroke	Suicides, self-inflicted injuries
Hepatitis	Pancreatitis	Homicides or shootings
Cirrhosis	Diseases of stomach, esophagus, and duodenum	Choking on food
Other liver damage	Cirrhosis of bile tract	Domestic violence
Excessive BAC		Rapes or date rapes
Accidental poisonings		
Seizure activity		

(Adapted from U.S. Department of Health and Human Services, Alcohol & Health, 1997)

myself and the alcohol just made it worse. It definitely made it worse."
Recovering 16-year-old alcoholic with major depression

Researchers from the Scripps Institute found that heavy drinking strips the brain of its natural chemical reactions that trigger feelings of well-being in the mesolimbic/dopinergic reward pathway (opioid peptides, dopamine, serotonin, and GABA) while raising the levels of chemicals that cause tension and depression, including norepinephrine, epinephrine, and serotonin (Koob, 1999). The brain tries to compensate for the depletion of neurotransmitters by releasing corticotropin-releasing factor, a stress chemical that, unfortunately, can induce depression. The depression can last for as long as a month after abstinence begins. This combination of decreased action of reward chemicals and excess stress chemical increases craving for alcohol.

MORTALITY

Drinking can affect a person's life span since heavy drinking increases the chances of dying from disease or trauma. For instance, the average life span is shortened 4 years by cancer, 4 years by heart disease, and from 9–22 years for alcoholic liver disease. In one study a difference in life span was found even between abstainers (defined as 12 drinks or less per year) and light drinkers (1–2 drinks per day) (Vaillant, 1995; U.S. Department of Health & Human Services, 1997).

FETAL ALCOHOL SYNDROME (FAS) & FETAL ALCOHOL EFFECTS (FAE)

Maternal Drinking

A survey of pregnant women in the United States found that 18.8% drank alcohol during pregnancy while 5.5% used illicit drugs at least once (NIDA, 1996). Alcohol use during pregnancy is the leading cause of mental retardation in the United States (Abel & Sokol, 1986; Cook et al., 1991). Alcohol overuse during pregnancy also increases the number of miscarriages and infant deaths; there are more problem pregnancies; and newborns are smaller and weaker. Certain specific toxic effects of alcohol on the developing fetus are known as "fetal alcohol syndrome" or FAS, a term first coined in 1973 (Jones & Smith, 1973). At first it was thought that the defects were the result of malnutrition but the toxicity of alcohol was recognized as the cause. Criteria for standardizing the diagnosis of FAS were standardized in 1980. The defects can range widely from obvious gross physical defects to behavioral problems. Not all women who drink heavily during pregnancy bear children with FAS. There is as yet no definitive test for confirming FAS at birth and only the most severe cases are diagnosable at birth. The minimal standards for a diagnosis of FAS are

◊ retarded growth before and after birth, including height, weight, head circumference, brain growth, and brain size;

◊ central nervous system involvement such as delayed intellectual development, neurological abnormalities, behavioral problems, visual problems, hearing loss, and balance or gait problems;

◊ facial deformities including shortened eye openings, thin upper lip, flattened midface, groove in the upper lip, and occasional problems with heart and limbs.

(Sokol & Clarren, 1989)

In addition children with FAS are liable for increased risks of other common birth defects including heart disease, cleft lip and palate, and spina bifida. A weak and irregular sucking response, jitteriness, trembling, and sleep disturbances have been reported in babies exposed to large doses of alcohol. If only a few of these FAS attributes are present, the diagnosis could be fetal alcohol effect (FAE) or alcohol-related birth defects (ARBD) (NIAAA, 1997).

Worldwide studies estimate that FAS births occur anywhere from 0.33 to 2.9 cases per 1,000 live births. In the United States, African Americans have about 6 FAS births per 1,000; Asians, Hispanics, and Whites, about 1 to 2; and Native Americans about 30, although rates from 10–120 births per 1,000 have been reported in various specific Native American and Canadian Indian communities. FAE rates are 1.7 to 3.6 while ARBD rates range from 3.4 to 6.0 (May, 1996; Hans, 1998).

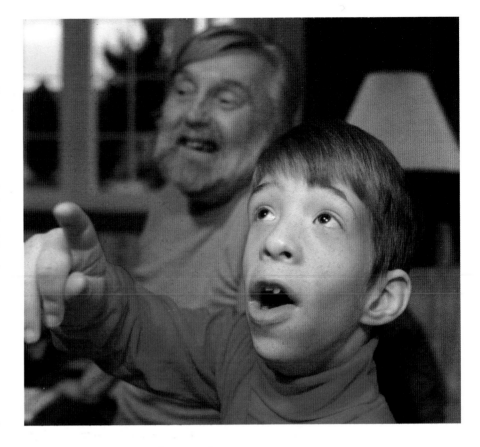

The physical abnormalities in a child with FAS are readily apparent.
© David H. Wells/CORBIS. Reprinted, by permission.

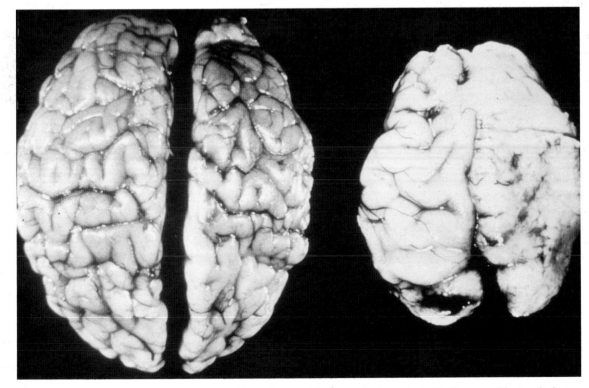

The greatest danger of alcohol use by a pregnant woman is brain damage. The larger brain on the left is the normal brain of a human newborn (that died in an accident). The smaller brain on the right is of a child born with FAS or fetal alcohol syndrome. The FAS brain is obviously small and malformed. Often the damage is more subtle and learning deficits don't show up until the children are six or seven years old.
Courtesy of Sterling K. Clarren, M.D., Children's Hospital, Seattle

Critical Period. Because the brain is among the first organs to develop and the last to finish, it appears to be vulnerable throughout pregnancy, however weeks three through eight, at the onset of embryogenesis (formation of the embryo), are crucial. For example, the corpus callosum, a crucial structure that connects the cerebral hemispheres, is extremely vulnerable to alcohol use during the sixth to eighth gestational weeks; damage to the basal ganglia affects fine motor coordination and cognitive ability (Rosenberg, 1996). The greatest behavioral damage results from early heavy fetal exposure to alcohol.

Critical Dose. Animal models suggest that peak blood alcohol concentration rather than the total amount of alcohol drunk determines the critical level above which adverse effects are seen. A pattern of rapid drinking and the resulting high BAC seem to be the most dangerous style of drinking.

How many drinks are safe during pregnancy? One study concludes that seven standard drinks per week by pregnant mothers are a threshold level below which most neurobehavioral effects are not seen. This might lead some health care professionals to feel that they need not recommend total abstinence. However seven drinks per week are an average and if a pregnant woman consumes a large number of those drinks at one sitting, the fetus may be much more at risk. Also some neurobehavioral tests are so sensitive that effects on the fetus can be found even with extremely low levels of exposure to alcohol. Further it is important to remember that even one drink per day has been associated with the development of breast cancer in women.

A new animal study showed that even one high-dose use episode of alcohol in rats, when the developing brain is creating neurons and neuronal connections at a furious pace, will also kill brain cells at a furious pace. In the experiment they showed that normally 1.5% of brain cells die during a certain period in a rat's growth but in rats exposed to alcohol during that critical period, 5% to 30% of neurons will die. When extrapolating these results to humans, the blood alcohol concentration would be .20, about twice the legal allowable limit for drivers and the crucial period would be six months into the pregnancy until two years after birth. During the brain growth spurt, a single prolonged contact with alcohol lasting for four hours or more is enough to kill vast numbers of brain cells (Ikonomidou, Bitigau, Ishimaru, et al., 2000).

One approach suggests that one standard drink every 10 days might be safe but there is still the potential for unobservable damage that could impair a child when stressed or when the child reaches adulthood and old age. The U.S. Surgeon General advises that pregnant women should not drink at all while pregnant since there is no way to determine which babies might be at risk from even very low levels of alcohol exposure. Current research simply does not permit us to know at what quantity alcohol begins to damage the fetus (Ernhart, Sokol, Martier, et al., 1987; NIAAA, 1997; Hans, 1998).

Paternal Drinking

As we have seen in Chapter 2, genetic transmission of alcoholism by fathers is strongly suspected. There is now growing evidence that the detrimental effects of alcohol on the fetus may also be transmitted by paternal alcohol consumption. Researchers are unable to say definitively whether paternal exposure to alcohol results in FAS or in some other syndrome. In laboratory tests, alcoholic-sired rats of nonalcohol-using mothers produced male offspring with disturbed hormonal functions and spatial learning impairments. Adolescent male rats subjected to high alcohol intake produced both male and female offspring suffering from abnormal development.

Observations of alcoholic-sired human males indicate no gross physical deficits but do show an association with intellectual and functional deficits in offspring. In addition to the deficits in verbal, thinking, and planning skills of children of alcoholics (COAs), sons of male alcoholics (SOMAs) exhibit further deficiencies in visual/spatial skills, motor skills, memory, and learning (NIAAA, 1997).

Preliminary explanations of the causes of these abnormalities suggest that alcohol may mutate genes in sperm, kill off certain kinds of sperm, or biochemically and nutritionally alter semen and influence sperm.

ADVERSE SOCIAL CONSEQUENCES

Aggression & Violence

"On a typical Friday night, at least 50% of our calls will be some kind of alcohol and drug violent behavior situation whether it be a shooting, stabbing, or a beating. A lot of those involve significant others, a spouse, or cohabitants."

Emergency medical technician, San Francisco, 1997

In the past 15 years almost every major league baseball park and professional football stadium has stopped selling beer in the spectator seats. Alcohol and beer must now be purchased only at the concession stands where a customer is limited to two drinks at a time and no sales are allowed after the seventh inning or third quarter. These changes have sharply reduced rowdiness, violence, and fights. In England and other countries where such a ban is rare, fan violence, especially at soccer matches, is still a major problem.

Alcohol itself usually does not cause a person to be violent but it can magnify existing traits and susceptibility and contribute to or trigger interpersonal and criminal violence.

"The use of alcohol would really bring out the hit man in me. I mean, I could talk to my partner or whoever fairly good if I was sober but after I started drinking, the deep emotions really would come out."

28-year-old male in domestic violence prevention class

Based on victim reports, 15% of robberies, 27% of aggravated assaults, 50% of all homicides, and 37% of rapes and sexual assaults involved alcohol use (U.S. Department of Justice, 1998; Roizen, 1997). About 1/3 of the 5.3 million convicted offenders under the jurisdiction of corrections agencies in 1996 were drinking at the time of their offense.

There are some relatively fixed and unalterable pharmacological causal connections between alcohol and violence. Alcohol has been shown to increase aggression by interfering with GABA, the main inhibitory neurotransmitter, in ways that may encourage intoxicated people with preexisting aggressive tendencies to become aggressive. Also, in some people alcohol can increase dopamine, which stimulates aggression. Alcohol also decreases the action of serotonin that may cause drinkers to use aggression to gain pleasure and avoid punishment and to

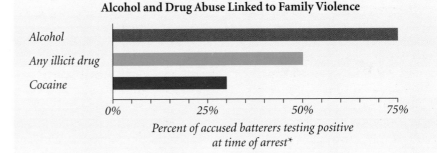

Alcohol and Drug Abuse Linked to Family Violence

Percent of accused batterers testing positive at time of arrest*

*Figures do not add to 100% since many abuse more than one substance.

Figure 5-7 •

Three out of four of those arrested for family violence tested positive for alcohol. Half had used some illicit drug and more than one in four tested positive for cocaine.
The National Research Council, 1993

be less able to stop drinking once it has started (Gustafson, 1994).

There are also some variable causes of alcohol-related violence that are complex and involve personality, occasion (setting), social and cultural factors, and economic conditions.

Experiments have shown that the expectation that alcohol will make one braver leads people to be more aggressive even if they are drinking a nonalcoholic beverage that they believe contains alcohol (Bushman, 1997). Also, along with increases in the divorce rate,

Drink began day that ended in murder

By MARK FREEMAN
of the Mail Tribune

Ruben Landeros awoke at 10:30 a.m. Saturday and, as was his custom, poured a smidgeon of orange juice into a glass that he then filled with whiskey from a half-gallon plastic bottle.
The whiskey and orange juice...

more money than him. How she was leaving him for good.

Ten hours and a half-bottle of whiskey later, Ruben Landeros ended his marital dilemmas, but this time with the family pistol, family members say.

He shot Bobbi Jo dead inside her North...

"She (Bobbi Jo) loved Ruben with all her heart," said Brenda Landeros, Ruben's sister-in-law and the dead woman's cousin, as she poured the last swig of whiskey from Ruben's bottle onto the ground Monday outside their Tripp Street apartment.
"The bottle took the best...

Office.

Prosecutors on Monday planned to issue formal arrest warrants for Ruben on charges of murder and attempted murder, and on Jose, 32, for hindering prosecution, said Doug McGeary, an assistant district attorney... Jackson County.

...pair won't be charged until prosecutesent the case to a Jackson County... McGeary said. No grand jury

Alcohol Linked to 40 Percent of Violent Crimes

Associated Press Writer

Washington
Although declining as a cause of death, alcohol remains a factor in nearly 40 percent of violent crimes, the Justice Department reported yesterday.
Alcohol is an even bigger factor in violence by a...

Of the 5.3 million convicted adult offenders in prison, jail or on parole or probation in 1996, 36 percent reported they had been drinking at the time of the offense for which they were convicted, the report estimated.

The report also said... ictims of ...inancial ...age out-...

...inancial ...iolence, million,

since 1990. In the past decade, highway fatalities blamed on alcohol sank from 24,000 in 1986 to 17,126 in 1996.

Nevertheless, local police made 1,467 arrests nationwide in 1996, for driving under the influence of alcohol. That was down from the peak of 1.9 million arrests in 1983... 33 states permitted alcohol consumption before age 21. Since then, responding to federal highway funding requirements, every... has gone to a minimum drinking age...

The most common state laws define ...ication as 0.10 grams of alcohol per...

Student Barflies Take to Streets In Daylight-Saving Time Protest

Associated Press

Athens, Ohio
For the second year in a row, a rowdy crowd confronted police in this college town yesterday as bars closed early for the switch to daylight-saving time.
An estimated 2,000 people gathered outside downtown bars that cater to Ohio University students before the bars started closing at 2 a.m., half an hour earlier than usual because of the time change, authorities said.

No civilian Sheriff Dave... dispersed the...

Five offic... juries, and a... arrested, aut... rests were p... photograph... lice said.

One yea... change sen... to the stre... were arres... Those...

Teenage Beer Party Leads to Rape Arrests

By Sandy Kleffman
Chronicle Correspondent

Two Union City teenagers were in custody yesterday for allegedly raping a 15-year-old girl during an afternoon gathering at one boy's apartment.
Police arrested the boys, ages 16 and 14, on Thursday and took them to Alameda County Juvenile Hall in San Leandro.
The girl told police the rape oc-

on the bed she was undressed and raped by at least two of the boys who were present," Packard said.
The girl told police she drifted in and out of consciousness during the attack.
Later, the boys helped her get dressed and leave the apartment. She then went to a friend's house and called police at 10:45 p.m.

Domestic Abuse Linked To Alcohol, Job Stability

Male ethnicity is not a factor, study says

LOS ANGELES TIMES

Men's alcohol abuse and shaky ...nployment status rank among the ...ost important precipitating factors ...domestic violence against wom... ...while ethnicity plays virtually no ...e at all, according to one of the ...st comprehensive studies to date ...ssailants and their victims.

Fewer Drunk Drivers — Tough Sentences

More than 500,000 in jail or on probation

ASSOCIATED PRESS

WASHINGTON — Reflecting tougher punishm mix drinking and half a million probation or beh under the influe twice the level o

drunken driving problem."

Forty-six percent of DUI offenders on probation were in alcohol treatment programs in 1997, according to the bureau study.

Support for Schiavone's view that the half million drivers now under correctional supervision are "hardcore" includes:

— About half of DUI offenders in local jails reported consuming the

Study shows it takes time to catch drunken drivers

Los Angeles Times

A study of hard-core drunk drivers — repeat offenders whose blood-alcohol level is twice that allowed by law — has found that such people may drive under the influence more than 1,000 times before they are caught.

John C. Lawn, chairman of the Los Angeles-based Century Council, an anti-drunk driving gro

ing advocates. They said they applaud any indictment of repeat DUI offenders. But, they added, they worry that the distillery-funded study suggests that casual drinkers are a lesser threat.

"If a person at an office party drinks one too many and gets out there and drives, their very same behavior can be structive as d big-time Post, execu os Angeles inst Drunk

THURSDAY, AUGUST 25, 1994   **NATION**

Reckless Drivers Often High, Not Drunk, Study Finds

Chronicle Wire Services

Boston

More than half of all reckless drivers are high on cocaine or marijuana if they are not intoxicated on alcohol, a study has found.

"Our findings strongly suggest that (driving under the influence of drugs) is more common than previous arrest statistics would indicate," the team, led by Dr. Daniel Brookoff of Methodist Hospital in Memphis, Tenn., said in its report.

Police in Memphis gave urine tests to reckless drivers who did not appear drunk. They found that

same as that used by the federal government to measure recent drug use in the workplace.

Although a positive result often means that people have taken drugs in recent hours, those who regularly use very high amounts of cocaine or marijuana may flunk the tests even though they have been off drugs for days.

The results of the police experiment were written for today's issue of the New England Journal of Medicine by Brookoff.

Brookoff said he decided to get

involved in the issue of drugged driving after a man hit his friend's two daughters while driving on the wrong side of the road. The man was never tested for drugs, but Brookoff believes he was high on marijuana.

"The reality is, we think it's as big a problem, or maybe bigger, as drunk driving," Brookoff said.

Difficult to Diagnose

Police can often tell when drivers are drunk even before they give the breath test. But drugged driving is much harder to detect,

because there is no clear pattern of appearance. For instance, drivers on cocaine may act sleepy and slow, happy and talkative or combative and paranoid.

When asked to take the standard curbside sobriety test, which involves measuring coordination and attention, cocaine drivers can actually perform better than sober drivers.

"We saw people who did great on the sobriety test," said Brookoff. "The problem was, they were driving 90 miles an hour on the wrong side of the road with their

lights off."

He said drivers on cocaine were often glad to take the drug test, certain they would pass. They show poor judgment on the road, too. Typically they are wildly overconfident of their abilities, taking turns too fast or weaving through traffic.

"Diagonal driving," Cook calls this. "They are just as involved in changing lanes as in going forward."

The effects of cocaine can last for days. Those withdrawing from

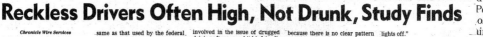

more women are victims of alcohol-influenced homicides.

Because alcohol reduces inhibitions, it can encourage someone with a tendency toward violence to release pent-up anger, hatred, and desires forbidden by society, and to act on them. Besides the homicides and rapes that occur each year due to alcohol, over seven million other crimes are committed under the influence. Alcohol can also undermine moral judgment and increase aggression. When a person drinks, the common sense that would keep a person out of trouble is often suppressed (Collins & Messerschmidt, 1993).

"Seems like alcohol is always referred to as this liquid courage, you know. And I guess it depends where you're at—courage to do what? Courage to ask a girl on a date that you hadn't had the courage to do before, or courage to dance like a fool on the floor, or is it courage to beat your wife or to beat your girlfriend cause you didn't have the guts to do it before?"

College counselor

Another mechanism that connects alcohol and violence is that alcohol can cause a drinker to misjudge social cues causing a person to perceive a threat where none exists. What occurs is that alcohol disrupts the judgment and reasoning center of the brain (Miczek, 1997). In some men alcohol can release their aggressive tendencies and they become violent when they drink but the violence was sitting in them and residing in their psyche way before they picked up that first drink.

"He beat me only when he was drunk. To me it was just an excuse, it was just an excuse of being drunk and doing it. So for me drinking and being violent is just an excuse. It is a coward that is doing it the way I'm seeing it."

43-year-old ex-wife of an alcoholic abuser

Serious & Fatal Injuries

Medical examiner reports indicate that alcohol increases the risk of injury.

◇ Emergency room studies confirm that from 15% to 25% of emergency room patients tested positive for al-

cohol or reported alcohol use, with relatively high rates among those involved in fights, assaults, and falls.

◇ Alcoholics are 16 times more likely than others to die in falls and 10 times more likely to become burn or fire victims.

◇ The Coast Guard reported that 31% of boating fatalities had a BAC of .10 or more.

◇ At work up to 40% of industrial fatalities and 47% of injuries involved alcohol.

(Bernstein & Mahoney, 1989; NCADI, 1999)

Motor Vehicle Accidents

"Drunken driver Henri Paul caused the 1997 car crash that killed Princess Diana, French judges ruled Friday in a report clearing photographers and her companion Dodi al Fayed of blame for the fatal accident. The 32-page ruling on the high-speed crash said Paul was inebriated and was taking antidepressants and consequently lost control of the limousine."

Reuters News Service, September 04, 1999

Whether it is the death of the Princess Diana or the death of 27 children in a school bus, drunk driving affects more than just the driver. According to the U. S. National Highway Traffic Safety Administration (NHTSA), more than one in four drivers get behind the wheel within two hours of drinking. This leads to relatively high rates of alcohol use for drivers involved in motor vehicle collisions.

◊ In one study more than 38% of motor vehicle fatalities in 1997 involved alcohol use.

◊ Alcoholics are five times more likely to die in motor vehicle crashes.

◊ Projections are that 3 out of every 10 persons in the United States will in some way be involved in an alcohol-related crash during their lifetime.

◊ On any weekend night 3 out of every 100 drivers exceed the legal BAC limit.

◊ Of those convicted of DWI, 61% drank beer only, 2% drank wine only, 18% drank liquor only, and 20% drank more than one type of alcoholic beverage.

◊ About 40% of first-time DUI offenders and 60% of multiple DUI offenders reported consuming five or more drinks compared with 10% of the adult male population.

◊ Approximately 1 in 7 intoxicated drivers who were involved in a fatal collision had a prior DWI (driving while intoxicated) conviction whereas only 1 in 34 sober drivers involved in a fatal collision had a prior DWI conviction.

(NHTSA, 1999, 1998, 1997, 1995; NIAAA, 1997)

Suicide

Among adult alcoholics, suicide rates are twice as high as for the general population and from 60–120 times greater than the nonmentally ill population—rates increase with age. One reason given for the increase in suicide with age is that the longer the alcoholism, the more social, health, and interpersonal problems there are. The alcoholic suicide victim is typically white, middle-aged, male, and unmarried with a long history of drinking. Additional risk factors for suicide include depression, loss of job, living alone, poor social support, other illnesses, and continual drinking.

EPIDEMIOLOGY

PATTERNS OF ALCOHOL CONSUMPTION

Global Consumption

It is difficult to get accurate, comparable, and consistent alcohol use data in other countries but as Table 5-5 points out, most European countries have higher per capita alcohol consumption rates than the United States while most Asian countries have lower per capita consumption. These differences result from a combination of physiological, cultural, social, religious, and legal factors.

Culture is one of the determinants of how a person drinks. Different drinking patterns are found in the so-called wet and dry drinking cultures in Europe. A wet drinking culture (e.g., Austria, Belgium, France, Italy, and Switzerland) sanction daily or almost daily use and integrate social drinking into everyday life. For example, in France children are served watered-down wine at the dinner table (Vaillant, 1995). France also has Europe's second highest per capita consumption of alcohol and second highest death rate from cirrhosis of the liver than any other European nation.

Dry drinking cultures (e.g., Denmark, Finland, Norway, and Sweden) restrict the availability of alcohol and tax it more heavily. Wet cultures consume more wine and beer, 5 times the amount of wine drunk in dry cultures. Dry cultures consume more distilled spirits, almost 1.5 times the amount in wet cultures, and are characterized by binge-style drinking, particularly by males on weekends (Eurocare, 1999). Countries like Canada, England, Ireland, the United States, Wales, and Germany exhibit combinations of wet and dry or mixed drinking cultures

TABLE 5–5 WORLDWIDE PER CAPITA USE OF ALCOHOL VS. INCIDENCE OF CHRONIC LIVER DISEASE

	Alcohol in Liters of Pure Ethanol	Cirrhosis Rate/100,000
Russian Federation	14.0 liters/person/year (1992)	15
France	12.6 liters/person/year (1996)	18
Germany	11.8 liters/person/year (1996)	23
Ireland	11.2 liters/person/year (1994)	2
Spain	9.3 liters/person/year (1996)	20
Greece	8.7 liters/person/year (1996)	8
Italy	8.1 liters/person/year (1996)	21
United States	8.1 liters/person/year (1995)	10
United Kingdom	7.6 liters/person/year (1996)	9
Japan	6.8 liters/person/year (1996)	—
Canada	6.4 liters/person/year (1996)	—
Poland	6.2 liters/person/year (1996)	12
Mexico	3.4 liters/person/year (1996)	—
Israel	2.0 liters/person/year (1996)	10
Algeria	0.4 liters/person/year (1996)	—

(Harkin, 1995; Eurocare, 1999)

where patterns such as binge drinking in social situations are common. A relatively higher incidence of violence against women is found in mixed drinking cultures than in dry or wet cultures, probably because binge drinking often occurs in social situations.

Chinese families generally don't drink much because of cultural pressures. However in Japan and South Korea, social pressures to drink are very powerful. In Japan most of the men and half the women drink, yet their alcoholism rate is half of that in the United States.

In Russia vodka is traditionally drunk between meals in large quantities. Alcoholism had become so rampant in Russia that in 1985, Premier Mikhail Gorbachev severely restricted the availability of alcohol, almost to the point of prohibition. Illegal stills and the consumption of anything with alcohol in it, such as shoe polish and insecticides, soared (Segal, 1990; Davis, 1994). Many of those restrictions have since been lifted. Currently 9% of Russian men and 35% of Russian women abstain from alcohol while 10% of the men and 2% of the women drink several times a week (Bobak, 1999).

In England a trip to the pub for warm beer and darts is a tradition, so 70% of Britons drink regularly. In a recent campaign to stem alcoholism, Britons were urged to reduce their average daily consumption to three drinks a day.

In the United States, a land of many different cultures and lifestyles and a mixed drinking culture, a variety of culturally influenced drinking customs are present. However, much drinking is done away from the lunch and dinner table.

POPULATION SUBGROUPS

Men

In all age groups men drink more per drinking episode than women do, regardless of country. Much of this difference has to do with the cultural acceptability of male drinking and the disapproval of female drinking in almost every country. The other reason

United States Consumption

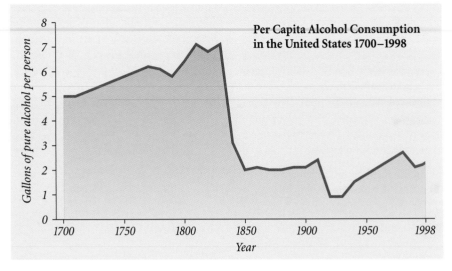

Figure 5-8 •

In the United States the per capita consumption of pure alcohol at present is 2.2 gallons but as this chart shows, the rate has varied wildly with the rise and fall of prohibition movements, health concerns, and the availability of a good water supply.

Adapted from David F. Musto's Alcohol in American History, *Scientific American,* April 1996

for the difference reflects the ability of men to be able to more efficiently metabolize higher amounts of alcohol. Unfortunately men also have more adverse consequences and develop problems with alcohol abuse or alcohol dependence (alcoholism) at a higher rate than women.

Women

For women alcohol problems become greater in their 30s, not in their 20s as for men (Blume, 1997). Alcohol-dependent women as a group drink

about 1/3 less alcohol than alcohol-dependent men (York, 1990).

Negative health consequences develop faster for women than for men. Proportionally, more women than men die from cirrhosis of the liver, circulatory disorders, suicide, and accidents. As mentioned female alcoholics have a 50–100% higher death rate than male alcoholics. But just as health problems develop after sustained heavy drinking, health disorders, especially reproductive problems, and depression may precede heavy drinking and even contribute to it. Also women get higher

TABLE 5–6   ALCOHOL ABUSE OR DEPENDENCE WITHIN PAST YEAR

	Males	Females	
Abstainers	28.0%	38.0%	
Light drinkers	58.7%	45.1%	(at least once a month)
Moderate drinkers	25.4%	9.6%	(at least once a week)
Binge drinkers	23.2%	8.6%	(5 or more drinks on the same occasion at least once in the last 30 days)
Heavy drinkers	9.7%	2.4%	(5 or more drinks per day at least 5 or more days in the last 30 days)

(SAMHSA, 1998)

TABLE 5–7   WOMEN & ALCOHOL PROBLEMS

More Likely to Have Drinking Problems	Less Likely to Have Drinking Problems
Younger women	Older women (60+)
Loss of role (mother, job)	Multiple roles (married, stable, work outside the home)
Never married	Married
Divorced, separated	Widowed
Unmarried and living with a partner	Children in the home
White women	Black women
Using other drugs	Hispanic women
Experiencing sexual dysfunction	Nondrinking spouse
Victim of childhood sexual abuse	

(NIDA, 1994)

BAC from the same amount of alcohol drunk than men and therefore have greater toxic effects from the same level of alcohol ingestion.

In terms of treatment, studies show that society has a double standard that more readily accepts the alcoholic male but disdains the alcoholic female. Thus women are less likely to seek treatment for alcoholism than men but are quicker to utilize mental health services when, in fact, their real problem is alcohol or other drugs. Women are also more likely to be driven to treatment when their physical or mental health is suffering whereas men are more likely to seek treatment when they have problems with their employment or with the law (Gomberg, 1991; Ross, 1989).

Alcohol, Students, & Learning

It used to be that only college students, away from the control of their parents, began heavy drinking. But in the late 1980s and '90s, the age of first use and heavy use dropped to where many students had done it all by the time they finished their senior year in high school. The problem is that since so much maturing and developing takes place during high school and college years, drinking can negatively affect learning and maturation.

"Often it's the style of drinking, not experimentation, that gets college students (as well as high school kids and young adults) in trouble. Many think the name of the game is to get drunk. They drink too fast, they drink without eating, they play drinking games or contests, or they binge drink. They drink heavily and hard on "hump day" [Wednesday] or over the weekend. But because they drink heavily only once or twice a week, they think that there is no problem. But there usually is a problem: lower grades, disciplinary action, or behavior they regret, which usually means sexual behavior. And both males and females talk to me about having been drunk and regretting the person they were with or their conduct with that person."
College drug and alcohol counselor

Forty-four percent of college students admit to binge drinking at least once every two weeks (Wechsler et al., 2000). Binge drinking is defined as having five or more drinks at one sitting for males, four for females. About half the students in one study who admitted to binge drinking also admitted that their grades fell in the C to F range as opposed to the A to C range of most students. Many binge drinkers missed classes on a regular basis. In a national study there was a startling, dramatic, and direct correlation between the number of drinks consumed per week and the grade point average.

Doonesbury

BY GARRY TRUDEAU

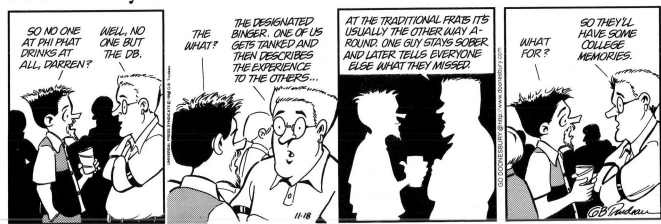

TABLE 5–8 AVERAGE NUMBER OF DRINKS PER WEEK, LISTED BY GRADE AVERAGE

Grade Average	Drinks Per Week		
	Males	Females	Overall
A	5.4	2.3	3.3
B	7.4	3.4	5.0
C	9.2	4.1	6.6
D or F	14.6	5.2	10.1

(College Core Study of 56 four-year and 22 two-year colleges by Southern Illinois University - Carbondale, 1993)

Notice that women's grades start to deteriorate at slightly less than half the level it takes for men's marks to go down. The National Household Survey on Drugs 1998 (Fig. 5-9) indicates that the higher the level of educational attainment, the more likely was the current use (not necessarily abuse) of alcohol. This seems a contradiction with the statistics about grade performance; however, the rate of heavy alcohol use in the 18–34 age group among those who had not completed high school was twice that of those who had completed college. In general, college students learn to moderate their drinking before they graduate.

Older Americans

"I visited my granddad in the retirement center/nursing home when he was 93 years old. He showed me the medicine cabinet. It was a small closet that, when opened by a nurse, revealed dozens of bottles of alcohol—whiskey, rum, scotch, vodka, and a variety of wines—each one with the name of one of the elderly residents. Depending on the health of the patient, they could have one or two drinks a day for their health. The tension and heart attack relief seemed to work quite as well as a sedative-hypnotic. He was still healthy at 96 when a fall killed him."

Doting 42-year-old grandson

People who are 65 years or older constitute the fastest growing segment of the U.S. population. About 6% to 21% of elderly hospital patients, 20% of elderly psychiatric patients, and 14% of elderly emergency room patients exhibit symptoms of alcoholism (AMA, 1996). One study indicates that approximately 2.5 million older adults have alcohol-related problems (Schonfeld & Dupree, 1991).

Research indicates that patterns of drinking persist into old age and that the amount and frequency of drinking are a result of general trends in society rather than the aging process. Hip fractures, one of the most debilitating injuries that occurs to the elderly, increase with alcohol consumption mainly due to decrease in bone density because of the deleterious effects of alcohol (Adams, Yuan, Barboriak, et al., 1993). In nursing homes as many as 49% of the patients have drinking problems although some nursing homes are used as a place to hospitalize problem drinkers, so the rate may seem higher than the general population (Joseph, 1997). Another problem is that the average American over 65 years old takes two to seven prescription medications daily and so alcohol-prescription drug interactions are quite common (Korrapati & Vestal, 1995).

About 1/3 of elderly alcohol abusers are of the late onset variety. Some older people may increase their drinking because of isolation, retirement, more leisure time, financial pressures, depression over health, loss of friends or a spouse, lack of a day-to-day structure, or simply the availability and access to alcohol in the home or at friends' homes. This increased drinking can lead to abuse and addiction problems. The elderly alcohol abuser is less likely to be in contact with the workplace, the criminal justice system, or treatment providers than those experiencing more visible mainstream problems. Thus it may be more difficult to identify elderly abusers and get them help.

One of the reasons diagnosis of drug or alcohol problems is difficult in the elderly is the coexistence of other physical or mental problems that become much more prevalent due to the aging process. Dementia, depression, hypertension, arrhythmia, psychosis, and panic disorder are just some of the conditions whose symptoms are mimicked either by drug use or withdrawal from drug use (Gambert, 1997).

However even with all the reasons and pressures to drink, people 65 and older have the lowest prevalence of problem drinking and alcoholism. There are several reasons for the lower rates.

◇ People who become alcohol abusers or alcoholics usually do so before the age of 65, suggesting a high degree of self-correction or spontaneous remission with age.

◇ Cutting down on drinking or giving up drinking may be related to the relatively high cost of alcohol for those on a fixed income, as well as to adverse health consequences or to the fear of adverse health consequences.

◇ The body is less able to handle alcohol since liver function declines with age. The general aging process

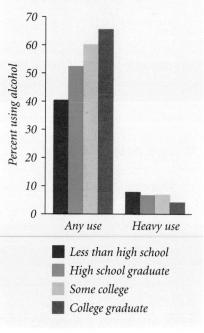

Alcohol Use in Past Month by Education in the United States – 1998

Figure 5-9 •

This chart compares the use and abuse of alcohol vs. the level of education.
SAMHSA, 1999

also decreases tolerance and slows metabolism, so the older drinker often has to limit intake.

◊ Since effects are increased if someone is ill or is taking medications, more severe side effects and greater toxic effects encourage drinkers to cut back as they age.

Homeless

For various reasons, some obvious, some not, it is hard to estimate the number of homeless in the United States. Varied sources suggest figures from 500,000 to 2 million with the average length of homelessness of 6 months. The breakdown of the homeless population is

◊ 46% are single males,

◊ 14% are single women,

◊ 36.5% are female heads of household with children,

◊ 25% are children.

Minorities are overrepresented:

◊ 56% are African American,

◊ 12% are Hispanics,

◊ 29% are Caucasian,

◊ 2% are Native Americans,

◊ 1% are Asians.

Finally it is estimated that

◊ 8% have HIV or AIDS (1/3 of prostitutes who are homeless have HIV or AIDS [Wallace, 1989]),

◊ 23% could be considered mentally ill,

◊ and a staggering 45% have serious substance abuse problems.

(U. S. Conference of Mayors, 1995)

Street young adult: "We wake up and we drink."

Street teenager #1: "Drink a beer."

Street teenager #1: "And we go to sleep right after we're done drinking at night. But we drink all day long, every day, all the time, constantly."

Street teenager #2: "Except for right now 'cause we don't have enough money for a beer."

Counselor: "How long have you been doing that?"

Street young adult: "All my life, pretty much since I was a teenager."

Counselor: "How old are you now?"

Street young adult: "Twenty eight ... and I've been living like this since I was 13. I take breaks. I'll get a job and shit but then I still drink then too. Don't get me wrong. I have money for beer even if I have to pawn stuff."

Interview with street people by a counselor from the Haight-Ashbury Clinic Youth Outreach Program

The reasons for homelessness vary widely. There are

◊ the situationally homeless who, because of job loss, spousal abuse, poverty, or eviction, find themselves on the street;

◊ the street people who have made the streets their home and have made an adjustment to living outside;

◊ the chronic mentally ill who have been squeezed out of inpatient mental facilities in the last three decades in favor of less costly out-

patient health facilities for treating their conditions;

◊ the homeless substance abusers, particularly alcohol abusers, whose lives center around their addiction that has made them incapable of living within the boundaries of normal society.

Within the last two groups are seen the mentally ill person who has begun to use drugs (often to self-medicate) and the drug user/abuser who has developed mental/emotional problems as a result of drug use. One of the keys to all these groups is to understand their lack of affiliation with any kind of support system. Services to identify and treat substance abuse or mental problems are hard to come by or shunned by the homeless person (Joseph & Paone, 1997).

A comprehensive program to alleviate the drug and mental problems of the homeless usually involves outreach that will bring services to the clients and eventually bring the clients to where the services are located. Many cities try to locate services at shelters and gathering places for the homeless but since a wide variety of services are needed to meet the wide variety of problems, budget constraints often become the deciding factor.

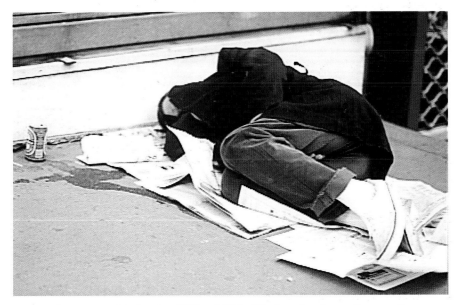

Depending on the survey, between 30% and 50% of the homeless have substance abuse problems and 23% have a diagnosable mental illness.

Courtesy of Simone Garlaund

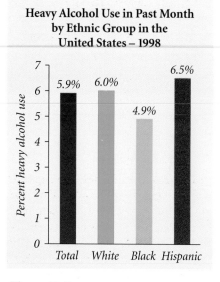

Heavy Alcohol Use in Past Month by Ethnic Group in the United States – 1998

Figure 5-10 •

In the United States during 1998, Caucasians continued to have a high rate of heavy alcohol use (5 or more drinks 5 or more times in the past month) at 6.0%. Rates for Hispanics were 6.5% and for African Americans, 4.9%.

SAMHSA, 1999

MINORITY POPULATIONS

Biological and neurochemical differences between different ethnic groups account for some of the different patterns of alcohol and drug use in different communities. However, diverse cultural traditions represented by ethnic minorities seem to make a greater contribution to alcohol use and abuse patterns as do the degree of assimilation into the drinking patterns of the dominant culture. Sensitivity to ethnic traditions and degrees of assimilation can help us understand how alcohol use affects the health, family life, and social interactions of various cultures and in turn, can contribute to more effective treatment and prevention. Generally a family history of alcoholism in both first- and second-generation relatives varies among ethnic groups in the United States.

African American Community

In the 1998 Household Drug and Alcohol Survey as in previous years, heavy use of alcohol was lower among African Americans than among Caucasians or Hispanics (4.9% vs. 6.0%) (Fig. 5-10). Use on a monthly basis in Black men is also less than White men (49% vs. 61%). The same patterns hold for use by Black women vs. White women (32% monthly use vs. 50%) (SAMHSA, 1998). On the other hand even though more Black women abstain than White women, there is greater heavy drinking among those Black women who do drink. Peak drinking for Blacks occurred after the age of 30 whereas drinking among Whites peaked at a younger age. Two reasons for the higher rate of abstention and the lower rate of heavy drinking among African Americans is their long history of spirituality, along with a strong matriarchal family structure, both of which look down upon heavy drinking.

One disturbing fact is that medical problems brought on by heavy drinking among African Americans are more severe (Caetano & Clark, 1998). This is probably due to less access to health care facilities, insurance programs, and prevention programs as well as a delayed entrance into treatment for alcoholism as compared to Whites (John, Brown, & Primm, 1997).

Hispanics

In 1999 there were 32 million Hispanics in the United States or about 11.6% of the total population (U.S. Bureau of the Census, 1999). One of the problems with examining Hispanic alcohol or drug use is the diversity of cultures involved: Mexican American, Cuban American, Puerto Rican, Colombian American, and a dozen other Spanish-speaking countries. In addition a single culture consists of anywhere from first- to tenth-generation immigrant Americans. About 60% of all Hispanics in the United States are of Mexican origin; 15% of the total are of Puerto Rican origin; and 5% are of Cuban origin (U.S. Bureau of the Census, 1999). The remaining 20% are from a variety of Latin countries. In a survey done in the early '80s, heavy alcohol use was highest in the Mexican American community, somewhat lower in the Puerto Rican community, and very low in the Cuban American community.

Drinking in the Hispanic community increases with both sexes as education and income increase. One of the problems with alcohol abuse and addiction in the Hispanic community is a lack of culturally relevant treatment facilities and personnel. Part of the severity of the problem has to do with the disruption of the family unit and the degree of assimilation.

"I think the cultural differences are crucial. To give you an example, I was in detox once and this woman came in, an Hispanic woman, and she was being interviewed by another counselor, and she was in an abusive relationship and the other counselor told her that she would have to leave her relationship if she wanted to stay clean. And I thought, 'this woman's going to bolt. She's not going to leave her family.' And I had to intervene in a delicate way because otherwise I felt we were going to lose her."

35-year-old female Hispanic drug counselor

The rate of alcohol use among female Hispanics has grown over the last 20 years possibly due to the different attitude towards women's rights, more female heads of household, or because of different cultural traditions. Generally women still drink considerably less than men. In treatment a strong involvement of the family is necessary plus an appreciation of the values of **dignidad, respeto, y cariño** (dignity, respect, and love) (Ruiz & Langrod, 1997).

TABLE 5–9   HISTORY OF ALCOHOLISM IN FAMILY

American Indians and Alaska Natives	(48%)
Caucasians	(23%)
African Americans	(22%)
Hispanics of Hispanic origin	(25%)
Non-Hispanics of Hispanic origin	(23%)

(NCADI, 1999)

TABLE 5–10   ALCOHOL USE BY HISPANIC COMMUNITIES, 1998

	Lifetime	Past Year	Past Month	Past Week	Heavy	% Reporting Dependence
Total	70.8%	58.56%	45.4%	15.6%	6.5%	7.0%
Hispanic males	80.4%	68.3%	56.8%	24.8%		
Hispanic females	60.8%	48.4%	33.6%	6.1%		

(SAMHSA, 1998)

Asian Americans & Pacific Islanders (API)

Asian Americans and Pacific Islanders (APIs) are the fastest growing ethnic minority in the United States and currently make up about four percent of the total population, approximately 11 million people. However because the label API encompasses dozens of distinct ethnicities throughout the Pacific basin, including Japanese, Chinese, Filipino, Korean, Vietnamese, Thai, Indonesian, Burmese, and Pacific Islanders, the diversity of Asian cultures is much greater than the differences between European cultures.

Asian Americans and Pacific Islanders are reported to have the lowest rate of drinking and drug problems in the United States. However as the APIs became more highly acculturated (more generations in America and increased ease with English), drinking increased (Zane & Kim, 1994). There are genetic factors that may help deter heavy drinking among APIs. The other major influence seems to be cultural (i.e., heavy drinking is strongly disapproved of in most API cultures). Surveys confirm that there are significant differences in drinking patterns among different national API groups (Johnson & Nagoshi, 1990). (Note that there are sometimes large differences between Asian and Asian American drinking patterns for the same country—the foreign-born vs. American-born Asians of the same ethnic origin and even among the same generation of Asian Americans in with identical ethnicities (Westermeyer, 1997).

In one study in Los Angeles (Table 5-11), Filipino Americans and Japanese Americans were twice as likely to be heavy drinkers as Chinese Americans but Chinese Americans were less likely to be abstainers. The Korean Americans have the highest number of abstainers. In general, Asian American males under 45 who are educated and in the middle class are most likely to drink but there is relatively little problem drinking even among this group (Makimoto, 1998).

As with other ethnic groups, treatment is much more effective when it is culturally relevant. For example, in San Francisco at the Haight-Ashbury Clinic, relatively few APIs came in for treatment, often because of the stigma involved in admitting that there was a problem. When research was done on the drug use patterns of the API communities in San Francisco, when more API counselors were hired, and when a specific treatment facility for Asian Americans was created, the API population in treatment vastly increased.

American Indians & Alaskan Natives

There are approximately 2.4 million American Indians and Alaskan Natives in the United States (U.S. Bureau of the Census, 1999). They are divided into more than 300 tribal or language groups. Stereotypes and old western movies seem to have influenced much of the thinking about Native Americans and drinking. The picture of the "Indian who can't hold his liquor" has been perpetuated for generations. One explanation is that although the rate of abstinence is quite high in many tribes, it is the pattern of heavy binge drinking among males in various tribes, especially on reservations, that accounts for the highly visible Native American alcoholic. (However in a survey of Sioux tribes, the women drank as much as the men.) The fact that many surveys are done on reservations where only 1/3 of the total Native American population lives, coupled with the grinding poverty found on many of those tribal reservations, is also a strong causative factor in heavy drinking (Beauvais, 1998).

Historically Native Americans only drank weak beers or other fermented beverages but usually just for ceremonial purposes. When distilled alcoholic beverages were introduced, most Native American cultures did not have time to develop ethical, legal, and social customs to handle the stronger drinks.

A study of a group of Native

TABLE 5–11   DRINKING PATTERNS OF 1,100 LOS ANGELES ASIAN AMERICANS

Group Drinking	Heavy Drinking	Moderate Drinking	Abstaining
Japanese Americans	25%	42%	33%
Chinese Americans	11%	48%	41%
Koreans Americans	14%	24%	62%
Filipino Americans	20%	29%	51%

(NIAAA, 1991)

Americans (Mission Indians) studied the inherited sensitivity to alcohol and found that they were not more sensitive to the effects of alcohol. Rather they were less sensitive and so had to drink more to get drunk (a sign of susceptibility to developing alcoholism) (Garcia-Andrade, Wall, & Ehlers, 1997).

Generally the abuse of alcohol accounts for 5 of the leading 10 causes of death in most tribes. Alcohol-related motor vehicle deaths are 5.5 times higher than for the rest of the U.S. population. Cirrhosis of the liver is 4.5 times higher; alcoholism, 3.8 times higher; homicide, 2.8 times higher; and suicide, 2.3 times higher. Although Native American women drink less than men, they are especially vulnerable to cirrhosis and account for almost half of the deaths from cirrhosis (Manson, Shore, Baron, et al., 1992).

In general, drinking patterns vary widely among the more than 300 tribes of Native American and Alaskan peoples who make up about 1% of the population of the United States. Some tribes are mostly abstinent; some drink moderately with few problems; and some have high rates of heavy drinking and alcoholism. One study in Oklahoma found alcohol-related causes of death varied from less than 1% up to 24% among the 11 tribes surveyed, compared with 2% for Blacks and 3% for Whites (Manson et al., 1992).

TABLE 5–12   THE MICHIGAN ALCOHOLISM SCREENING TEST (MAST) QUESTIONNAIRE

Points	Questions
2	*1. Do you feel you are a normal drinker?
2	2. Have you ever awakened the morning after some drinking and found that you could not remember a part of the evening before?
1	3. Does your wife (husband), girlfriend (boyfriend), and/or parents ever worry or complain about your drinking?
2	*4. Can you stop drinking without a struggle after one or two drinks?
1	5. Do you ever feel guilty about your drinking?
2	6. Do your friends or relatives think you are a normal drinker?
	7. Do you ever try to limit your drinking to certain times of the day or to certain places?
2	*8. Are you always able to stop drinking when you want to?
5	9. Have you ever attended a meeting of Alcoholics Anonymous (AA) because of your own drinking?
1	10. Have you gotten into fights when drinking?
2	11. Has drinking ever created problems with you and your wife (husband) or girlfriend (boyfriend)?
2	12. Has your wife (husband), girlfriend (boyfriend), or other family member ever gone to anyone for help about your drinking?
2	13. Have you ever lost friends because of your drinking?
2	14. Have you ever gotten into trouble at work because of drinking?
2	15. Have you ever lost a job because of drinking?
2	16. Have you ever neglected your obligations, your family, or your work for two or more days in a row because you were drinking?
1	17. Do you ever drink in the morning?
2	18. Have you ever been told you have liver trouble? Cirrhosis?
5	19. Have you ever had delirium tremens (DTs), severe shaking, heard voices, or seen things after heavy drinking?
5	20. Have you ever gone to anyone for help about your drinking?
5	21. Have you ever been in a hospital because of drinking?
2	22. Have you ever been seen at a psychiatric hospital or on a psychiatric ward of a general hospital where drinking was part of the problem?
5	23. Have you ever been seen at a psychiatric or mental health clinic, or gone to any doctor, social worker, or clergyman for help with an emotional problem related to drinking?
2 (for each arrest)	24. Have you ever been arrested, even for a few hours, because of drunken behavior?
2	25. Have you ever been arrested for drunk driving?

Scoring: For each "yes" for all questions except 1, 4, and 8, give yourself the points indicated. For questions 1, 4, and 8 (marked with an *) give yourself the points indicated if you give a "no" answer and zero points for a "yes" answer. A score of 12 or more indicates in most cases, that the client/patient has alcoholism.

Traditionally the cutoff score for determining alcoholism was 5 but this seemed to result in a high false positive rate of 33% to 59%. By using a cutoff of 12, the false positive dropped to 5% to 8%. Scores between 5 and 10 are suggestive of an alcohol problem, not necessarily alcoholism. Each clinician giving the test determines the cutoff best for his or her clients or patients. A person self-administering the test also has to judge whether a score of between 5 and 12 is reason for concern.

ASSESSMENT

The most widely used direct assessment tests are the Alcohol Severity Index and Addiction Severity Index or their modified shortened versions (*see Chapter 9*). In the past the most popular instrument was The Michigan Alcoholism Screening Test (MAST) Questionnaire. It was developed in 1971 by Selzer and updated in 1980 and 1981.

CONCLUSIONS

When surveys are done on the incidence of alcoholism and drinking problems, what is often lost is the idea that first, alcoholism is a progressive illness that will prove fatal if not treated. Second is that although the progression from experimentation to addiction can take 3 months or 30 years, if one continues to drink heavily and frequently, the biochemical and psychological changes become extremely difficult, if not impossible, to reverse. Finally, alcohol use is often involved in polydrug use, so any treatment has to include the other addictions as well.

CHAPTER SUMMARY

Overview

1. The majority of people in almost every country, except for Islamic countries, consume alcohol.

2. Two million people worldwide died last year due to alcohol.

3. Since the process of fermentation occurs naturally, alcohol was discovered by chance.

4. Over the centuries alcohol has been used as a food, as a medicine, as a sacrament, as a reward, as recreation, and to cover emotional and mental problems.

5. Because alcohol also causes the most health and societal problems, such as the Gin Epidemic in England, its use has often been restricted or banned by almost every country but presently, because of demand, most restrictions have been overturned.

Alcoholic Beverages

6. Though there are hundreds of different alcohols, ethyl alcohol (ethanol) is the main psychoactive ingredient in all alcoholic beverages.

7. When yeast is added to certain fruits, vegetables, or grains, they ferment into alcoholic beverages.

8. When grains ferment, beer is the result. When fruits ferment, wine is the result. More highly concentrated spirits are distilled from the original fermentation of grains, some vegetables such as potatoes (vodka), and from wine.

9. Most wine is 12% alcohol; most beer is 4% to 7% alcohol; and most liquors and whiskeys are about 35% to 45% alcohol.

Absorption, Distribution, & Metabolism

10. When alcohol is drunk, it is absorbed (even from the stomach in men), metabolized (mostly in the liver), and then excreted.

11. The rate of absorption depends on body weight, sex, health, and a dozen other factors. Women usually absorb alcohol faster and get a higher BAC from the same amount drunk in comparison to men, so the effects on women are more damaging.

12. About 2% to 10% of alcohol is excreted directly through the urine and lungs. The rest is metabolized and then excreted as carbon dioxide and water.

13. Alcohol is metabolized at a defined continuous rate, so it is possible to determine what level of drinking will produce a certain blood alcohol concentration (BAC). A BAC of .08 to .10 defines legal intoxication in all 50 states.

Desired Effects, Side Effects, & Health Consequences

14. The six levels of alcohol use are abstention, experimentation, social/recreational use, habituation, abuse, and addiction (alcoholism).

Low- to Moderate-Dose Episodes

15. Small amounts of alcohol or occasional episodes of intoxication episodes are usually not harmful and have some positive cardiovascular benefits, mostly for men.

16. The negative side of low to moderate drinking is accidents, unwanted pregnancies, sexually transmitted diseases, or legal problems.

17. People who are pregnant or who have preexisting physical or mental health problems, allergies to alcoholic beverages, high genetic/environmental susceptibility to addiction, and preexisting abuse problems should avoid alcohol.

18. Low-dose use can help digestion, promote relaxation, and slightly lower the risk of heart attacks or coronary artery disease (CAD).

19. The psychological effects depend on the mood of the drinker and the setting where the alcohol is consumed.

20. Since alcohol is a disinhibitor, low-dose use can increase self-confidence, sociability, and sexual

desire. The disinhibition is mostly due to GABA, an inhibitory neurotransmitter.

21. As the amount consumed increases, the initial desirable effects are often offset by unwanted side effects, such as physical and mental depression.

High-Dose Episodes

22. Intoxication is a combination of blood alcohol concentration, psychological mood, expectation, and drinking history.

23. As the blood alcohol concentration rises, effects go from lowered inhibitions and relaxation, to decreased alertness and clumsiness, to slurred speech and inability to walk, to unconsciousness and death.

24. Blackouts are caused by heavy drinking and marked by loss of memory even though the drinker is awake and conscious.

25. Hangovers are a withdrawal symptom of high-dose use.

Chronic High-Dose Use

26. About 10% to 12% of drinkers progress to frequent, high-dose use; two to three times more men than women have a major problem with alcohol.

27. Heredity, environment, and frequency of consumption help determine if a person will have a problem with their drinking.

28. Tolerance and tissue dependence occur as the body, especially the liver, attempts to adapt to ever-increasing amounts of alcohol.

29. Withdrawal after cessation of frequent high-dose use can be life threatening. Delerium tremens (DTs) is a life-threatening form of severe withdrawal that includes hallucinations and convulsions.

Addiction (alcoholism)

30. About 10% to 12% of 140 million adult drinkers in the United States have developed alcohol addiction (alcoholism).

31. Just 20% of drinkers consume 80% of all alcohol.

Classification

32. There have been numerous attempts to classify alcoholism so the condition can be studied more systematically and strategies for treatment can be more realistic.

33. Classifications vary from E. M. Jellinek's gamma and delta alcoholics, to type I and II alcoholics, to type A and B alcoholics, and finally to the disease concept of alcoholism.

34. Most current concepts look at addiction as a progressive disease that is caused by a combination of hereditary and environmental influences that are triggered and aggravated by the use of alcohol or other drugs.

Long-Term Effects of Addiction (alcoholism)

35. The liver is the organ most severely affected. Problems include a fatty liver, alcoholic hepatitis, and cirrhosis (which is a scarring of the liver and is eventually fatal).

36. Digestive effects of chronic drinking include ulcers, diarrhea, pancreatitis, bleeding, and malnutrition.

37. Enlarged heart, high blood pressure, intracranial bleeding, and stroke are seen with frequent high-dose use.

38. Heavy drinking can cause large loss of brain cells since alcohol is toxic to all cells. Dementia is also a possible effect.

39. Alcohol can lower inhibitions and increase desire but as use increases, the physical ability to perform sexually is depressed.

40. In moderate to heavy drinkers, the chance of breast cancer in women as well as the chance of mouth, throat, and esophageal cancer increase in both men and women especially if they also smoke.

Polydrug Abuse

41. Most drug abuse involves more than one substance, especially al-

cohol, so the problems can by synergistic not just additive.

Other Problems

42. Many people use alcohol to self-medicate their emotional depression but as drinking continues, it can induce depression.

43. A large percentage of homicides, suicides, and accidents involve alcohol.

44. Heavy drinking during pregnancy can cause birth defects, most notably fetal alcohol syndrome (FAS), that involves abnormal growth and mental problems. It is not known what level of drinking, if any, is safe during pregnancy.

45. Alcohol is heavily involved in aggression, violence, and sexual assault, mostly from the lowering of inhibitions. The mood of the drinkers and the setting also affect violence.

Epidemiology

46. Alcohol consumption varies from 3.1 gallons of pure alcohol a year in France, to 2.2 gallons in the United States, down to 0.1 gallons in a Moslem country, such as Algeria.

47. Men drink more per episode than women and have a higher level of addiction. This is because of a combination of physiological differences and cultural mores.

48. Given the same blood alcohol concentration (BAC), women have more health problems than men.

49. The amount and frequency of alcohol consumption directly affects grades. About 28% of high school students and 45% of college students have five or more drinks at one setting.

50. About 2.5 million older Americans have alcohol-related problems. As the drinker ages, the liver is less able to handle alcohol but even so, the elderly have the lowest prevalence of problem drinking and alcoholism.

51. About 45% of the homeless have serious substance abuse problems,

23% have a mental illness, and 8% are infected with HIV or AIDS. Treatment must be brought to the homeless rather than expecting they will come in for treatment.

52. Each ethnic group in the United States has unique drinking problems due to physiology and culture.

53. Heavy drinking is lower in the African American community than the Caucasian or Hispanic communities. The Asian community has so many components that it is hard to make generalizations. There is also a wide variation in the Native American communities although in some groups, 5 of the 10 leading causes of death are due to alcohol.

Assessment

54. The most widely used direct assessment tests for drug and alcohol problems are the Alcohol Severity Index and Addiction Severity Index. The Michigan Alcoholism Screening Test (MAST) used to be the most widely used screening test.

Conclusions

55. The road to alcoholism can take 3 months, 30 years, or it may never occur. One has to recognize that alcohol is a psychoactive drug and can cause irreversible physiological changes that make one susceptible to alcoholism.

REFERENCES

Abel, E. L., & Sokol, R. J. (1986). Fetal alcohol syndrome is now leading cause of mental retardation. *Lancet, 2*, 1222.

Adams, W. L., Yuan, Z., Barboriak, J. J., et al. (1993). Alcohol-related hospitalizations of elderly people. *JAMA, 270*(10), 1222–1225.

AHA (American Heart Association). (1996). Dietary guidelines for healthy American adults. *American Heart Association, Nutrition Committee statement.*

Alcohol Alert. (1992). Moderate drinking: Benefits and risks. *Alcohol Alert, 16.*

AMA (American Medical Association). (1996). Alcoholism in the elderly. AMA Council on Scientific Afairs. *JAMA, 275*(10), 797–801.

Amerine, M. A. (1985). Wine making. *Encyclopaedia Britannica* (Volume 19, pp. 875–884). Chicago: Encyclopaedia Britannica.

Anthenelli, R. M., & Schuckit, M. A. (1998). Genetic influences in addiction. In A. W. Graham & T. K. Schultz (Eds.), *Principles of Addiction Medicine* (2nd ed., pp. 41–51). Chevy Chase, MD: American Society of Addiction Medicine, Inc.

APA (American Psychiatric Association). (1994). *Diagnostic and Statistical Manual of Mental Disorders* (4th ed.). Washington, DC: Author.

Babor, T. F. (1995). The classification of alcoholics. In *Typology: The Classification of Alcoholism. Alcohol World: Health & Research.* Bethesda, MD: NIAAA.

Babor, T. F., Dolinsky, Z. S., Meyer, R. E., Brock, M., Hofmann, M., & Tennen, H. (1992). Types of alcoholics: Concurrent and predictive validity of some common classification schemes. *British Journal of Addiction, 87,* 1415–1431.

Bailey, W. J. (1995). Alcohol doses, measurements, and blood alcohol levels. *Indiana Prevention Resource Center.* http://www.drugs.indiana.edu.

Beauvais, F. (1998). American Indians. *Alcohol Health & Research World, 22*(4).

Becker, H. C. (1998). Kindling in alcohol withdrawal. *Alcohol Health & Research World: Alcohol Withdrawal, 22*(1), 25–33.

Begleiter, H. (1980). *Biological Effects of Alcohol.* New York: Plenum Press.

Bernstein, M., & Mahoney, J. J. (1989). Management perspectives on alcoholism: The employer's stake in alcoholism treatment. *Occupational Medicine, 4*(2), 223–232.

Blot, W. J. (1992). Alcohol and cancer. *Cancer Research Supplement, 52,* 2119s–2121s.

Blum, K., Braverman, E. R., Cull, J. G., Holder, J. M., Luck, R., Lubar, J., Miller, D., & Comings, D. E. (2000). "Reward deficiency syndrome" (RDS): A biogenetic model for the diagnosis and treatment of impulsive, addictive, and compulsive behaviors. *Journal of Psychoactive Drugs, 32*(1).

Blum, K., Cull, J. G., Braverman, E. R., & Comings, D. E. (1996). Reward deficiency syndrome. *American Scientist, 84,* 132–145.

Blum, K., & Payne, J. E. (1991). *Alcohol and the Addicted Brain.* New York: The Free Press, 165.

Blume, S. (1997). Women: Clinical aspects. In J. H. Lowinson, P. Ruiz, R. B. Millman, & J. G. Langrod, (Eds.), *Substance Abuse: A Comprehensive Textbook* (3rd ed., pp. 645–654). Baltimore: Williams & Wilkins.

Bobak, M. (1999). Alcohol consumption in a national sample of the Russian population. *Addiction, 94*(6), 857–866.

Boffetta, P., & Garfinkel, L. (1990). Alcohol drinking and mortality among men enrolled in an American Cancer Society prospective study. *Epidemiology, 1,* 342–348.

Bohman, M., Sigvardson, S., & Cloniger, C. G. (1981). Maternal inheritance of alcohol abuse: Cross-fostering analysis of adopted women. *Archives of General Psychiatry, 38,* 965–969.

Bosron, W. F., Ehrig, T., & Li, T. K. (1993). Genetic factors in alcohol metabolism and alcoholism. *Seminars in liver disease, 13*(2), 126–135.

Bowlin, S. J. (1997). Alcohol intake and breast cancer. *International Journal of Epidemiology, 26,* 915–923.

Bureau of Alcohol, Tobacco, and Firearms. (1998). Monthly (Tax) statistical release: Wines, beer, distilled spirits. *Bureau of Alcohol, Tobacco, and Firearms.* http://www.atf.treas.gov.

Bushman, B. J. (1997). Effects of alcohol on human aggression. In M. Galanter (Ed.), *Recent Developments in Alcoholism* (Vol. 13, pp. 227–243). New York: Plenum Press.

Caetano, R., & Clark, C. L. (1998). Trends in alcohol-related problems among whites, African Americans, and Hispanics: 1984–1995. *Alcoholism: Clinical and Experimental Research, 22*(2), 534–538.

Cloninger, C. R., Bohman, M., & Sigvardson, S. (1996). Type I and type II alcoholism: An update. *Alcohol Health and Research World, 20*(1), 18–23.

Collins, J. J., & Messerschmidt, P. M. (1993). Epidemiology of alcohol-related violence. *Alcohol Health and Research World, 17*(2), 93–100.

Cook, P. S. et al. (1990). *Alcohol, Tobacco and Other Drugs May Harm the Unborn. UADHHS Pub. No. (ADM) 90–1711*, 17.

Davis, R. (1994). Drug and alcohol use in the former Soviet Union, selected factors and future considerations. *International Journal of the Addictions, 29*(3), 88–89.

Dawson, A. Bigby, B. G., Poceta, J. S., & Mitler, M. M. (1993). Effect of bedtime ethanol on total inspiratory resistance and respiratory drive in normal nonsnoring men. *Alcoholism: Clinical and Experimental Research,* 17(2), 256–262.

DeBakey, S. F., Stinson, F. S., Grant, B. F., & Dufour, M. C. (1996). Liver cirrhosis mortality in the United States, 1970–1993. *Surveillance Report #41.* Bethesda, MD: National Institute on Alcohol Abuse and Alcoholism.

Devantag, F., Mandich, G., Zaiotti, G., & Toffolo, G. G. (1983). Alcoholic epilepsy: Review of a series and proposed classification and etiopathogenesis. *Harvard Journal of Neurologic Science, 4,* 275–284.

Ellison, R. C. (1999). Breast cancer risk not increased by light drinking. *American Journal of Epidemiology. January 18, 1999.*

Ernhart, C. B., Sokol, R. J., Martier, S., et al. (1987). Alcohol teratogenicity in the human: A detailed assessment of specificity, critical period, and threshold. *American Journal of Obstetrics and Gynecology, 156*(1), 33–39.

Eurocare. (1999). *Report on European Alcohol Use.* http://www.eurocare.org/profiles.htm.

Gambert, S. R. (1997). The elderly. In J. H. Lowinson, P. Ruiz, R. B. Millman, & J. G. Langrod, (Eds.), *Substance Abuse: A Comprehensive Textbook* (3rd ed., pp. 693–699). Baltimore: Williams & Wilkins.

Garcia-Andrade, C., Wall, T. L., & Ehlers, C. L. (1997). The firewater myth and response to alcohol in Mission Indians. *American Journal of Psychiatry, 154,* 983–988.

Geller, A. (1997). Neurological effects. In A. W. Graham & T. K. Schultz (Eds.), *Principles of Addiction Medicine* (2nd ed., pp. 775–784). Chevy Chase, MD: American Society of Addiction Medicine, Inc.

Goedde, H. W., Harada, S., & Agarwal, D. P. (1979). Racial differences in alcohol sensitivity: a new hypothesis. *Human Genetics, 51,* 331–334.

Goldstein, A. (1994). *Addiction: From Biology to Drug Policy.* New York: W.H. Freeman and Company.

Gomberg, E. A. L. (1991). Alcoholic women in treatment: New research. *Substance Abuse 12*(1), 6–12.

Goodwin, D. W., & Gabrielli, W. F. (1997). Alcohol: Clinical aspects. In J. H. Lowinson, P. Ruiz, R. B. Millman, & J. G. Langrod, (Eds.), *Substance Abuse: A Comprehensive Textbook* (3rd ed., pp. 142–147). Baltimore: Williams & Wilkins.

Greenfield, T. K., & Rogers, J. D. (1999). Who drinks most of the alcohol in the U.S.? The policy implications. *Journal of Studies on Alcohol,* in press.

Gustafson, R. (1994). Alcohol and aggression. *Juvenile Offender Rehabilitation, 21*(3/4), 41–80.

Hans, S. L. (1998). Developmental outcomes of prenatal exposure to alcohol and other drugs. In A. W. Graham & T. K. Schultz (Eds.), *Principles of Addiction Medicine* (2nd ed., pp. 1223–1237). Chevy Chase, MD: American Society of Addiction Medicine, Inc.

Harkin, A. M., Anderson, P., & Lehto, J. (1995). *Alcohol in Europe A health perspective.* Copenhagen: World Health Organization (WHO).

Heath, D. B. (1995). Alcohol: History. *Encyclopedia of Drugs and Alcohol* (Vol.1, pp. 70–78). New York: Simon & Schuster Macmillan.

Heinz, A. Ragan, P., Jones, D. W., et al. (1998). Reduced central serotonin transporters in alcoholism. *The American Journal of Psychiatry, 155,* 1544–1549.

Helzer, J. E., & Pryzbeck, T. R. (1988). The co-occurrence of alcoholism with other psychiatric disorders in the general population and its impact on treatment. *Journal of Studies on Alcohol, 49*(3), 219–224.

Ikonomidou, C., Bitigau, P., Ishimaru, M. J. et al. (2000). Ethanol-induced apoptotic neurodegeneration and fetal alcohol syndrome. *Science, 287,* 1056–1060.

Jellinek, E. M. (1961). *The Disease Concept of Alcoholism.* New Haven, CT: College & University Press.

John, S., Brown, L. S. Jr., & Primm, B. J. (1997). African Americans: Epidemiologic, Prevention, and treatment issues. In J. H. Lowinson, P. Ruiz, R. B. Millman, & J. G. Langrod, (Eds.), *Substance Abuse: A Comprehensive Textbook* (3rd ed., pp. 699–705). Baltimore: Williams & Wilkins.

Johnson, R. C., & Nagoshi, C. T. (1990). Asians, Asian Americans and alcohol. *Journal of Psychoactive Drugs. 22*(1), 45–52.

Jones, A. W., & Pounder, D. J. (1998). Measuring blood-alcohol concentration for clinical and forensic purposes. In S. B. Karch (Ed.), *Drug Abuse Handbook* (pp. 181–184). Boca Raton, FL: CRC Press. 327–355.

Jones, K. L., & Smith, D. W. (1973). Recognition of the fetal alcohol syndrome in early infancy. *Lancet, 2,* 999–1001.

Joseph, C. L. (1997). Misuse of alcohol and drugs in the nursing home. In A. M. Gumack (Ed.), *Older Adults' Misuse of Alcohol, Medicines, and Other Drugs: Research and Practice Issues.* New York: Springer.

Joseph, H., & Paone, D. (1997). The homeless. In J. H. Lowinson, P. Ruiz, R. B. Millman, & J. G. Langrod, (Eds.), *Substance Abuse: A Comprehensive Textbook* (3rd ed., pp. 733–743). Baltimore: Williams & Wilkins.

Justice Department. (1998). *Alcohol and Crime: An Analysis of National Data on the Prevalence of Alcohol Involvement in Crime.*

Keller, M. (1984). Alcohol consumption. *Encyclopaedia Britannica* (Vol. 1, pp. 437–450). Chicago: Encyclopaedia Britannica.

Klatsky, A. L. (1988). The cardiovascular effects of alcohol: *Alcohol, 22* (1), 1178–1204.

Knop, J., Goodwin, D. W., Teasdale, T.W., Mikkelsen, U., & Schulsinger, F.A. (1984). A Danish prospective study of young males at high risk for alcoholism. In Goodwin, D.W., Van Dusen, K., Mednick, S.A., (Eds.), *Longitudinal research in alcoholism.* Boston: Kluwer-Nijhoff.

Koob, G. (8/23/99). Alcohol stimulates release of stress chemicals. *Speech to American Chemical Society meeting in New Orleans.*

Korrapati, M. R., & Vestal, R. E. (1995). Alcohol and medications in the elderly: Complex interactions. In T. Beresford and E. Gomberg (Eds.), *Alcohol and Aging* (pp. 42–55). New York: Oxford University Press.

Kurose, I., Higuchi, H, Kato, S, Miura, S., & Ishii, H. (1996). Ethanol-induced oxidative stress in the liver. *Alcoholism: Clinical and Experimental Research, 20*(1), 77A–85A.

Kushner, M. G., Mackenzie, T. B., Flazdon, J., et al. (1996). The effects of alcohol consumption on laboratory-induced panic and state anxiety. *Archives of General Psychiatry, 53,* 264–270.

Landolt, H. P. et al. (1996). Late-afternoon ethanol intake affects nocturnal sleep and the sleep EEG in middle-aged men. *Journal of Clinical Psychopharmacology, 16*(6), 428–436.

Langton, P. A. (1995). Temperance movement. *Encyclopedia of Drugs and Alcohol* (Vol. 3, pp. 1019–1023). New York: Simon & Schuster Macmillan.

Lee, J. A. (1987). Chinese, Alcohol and Flushing: Sociohistorical and Biobehavioral Considerations. *Journal of Psychoactive Drugs, 19*(4), 319–327.

Li, T. K., Lumeng, L., McBride, W. J., Waller, M. B., & Murphy, J. M. (1986). Studies on an animal model of alcoholism. In M. C. Braude, J. M. Chao (Eds.), *Genetic and Biological Markers in Drug Abuse and Alcoholism. NIDA Research Monograph 66.* Rockville, MD: Department of Health and Human Services.

Lichine, A. (1990). Distilled Spirits. *Encyclopedia Americana* (pp. 188–190).

Lieber, C. S. (1998). Hepatic disorders. In A. W. Graham & T. K. Schultz (Eds.), *Principles of Addiction Medicine* (2nd ed., pp. 755–771). Chevy Chase, MD: American Society of Addiction Medicine, Inc.

Longenecker, G. L. (1994). *How Drugs Work: Drug Abuse and the Human Body.* Emeryville, CA: Ziff-Davis Press.

Lukas, S. E. (1995). Beer. *Encyclopedia of Drugs and Alcohol* (Vol.1, pp. 146–149). New York: Simon & Schuster Macmillan.

Maher, J. (1997). Exploring alcohol's effects on liver function. *AHRW, 21*(1), 10.

Makimoto, K. (1998). Drinking patterns and drinking problems among Asian Americans and Pacific Islanders. *Alcohol Health & Research World, 22*(4), 265–269.

Manson, S. M., Shore, J. H., Baron, A.E., et al. (1992). Alcohol abuse and dependence among American Indians. In J. E. Helzer, & G. J. Canino (Eds.), *Alcoholism in North America, Europe, and Asia* (pp. 113–130). New York: Oxford University Press.

Matthews, J. (1995). *Beer, Booze and Books: A Sober Look at Higher Education.* Peterborough, NH: Viaticum Press.

May, P. A. (1996). Research issues in the prevention of fetal alcohol syndrome and alcohol-related birth defects. *Research Monograph 32, Women and Alcohol: Issues for Prevention Research.* Bethesda, MD: National Institute on Alcohol Abuse and Alcoholism.

Mayo-Smith, M. (1998). Management of alcohol intoxication and withdrawal. In A. W. Graham & T. K. Schultz (Eds.), *Principles of Addiction Medicine* (2nd ed.). Chevy Chase, MD: American Society of Addiction Medicine, Inc.

Miczek, K. A. et al. (1997). Alcohol, GABA-benzodiazepine receptor complex and aggression. In M. Galanter (Ed.), *Recent Developments in Alcoholism,* (Vol. 13, pp. 139–171). New York: Plenum Press.

Miller, M. M. et al. (1988). Bedtime ethanol increases resistance of upper airways and produces sleep apneas in asymptomatic snorers. *Alcohol Clinical Experimental Research, 12*(6), 801–805.

Miller, N. S., Klamen, D., Hoffman, N. G., & Flaherty, J. A. (1995). Prevalence of depression and alcohol and other drug dependence in addictions treatment populations. *Journal of Psychoactive Drugs, 28*(2), 111–124.

Moddrey, W. C. (1988). Alcoholic hepatitis: Clinicopathologic features and therapy. *Seminars in Liver Disease, 8*(1), 91–102.

Morse, R. M., Flavin, D. K., et al. (1992). The definition of alcoholism. *JAMA, 268,* 1012–1014.

NCADI (National Council on Alcohol and Drug Information). (1999). Online statistics. *http://www.NCADI.com.*

NHTSA (National Highway Transportation and Safety Administration). (1999, 1998, 1997, 1995). *Traffic Fatality Statistics.*

NIAAA/Congress. (1997). *Ninth Special Report to U.S. Congress on Alcohol and Health.* Bethesda, MD: U.S. Department of Health and Human Services.

NIAAA (National Institute on Alcohol Abuse & Alcoholism). (1990). Alcohol and women. *Alcohol Alert No. 10.*

NIAAA. (1991). Alcohol & Asian Americans. *Alcohol Health & Research World, 2*(2), 41.

NIAAA. (1993). Alcohol and the liver. *Alcohol Alert No. 19.*

NIAAA. (1997). Alcohol metabolism. *Alcohol Alert No. 35.*

NIAAA. (1998). Alcohol and tobacco. *Alcohol Alert No. 39.*

NIAAA. (1999). *Apparent Per Capita Alcohol Consumption: National, State, And Regional Trends, 1977–96. Surveillance Report #47.* Bethesda, MD: U. S. Department of Health and Human Services.

NIDA (National Institute on Drug Abuse). (1996). *National Pregnancy and Health Survey. NIH Publication 96–3819,* xxi–xxii. Bethesda, MD: U.S. Department of Health and Human Services.

NIDA. (1994). *Women and Drug Abuse: You and your community can help. http://www.DEA.gov.*

Noble, E. P., Blum, K., Montgomery, A., & Sheridan, P. J. (1991). Allelic association of the D2 dopamine receptor gene with receptor-binding characteristics in alcoholism. *Archives of General Psychiatry, 48,* 648–654.

Nutt, D. J. (1998). The Neurochemistry of Addiction. In A. W. Graham & T. K. Schultz (Eds.), *Principles of Addiction Medicine* (2nd ed.). Chevy Chase, MD: American Society of Addiction Medicine, Inc.

O'Brien, R., & Chafetz, M. (1991). *The Encyclopedia of Alcoholism* (2nd ed.). New York: Facts on File.

Olds, J., & Milner, P. (1954). Positive reinforcement produced by electrical stimulation of septal area and other regions of rat brain. *Journal of Comprehensive Physiology and Psychology, 47,* 419–427.

Olds, J. (1956). Pleasure centers in the brain. *Scientific American, 195*(4), 105–116.

Peele, S. (1995). Controlled Drinking Versus Abstinence. *Encyclopedia of Drugs and Alcohol* (Vol. 1, pp. 92–97). New York: Simon & Schuster Macmillan.

Prescott, C. A., & Kendler, K. S. (1999). Genetic and environmental contributions to alcohol abuse and dependence in a population-based sample of male twins. *The American Journal of Psychiatry, 156,* 34–40.

Presley, C. A. et al. (1997). *Alcohol and Drugs on American College Campuses; Issues of Violence and Harassment.* Carbondale IL: Southern Illinois University at Carbondale.

Roizen, J. (1997). Epidemiological issues in alcohol-related violence. In M. Galanter (Ed.), *Recent Developments in Alcoholism* (Vol. 13). New York: Plenum Press.

Rosenberg, A. (1996). Brain damage caused by prenatal alcohol exposure. *Science & Medicine, 3*(4), 43–51.

Ross, H. E. (1989). Alcohol and drug abuse in treated alcoholics: A comparison of men and women. *Alcohol Clinical & Experimental Research, 13,* 810–816.

Ruiz, P., & Langrod, J. G. (1997). Hispanic Americans. In J. H. Lowinson, P. Ruiz, R. B. Millman, & J. G. Langrod, (Eds.), *Substance Abuse: A Comprehensive Textbook* (3rd ed., pp. 705–711). Baltimore: Williams & Wilkins.

Sacco, R. L., Elkind, M., Boden-Albala, B., et al. (1999). The protective effects of moderate alcohol consumption on ischemic stroke. *JAMA, 281*(1).

SAMHSA (Substance Abuse and Mental Health Services Administration). (1998). *Summary of Findings from the 1998 National Household Survey on Drug Abuse.* Rockville, MD: SAMHSA.

Schonfeld, L., & Dupree, L. W. (1991). Antecedents of drinking for early- and late-onset elderly alcohol abusers. *Journal of Studies of Alcohol, 52,* 587–592.

Schuckit, M. A., & Smith, T. L. (1996). An 8-year follow-up of 450 sons of alcoholic and control subjects. *Archives of General Psychiatry, 53*(3).

Segal, B. (1990). *The Drunken Society: Alcohol Abuse and Alcoholism in the Soviet Union.* New York: Hippocrene Books.

Shiffman, S., & Balabanis, M. (1995). Associations between alcohol and tobacco. In J. B. Fertig & J. P. Allen (Eds.), *Alcohol and Tobacco: From Basic Science to Clinical Practiced, NIAAA Research Monograph No. 30* (pp. 17–36). Washington, DC: U.S. Government Printing Office.

Sokol, R. J., & Clarren, S. K. (1989). Guidelines for use of terminology describing the impact of prenatal alcohol on the offspring. *Alcoholism: Clinical and Experimental Research, 13*(4), 597–509.

Span, S. A., & Earleywine, M. (1999). Familial risk for alcoholism and hangover symptoms. *Addictive Behaviors, 24*(1), 121–125.

Sue, D. (1987). Use and abuse of alcohol by Asian Americans. *Journal of Psychoactive Drugs, 19*(1), 57–66.

Surgeon General (U. S. Department of Health and Human Services). (1992). *Youth and Alcohol: Dangerous and Deadly Consequences: Report to the Surgeon General.* Bethesda, MD: SAMHSA.

Swift, R., & Davidson, D. (1998). Alcohol hangover: Mechanisms and mediators. *Alcohol Health & Research World, 22*(1), 54–60.

Tabakoff, B., Cornell, N., & Hoffman, P. L. (1992). Alcohol tolerance. *Annals of Emergency Medicine, 15*(9), 1005–1012.

Teng, Y. S. (1981). Human liver aldehyde dehydrogenase in Chinese and Asiatic Indians: Gene deletion and its possible implications in alcohol metabolism. *Biochemical Genetics, 19,* 107–114.

Thun, M. J., Peto, R., Lopez, A. D., Monaco, J. H., Henley, S. J., Heath, C. W., & Doll, R. (1997). Alcohol consumption and mortality among middle-aged and elderly U.S. adults. *New England Journal of Medicine, 337*(24), 1711.

Trice, H. M. (1995). Alcoholics Anonymous. In D. B. Heath, D. B. (Ed.), Alcohol: History. *Encyclopedia of Drugs and Alcohol* (Vol.1, pp. 85–92). New York: Simon & Schuster Macmillan.

U.S. Bureau of the Census. (1999). *http://www.census.gov/population/estimates/nation/intfile3-1.txt.*

U.S. Department of Justice. (1998). *Alcohol and Crime.* Bureau Justice Statistics, Washington, DC.

University of Michigan. (1999). *Monitoring the Future Study.* Rockville, MD: SAMHSA. *http://www.MonitoringThe Future.org.*

Vaillant, G. E. (1995). *The Natural History of Alcoholism Revisited.* Cambridge: Harvard University Press.

Valenzuela, C. F., & Harris, F. A. (1997). Alcohol: Neurobiology. In J. H. Lowinson, P. Ruiz, R. B. Millman, & J. G. Langrod, (Eds.), *Substance Abuse: A Comprehensive Textbook* (3rd ed., pp. 119–141). Baltimore: Williams & Wilkins.

Vitiello, M. V. (1997). Sleep, alcohol, and alcohol abuse. *Addiction Biology, 2,* 151–158.

Vogel-Sprott, M., Rawana, E., & Webster, R. (1984). Mental rehearsal of a task under ethanol facilitates tolerance. *Phar-*

macology, *Biochemistry & Behavior, 21*(3), 329–331.

Volkow, N., Wang, G. J., & Doria, J. J. (1995). Monitoring the brain's response to alcohol with positron emission tomography. *Alcohol World: Health and Research: Imaging in Alcohol Research, 19*(4).

Wallace, G. I. (1989). *New York City streetwalker data.* New York: Foundation for Research on Sexually Transmitted Disease.

Waugh, A. (1968). *Wines and Spirits.* New York: Time-Life Books.

Wechsler, H., Lee, J. E., Kuo, M., & Lee, H. (2000). College Binge Drinking in the 1990s: A continuing problem. *Journal of American College Health, 48*(3).

Westermeyer, J. (1997). Native Americans, Asians, and new immigrants. In J. H. Lowinson, P. Ruiz, R. B. Millman, & J. G. Langrod, (Eds.), *Substance Abuse: A Comprehensive Textbook* (3rd ed., pp. 712–716). Baltimore: Williams & Wilkins.

WHO (World Health Organization). (1999). Health and development in the twentieth century. *The World Health Report, 1999* (p. 16). Geneva: WHO.

Wilson, G. T., & Lawson, D. M. (1976). Effects of alcohol on sexual arousal in women. Journal of Abnormal Psychology, 85, 489–497.

Woodward, J. J. (1998). The pharmacology of alcohol. In A. W. Graham & T. K. Schultz (Eds.), *Principles of Addiction Medicine* (2nd ed., pp. 103–116). Chevy Chase, MD: American Society of Addiction Medicine, Inc.

York, J. L. (1990). High blood alcohol levels in women (Letter). *New England Journal of Medicine, 323*(1), 59–60.

Zane, N. W., & Kim, J. C. (1994). In N. W. Zane, D. T. Takeuchi, and K. N. J. Young (Eds.), *Confronting Critical Health Issues of Asian and Pacific Islander Americans.* Thousand Oaks, CA: Sage Publications.

Zhang, Y., Schatzkin, A., Kreger, B. E., Dorgan, J. F., Splansky, G. L., Cupples, L. A., & Ellison, R. C. (1998). Alcohol consumption and risk of breast cancer: The Framingham study revisited. *American Journal of Epidemiology, 3.*

All Arounders

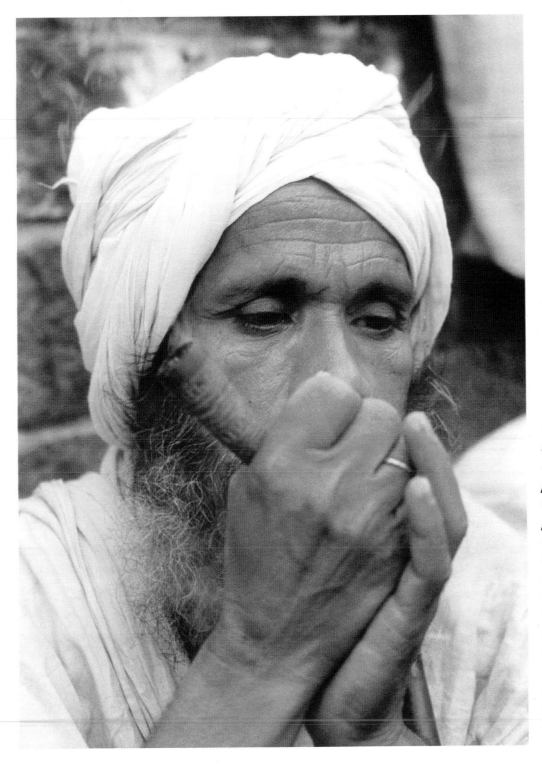

*I*n India, ganja, the stronger leaves and flowering tops of the Cannabis plant, are smoked in chillums, hollow cone-shaped pipes. The smoker cups his hands over the opening at the bottom of the pipe and draws the smoke in through his hands. Charas, the concentrated resin of the marijuana plant, is also called "hashish." "Bhang," the stems and weaker leaves of the Cannabis plant, can also be smoked in a chillum.
Courtesy of Simone Garlaund

- **History:** All arounders have been around since the origin of man; virtually all are found in plants.

- **Classification:** LSD, MDMA, ketamine, psilocybin mushrooms, DMT, PCP, peyote, and especially marijuana are the most commonly used all arounders (also called "hallucinogens" or "psychedelics").

- **General Effects:** Psychedelics cause intensified sensations, crossed sensations (e.g., visual input becomes sound), illusions, delusions, hallucinations, stimulation, impaired judgment, and distorted reasoning.

- **LSD, Psilocybin Mushrooms, & Other Indole Psychedelics:** LSD, an ergot alkaloid, is very potent; it causes stimulation and can induce hallucinations and illusions. Psilocybin mushrooms cause nausea and induce hallucinations. Ibogaine and yage, two other indole psychedelics, are much less widely used.

- **Peyote, MDMA, & Other Phenylalkylamine Psychedelics:** Peyote cacti (mescaline), used in sacred rituals and ceremonies, cause more hallucinations than LSD. Designer psychedelics like MDMA ("ecstasy") are similar to amphetamines but also have calming and psychic effects.

- **Belladonna & Other Anticholinergic Psychedelics:** Plants such as belladonna, jimsonweed, and henbane have been used for more than 3,000 years in ancient cultures, often in rituals and ceremonies.

- **Ketamine, PCP, & Other Psychedelics:** Ketamine is an anesthetic used mainly for animals and occasionally humans. It causes mind-body disassociation, a sensory-deprived state, and hallucinations. PCP is similar to ketamine and produces many of the same effects. It predates ketamine in street popularity. PCP and ketamine are also known as "disassociative anesthetics." Amanita mushrooms, nutmeg, and mace are also psychedelics but rarely used in Europe and the United States.

- **Marijuana & Other Cannabinols:** Marijuana is the most popular illicit psychoactive drug. It magnifies existing personality traits of users. Effects often depend on the mind-set of the user and the setting where used. Recently there has been an intense social and legal battle over the use of marijuana for medical purposes. The 1999 report *Marijuana and Medicine, Assessing the Science Base* from the National Academy of Sciences' Institute of Medicine examines the scientific basis for medical marijuana.

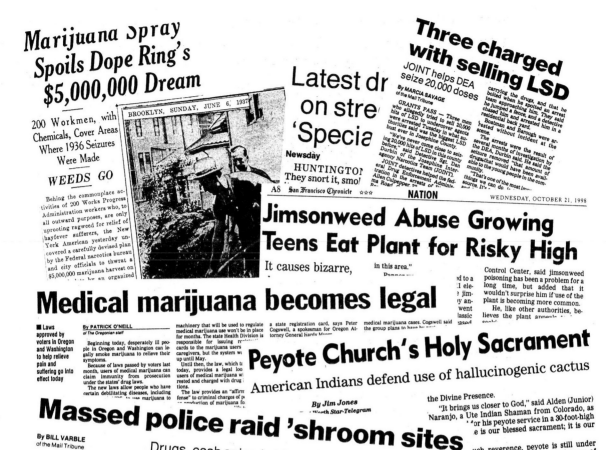

Behind the commonplace activities of 200 Works Progress Administration workers who, to all outward purposes, are only uprooting ragweed for relief of hayfever sufferers, the New York American yesterday uncovered a carefully devised plan by the Federal narcotics bureau and city officials to thwart a $5,000,000 marijuana harvest on ...

Marijuana Spray Spoils Dope Ring's $5,000,000 Dream

200 Workmen, with Chemicals, Cover Areas Where 1936 Seizures Were Made

WEEDS GO

BROOKLYN, SUNDAY, JUNE 6, 1937

Latest dr on stre 'Specia

Newsday

HUNTINGTOI
They snort it, smol

A8 San Francisco Chronicle ☆☆☆

Three charged with selling LSD

JOINT helps DEA
seize 20,000 doses

By MARCIA SAVAGE
of the Mail Tribune

GRANTS PASS — Three men who allegedly tried to sell 20,000 hits of LSD to undercover agents were arrested Tuesday in what authorities said was the biggest LSD bust ever in Josephine County.

"We've never come close to seizing 20,000 hits of LSD in this county before," said Detective Sgt. Dan Durbin of the Josephine County Narcotics Team (JOINT).

JOINT detectives helped the federal Drug Enforcement Administration in the arrests of Allen Culpepper ...

...carrying the drugs, and that he bolted when he spotted an arrest team approaching him. They said he jumped a fence, and a detective chased him and arrested him in a residential back yard.

Boatman and Barough were arrested without incident at the scene.

The arrests were the result of several months of investigation by the DEA, Durbin said. He said the seizure removed "that amount of drugs that would have been available to the young people in the community."

"That's one of the most important things we can do ... source. It's ...

NATION WEDNESDAY, OCTOBER 21, 1998

Jimsonweed Abuse Growing
Teens Eat Plant for Risky High

It causes bizarre, in this area."

...ed to a
...l ele-
...e Jim-
...y an-
went
...lassic
...ased

Control Center, said jimsonweed poisoning has been a problem for a long time, but added that it wouldn't surprise him if use of the plant is becoming more common.

He, like other authorities, believes the plant appeals ...

Medical marijuana becomes legal

■ Laws approved by voters in Oregon and Washington to help relieve pain and suffering go into effect today

By PATRICK O'NEILL
of The Oregonian staff

Beginning today, desperately ill people in Oregon and Washington can legally smoke marijuana to relieve their symptoms.

Because of laws passed by voters last month, users of medical marijuana can claim immunity from prosecution under the states' drug laws.

The new laws allow people who have certain debilitating diseases, including ...

machinery that will be used to regulate medical marijuana use won't be in place for months. The state Health Division is responsible for issuing re... cards to the marijuana users caregivers, but the system w... up until May.

Until then, the law, which t... today, provides a legal loo... users of medical marijuana wi... rested and charged with drug i... tions.

The law provides an "affirm... fense" to criminal charges of p... ...production of marijuana fo...

a state registration card, says Peter Cogswell, a spokesman for Oregon Attorney General Hardy My...

medical marijuana cases. Cogswell said the group plans to have b...

Peyote Church's Holy Sacrament

American Indians defend use of hallucinogenic cactus

By Jim Jones
Worth Star-Telegram

the Divine Presence.

"It brings us closer to God," said Alden (Junior) Naranjo, a Ute Indian Shaman from Colorado, as ...or his peyote service in a 30-foot-high ...e is our blessed sacrament; it is our

Massed police raid 'shroom sites

By BILL VARBLE
of the Mail Tribune

Drugs, cash seized at 20 locations

More than 100 federal and local law enforcement officers swooped down Thursday on at least 20 Josephine County locations suspected of being part of the largest psilocybin mushroom growing and distributing system in the country.

Police spokesmen in Jackson and Josephine counties were tight-lipped about the operation Thurs...

only one person had been arrested, he said.

"It's all federal search warrants," he said. "The feds aren't arresting people at these locations. They're gathering evidence, and down the road they'll present it to a grand jury."

"It's not the way we do business," he said. "We'd arrest everybody ...

for three years, during which some 250 pounds of hallucinogenic mushrooms have been seized in rural Oregon and locations in California, Kansas and Vermont.

Officers have seized approximately $195,000 in cash from three suspects and smaller amounts from others during the investigation, Daniel said.

Roseburg and Brookings in addition to Oregon State Police and the U.S. Attorney's Office in Eugene.

Daniel said officials believe Josephine County is a center for the largest growing and distribution system for hallucinogenic mushrooms in the United States.

"I don't how we get this kind of designation," he said.

Warrants stemming from the investigation earlier led to raids and ...

uch reverence, peyote is still under ...troversial hallucinogen, the source of ...s and legal disputes for decades. Even ...e American tribes are skeptical of its

...nforcement officials classify peyote, a ...oice for hippies in the '60s, in the same

---

HISTORY

"I got into marijuana and particularly LSD in the university setting in the late 1960s where we all felt it was a spiritual thing. We went to Dead concerts, Grateful Dead that is. We traveled around to wherever they were playing. Also I went to about 20 Santana concerts. Later on we got out of it because everybody started doing it and doing it just to get loaded—no spirituality there. Some could maintain while they were taking LSD, some

just became idiots. I started just after my 17th birthday. Nowadays kids get into it when they're 12."

48-year-old former psychedelic abuser

The headlines that concern psychedelics (hallucinogens) usually focus on marijuana, LSD, MDMA ("ecstasy"), and ketamine. The articles talk about the legacy of the 1960s, unusual effects, medical uses, availability, and dangers. Psychedelics have probably been used since the origin of man due to the fact that so many are found in plants. Plant fossils 3.2 billion years old have been found, so it is reasonable

to assume that plants that could affect animal and human brains to induce hallucinations and illusions were also around and predated the dinosaurs (Schultes & Hofmann, 1992). When primitive man and woman came on the scene a few million years ago, they probably stumbled across these plants, tried them as food, and had hallucinogenic experiences (Siegel, 1985).

Over the years Neanderthal men and women and eventually shamans, witches, and healers experimented with different methods of ingestion: boiling and drinking, smoking, eating, or absorbing (through the nasal passages, the gums, or the skin). Even

THE FAR SIDE   By GARY LARSON

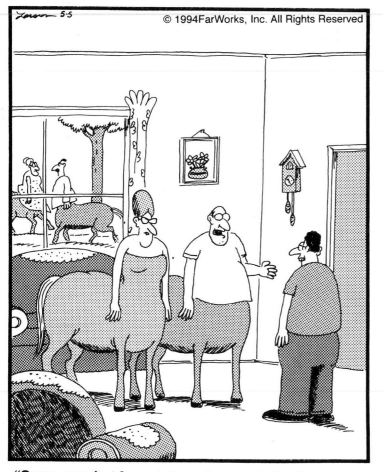

"Sorry, son, but for you to understand what happened, you have to first understand that back in the '60s we were all taking a lot of drugs."

after the hypodermic needle was invented 150 years ago, hallucinogens were rarely injected since the object of using them was to alter one's consciousness and perception of reality rather than to induce a rush or euphoria.

Historically amanita mushrooms were eaten in India and pre-Columbian Mexico, belladonna was drunk in ancient Greece and medieval Europe, marijuana was inhaled and eaten in ancient China and Scythia, and poisonous ergot, found in rye mold (a natural form of LSD), was accidentally eaten in renaissance Europe. No matter where explorers and anthropologists ventured, they found that every culture had discovered and was using a psychoactive substance from some natural source (Goldstein, 1994).

In the twenty-first century, even though psychedelics can still be found in every country, the majority of these drugs are grown and used in the Americas, Europe, and Africa (the major exception is marijuana, which is grown in most countries). Hundreds of primitive tribes in the Americas, such as the Aztecs and Toltecs in the past and the Kiowas and Huichols in the present, have used peyote, psilocybin mushrooms, yage, and morning glory seeds among others for religious, social, ceremonial, and medical reasons (Diaz, 1979; Efferink, 1988).

Recently there has been an upsurge of interest in psychedelics; LSD, MDMA ("ecstasy," "rave"), and even psilocybin mushrooms ("'shrooms") are found in colleges, high schools, and even middle schools throughout the United States. The percentage of high school seniors who used LSD in the past month surged in 1994 and 1995 and has leveled off since then (2.7% used LSD in 1999). It is about the same percentage that used cocaine in the past month (2.6% in 1999). Interest in marijuana, the most widely used psychedelic, had been declining since 1979 but in the past few years, use has begun to rise again (23.1% of high school seniors used in the past month in 1999, double the amount in 1992) (University of Michigan, 1999). Psychedelic use, as in the 1960s and '70s, was and still is most popular among young White users, then Hispanic users, and finally, the lowest per capita use, the Black community (SAMHSA, 1999; National Institute of Justice, 1997).

CLASSIFICATION

Uppers stimulate the body and downers depress it. All arounders usually act as stimulants and occasionally as depressants but mostly they distort a user's perception of the world and create a world in which logic takes a back seat to intensified confused sensations (Weil & Rosen, 1993). From alphabet soup psychedelics (LSD, PCP, MDMA) to naturally occurring plants used socially or in religious ceremonies (marijuana, peyote, mushrooms, belladonna), all arounders represent a diverse group of substances.

The five main classes of psychedelics are (1) the indole psychedelics (e.g., LSD and psilocybin); (2) the phenylalkylamines (e.g., mescaline and "ecstasy"); (3) the anticholinergics (e.g., belladonna); (4) those in a class by themselves (e.g., PCP); and (5) the cannabinols found in marijuana (*Cannabis*) plants.

TABLE 6–1 ALL AROUNDERS (PSYCHEDELICS)

Common Names	Active Ingredients	Street Names
INDOLE PSYCHEDELICS		
LSD (LSD-25 & -49) (schedule I)	Lysergic acid diethylamide	Acid, sugar cube, window pane, blotter, illusion, boomers, yellow sunshine
Mushrooms (schedule I)	Psilocybin	'Shrooms, magic mushrooms
Tabernanthe iboga (schedule I)	Ibogaine	African LSD
Morning glory seeds or Hawaiian woodrose	Lysergic acid amide	Heavenly blue, pearly gates, wedding bells, ololiuqui
DMT (synthetic or from yopo beans, epena, or Sonoran Desert toad) (schedule I)	Dimethyltryptamine	Businessman's special, cohoba snuff
Yage, ayahuasca, caapi	Harmaline (also mixed with DMT)	Visionary vine, vine of the soul, vine of death, mihi, kahi
PHENYLALKYLAMINE PSYCHEDELICS		
Peyote cactus (schedule I)	Mescaline	Mesc, peyote, buttons
STP (DOM) (synthetic) (schedule I)	4 methyl 2,5 dimethoxy-amphetamine	Serenity, tranquillity, peace pill
STP-LSD combo	Dimethoxy-amphetamine with LSD	Wedge series, orange and pink wedges, Harvey Wallbanger
Designer psychedelics, e.g., MDA, MDMA (MDM), MMDA, MDE (schedule I)	Variations of methylene-dioxy amphetamines	Ecstasy, rave, love drug, XTC, Adam, Eve
2CB or CBR (schedule I)	4 bromo 2,5 dimethoxy phenethylamine	Nexus
U4Euh (schedule I)	4 methyl pemoline	Euphoria
ANTICHOLINERGICS		
Belladonna, mandrake, henbane, datura (jimson weed, thornapple), wolfbane (schedule I)	Atropine, scopolamine, hyoscyamine	Deadly nightshade
Artane®	Trihexypheneidyl	
Cogentin®	Benztropine	
Asmador® cigarettes	Belladonna alkaloids	
OTHER PSYCHEDELICS		
PCP (schedule II)	Phencyclidine	Angel dust, hog, peace pill, krystal joint, ozone, Sherms, Shermans
Ketamine (schedule II)	Ketajet®, Ketalar®	Special K, K, vitamin K, super-K
Nutmeg and mace	Myristicin	
Amanita mushrooms (fly agaric) (schedule I)	Ibotenic acid, muscimole	Soma
Kava root	Alpha pyrones	Kava-kava
CANNABINOLS		
Marijuana (schedule I) (Marinol® is legal	Δ-9-tetrahydrocannabinol (THC)	Grass, pot, weed, Mary Jane, joint, reefer, dank, dubie, mota, prescription THC, blunt, honey blunt, chronic, sens, stink weed, herb, charas, ganja, grifa, the kind, bhang, ditch weed, Colombian, Canadian black
Sinsemilla (schedule I)	High potency, seedless flowering tops female marijuana plant	Sens, skunk weed, ganja
Hashish, hash oil (schedule I)	THC (pressed resin or extracted resin of marijuana)	Hash

GENERAL EFFECTS

ASSESSING THE EFFECTS

Unlike stimulants and depressants that have been well researched, psychedelics are manufactured or grown illegally, so with the exception of marijuana, much of the information about the effects is anecdotal or the result of surveys rather than extended scientific testing. Since many psychedelics contain more than one active ingredient, it is hard to say which chemical is causing certain effects. Also many drugs that are sold as one psychedelic may actually be another cheaper psychedelic, so even the anecdotal information can be incorrect. Some common examples of misrepresentation are PCP sold as THC (the active ingredient in marijuana) or regular mushrooms sprinkled with LSD and sold as psychedelic mushrooms (Weil & Rosen, 1993).

The effects of many psychedelics are dependent on the specific toxicity of the substance and especially on the amount of drug ingested. A drug like LSD is thousands of times more powerful by weight than a similar amount of peyote. The effects of a 25-microgram dose of LSD are quite different than the effects of a 250-microgram dose.

Experience with the drug, the basic emotional makeup of the user, the mood and mental state at the time of use, any preexisting mental illnesses, and the surroundings in which the drug is taken are also crucial to the kind, duration, and intensity of the effects. For instance a first- or second-time psychedelic user may become nauseous, extremely anxious, depressed, and totally disoriented, whereas an experienced user may only experience euphoric feelings or some mild illusions. A user with a tendency towards schizophrenia or major depression could get a severe reaction from LSD because it might trigger any unstable tendencies. Someone who is basically aggressive might become violent when using PCP, whereas a young and immature user of marijuana could become more child-like.

PHYSICAL & MENTAL EFFECTS

LSD and most other hallucinogens stimulate the sympathetic nervous system. This stimulation results in a rise in pulse rate and blood pressure. Many psychedelics can trigger sweating, palpitations, or nausea.

Generally psychedelics interfere with neurotransmitters such as dopamine, norepinephrine, acetylcholine, anandamide, and especially serotonin. Because serotonin neurons are amply represented in the limbic system, the emotional center of the brain, most psychedelics greatly affect mood. Serotonin S2 receptors are especially affected by the indole psychedelics such as LSD. The strength of most psychedelics is related directly to their influence of the S2 receptors (Snyder, 1996).

The stimulation of the brainstem, and specifically the reticular formation, can overload the sensory pathways, making the user very conscious of all sensation. Disruption of visual and auditory centers can confuse perception. An auditory stimulation such as the sound of music might jump to a visual pathway, causing the music to be "seen" as shifting light patterns, or visual impulses might shift to auditory neurons, resulting in strange sounds. This crossover or mixing of the senses is known as "**synesthesia.**" Some practitioners of Buddhism, Christianity, and other religions or other forms of mysticism say that many psychedelic experiences are similar to the transcendental state of mind achieved through deep meditation (Snyder, 1996).

It is important to note the differences between an illusion, a delusion, and a hallucination. An **illusion** is a mistaken perception of a real stimulus (synesthesia). For example, a rope can be misinterpreted as a snake or smooth skin as silk. A **delusion** is a mistaken idea that is not swayed by reason. An example is someone who thinks he can fly or thinks he has become deformed or ugly. A **hallucination** is a sensory experience that doesn't relate to reality, such as seeing a creature or object which doesn't exist. With LSD and most psychedelics, illusions and delusions are the primary experiences. With mescaline, psilocybin, and PCP, hallucinations are the primary experience.

LSD, PSILOCYBIN MUSHROOMS, & OTHER INDOLE PSYCHEDELICS

LSD (lysergic acid diethylamide)

History (*also see Chapter 1*)

"LSD was very colorful, a super rush, magical, trippy, giggly, sometimes scary. I was called the 'King of Acid' because I always had a very good trip unlike some friends who took it every day. I waited at least three or four days in between trips because your body needs some time to recover. My friends who used it daily, they got pretty burnt out with insomnia, grinding teeth, and exhaustion because of the total nerve action."
48-year-old accountant, former "Deadhead"

"Acid," "blotter," "barrels," "sunshine," "illusion," and "window panes" are just some of the street names for LSD, a semisynthetic form of the chemicals produced by *Claviceps purpurea,* an ergot fungus toxin that infects rye and other cereal grasses. The active ingredient in ergot contains lysergic acid diethylamide (LSD). Historically many outbreaks of ergot poisoning (ergotism) occurred when people accidentally ate the infected grain, particularly in Europe and Russia. Thousands died from the symptoms caused by ingesting large amounts of the brownish-purple fungus. There are two types of ergotism, gangrenous and convulsive. **Gangrenous ergotism,** also known as "St. Anthony's Fire," is marked by feverish hallucinations and falling away of gangrenous extremities of the body. The gangrene is caused by the extreme vasoconstriction of small blood vessels that causes the unnourished tissues to die. **Convulsive ergotism** is marked by visual and auditory hallucinations, painful muscular contractions, vomiting, diarrhea, headaches, disturbances in sensation, mania, psychosis, delirium, and convulsions (Siegel, 1985).

LSD was first derived in 1938 at Sandoz Pharmaceuticals by Dr. Albert Hoffman when he and Dr. Arthur Stoll were investigating the alkaloids of *Claviceps purpurea*. LSD (technically LSD-25) was the 25th derivative the doctors tried. Five years later Dr. Hoffman discovered the hallucinogenic properties of the new drug when he accidentally ingested a dose of LSD while developing a new way to chemically synthesize it in his laboratory.

"I suddenly became strangely inebriated. The external world became changed as in a dream. Objects appeared to gain in relief; they assumed unusual dimensions; and colors became more glowing. Even self-perception and the sense of time were changed. When the eyes were closed, there surged upon me an uninterrupted stream of fantastic images of extraordinary plasticity and vividness and accompanied by an intense, kaleidoscope-like play of colors. After about two hours, the not unpleasant inebriation, which had been experienced whilst I was fully conscious, disappeared.

[Another time] I lost all control of time; space and time became more and more disorganized and I was overcome with fears that I was going crazy. The worst part of it was that I was clearly aware of my condition though I was incapable of stopping it. Occasionally I felt as being outside my body. I thought I had died."

Albert Hoffman in 1943 describing one of his experiences with LSD (Stafford, 1992)

LSD was investigated as a therapy for mental illnesses, as a key to investigating thought processes, and as a possible weapon for chemical warfare and mind control (Marnell, 1997). In the early 1950s the CIA conducted a number of experiments with LSD as a truth drug or mind-control drug in a program code-named "MK-ULTRA." The drug did not do what was expected and the program was discontinued in the mid-1960s (Stafford, 1985).

LSD-25 was popularized by Drs. Timothy Leary and Richard Alpert, psychologists at Harvard who did psilocybin and LSD research in the 1960s as a way to explore consciousness and feelings. They emphasized the mind-expanding qualities of the drug and looked on use as something other than just getting loaded. Dr. Leary's first experience with a large amount of LSD kept him "unable to speak for five days." He wrote that he never recovered from that mind-shattering experience. He even started a religion called the "**L**eague for **S**piritual **D**iscovery"

(Stafford, 1992). Dr. Leary's slogan, "Turn on, tune in, and drop out," was used in endless newspaper articles and TV news shows as the rallying cry for youth of the 1960s and 1970s. (It led to the suspicion that the media was as much responsible for the rise and fall of LSD as was its identification and subsequent vilification as the drug of the hippie generation).

In 1965 the Federal Drug Abuse Control Amendments made LSD illegal starting February 1, 1966. In 1966 Sandoz Pharmaceuticals withdrew Delysid® (the trade name for LSD-25). In 1974 the National Institute of Mental Health concluded that LSD had no therapeutic use (Henderson & Glass, 1994). Scientific research virtually ceased in the early 1970s and it wasn't until recently that any research on LSD or psychedelics in general was renewed. LSD use continued to decline in the 1980s but in the '90s there was a resurgence in its popularity.

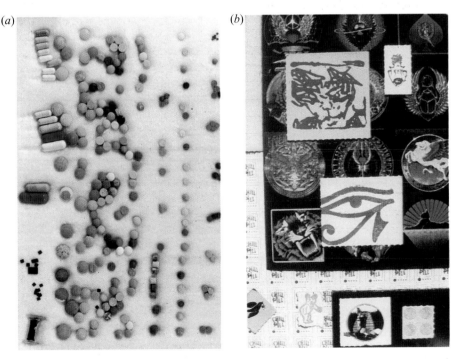

(a)   *(b)*

The effective dose of LSD is so small that it can be delivered in many guises. In the past, tablets, capsules, microdots, a drop on a sugar cube, a saturated bit of gelatin, or a drop on a piece of blotter paper were used (a). Presently "blotter acid" is the preferred method of use (b). Liquid LSD is deposited on a sheet of blotter paper. Each perforated square contains anywhere from 30–50 micrograms of the drug. In the 1960s and '70s, they contained 100–300 micrograms.

Epidemiology

Younger and younger Americans are currently using LSD. Anecdotal reports at the Haight-Ashbury Clinic indicate that low doses of LSD are abused on occasion by junior high and high school students while they are sitting in class. This is because low-dose use results in less detectable physical symptoms (e.g., stimulation) than alcohol or marijuana, only mild psychedelic effects, and low costs—one dollar to five dollars a hit. In the 1960s "acidheads" were usually in their early '20s and many were searching for a quasi-religious experience. In the 1990s younger teenagers said they mostly just wanted to get high and escape harsh realities.

Besides the usual reasons for using a drug like LSD (experimentation, peer pressure, availability, and curiosity), there are three other factors that have spurred current usage. One is the proliferation of "rave" clubs and parties where MDMA, LSD, ketamine, GHB, and amphetamines are utilized (Pechnick & Ungerleider, 1997). Another reason is that standard drug testing usually does not test for LSD and even when tested for, the effective dose is so small that it is almost impossible to detect. Finally low-dose "blotter acid," 30–50 micrograms of LSD, results in less toxic reactions than in the past, so some users take it on a daily basis.

Manufacture of LSD

"We had Palo Alto Owsley stuff—Augustus Stanley Owsley. He ran the sound for the Grateful Dead for years.

He made pure LSD and no additives or bad chemistry. I started with 200 'mics' then up to 400. The best dose was 100 to 150. If we were out of doors, we would only take 50, so we'd still be able to navigate. Back in 1969 and the early '70s, it cost about one to three dollars a hit."

48-year-old former LSD user

The majority of LSD is manufactured in northern California, mostly in the San Francisco Bay area, although there is some secondary manufacture in Los Angeles by street gangs (NIDA Advisory Council, 1999). The labs are hard to find since the quantities of raw material needed to make the drug are very small. Indeed the entire U.S. supply for one year could be carried by one person. For example, 60 pounds of ergotamine tartrate, the basic synthetic raw ingredient for LSD, could produce 11 pounds of LSD, the nation's annual consumption (Marnell, 1997). LSD can also be synthesized from morning glory plants that contain lysergic acid amide. The production of LSD is tedious and involves volatile and dangerous chemicals. Crystalline LSD, the end product of the initial synthesis, is dissolved in alcohol and drops of the solution are put on blotter paper and chewed or swallowed. It has also been put into microdots or tiny squares of gelatin and eaten or dropped onto a moist body tissue and absorbed (Stafford, 1992).

To reach the younger group of potential users, illegal manufacturers even

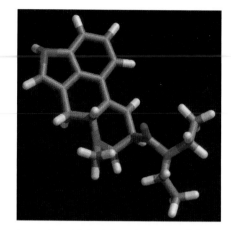

Lysergic acid diethylamide is derived from chemicals in the ergot fungus or from synthetic ergotamine tartrate.

Courtesy of the Molecular Imaging Department, University of California Medical Center, San Francisco

use Mickey Mouse, Donald Duck, a teddy bear, and other characters printed on the blotter paper. In 1999 about 2.7% of high school seniors said they use it on a monthly basis.

Pharmacology

LSD ($C_{20}H_{25}N_3O$) is remarkable for its potency. Doses as low as 25 micrograms (mics) or 25 millionths of a gram, can cause mental changes (spaciness, decreased perception of time, mild euphoria) and mild stimulatory effects. One pound of LSD is sufficient to make up to 9 million hits of the drug.

Effects appear 15 minutes to 1 hour after ingestion and last 6–8 hours. The usual psychedelic dose of LSD is 150–300 mics. Low-dose use of 30–50 mics acts more like a stimulant than a psychedelic. The DEA reports that the current strength of LSD street samples ranges from 20–80 mics and each dose costs $1 to $10. In the late 1960s and '70s, samples ranged from 100–200 mics or more (NIDA INFOFAX, 1998). Tolerance to the psychedelic effects of LSD develops very rapidly. Within a few days of daily use, a person can tolerate a 300-mic dose without experiencing any major psychedelic effects. The tolerance is lost rapidly after cessation of use—usually within a few days. Some cross-tolerance can also develop

TABLE 6–2 30-DAY PREVALENCE OF LSD AMONG 8th, 10th, & 12th GRADERS

	1975	1985	1991	1993	1995	1997	1999
8th Grade	—	—	0.6%	1.0%	1.4%	1.5%	1.1%
10th Grade	—	—	1.5%	1.6%	3.0%	2.8%	2.3%
12th Grade	2.3%	1.6%	1.9%	2.4%	4.0%	3.1%	2.7%

The use of LSD by high school students in general started climbing in 1991 after years of decline. The use of LSD for those who have been arrested is double the above figures (University of Michigan, 1999).

to the effects of mescaline and psilocybin but there is little cross-tolerance between LSD and DMT (Pechnick & Ungerleider, 1997).

"When we took it every day, we got off less 'cause we depleted our brain chemistry, and you just get burned out, and you have to take twice as much. Some had to take five times as much, about 2,000 mics to get any reaction, like a depleted 'speed' freak, like in a cloud."
28-year-old former LSD user

Withdrawal after LSD use is usually more mental and emotional than physical—a psychedelic hangover.

"Withdrawal was like the next day; the Germans call it 'Katzenjammer,' which is like a chemical depletion of mind and body, similar to a really bad hangover. You're still psychedelically spaced the next day and you're dealing with all the revelations. Dependence was more of a social urge to do it rather than a private urge."
24-year-old former LSD user

Several years ago a new version of the drug called "LSD-49" (instead of the old designation, LSD-25) appeared on the streets. Called "illusion," it seems to give more intense visual effects than an equal amount of the original LSD-25. It is still unclear whether LSD-49 really exists or if it is just a new street name for LSD-25.

Physical Effects

LSD can cause a rise in heart rate and blood pressure, a higher body temperature, dizziness, dilated pupils, and some sweating, much like amphetamines. Users see many light trails, like after-images in cheap televisions where there is always an after-image of whatever is happening on camera (this after-effect is known as the "trailing phenomena").

"In a real strong 'acid' you'll see the walls melting like candles and water running down the wall. That kind of distortion is not a complete hallucination or anything real solid like a bottle where you wonder whether it's there or not. The thing that got me really crazy was hearing a dog or airplane or passenger car miles away and you didn't know whether that was real or an illusion. There was also what we called the psychedelic hummmmmm that we thought we heard."
Recovering 38-year-old LSD and marijuana user

Mental Effects

Mentally LSD overloads the brainstem, the sensory switchboard for the mind, causing sensory distortions (seeing sounds, feeling smells, or hearing colors), dreaminess, depersonalization, altered mood, and impaired concentration and motivation. The locus coeruleus is activated to release extra amounts of norepinephrine, which greatly enhances alertness. This heightened awareness of the senses is possibly responsible for the introspection and awareness of the inner self that is common with LSD users (Snyder, 1996).

It becomes difficult to express oneself verbally while on LSD. Single word answers and seemingly nonassociated comments (non-sequiturs) are common. A user might experience intense sensations and emotions but find it difficult to tell others what he or she is feeling.

One of the greatest dangers of LSD is the loss of judgment and impaired reasoning. This, coupled with slowed reaction time and visual distortions, can make the driving of a car or a simple camping trip risky.

"I stuck my hand in this flame and then I went, 'Uh-oh, my hand is in the flame,' and I pulled it out and I thought it didn't burn but later that night, my hand started blistering and I'm going, 'Oh no, I got burned.'"
43-year-old former LSD user

Bad Trips (acute anxiety reactions)

Because LSD affects the emotional center in the brain and distorts reality, a user, particularly a first-time user, is subject to the extremes of euphoria and panic. Depersonalization and lack of a stable environment can trigger acute anxiety, paranoia, fear over loss of control, and delusions of persecution or feelings of grandeur leading to dangerous behaviors. One survivor of a jump from the Golden Gate Bridge claimed he was jumping through a golden hoop. (*See Chapter 9 concerning treatment for bad trips.*)

"I've done 'acid' one time. I took a couple of hits, you know, little tabs, and walls started melting and everything like that. Everybody started looking like monsters and just weird crazy shit, man. I was freaking out. I had a real bad trip that time, worse than the "shrooms.' I was too scared to do that ever again."
15-year-old polydrug abuser in recovery

Mental Illness & LSD

Much of the research, as well as enthusiasm for LSD as an adjunct to psychotherapy, has decreased over the years. Proponents of psychotherapeutic use claim that drug-stimulated insights afford some users a shortcut to the extended process of psychotherapy where uncovering traumas and conflicts from the unconsciousness helps to heal the patient. Opponents of this kind of therapy say that the dangerous side effects of LSD more than outweigh any benefit.

The popular picture of someone using LSD just one time and becoming permanently psychotic or schizophrenic is incorrect. It is an unusual occurrence. What usually happens is that in people with a preexisting mental instability, LSD use nudges those tendencies into more severe mental disturbances. Use can also cause people to experience their mental illness at an earlier age or it may provoke a relapse in someone who has previously suffered a psychotic disorder or a major depression.

"The whole thing started with my schizophrenia. That always plays a part. And any time I get too involved in the music scene, the 'acid' starts to trigger the schizophrenia, like flashbacks, and sometimes it makes me want to use. But I'm drawn to it like a moth drawn to a light."
Recovering LSD user with schizophrenia

Also some otherwise normal users can be thrown into a temporary but prolonged psychotic reaction or severe depression that requires extended treatment. In addition prolonged trips (extended LSD effects) devoid of other psychiatric symptoms have also occurred. Though very rare these reactions can be emotionally crippling and may last for years.

A number of users experience mental flashbacks of sensations or a bad trip they had when under the influence of LSD even when they have not used any drugs in several months or even years. The flashbacks, which can be triggered by stress, the use of another psychoactive drug, or even exercise, recreate the original experience (much like the posttraumatic stress phenomenon). This sensation can also cause anxiety and even panic since it is unexpected and the user seems to have little control over its recurrence. Most flashbacks are provoked by some sensory stimulus: sight, sound, odor, or touch. It has been estimated that flashbacks occur in about 23% to 64% of regular LSD users (Hollister, 1984; Carroll & Comer, 1998; Jaffe, 1989). Although the LSD flashback appears to be similar to a posttraumatic stress disorder, recent case reports suggest that medications like sertraline and naltrexone may be useful in treating this problem (Wilkins, Gorelick & Conner, 1998; Young, 1997; Lerner, Oyffe, Issacs & Sigal, 1997).

Dependence

Since LSD does not produce compulsive drug-seeking behavior, it is not considered addictive though some use it frequently. Five hundred LSD trips or more are reported by some users—a psychological dependence rather than a physical dependence, although tolerance does develop rapidly.

"MAGIC MUSHROOMS" (psilocybin & psilocin)

"We tried strawberry psilocybin or rather psilocin, a synthetic version of psilocybin. The second batch we got was pink and we called that 'pink silly.' Then we tried 'Czeckoslovakian microdot.' The psilocybin was very similar to LSD. There was a lot of romantic adventure. I remember eating rhododendron flowers in the park. All the flowers were smiling. After concerts the music would continue in my head for hours. There wasn't much difference but you didn't know if the psilocin was really LSD."
48-year-old refugee from the 1960s

Psilocybin and psilocin are the active ingredients in a number of psychedelic mushrooms found in Mexico, the United States, South America, Southeast Asia, and Europe. These mushrooms, originally called *"Teonanacatl"* (divine flesh) by the Aztecs, were especially important to Indian cultures in Mexico and some other areas in the pre-Colombian Americas and were used in ceremonies dating as far back as 1000 B.C. More than 200 stone sculptures of mushrooms have been found in El Salvador, Guatemala, and parts of Mexico (Furst, 1976). The existence of a mushroom cult that flourished from 100 B.C. to A.D. 400 has been found in northwestern Mexico (Schultes & Hofmann, 1992). They are still used today, although persecution by the Spaniards, who conquered much of Central and South America in the sixteenth and seventeenth centuries, drove the ceremonial use of mushrooms underground for hundreds of years. It wasn't until the 1950s that much was known about the ceremonies conducted

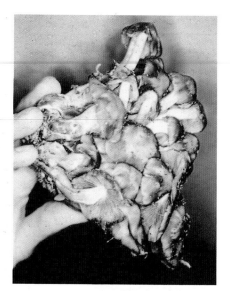

One of the 75 species of mushrooms containing psilocybin or psilocin. The "shrooms" can be used fresh or dried, although fresh psilocybin mushrooms are more potent than dried ones.
Courtesy of the Allan Richardson Estate

by Mazatec, Chol, and Lacandon Mayan shamans or curanderas (medicine women or men). The ceremonies include eating or drinking the extracted psychedelic substances in order to get intoxicated, along with hours of chanting, all to induce visions that will help treat illnesses, solve problems, or get in contact with the spirit world.

The famous Mazatec shaman María Sabina wrote,

"The sacred mushroom takes me by the hand and brings me to the world where everything is known. It is they, the sacred mushrooms, that speak in a way I can understand. When I return from the trip that I have taken with them, I tell what they have told me and what they have shown me."
María Sabina (Schultes & Hofmann, 1992)

Pharmacology

In 1956 the active psychedelic ingredients psilocybin and psilocin were isolated by mycologist (mushroom expert) Roger Heim and researcher Dr. Albert Hoffman, the same scientist at

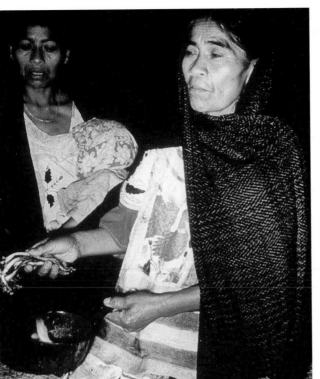

The Mazatec curandera (shaman) María Sabina blesses psylocybin mushrooms before a ceremony.
Courtesy of the Allan Richardson Estate

There is a small market for mail order kits containing spores for growing mushrooms in a closet or basement. Some users also tramp the countryside looking for a certain species. The major danger in "'shroom" harvesting is mistaking poisonous mushrooms for those containing psilocybin. Some poisonous mushrooms (e.g., *Amanita phalloides*) can cause death or permanent liver damage within hours of ingestion. Further, grocery-bought mushrooms are then laced with LSD or PCP and often sold to those seeking the "magic mushroom" experience.

OTHER INDOLE PSYCHEDELICS

Ibogaine

Produced by the African *Tabernanthe iboga* shrub and some other plants, ibogaine is a long-acting psychedelic and stimulant. In low doses it acts as a stimulant and in higher doses it can produce psychedelic effects and a self-determined catatonic reaction that can be maintained up to two days. It is rarely found in the United States, although it has been synthesized in laboratories. Its use is generally limited to native cultures in western and central Africa such as the Bwiti tribe of Gabon. They use it to help them stay alert and motionless while hunting (O'Brien, Cohen, Evans, & Fine, 1990). They also claim to experience ancestral visions while using it.

Recently there has been research into the use of ibogaine to treat heroin addiction. Anecdotal reports, as well as a few limited studies, claim that just a few treatments eliminated withdrawal symptoms and craving for opioids. However, several deaths have been associated with ibogaine administration. Also animal studies indicate cerebellum neurotoxicity results from ibogaine use. These concerns have effectively limited further research into ibogaine as a medical treatment of heroin dependence (Wilkins, 1998).

Morning Glory Seeds (ololiuqui)

These seeds from the *Turbina* plant (morning glory plant also called the

Sandoz Pharmaceutical who had discovered LSD-25. Psilocybin and psilocin are found in about 75 different species of mushroom from 4 genera: *Psilocybe, Panaeolus, Stropharia,* and *Conocybe* (Schultes & Hofmann, 1992). Fifteen species have been identified in the U.S. Pacific Northwest. Psychic effects are obtained from doses of 10 mg to 60 mg and generally last for three to six hours.

Both wild and cultivated mushrooms vary greatly in strength, so a single potent mushroom might have as much psilocybin as 10 weak ones. When the caps and stems are ingested, either fresh or dried, the psilocybin is converted to psilocin. However, psilocybin is more plentiful and is almost twice as potent as psilocin. It also crosses the blood-brain barrier more readily. Its chemical structure is similar to that of LSD.

Effects

Most mushrooms containing psilocybin cause nausea and other physical symptoms before the psychedelic effects take over. The psychedelic effects include visceral sensations, changes in sight, hearing, taste, and touch, and altered states of consciousness. There seems to be less disassociation and panic than with LSD. Prolonged psychotic reactions are rare. However, these effects are not consistent with every user and depend on the setting in which the drug is taken. As with LSD and other indole psychedelics, many of the effects are caused by disruption of the neurotransmitters serotonin and dopamine, along with the sudden release of norepinephrine, a stimulatory neurotransmitter that supersensitizes the senses (Pechnick, 1997).

"We were living in an Indian village in the mountains of central Mexico where the 'hongos' [mushrooms] grow. One night when it rained, the locals were shouting, 'hongos mañana' and they were right. We got some and it made all the colors seem softer and more pastel. My body felt like there was a river running through it and all sorts of visceral feelings were let loose. The environment was fortunately non-threatening."

Former psychedelic user

"Hawaiian woodrose") contain several LSD-like substances, particularly lysergic acid amide, which is about 1/10 as potent as LSD. The lysergic acid amide can be used to make lysergic acid diethylamide (LSD). Used by Indians in Mexico before the Spanish arrived, several hundred seeds have to be taken to get high, so the nauseating properties of the drug are magnified. In sufficient quantities the seeds cause LSD-like effects but they are not particularly popular among those who use psychedelics. Along with sensory disturbances and mood changes come the nausea, vomiting, drowsiness, headaches, chills, and other physical disturbances. Effects last up to six hours and LSD-like flashbacks are somewhat common. Morning glory seeds are sold commercially but to prevent misuse, many of these seeds are dipped in a toxic substance that induces vomiting (O'Brien et al., 1990). The seeds have street names such as "heavenly blue" and "pearly gates."

DMT (dimethyltryptamine)

Dimethyltryptamine is a naturally occurring, easily synthesized psychedelic substance similar in structure to psilocin. Since digestive juices destroy the active ingredients, the drug, which is usually a white, yellow, or brown powder, is snorted or injected but usually smoked. South American tribes have used it for at least 400 years. They prepare it from several different plants as a snuff called "yopo," "cohoba," "vilca," "cebil," or "epena." They blow it into each other's noses through a hollow reed and then dance, hallucinate, and sing. The synthetic form can be made in basement laboratories (Schultes & Hofmann, 1992).

DMT causes intense visual rather than auditory hallucinations, intoxication, and often a loss of awareness of surroundings lasting about 30–60 minutes or less. The short duration of action gave rise to the nickname "businessman's special" because the white-collar worker can get high and almost sober during lunch.

Newspaper reports have sensationalized a variant of DMT, 5-MeO-DMT, the venom of the Sonoran Desert toad. Contrary to anecdotes about people licking the toad to get high, the substance is milked onto cigarettes, dried, and smoked (Lyttle, Goldstein, & Gartz, 1996; Chilton, Bigwood, & Jensen, 1979).

Yage

Yage or ayahuasca is a psychedelic drink made from the leaves, bark, and vines of *Banisteriopsis caapi* and *Banisteriopsis inebrians,* Amazon Jungle vines. Drinking this preparation causes intense vomiting, diarrhea, and then a dreamlike condition that usually lasts up to 10 hours. The Chama, Tukanoan, and Zaparo Indians of Peru, Brazil, and Ecuador use it for prophecy, divination, sorcery, and medical purposes. They believe that yage frees the soul to wander at will and return at will and communicate with ancestors (Schultes & Hofmann, 1992).

The active ingredient is harmaline, an indole alkaloid found in several other psychedelic plants, such as the Syrian rue herb from China. Native cultures often mix yage with DMT plant extracts in order to intensify the effects of their psychedelic beverage. It has been recently discovered that harmaline protects the DMT from being deactivated by gastric enzymes, thus allowing DMT to be effective when taken orally.

In the last few years, cults using ayahuasca as the focus of their beliefs have sprung up in Brazil. The use has spread to the United States and other countries.

PEYOTE, MDMA, & OTHER PHENYLAL-KYLAMINE PSYCHEDELICS

This class of psychedelics is chemically related to adrenaline and amphetamine, although many of the effects are quite different. Whereas the effects of amphetamines will peak within half an hour, much sooner if smoked, the phenylalkylamines take several hours to reach their peak. Effects of phenylalkylamines also take longer to reach their peak than effects of indole psychedelics, like LSD.

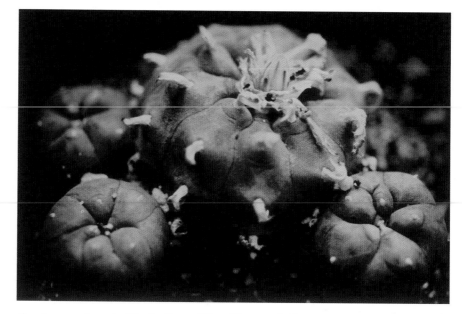

A mature peyote cactus (Lophophora williamsii) *is ripe for harvesting. Each button (the top of the cactus) contains about 50 mg of mescaline. It can take from 2–10 buttons to get high.*

PEYOTE (mescaline)

Mescaline is the active component of the San Pedro cactus (*Trichocereus pachanoi*) and the peyote cactus (*Lophophora williamsii*). San Pedro cacti have been depicted in 3,000-year-old Chavin art from coastal Peru. The use of the peyote cacti stretches as far back as 300 B.C. Over the centuries the Aztecs, Toltecs, Chichimecas, and several Meso-American cultures included it in their rituals. When the Spaniards invaded the New World and encountered the use of peyote, they regarded it as evil and the hallucinations as an invitation from the devil. They tried to abolish it but never succeeded. In the 1800s its use spread north to the United States where about 50 North American tribes were still using it by the early 1900s (Furst, 1976).

Peyote cacti are still eaten in ritual ceremonies by the northern Mexican tribes, such as the Huichol, Tarahumara, and Cora Indians, and by the Southwest Plains Indian tribes, including the Comanches, Kiowas, and Utes. In addition the Native American Church of North America, with a claimed membership of 250,000, also uses the peyote cactus as part of their ceremonies, supposedly to build spirituality and community.

In the 1950s and '60s peyote buttons were available by mail order. Presently they are still available by mail but one has to file documentation of membership in the Native American Church. About 2 million buttons are harvested in Texas each year. Heavy active users might consume up to 1,000 buttons a year. There are nine licensed distributors of peyote in the United States (Marnell, 1997; DEA, 1997).

"I took three dried buttons and had to clean them out like an artichoke. You let them soften in your mouth and then you chew them. It takes a real long time to get off. What I remember is waterfalls of green fire and the campfire experience. I did have some nausea but I didn't throw up."
38-year-old accountant

Effects

The gray-green crowns of the peyote cactus are cut at ground level or uprooted. They are eaten fresh or dried into peyote or mescal buttons and then ingested. The bitter nauseating substance is either eaten (seven to eight buttons is an average dose) or boiled and drunk as a tea. They can also be ground and eaten as a powder (Schultes & Hofmann, 1992). Synthetic mescaline, which was isolated in 1890, is a thin needlelike crystal that is sold in capsules. The effects of mescaline last approximately 12 hours and are very similar to LSD with an emphasis on colorful visions. Users term it the "mellow LSD" but real hallucinations are more common with mescaline than with LSD. Each use of peyote is usually accompanied by a severe episode of nausea and vomiting, although some users can develop a tolerance to these effects. As with most psychedelics, tolerance to the psychedelic effects can also develop rapidly (LaBarre & Weston, 1979).

A peyote ceremony might consist of ingesting the peyote buttons, then singing, drumming, chanting hymns, and trying to understand the psychedelic visions in order to have spiritual experiences. Many participants also have hallucinatory visions of a deity or spiritual leader whom they are able to converse with for guidance and understanding (Furst, 1976).

"When you get fresh buttons, they go down easier. No doubt about it, peyote is the worst taste I've ever experienced. Whenever I took it I got into projectile vomiting. It would happen as I was coming on to it. My reaction was intensely visual but it was different than LSD in that my mind could work and I could have a conversation."
Former psychedelic user

Since the reaction to many psychedelics depends on the mind-set and setting almost as much as on the actual properties of the drug, use of a mind-altering substance in a structured cere-monial setting can induce more spiritual feelings than if it's used at a rock concert.

Many challenges have been made concerning the legality of using a psychedelic substance for a religious ceremony. In 1990 the U.S. Supreme Court ruled that the use of a psychoactive drug, such as peyote, during religious ceremonies is not protected by the Constitution and that states can ban its use. For this reason many ceremonies are held in secret.

DESIGNER PSYCHEDELICS (MDA, MDMA, MMDA, MDM, MDE, et al.) & CLUB DRUGS

This set of synthetic drugs uses laboratory variations of the amphetamine molecule. First synthesized in 1910 (MDA) and 1914 (MDMA), the drugs can cause feelings of well-being and euphoria, along with some stimulatory effects, side effects, and toxicity similar to amphetamines. The differences among the more than 150 compounds of these stimulant psychedelics in common use (thousands more are not in common use) have to do with duration of action, extent of delusional effects, and degree of euphoria. MDA was the first of these compounds to be widely abused (in the late 1960s, '70s, and early '80s). It was called the "love drug" but research that showed damage to serotonin-producing neurons in the brain, overdose deaths, and increased legal scrutiny dampened its popularity and by the mid-1980s, MDMA had taken over as the designer psychedelic of choice.

MDMA ("ecstasy," "rave," "XTC," "X," "Adam," "Eve," et al.)

Just before Christmas in December 1999, Customs and DEA agents seized 700 pounds of "ecstasy" (MDMA) in Southern California. The $30-million (wholesale) bust was the biggest MDMA bust ever. It was a sign that the traffic in this hallucinogenic stimulant had reached unprecedented proportions. The Monitoring the Future Survey found that in 1999, about 5.6% of high school seniors had used MDMA and about 1/2 that amount used on a

The Mail Tribune, Friday, Dec. 24, 1999

U.S. Customs agents bust 'Ecstacy' drug traffickers

By TOM GORMAN
Los Angeles Times

LOS ANGELES — Drug agents seized 700 pounds of the hallucinogenic stimulant known as Ecstasy — popularly used at raves and other all-night dance parties — and arrested six people who they said were responsible for its wholesale distribution in Southern California, federal authorities announced Thursday.

arrival of about 100 pounds of Ecstasy from France at a Federal Express shipment center in Memphis, Tenn.

With the cooperation of Fed Ex officials, the shipment was tracked to a beauty salon in Upland and then followed to various undisclosed locations in Los Angeles.

On Wednesday, federal, state and San Bernardino County drug agents believed they had followed the

Notice that "ecstasy" is misspelled in the headline.

• •

monthly basis (University of Michigan, 1999). The compound MDMA, chemical name 3,4 methylenedioxymethamphetamine, is shorter acting than MDA (4–6 hrs. vs. 10–12 hrs.) and can be swallowed, snorted, or injected, much like amphetamines, though it is usually sold as a white capsule or tablet or as a white, reddish, or brownish powder. A capsule, tablet, or equivalent powder packet (100–150 mg) costs anywhere from $10 to $25 and has been manufactured illegally since it was banned in 1987 by the U.S. federal government (Morgan, 1997).

Physical Effects. MDMA has many stimulant effects similar to amphetamines, such as increased heart rate, faster respiration, excess energy, and hyperactivity. Some claim that it has the opposite effect and calms these bodily functions. Part of this contradiction has to do with the amount ingested. The more that is used, the greater the physical effects. MDMA can trigger nausea, loss of appetite, and the clenching of jaw muscles. Though some report more sexual desire, prolonged use decreases orgasm in men and sexual arousal in women (DuPont, 1997). Since MDMA releases less adrenaline than most amphetamines, a user doesn't receive quite as much sympathetic nervous stimulation of heart rate and blood pressure. However, tolerance to its mental effects develops rapidly, so users increase doses that can result in greater physical harm.

Mental Effects. Twenty minutes to one hour after ingestion and continuing for three to four more hours, MDMA causes stimulation and mild distortions of perception but most often, according to some users, it has a calming effect and increases empathy with others. Users also claim that it heightens their awareness and induces a desire to dance. Many of the psychic effects are probably due to serotonergic activity. It doesn't give the visual illusions most often associated with psychedelics (Snyder, 1996). Physical dependency is generally not a problem but, as with amphetamines and cocaine, psychological dependence can cause compulsive use. If used daily, tolerance develops rather quickly, as with the amphetamines (Markert & Roberts, 1991).

"I remember we had some MDMA. This friend snorted this whole big line. We stuck him in the bath to cool him down. It took about an hour and a half to mellow him out."

24-year-old "raver"

Toxicity. Major problems seen with MDMA abuse consist of a high body temperature resulting from the effects of the drug plus dehydration caused by physical exertion, the combination of which has caused death in some users. High-dose use also results in high blood pressure and seizure activity, much like that seen in amphetamine overdose. Following an "ecstasy"

experience, users have also been known to become extremely depressed and suicidal. Despite the claim that the drug does not produce major psychedelic reactions, high-dose use has resulted in an acute anxiety reaction ("bum trip"), prolonged reaction, and even flashbacks (Carroll & Comer, 1998). MDMA is often taken at "raves" and "rave" clubs (dance and party clubs where drug taking is common) because users claim it creates a strong desire to dance.

In recent animal experiments (rats and monkeys), it was found that MDMA damaged serotonin-producing neurons in the brain in much the same way that MDA was proven to do in humans. Much of the damage remained even 12–18 months after use (Fischer, Hatzidimitriou, Wlos, et al., 1995).

"Rave" Clubs. One of the dangerous effects of MDMA, becoming overheated and dehydrated, has much to do with the way the drug is being used. Starting in 1990 in Europe, particularly in the Netherlands and England, and quickly spreading to the United States, there has been an upsurge in "rave" clubs. Anywhere from a few hundred to thousands of young people attend these "rave" gatherings. Some of the clubs are legal and some are nomadic. Flyers are handed out during the week for a party at an empty warehouse that weekend. "Rave" clubs are so popular that they have become a big business enterprise often charging as much as $20 to $50 per admission (DuPont, 1997).

These clubs hark back to the psychedelic ballrooms of the 1960s where not only light shows, the music of the times, and current hip fashions were on display but where marijuana, LSD, amphetamine, MDA, and almost any other abused drug were common. In the "rave" clubs of the '90s, the drugs of choice were MDMA, LSD, amphetamines, marijuana, volatile nitrites, and of course alcohol. Combinations of these drugs are also being used, e.g., "ecstasy" and LSD called "Xs and Ls," "flip flops," or "candy snaps"; "speedballs" of "ecstasy" and heroin; "ecstasy" and methamphetamine; "ec-

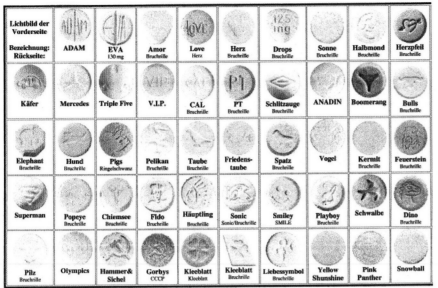

Lichtbild der Vorderseite								
Bezeichnung: Rückseite:	ADAM	EVA 130 mg	Amor Bruchrille	Love Herz	Herz Bruchrille	Drops Bruchrille	Sonne Bruchrille	Halbmond Bruchrille	Herzpfeil Bruchrille
Käfer	Mercedes	Triple Five	V.I.P.	CAL Bruchrille	PT Bruchrille	Schlitzauge Bruchrille	ANADIN	Boomerang	Bulls Bruchrille
Elephant Bruchrille	Hund Bruchrille	Pigs Ringelschwanz	Pelikan Bruchrille	Taube Bruchrille	Friedens-taube	Spatz Bruchrille	Vogel	Kermit Bruchrille	Feuerstein Bruchrille
Superman	Popeye Bruchrille	Chiemsee Bruchrille	Fido Bruchrille	Häuptling Bruchrille	Sonic Sonic/Bruchrille	Smiley SMILE	Playboy Bruchrille	Schwalbe	Dino Bruchrille
Pilz Bruchrille	Olympics	Hammer& Sichel	Gorbys CCCP	Kleeblatt Kleeblatt	Kleeblatt Bruchrille	Liebessymbol Bruchrille	Yellow Shunshine	Pink Panther	Snowball

(Fotomaterial: Bundeskriminalamt Wiesbaden)

These are some MDMA ("ecstasy") tablets confiscated in Europe by various police agencies and Interpol. Seizures by the U.S. Customs Service have soared from 400,000 pills in 1997 to 3 million in 1999. About 90% of "ecstasy" comes from Northern Europe, mainly the Netherlands and Belgium.

Courtesy of the Bundeskriminalant Wiesbaden, U.S. Customs Service, and Trinka Porrata

stasy" and the so-called "smart drugs" or "smart drinks," such as ephedrine or vasopressin or amino acids. Further there has been an increasing use of other psychedelic drugs at these "raves," including "euphoria," 2CB ("nexus"), CBR, GHB, "illusion," DMT, and ketamine.

A recent variation of the nomadic "raves" are "desert raves." Invitations are passed out during the week designating a location in the desert or some isolated piece of property. Hundreds of "ravers" show up to party and take drugs. There have been problems with environmental damage from so many people on an ecologically sensitive piece of land. Medically "desert ravers" have suffered from overheating or hypothermia from the hot daytime sun and the cold night desert air, aggravated by the effects of certain drugs on body temperature (e.g., alcohol causes heat loss).

STP (DOM) (4 methyl 2,5 dimethoxy amphetamine)

STP, also called the "serenity, tranquillity, and peace pill," is similar to MDA. It causes a 12-hour intoxication characterized by intense stimulation and several mild psychedelic reactions. There are, however, reports that it is a thicker duller trip than those experienced from mescaline or LSD, although it is 80 times more active than mescaline (Smith, 1981). The combination of STP and LSD, called "pinks" and "purple (or "orange") wedges," was popular in the late 1960s but is rarely seen currently because of the high incidence of bad trips.

BELLADONNA & OTHER ANTICHOLINERGIC PSYCHEDELICS

BELLADONNA, HENBANE, MANDRAKE, DATURA (jimsonweed, thornapple)

From ancient Greek times through the Middle Ages and the Renaissance, these plants, which contain scopolamine, hyoscyamine, and atropine, have been used in magic ceremonies, sorcery, witchcraft (black mass), and religious rituals. They've also been used as a poison, to mimic insanity, and even as a beauty aid by ancient Greek, Roman, and Egyptian women because they dilate pupils (Ott, 1976). In fact *belladonna* in Latin means "beautiful woman." Datura is more widely grown and references to it are found in Chinese, Indian, Greek, and Aztec history.

One of the effects of these plants is to block acetylcholine receptors in the central nervous system. Acetylcholine helps regulate reflexes, aggression, sleep, blood pressure, heart rate, sexual behavior, mental acuity, and attention. This disruptive effect can cause a form of delirium, make it hard to focus vision, speed up the heart, create an intense thirst, and raise the body temperature to dangerous levels. Anticholinergics also create some hallucinations, a separation from reality, and a deep sleep for up to 48 hours (Schultes & Hofmann, 1980). They are still used today by some native tribes in Mexico and Africa. Synthetic anticholinergic prescription drugs, like Cogentin® and Artane® that are used to treat the side effects of antipsychotic drugs and Parkinson's disease symptoms, are diverted from legal sources and abused for their psychedelic effects. Further, even belladonna cigarettes (Asmador®), used to treat asthma, are abused by youth in search of a cheap high (Smith, 1981).

KETAMINE, PCP, & OTHER PSYCHEDELICS

KETAMINE (Ketalar®, Ketajet®, "special-K")

Ketamine, an animal and human anesthetic that is used to control pain, is also a psychedelic drug. It has become popular in recent years with the decline in the popularity of PCP, another animal anesthetic that was also widely used illegally as a psychedelic. Ketamine, called "K" or "special-K," is available through diversion from medical and veterinary supplies. When used clinically, it is usually injected;

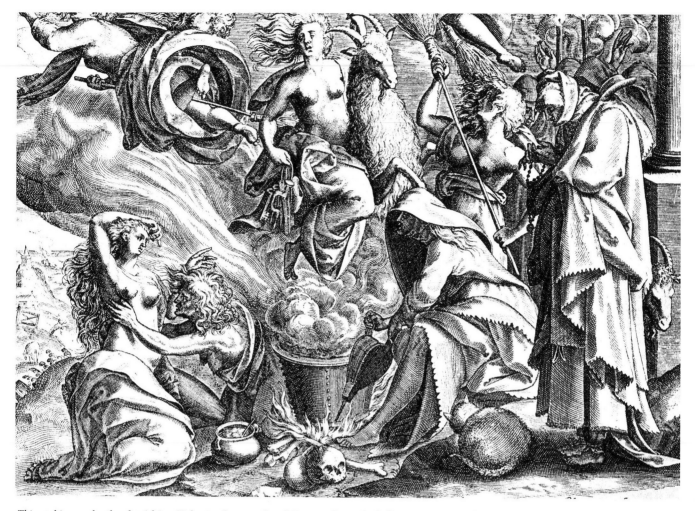

This etching on leather by Adrien Hubertus from medieval Europe shows the hallucinations caused by the hexing herbs, along with visions of sexual activity and death.

Reprinted, by permission, EMB Service for Publishers.

when used on the street, it is heated and evaporated to form solid crystals. It is then smoked, powdered and snorted, or mixed into drinks and swallowed. These crystals are smoked like "crack" or PCP, making it easy to abuse.

Users experience a disassociative effect that separates the mind from the body senses. They enter a dreamlike state, often filled with a mild euphoria, illusions, and even hallucinations, which last for about six hours. According to some users, music sounds different when high on ketamine and there is selective loss of some frequencies. They are also impervious to pain, including injuries sustained by rough activities, such as fighting or dancing in a "mosh pit" at rock concerts where peo-

ple bang against each other. Because of these effects, ketamine is popular as a "rave" club drug. Its side effects are similar to those of PCP, including toxic reactions such as coma, convulsions, and combative or belligerent behavior.

The retail price of ketamine for veterinarians is about $7 per vial. Middle-level street dealers pay $30 to $45 per vial and the users may pay $100 to $200 per vial. A vial contains about 1 gram of powder. A smaller amount, a "bump" or 0.2 grams costs about $20. A dose of .07 grams can cause mild intoxication, 0.2 grams can induce a mellow colorful wonder world, while 0.5 grams can produce a "K-hole" or out-of-body near-death experience (DEA, 1997).

Several researchers have used keta-

mine to treat alcoholism in a technique known as "ketamine-assisted psychotherapy." The ketamine is injected intramuscularly supposedly to make the brain more accessible to emotions and dialogue. The researchers reported that about 2/3 of their clients treated this way stayed abstinent for more than a year compared to 1/4 of a control group that tried conventional treatment (Krupitsky & Grinenko, 1997).

PCP

PCP (phencyclidine hydrochloride) was originally created during the 1950s by Parke-Davis (under the trade name Sernyl®) as a new type of disassociative general anesthetic for humans. However, the frequency and severity of toxic and hallucinogenic effects soon limited its use to veterinary medicine starting in 1965 (Petersen, 1980; Zukin, Sloboda, & Javitt, 1997). Eventually use of PCP was even discontinued in veterinary medicine. Now the only supplies are illegal ones. It is fairly easy to manufacture in a home laboratory, although the pungent odor of manufacture is easily detectable. PCP can be smoked in a "joint," snorted, swallowed, or injected. It appears to distort sensory messages sent to the central nervous system. PCP stifles inhibitions, deadens pain, and results in an experience that has been described by users as a separation of the mind from the body (O'Brien, 1992). In one study, almost 3/4 of the users reported forgetfulness, difficulty concentrating, aggressive and violent behavior, depersonalization, and/or estrangement while a smaller amount, about 40% of users, reported hallucinations (tactile, visual, or auditory) (Siegel, 1989).

Phencyclidine or PCP, also called "angel dust," "peep," "KJ," "Shermans," or "ozone," is often misrepresented as THC, mescaline, or psilocybin. Two other names used for PCP are "ice" and "krystal," (which are also the street names for methamphetamine). Phencyclidine was first synthesized in 1959 and patented in 1963 but didn't become popular as a street drug until 1967 and 1968 as a PeaCe Pill (ergo, PCP) in the "Summer of Love" in San Francisco (Longenecker, 1994).

"When I smoke PCP, I feel just like on top of the world, you know. You don't feel pain. You don't think about your past. It's a good drug if you want to cover up your feelings, you know? You feel like Superman. It's like 'acid' without the mind trip. A couple of times I got scared on it though, 'cause I smoked too much. And it was just like a scary experience—like a nightmare, you know? Weird."
Recovering PCP user

Since PCP is so strong, particularly for first-time users, the range between a

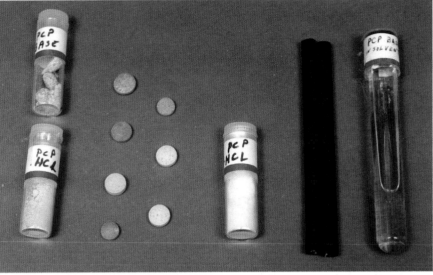

PCP ("angel dust") comes in liquid, crystal, or a powder. It is often smoked in a Sherman® cigarette or sprinkled onto marijuana in a "joint." It can also be snorted, swallowed, or injected and is often misrepresented as THC, the active ingredient in marijuana.

dose that produces a pleasant sensory deprivation effect and one that induces catatonia, coma, or convulsions is very small. Low dosages (2–5 mg) first produce mild depression, then stimulation. Moderate doses (10–15 mg) can produce a more intense sensory-deprived state. They can also produce extremely high blood pressure and very combative behavior. Other adverse reactions to moderate doses include an inability to talk, rigid or robotic movements, tremors, confusion, agitation, and paranoid thinking. Dosages just a little higher, above 20 mg, can cause catatonia, coma, and convulsions. Large PCP doses have also produced seizures, respiratory depression, rigidity of muscles, cardiovascular instability, and even kidney failure. PCP also induces amnesia in people under its influence (Jaffe, 1989).

"I've had seizures before on it and banged my head really hard—continually on hard objects—and got lots of bumps and everything and felt them the next few days but never realized I was doing it and never felt hurt from it."
Recovering PCP user

The effects of a small dose of PCP will last 1–2 hours, a moderate dose 4–6 hours, but the effects of a large dose can last up to 48 hours, much longer than effects produced by a similar dose of LSD. Further, current evidence shows that the body retains PCP for several months in fatty cells. The PCP stored in fat can be released during exercise or fasting, resulting in a true chemical PCP flashback. The flashback also results because of the drug's recirculation from the brain, to the blood, to the stomach, to the intestines, then back to the blood and brain. This is called "enterogastric recirculation" (Balster, 1995).

PCP was not widely used by the general drug-using population because of the frequency of bad trips associated with it. PCP is often sold as THC or mescaline to unsuspecting drug users. When the psychedelic effects kick in, surprised users can have a bad trip and often do not even remember what happened during the trip. This type of amnesia, which occurs after the use of PCP, is called "anterograde amnesia" and is frequently seen with "date rape" drugs like Rohypnol® and GHB. Sometimes PCP users even forget that they used the drug. PCP can also cause an emotional addiction resulting in high levels of abuse in certain populations.

AMANITA MUSHROOMS

Although many members of this family of mushrooms are deadly, the *Amanita muscaria* (fly agaric) and the *Amanita pantherina* (panther mushroom) have been used as psychedelics for many centuries. The *Amanita muscaria,* a large mushroom that has an orange, tan, red, or yellow cap with white spots, can cause dreamy intoxication, hallucinations, delirious excitement, and deadly physical toxic effects as well. The effects start a 1/2 hour after ingestion and can last for 4–8 hours (Schultes & Hofmann, 1992). The active ingredients are ibotenic acid and the alkaloid muscimole, substances that resemble the inhibitory neurotransmitter GABA. The *Amanita pantherina* contains more of the active ingredients and taking too much of the mushroom can make the user sick for up to 12 hours (Weil & Rosen, 1993).

The *Amanita* mushroom is mentioned in sacred writings in India in 1500 B.C. where it is referred to as the god Soma. *Amanita* has also been used by native tribes in Siberia but its use is limited in the modern age because of the unpredictability of its effects and because many even more deadly mushrooms can be mistaken for it. The use of *Amanita muscaria* in ancient ritual ceremonies is still practiced today by some Ojibway Indians in Michigan (Ott, 1976).

NUTMEG & MACE

At the low end of the desirable psychedelic drug spectrum, nutmeg and mace—both from the nutmeg tree (*myristica fragrans*)—can cause varied effects from a mild floating sensation to a full-blown delirium. So much has to be consumed (about 20 grams) that the user is left with a bad hangover and a severely upset stomach. The active chemicals in nutmeg and mace are variants of MDA (methylenedioxyamphetamine) (Marnell, 1997). Since this dose

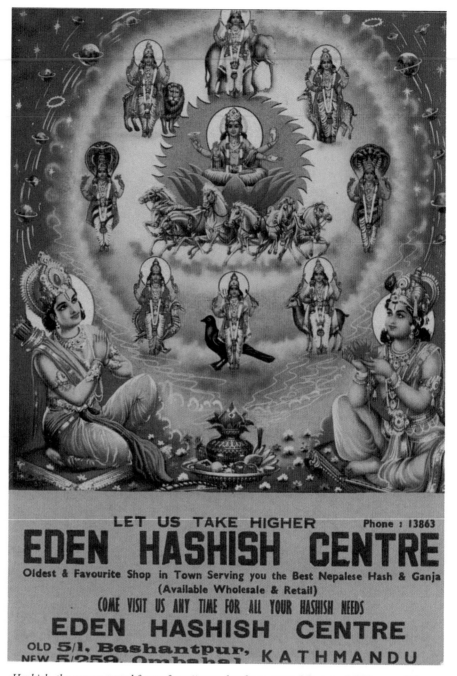

Hashish, the concentrated form of marijuana, has been around for over 1,000 years. It has been smoked or eaten in religious ceremonies and used as a recreational intoxicant and psychedelic. Its use is officially banned in almost every country but in some, a blind eye is turned to its existence. The Hindu god Shiva likes hashish and so there is a yearly festival of Shiva Ratri that is partially celebrated by devotees smoking hashish. The Eden Hashish Centre in Katmandu, Nepal is closed but hashish is still available.

exposes a user to the nauseating and toxic effects of other chemicals in nutmeg, its abuse is extremely rare outside of prisons where convicts are driven to use it since they have limited access to other psychedelics.

MARIJUANA & OTHER CANNABINOLS

The *Cannabis* or hemp plant, also called "marijuana," produces fibers used to make rope, cloth, roofing materials, and floor coverings. It grows edible seeds (*akenes*); it has an oil that is used as a fuel and lubricant; it contains a number of other active ingredients that have been used to treat illnesses; and it produces a psychedelic resin that can alter consciousness.

"The marijuana high—it's relaxing, it's pleasant. It opens the other side of the mind. It's like the left side saying 'Hi,' to the right and they're saying, 'Hey, we're together. We're having fun.'"

50-year-old marijuana smoker

Marijuana is also written about endlessly, researched in dozens of laboratories, smoked in hundreds of countries, and forbidden by thousands of laws. And in spite of the fact that research has led to the discovery of neurotransmitters and receptor sites that are specific for marijuana, uncertainty is still prevalent in many medical, political, legal, and user circles as to the real benefits and dangers of the drug.

HISTORY OF USE

The relationship between *Cannabis* and man has existed for at least 10,000 years. From its probable origin in China or central Asia in Neolithic times, hemp cultivation has spread to almost every country in the world. There are a variety of species. Some are better for fiber, some for food, and some for inducing psychedelic effects.

The first use of the plant was probably as a source of nutrition since Neolithic man (after 6500 B.C.) was always searching for food. When parts of the plant were eaten, our ancient ancestors undoubtedly experienced some psychedelic effects, particularly if the species had a high enough concentration of psychedelic chemicals. Next, *Cannabis* was most likely tried as a source of fiber. After that, various holy men and medicine men, especially the semilegendary Chinese emperor Shen Nung (c. 2700 B.C.), experimented with *Cannabis* for its medicinal benefits.

Finally, different ways to extract and consume psychedelic parts of the plant were discovered (around 200 B.C. the Chinese wrote about the hallucinations caused by excess use) (Aldrich, 1997).

The Indian *Vedas* (sacred writings), around 1500 B.C., described *Cannabis* as a divine nectar that could deter evil, bring luck, and cleanse man of sin. It was listed as one of the five sacred plants to bring about freedom from stress (Atharva Veda, 1400 B.C.). Indian writings also described its medicinal use to relieve headaches, control mania, counteract insomnia, treat venereal disease, cure whooping cough, and even arrest tuberculosis (Touw, 1981).

Galen, the Father of Medicine, wrote in A.D. 200 that it was sometimes customary to give *Cannabis* to guests to induce enjoyment and mirth. Ropes and sails were made from the fiber in third-century Rome. Medieval physicians recommended weedy hemp to treat cancer and cultivated hemp for the treatment of jaundice and coughs. Because *Cannabis* was not specifically banned in the Koran by the Prophet Mohammed, Islamic cultures spread its use to Africa and Europe. In Africa, starting about six centuries ago, it was used in social and religious rituals and in medicinal preparations to treat dysentery, fevers, asthma, and even the pain of childbirth (DuToit, 1980).

Starting in the fifteenth century, the Age of Exploration increased the need for rope, sails, and paper, so many colonies were introduced to *Cannabis* and encouraged to grow and export the more fibrous variants (hemp). Even George Washington had large fields of it growing on his plantation to produce hemp. *Cannabis* was widely cultivated in the Americas until the nineteenth century when the end of slavery made it less profitable to grow.

Over the centuries the medical profession has examined the use of marijuana and its extracts as a medicine. Since there were few other medications available, substances that had a real effect were prized. In a report to the Ohio State Medical Society in 1860, Dr. R. R. McMeens said he was convinced of its immense value because of the immediate action of the drug in appeasing the appetite for chloral hydrate or opium and restoring the ability to appreciate food. He also recommended it as a treatment for disordered bowels, as a diuretic, and as a sleeping tonic (McMeens, 1860). The concentration of THC was probably fairly high, approaching that of hashish. As in the present day, there were also warnings about the dangers of marijuana. For example, in 1890 Dr. J. Russel Reynolds in writing about his 30 years of experience using *Cannabis* medicinally said the problems included

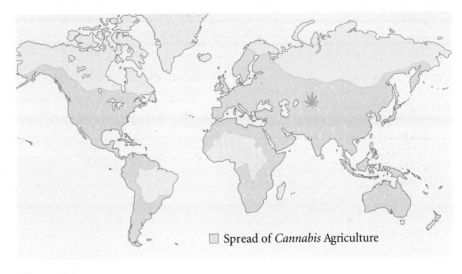

☐ Spread of *Cannabis* Agriculture

Figure 6-1 •

From its origin in central Asia, Cannabis *has spread to almost every country even though it is also illegal in almost every country.*

a wide variation in the strength of any *Cannabis indica* preparation, that people vary widely in their reaction to the same dose, and that if high concentrations are taken, severe reactions are quite possible (Reynolds, 1890).

Mexican laborers who worked in the United States introduced Americans to the habit of smoking marijuana for its psychedelic and psychoactive effects after World War I. Initially its use was confined to poor and minority groups but in the 1920s the use of *Cannabis* as a substitute for alcohol that had been prohibited by the Eighteenth Amendment spread its popularity. Marijuana "tea pads," similar to opium dens, became popular. It is estimated that there were more than 500 "tea pads" in New York by the beginning of the 1930s (O'Brien, 1992). This expanded use of marijuana alarmed prohibitionists who were left without a cause when the Eighteenth Amendment was repealed and may have contributed to prohibitions against marijuana. Marijuana, the Mexican word for *Cannabis,* was popularized by the Hearst newspapers in a series of crusading articles against use of the drug. The use of *Cannabis* (except for sterilized bird seed and medical

treatment) was banned by the Marijuana Tax Act of 1937. Although medical use was still permitted, any prescribing of the substance was actively discouraged. Pharmaceutical manufacturers removed *Cannabis* from 28 medications that were being prescribed at the time (Walton, 1938).

The fear of an interruption in the importation of hemp fiber to America during World War II temporarily lifted the ban on growing the plant but since the end of the war, its use has been illegal in the United States as well as in most other countries worldwide. The level of prohibition varies widely from country to country. In spite of restrictions, marijuana is used in some form by 200–300 million people worldwide. In addition several countries are cultivating a fibrous variant of the *Cannabis* plant to supply pulp and fiber to make paper, textiles, and rope. France, Italy, Yugoslavia, and to a lesser extent England and Canada now permit the growing of hemp.

EPIDEMIOLOGY

"My parents were hippies, so having drugs around wasn't like a bring down or anything, and this was in the '70s when it was peace, love, and everything was happening on a cool mellow level. So, you know, I enjoyed being the little kid around with a bunch of partying hippies in their 20s just having a good time. So I was very much accustomed to having 'pot' and smoking it."
30-year-old marijuana smoker

In 1960 only two percent of people in the United States (34 million) had tried any illegal drug. By the mid-'60s the growth of the counterculture, fueled by the baby boom, greatly increased the psychedelic use of marijuana and other illicit drugs. By 1979, 68 million people in the United States had tried marijuana and 23 million were using it on a monthly basis. The popularity of the drug led 10 states to decriminalize possession of small amounts of the drug for personal use but by the '90s, the resurgence of the concept of complete prohibition had recriminalized use of the drug in most states. It also greatly increased the number of people in prison for marijuana possession and use. By 1992 the monthly rate of use had dropped to 1/3 of its 1979 peak level of use but recently those levels have begun to climb, particularly among teenagers. By 1999 more than 11 million Americans (about four percent of the U.S. population) were using marijuana at least once a month (SAMHSA, 1999).

"Coming into high school, there's a lot of pressures and stuff socially and academically and it's like a break for me. Me and my friends would run out of school Friday and smoke. It was like a little vacation for a night."
16-year-old marijuana smoker

BOTANY

There is much confusion over the various terms used to describe the *Cannabis* plant. Terms such as *vulgaris, pedemontana, lupulus, mexicana,* and *sinensis* have been used in the last hundred years but there is a growing con-

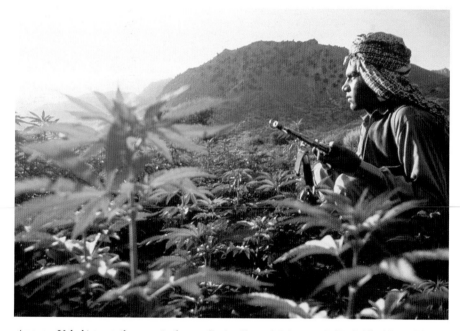

A young Uzbekistan tribesman in former Soviet Central Asia guards his field of Cannabis.
Reprinted, by permission, Alain Labrousse, Observatoire Geopolitique Des Drogues.

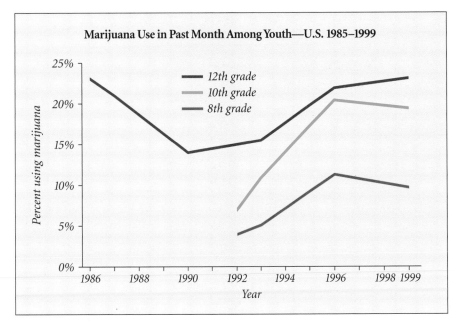

Marijuana Use in Past Month Among Youth—U.S. 1985–1999

Figure 6-2 •

In 1978, 37% of high school seniors used marijuana at least once a month. By 1992 that percentage had dropped to 12% but by 1997 it had risen back to 23.7% and stayed about the same for the last few years. Daily use for high school seniors rose from 1.9% in 1992 to 6.0% in 1999. This rise in monthly and daily use is also apparent in the 8th and 10th grades (University of Michigan, 1999).

"Most of the marijuana in the late '60s was 'brown Mexican' but we also had access to 'Colombian gold,' 'Panama red,' 'Acapulco gold,' and 'Thai sticks,' so we had plenty of concentration of THC. We also had connections for Vietnamese 'pot.' They didn't check the GIs' duffel bags. A lot of 'pot' nowadays just makes you incapacitated or you munch and go to sleep or have just a 20-minute mystery trip or rush, then you munch, then crash out."

48-year-old former marijuana smoker

Species

Marijuana (the psychedelic *Cannabis* plant) has many street names: "pot," "buds," "herb," "chronic," "dank," "the kind," "grass," "ganja," "charas," "sens," "weed," and "dope." There are also hundreds of strains that sound like brand names: "Maui wowie," "Humboldt green," "British Columbia bud," and "Buddha Thai." Constant experimentation by growers has resulted in variations in the size, concentration of psychoactive resin, and even shape of the leaf. Some botanists say that *Cannabis sativa*

sensus about terminology. *Cannabis* is the botanical genus of all these plants. Hemp is generally used to describe *Cannabis* plants that are high in fiber content, whereas marijuana is used to describe *Cannabis* plants that are high in psychoactive components (Schultes & Hofmann, 1992; Stafford, 1992).

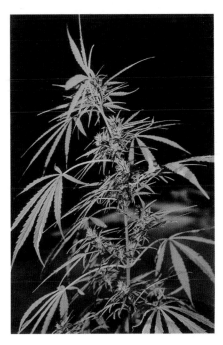

Female flowering top of Cannabis sativa *with relatively long slender leaf projections.*

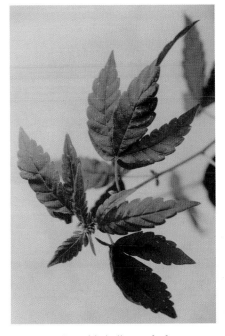

Immature Cannabis indica *with shorter stout leafs.*

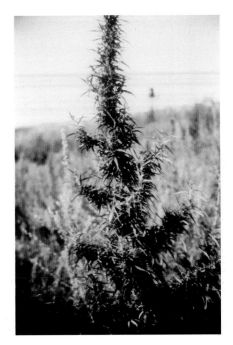

Cannabis ruderalis from southern Sibera has relatively little THC content.

is the only true species. Many other botanists think that there are three distinct species but all agree that there are hundreds of unique variants of the various *Cannabis* species. Unfortunately, intensive hybridization and cultivation has made them hard to identify. In this book we will designate three species: *Cannabis sativa, Cannabis indica,* and *Cannabis ruderalis* (Stafford, 1992).

The most common species type is **Cannabis sativa,** grown in tropical, subtropical, and temperate regions throughout the world. Variations of *Cannabis sativa* have sufficient quantities of active resins to cause psychedelic phenomena while other variations have a high concentration of fiber and are used for hemp. The average plant will grow from 5–12 feet tall but can grow up to 20 feet. There are generally five thin serrated leaves on each stem. A typical plant will produce between one to five pounds of buds and smokable leaves, both of which contain the highest concentration of the psychedelic resin. The second species, **Cannabis indica,** is a shorter bushier plant with fatter leaves and is generally not used for its fibers. It is especially plentiful in the Middle East and India and is the source of most of the world's hashish. Modifications of *Cannabis indica* have resulted in a stronger smellier variety of this plant nicknamed "skunk weed." Many illegal growers have come to prefer *Cannabis indica* as the base plant on which to use the sinsemilla-growing technique in the mistaken belief that *indica* is legal since the law as written prohibits only *Cannabis sativa.* Legal challenges have resulted in the interpretation that it is marijuana that's illegal regardless of the specific species. **Cannabis ruderalis,** a small thin species, has few psychoactive components and is especially plentiful in Siberia and Western Asia (Stafford, 1992; Emboden, (1981).

Sinsemilla

The **sinsemilla-growing technique,** used with both *Cannabis indica* and *Cannabis sativa* plants, increases the potency of the marijuana plant. The sinsemilla technique involves separating female plants from male plants be-

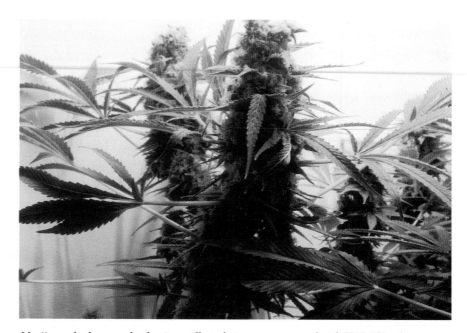

Marijuana buds grown by the sinsemilla technique are saturated with THC. This plant was grown at one of many coffeehouses in Amsterdam in the Netherlands where marijuana is illegal but the government virtually ignores enforcement.
Courtesy of Simone Garlaund

fore pollination. Female plants produce more psychoactive resin than male plants especially when they are unpollinated and therefore bare no seeds. *Sinsemilla* means "without seeds" in Spanish. The term "commercial grade" refers to marijuana that is not grown by the sinsemilla technique (Marnell, 1997).

Dried marijuana buds, leaves, and flowers can be crushed and rolled into "joints." They can also be smoked in pipes. In India and some other countries, marijuana in its various forms is smoked in chillums, which are cone-shaped pipes made out of clay, stone, or wood. They can also be used in food and in drinks or the leaves can be chewed. In India marijuana is divided into three different strengths, each one coming from a different part of the plant. **Bhang** is made from the stems and leaves and has the lowest potency. **Ganja** is made from the stronger leaves and flowering tops. **Charas** is the concentrated resin from the plant and is the most potent (Stafford, 1992; Blum, 1984).

When charas, the sticky resin that contains most of the psychoactive ingredients, is collected and pressed into cakes it is called **"hashish."** This con-

centrated form of *Cannabis* is usually smoked in special pipes, called "bongs" or "hookahs," or it can be added to a marijuana cigarette ("joint") to enhance the potency of weaker leaves. Bongs can also be used to smoke the less-concentrated parts of the marijuana plant. In India, Nepal, and other countries in the area, hashish use has been widespread. An early writer in the nineteenth century described five or six methods for collecting the resin and another dozen methods of preparing it for use, including pressed cakes, small pills, candies, or simply tiny balls of the dark brown resin (Bibra, 1855).

Hash oil can be extracted from the plant (using solvents) and added to foods. Most often it is smeared onto rolling paper or dripped onto crushed marijuana leaves to enhance the psychoactive effects of marijuana cigarettes.

Growers

The majority of the marijuana used in the United States comes from Mexico and Columbia according to the DEA. In addition tens of thousands of

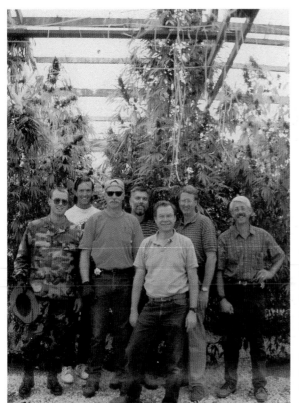

This indoor marijuana-growing operation was busted by JACNET, a drug task force run by the Sheriff's Department in Jackson County, Oregon. Growers can use grow lights or filtered sunlight to avoid detection by law enforcement agencies or passers-by.

Americans grow their own marijuana, either a few plants for their own use or hundreds, even thousands for large-scale dealing. Because of stiffer penalties and greater surveillance by law enforcement agencies, more growers are moving their operations indoors.

The indoor and even hydroponic (in water) growing of marijuana has led to very high-potency plants grown all over the United States, from Maine to Alaska (Marnell, 1997). Worldwide, marijuana production is widespread. Some of the major growing countries in the western hemisphere besides Mexico, Columbia, Canada, and the United States are Jamaica, Brazil, Belize, Guatemala, Trinidad, and Tobago. In Asia, Thailand, Laos, Cambodia, and the Philippines are big growers. In Africa and the Middle East, Morocco, Lebanon (greatly reduced in recent years), Nigeria, and South Africa produce mostly *Cannabis indica.* In southwest and central Asia, Pakistan and Afghanistan are the big producers (DEA, 1998).

The average street price of marijuana in the United States rose steadily from about $6 per gram in 1981 to a peak of about $18 per gram in 1991 (Fig. 6-3). Retail prices fell over the next decade but began to level off to about $10 per gram from 1996 to 1998. Since the common unit of sale for marijuana is one ounce (called a "lid"), the average street price by the end of the 1990s was about $300 per "lid" (ONDCP, 1999; Marnell, 1997).

PHARMACOLOGY

At last count researchers had discovered some 360 chemicals in a single *Cannabis* plant. At least 30 of these chemicals called "cannabinoids" have been studied for their psychoactive effects. The most potent psychoactive chemical is considered to be the cannabinoid called "Δ-9-tetrahydrocannabinol" or "THC." When smoked or ingested, this potent psychoactive chemical is converted by the liver into over 60 other metabolites, some of which are also psychoactive. In addition the widespread use of the sinsemilla-growing technique has increased the average concentration of THC from 1–3% in the 1960s to 6–14% in the late '70s, '80s, and '90s (DEA, 1997). High-concentration THC marijuana has been around for many years—it just hasn't been so readily available. What this means is that a user would have to smoke 5 to 14 of the weak "joints" from the 1960s to equal just 1 of the stronger "joints" available in the 1990s. Unfortunately many of the early studies on marijuana and many of the attitudes of the counterculture about the effects of the drug were based on the weaker plants. Luckily there has been a great increase in research over the last few years using the higher-potency marijuana.

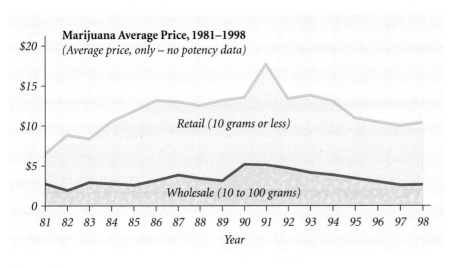

Marijuana Average Price, 1981–1998
(Average price, only – no potency data)

Retail (10 grams or less)

Wholesale (10 to 100 grams)

Year

Figure 6-3 •

Marijuana became so expensive in the 1990s that heroin was used as a means to spike cheap marijuana "joints," so the buyer thinks it is the more potent variety (ONDCP, 1999).

"I would sit there with a nice little metal pipe and a nice sack of big 'chronic bud' and try to see how much of it I could smoke and basically I get to the point where I realize I'm laying on the floor. I've got the pipe in my hand, I can barely keep my eyes open, and I assume that that's as high as I'm going to get."

24-year-old recovering user

Marijuana Receptors & Neurotransmitters

In 1990 at Johns Hopkins University, receptor sites in the brain that were specifically reactive to the THC in marijuana were discovered (Howlett, Evans, & Houston, 1992). This discovery implied that the brain had its own natural neurotransmitters that fit into these receptor sites that affected the same areas of the brain as marijuana.

In 1992 researchers at the National Institute on Drug Abuse announced the discovery of anandamide, the natural neurotransmitter that fits into the receptor sites (Devane, Hanus, Breuer, et al., 1992). Receptors for anandamide were found in several areas of the limbic system including the reward-pleasure center. Other parts of the brain with anandamide receptor sites are those regulating the integration of sensory experiences with emotions as well as those controlling functions of learning, motor coordination, and some automatic body functions. The presence of anandamide receptors means that these are the areas of the brain most affected by marijuana. It is important that there are less anandamide receptors in the brainstem for marijuana, compared to enkephalin receptors for opioids, and norepinephrine receptors for cocaine in that part of the CNS (central nervous system). Since involvement of this area of the brain that controls heart rate, respiration, and other body functions is the reason dangerous overdoses can occur with cocaine and opioids, it helps explain why it is so difficult to physically overdose with marijuana (Smith et al., 1994).

SHORT-TERM EFFECTS

Physical Effects

The immediate physical effects of marijuana often include physical relaxation or sedation, bloodshot eyes, coughing from lung irritation, an increase in appetite, and a loss in muscular coordination. Other physical effects include an increased heart rate, decreased blood pressure, decreased pressure behind the eyes (Marinol® capsules or marijuana "joints" are used as a treatment for glaucoma), increased blood flow through the mucous membranes of the eye resulting in conjunctivitis or red eye, and decreased nausea (capsules and "joints" are also used for cancer patients undergoing chemotherapy).

Marijuana impairs tracking ability (the ability to follow a moving object, such as a baseball) and causes a trailing phenomenon where one sees an after-image of a moving object. Impaired tracking ability, the trailing phenomena, and sedating effects make it more difficult to perform tasks that require depth perception and good hand-eye coordination, such as flying an airplane, catching a football, or driving a car.

Marijuana can act as a stimulant as well as a depressant depending on the variety and amount of chemical that is absorbed in the brain, the setting in which it is used, and the personality of the user.

"Marijuana is not a downer for me, it's a speed thing. I have plenty of friends who smoke marijuana and become quiet. They can't speak. They become immobile. They're total veggies, you know, sitting around and cannot move, whereas I become more active."

Marijuana smoker

Marijuana also causes a small temporary disruption of the secretion of the male hormone testosterone. That might be important to a user with hormonal imbalance or somebody in the throes of puberty and sexual maturation. The testosterone effect also results in a slight decrease in both sperm count and sperm motility in chronic "pot" users (Wilkins et al., 1998; Joy, Watson, & Benson, 1999; Marnell, 1997).

Mental Effects

Within a few minutes of smoking marijuana, the user becomes a bit confused and mentally separated from the environment. It produces a feeling of deja vu where everything seems familiar but really isn't. Additional effects include detachment, an aloof feeling, drowsiness, and difficulty concentrating.

"It's kind of like life without a coherent thought. It's kind of like an escape. It's like when you go to sleep, you forget about things. It's like everything's dreamlike and there are no restraints on anything. You can have freedom to say what you want to say."

16-year-old marijuana smoker

Stronger varieties of marijuana can produce giddiness, stimulation with increased alertness, and major distortions and perceptions of time, color, and sound. Very strong doses can even produce a sensation of movement under one's feet, visual illusions, and even hallucinations. One of the most frequently mentioned psychological problems with smoking marijuana is paranoia and a deeper depersonification (detachment from one's sense of self).

"I'd keep smoking, and keep smoking, and keep smoking, and I'd get paranoid. If you're not relaxed and having fun, it seems really insane to keep doing it. And I did keep doing it for a long time after I had started developing fear."

35-year-old marijuana user

Like most psychedelics the mental effects of marijuana are very dependent on the mood of the smoker and the surroundings. Marijuana acts somewhat as a mild hypnotic. Charles Baudelair, the nineteenth century French poet, referred to it as a "mirror that magnifies." It exaggerates mood and personality and makes smokers more empathetic to others' feelings but also makes them more suggestible.

"I mean sometimes, in some relationships, it helps me to think about it and maybe I come up with a solution for my problem or whatever but sometimes it wouldn't, so it's a very back and forth type deal. It could go either way."
17-year-old recovering compulsive marijuana user

Marijuana disrupts short-term memory but not long-term memory.

"I'd be doing the job and all of a sudden I'd look up and freeze and not know what to do. I would have a handful of checks in my hand and just look at the machine for a while and just think to myself, 'What is this and what do I do with it?'"
42-year-old recovering marijuana addict

The loss of a sense of time is responsible for several of the perceived effects of marijuana. Dull repetitive jobs seem to go by faster. In Jamaica some cane field workers smoke "ganja" (marijuana) to make their hard monotonous work pass by more quickly. On the other hand students who smoke marijuana while studying get easily bored and often abandon their books.

The effects of mental confusion, distortion of the passage of time, impaired judgment, and short-term memory loss result in a user's inability to perform multiple and interactive tasks, like programming a VCR, while under the influence of marijuana (Wilkins, Conner, & Gorelick, 1998; Joy et al., 1999; Marnell, 1997; Stafford, 1992).

LONG-TERM EFFECTS

Respiratory Problems

THC is a bronchodilator; it opens up the airways, at least initially. As smoking becomes chronic, so does irritation to the breathing passages. Because marijuana is grown under a wide variety of conditions and is unrefined, the "joints" made from the buds and/or leaves are harsh, unfiltered, irregular in quality, and composed of many different chemicals. Therefore, when it is inhaled and held in the lungs, smoking four to five "joints" gives the same harmful exposure to the lungs and mucous membranes as smoking a full pack of cigarettes according to studies by Dr. Donald Tashkin at UCLA (Tashkin, Simmons, & Clark, 1988, 1997). For these and other reasons, a major concern of health professionals is the damaging effect that marijuana smoking has on the respiratory system. Marijuana smoking on a regular basis leads to symptoms of acute and chronic bronchitis. In microscopic studies of these mucous membranes, Dr. Tashkin has found that most damage occurs in the lungs of those who smoke both cigarettes and marijuana. This is significant because most marijuana smokers also smoke cigarettes.

"It's just like cigarettes. I started smoking cigarettes at the age of 13

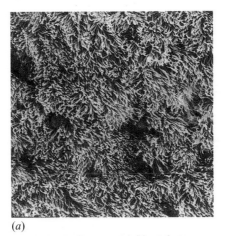
(a)

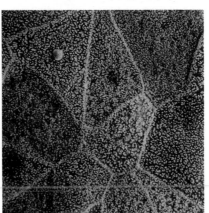
(c)

right behind the marijuana. As soon as I got done with a 'joint' or two, I'd smoke a cigarette to get rid of the smell. Then I'd hide it from my wife and go outside and smoke outside on the porch or outside in my woodshed."
32-year-old recovering compulsive marijuana smoker

In the series of slides, the normal ciliated surface epithelial cells in the mucous membranes of a nonsmoker of either cigarettes or marijuana (Fig. 6-4a) show healthy densely packed cilia that clear the breathing passages of mucous, dust, and debris.

The breathing passage of a chronic smoker of only marijuana (Fig. 6-4b) shows increased numbers of mucous-secreting surface epithelial cells that do not have cilia, so phlegm production is increased but is not cleared as readily from the breathing passages. The result is increased coughing and chronic bronchitis. Some of the changes involve the cell nucleus, suggesting that malig-

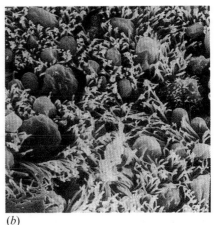
(b)

Figure 6-4 •

(a) Healthy mucous membrane of non-smoker.

(b) Mucous membrane of a marijuana smoker.

(c) Mucous membrane of a marijuana and cigarette smoker.

Courtesy of Dr. Donald Tashkin, Chief, Pulmonary Research Department, UCLA Medical Center, Los Angeles

nancy may be a consequence of regular marijuana smoking since some of these changes are precursors of cancer.

"I'm sure I've done some damage to my lungs. I mean, you can't put that kind of tar down in your system, heated tar going into your system constantly for 23 years and sit here and say there's nothing wrong and nothing had happened. Surely something has happened."
39-year-old marijuana smoker

Finally the breathing passage of a chronic marijuana and cigarette smoker (Fig. 6-4c) shows that the normal surface cells have been completely replaced by nonciliated cells resembling skin, so the smoker has to cough to clear mucous from the lungs since the ciliated cells are gone. This leads to acute and chronic bronchitis. Marijuana and cigarette smokers also have a greatly increased risk for developing cancer of the tongue, cancer of the larynx, and cancer of the lung (Joy et al., 1999; Tashkin, 1999; Tashkin, 1987; Wilkins et al., 1998).

Immune System

Some evidence suggests that heavy use of marijuana can depress the immune system making users more susceptible to a cold, the flu, and other viral infections. If such were the case, it would be a mistake for people who are already immune depressed, either as a result of AIDS or as a result of chemotherapy for cancer, to smoke marijuana for therapeutic purposes. The smoker is further suppressing an already depressed immune system and exposing the lungs to pathogens, such as fungi and bacteria, found in marijuana smoke. However, the health impact of marijuana on the immune system remains unclear from lack of definitive research (Joy et al., 1999; Hollister, 1992).

Learning & Emotional Maturation

"If you go home and have homework to do that night and you say, 'O.K. I'm going to get stoned before I do my homework,' you're never going to get your homework done."
High school student

Marijuana has been shown to slow learning and disrupt concentration. Part of this influence comes from marijuana's effect on short-term memory. Short-term memory, in contrast to long-term memory, is a processing of information to be retained for only a short period of time, such as a grocery list, a proper assortment of tools for a certain job, or facts crammed into the head for an upcoming exam. Marijuana greatly impairs a person's ability to retain this information. However, it has very little effect on long-term memory, which is the processing and storing of information for a long period of time, such as a theory in physics that has been studied for several weeks. This explains why some students have been able to maintain good grades while using marijuana on a regular basis while others end up flunking out (Brown & Massaro, 1996).

Although more research is needed into what some researchers call an "amotivational syndrome," a number of patients treated at the Haight-Ashbury Clinic for marijuana addiction do show a lack of motivation. They have a tendency to avoid problems.

"You know how they tell you go to school to get an education so you can get a good job? They did tell me how to get a job, so that's eight hours a day. I knew how to sleep, that's eight hours a day. I had another eight hours a day that I didn't know how to fill and I used marijuana to fill those eight hours. Period."
38-year-old recovering compulsive marijuana smoker

The way this mechanism operates is similar to the effects of other psychoactive drugs. What happens is that a drug can be used as a shortcut to a pleasing physical sensation or as a way to counteract boredom or emotional pain.

"Well when I used 'weed,' you know, like I was really depressed. I was just really angry at everybody—like my dad, myself, you know, I was just angry at the world. I hated myself. I wanted to commit suicide I was so bad. So I just smoked 'weed' just to get rid of it. I'd steal my dad's 'weed' or he'd give it to me."
18-year-old recovering marijuana smoker

If users then come to depend on this method for gaining pleasure or avoiding pain rather than learning how to receive pleasure and satisfaction naturally or face up to and deal with painful situations directly, they will habituate their minds and bodies to this chemical solution.

"I liked to do it so much that, it's like, why not do it? I couldn't find a reason for not doing it. It was too enjoyable. It was like going and looking in your refrigerator and seeing a thing of ice cream and a thing of Hershey's® chocolate syrup and going, 'No, I'm going to have a bran muffin instead.' Why? You can have ice cream and the chocolate syrup, man. That's what you want. Why don't you have it?"
17-year-old marijuana smoker

Since marijuana can be "the mirror that magnifies," smoking often exaggerates natural tendencies in the user. Thus if a person really isn't interested in working, studying, having a relationship, or reading a book and smokes marijuana, his or her primitive brain is given the edge over the new brain and says, "You don't have to do those things." So rather than the new brain, the neocortex, giving guidance and saying, "These are necessary things that you're going to have to do," the primitive brain takes over and says, "Forget it, let's not do this."

"When I got high I thought I was the smartest person in the world. I knew I had the answer to everything and one

day, I sat down with the tape recorder and I started rattling off all this brilliance that I had and the next day when I woke up in the morning and I played it back, it was almost like I wasn't even speaking English."

38-year-old recovering compulsive marijuana smoker

With marijuana many thoughts and feelings are internalized. Long-term marijuana smokers feel that they're thinking, feeling, and communicating better but often they're not.

"When I have worked with couples where one of the principal partners in the relationship has been using marijuana for a long period of time, the biggest complaint is that 'He never says anything' or 'She never says anything. We don't talk. We don't communicate.' But for the marijuana user, that person feels when they're under the influence that they are trying to communicate. So the intentions are there, the feelings are there, and the emotions are there but it's all internal. It never gets out to the other person."

John DeDomenico, counselor, Haight-Ashbury Detox Clinic

Acute Mental Effects

Lasting mental problems from short-term use are unusual but in someone with preexisting mental problems or with latent emotional problems, particularly if marijuana with high THC levels is smoked, acute anxiety or temporary psychotic reactions can occur (NIH, 1997). Individuals believe that they have lost control of their mental state. There's often paranoia or a belief that they have severely damaged themselves or that their underlying insecurities are insurmountable. These acute problems are usually treatable but what is problematic is when the symptoms persist. Counselors at the Haight-Ashbury Clinic have seen a number of cases of what medicine calls a "post-hallucinogenic drug perceptual disorder" where peo-

ple who, after experiencing a bad trip, don't come all the way down and may have problems going on with their lives. They experience continued confusion, concentration difficulty, memory problems, and feel as if their mind is always in a fog.

"I was working with a 13-year-old client who had no premorbid symptoms that could be identified prior to his 13th birthday when his friends turned him on to a 'honey blunt,' which is a cigar packed with marijuana soaked in honey and dried. It happened to be very strong sinsemilla and he experienced an acute anxiety reaction followed by a post-hallucinogenic drug perceptual disorder including a profound depression and an inability to concentrate. We don't know how long these problems will last."

Counselor, Haight-Ashbury Detox Clinic

Even seasoned veteran smokers who've been smoking some low-grade "pot" and then get some strong "Buddha Thai" sinsemilla may feel that somebody has slipped them a psychedelic like PCP or LSD. They begin to experience anxiety and paranoia that then create more anxiety than what they were feeling. Eventually they could have an acute psychotic break.

TOLERANCE, WITHDRAWAL, & ADDICTION

Tolerance

Tolerance to marijuana occurs in a rapid and dramatic fashion. Although high-dose chronic users can recognize the effects of low levels of THC in their systems, they are able to tolerate much higher levels without some of the more severe emotional and psychic effects experienced by a first-time user.

One great concern about marijuana is that it persists in the body of a chronic user for up to three months though the major effects last only four to six hours after smoking. These residual amounts in the body can disrupt

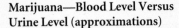

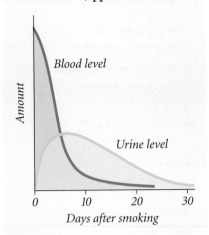

Figure 6-5 •

This chart shows the blood and urine levels of marijuana over time. The marijuana persists in the urine longer. Most drug testing usually only measures marijuana in the urine.

some physiological, mental, and emotional functions for a longer period.

Withdrawal

Because there is not the rapid onset of withdrawal from marijuana as with alcohol or heroin, many people deny that withdrawal occurs. The withdrawal from marijuana is more drawn out because most of the THC has been retained in the fat cells and only after a period of abstinence will the withdrawal effects appear.

"Sometimes people who've been smoking for five years decide to quit. They stop one, two, three days, even a week, and they say (especially those who think marijuana is benign), 'Wow, I feel great. Marijuana's no problem. I have no withdrawal. It's nothing at all.' Then they start up again. They never experience withdrawal. We see that withdrawal symptoms to marijuana are delayed sometimes for several weeks to a month after a person stops."

Counselor, Haight-Ashbury Detox Clinic

The delayed withdrawal effects of marijuana include

◇ anger or irritability and aggression;

◇ aches, pains, chills;

◇ depression;

◇ inability to concentrate;

◇ slight tremors;

◇ sleep disturbances;

◇ decreased appetite;

◇ sweating;

◇ craving.

Not everyone will experience all of these effects but everyone will experience some of them, especially craving. Recent human research demonstrated that irritability, anxiety, aggression, and even stomach pain caused by marijuana withdrawal occurred within three to seven days of abstinence (Kouri et al., 1999; Haney et al., 1999).

"I would break into a sweat in the shower. I could not maintain my concentration for the first month or two. To really treasure my sobriety, it took me about three or four months before I really came out of the fog and really started getting a grasp of what was going on around me."
38-year-old recovering marijuana addict

The discovery by French scientists in 1994 of an antagonist that instantly blocks the effects of marijuana enabled researchers to search for true signs of tolerance, tissue dependence, and withdrawal symptoms in long-term users. Experiments demonstrated that cessation of marijuana use could cause true physical withdrawal symptoms. Dr. Billy Martin of the Medical College of Virginia gave the THC antagonist SR14176A to rats who had been exposed to marijuana for four days in a row. The antagonist negated the influence of the marijuana. Within 10 minutes the rats exhibited immediate physical withdrawal behaviors that included "wet dog shakes" and facial rubbing, which is the rat equivalent of withdrawal. These experiments indicated

that marijuana dependence occurs more rapidly than previously suspected. This experiment, which compressed the withdrawal to minutes instead of weeks, allowed the addictive potential of cannabinoids to be more clearly understood. (Aceto, Scates, Lowe, & Martin, 1995; Rinaldi-Carmona et al., 1994; Tsou, Patrick, & Walker, 1995; NIDA, 1995).

Further, human studies have demonstrated rapid eye movement (REM) sleep changes similar to those seen in other drug addictions. They include decreased REM while smoking marijuana and increased REM during withdrawal.

Addiction

"I thought I could control it because when I woke up in the morning, I didn't get high for the first hour and a half. I figured an hour and a half— that proves that I'm not hooked on this stuff because I don't really need it. By the same token, once I smoked that first 'joint,' I did not come back down until I woke up."
Recovering user in Marijuana Anonymous 12-step program

The 1990s have made us take a different view of the addiction potential of this substance. Today many people smoke the drug in a chronic, compulsive way and have difficulty discontinuing their use. Like cocaine, heroin, alcohol, nicotine, and other addictive drugs, marijuana does have the ability to induce compulsive use in spite of the negative consequences it may be causing in the user's life.

"Why am I doing this? What's wrong with me? Why do I have to keep doing this? And I did this for a good 8–10 years. I used to buy it by the pound and then I found after a while that I wanted to make it harder on myself to smoke. So I started buying dime bags, figuring it would cost a lot more, and then eventually, I got to the point where it didn't work. I just kept on

buying. But, yeah, with me, I just could not stop."
38-year-old recovering marijuana addict

Finally all available research on marijuana was based on a THC calculation of 20 mg per marijuana cigarette (considered in the 1960s to be a high-dose exposure). Current marijuana "joints" used for research contain 40 mg of THC, still below most good quality street "joints" but closer than in the past. (The marijuana for these experimental "joints" is grown at a government farm in Mississippi.)

"The main problem we're dealing with is that today's potent form of marijuana is causing a lot more problems than we saw in the 1960s. I never treated a single marijuana self-admitted addict in the Clinic throughout the '60s nor the '70s and pretty much through the '80s but by the late '80s, we started seeing people coming in. Everyone of them came in on their own volition, saying, 'Help me. I want to stop smoking 'pot.' It is causing me these problems, causing me to have memory problems, causing me to be too spaced out, not to function in my work. I can't complete tasks. It's causing me to be sick in the morning and cough. I have withdrawal symptoms. I want to stop and I can't stop.' At our program in San Francisco, we now have about 100 patients every month who are in treatment specifically for marijuana addiction. So people who claim that marijuana is harmless have to sit down and listen to those people who are the wounded, what we call the walking wounded or the casualties from marijuana use. For them marijuana has caused some problems— not propaganda or other people telling them it's causing problems but they themselves saying it's so."
Darryl Inaba, Pharm.D., CEO, Haight-Ashbury Free Clinics

Is Marijuana a Gateway Drug?

In antidrug movies like *Reefer Madness* and *Marijuana, Assassin of Youth,* the claim was that marijuana physically and mentally changed users, so they started using heroin and cocaine and became helpless addicts. The exaggeration of this idea led to an undermining of drug education because people who smoked marijuana didn't become raving lunatics or depraved dope fiends. The experimenters who had tried marijuana said, "I tried marijuana and that didn't happen, so I guess they're lying about all the drugs."

This exaggeration and resultant ridicule, particularly by the younger generation, of propagandistic or scare films and books probably caused more drug abuse than it prevented. It also obscured an important idea, that is, the real role marijuana use plays in future drug use and abuse.

"I've been in a 12-step program [Narcotics Anonymous] for a little over six years and I'm not going to say like one and one equal two but just about everybody I meet in the 12-step program started out with either marijuana or alcohol."
Recovering marijuana addict

Marijuana is a gateway drug in the sense that if people smoke it, they will probably hang around others who smoke marijuana or use other drugs, so the opportunities to experiment with other drugs are greater. Incidentally the history of most addicts clearly demonstrates that the first drug they ever used or abused was either tobacco or alcohol—the more usual gateway drugs.

No two people will have the exact same reaction to marijuana but what has been observed is that those who continue to use it regularly establish a pattern of use and begin to find opportunities where drugs other than marijuana are available.

"The majority of people that I know, that I hang around with, if they ain't

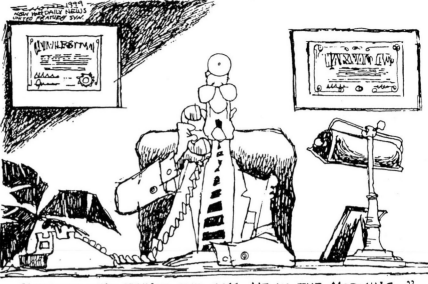

"SMOKE TWO JOINTS AND CALL ME IN THE MORNING..."

BILL SCHORR Reprinted, by permission of United Feature Syndicate, Inc.

smoking 'weed,' they're smoking 'crack,' or drinking. I'm not saying that they are bad people but that's just how it is."
30-year-old polydrug user who started smoking marijuana at the age of 13

Viewed from this perspective, it is not surprising that most users of other illicit drugs have used marijuana first but only after they began using alcohol and or nicotine (Joy et al., 1999; Kandel & Yamaguchi, 1993; Kandel, Yamaguchi, & Chen, 1992).

MARIJUANA (*Cannabis*) & THE LAW

Marijuana is one of the drugs that has never been out of favor and is still popular at the start of the twenty-first century. Internationally, marijuana is the most widely used illicit drug in countries such as Canada, Mexico, Costa Rica, El Salvador, Panama, Australia, and South Africa (NIDA, 1998). The biggest change in this drug is the increase in the availability of highly potent marijuana (up to 14 times as strong as varieties available in the '70s) and the increase in price that has gone up 10- to 30-fold since the early '70s. (Higher-potency marijuana was always available

but it was just not very plentiful.) Just as the refinement of coca leaves into cocaine and opium into heroin led to greater abuse of the drugs, so have better cultivation techniques increased the compulsive liability of marijuana use. There is also an increase in the practice of mixing marijuana with other drugs like cocaine, amphetamine, and PCP. Some users even smoke "joints" that have been soaked in formaldehyde and embalming fluid ("clickems") or even sprayed with Raid Roach Killer® ("canaid") for a bigger kick.

Marijuana, Driving, & Drug Testing

In more and more arrests for reckless driving or tests at the scene of an accident, the driver is tested for marijuana and other drugs. Four of the problems testing for marijuana are that

◇ it persists for a number of days in the body and can still be detected days after use;

◇ the elimination rate varies radically compared to alcohol that has a defined rate of metabolism;

◇ there is a scarcity of good data about the level of marijuana in the blood and the level of impairment;

◇ and most important (and most often), there is another drug besides marijuana in the system, especially alcohol, so even if marijuana has a relatively small effect, it is magnified by polydrug use and abuse.

Added to the fact that 65% of heavy drinkers also use marijuana (SAMHSA, 1999), it's no wonder that positive polydrug test results are the rule and not the exception in drivers arrested for DUI or DWI (Gieringer, 1988).

As with alcohol, driving impairment is directly related to the amount of THC in the body. One study found that 60% of smokers failed a field-sobriety test 2 1/2 hours after smoking moderate amounts, while other tests have shown some impairment 3–7 hours after smoking, while even others showed minimal impairment 3–8 hours later (Reeve et al., 1983; Smiley, 1986; Hollister, 1986). Testing machines can measure minute amounts of THC but are generally calibrated to start registering at 50 nanograms per milliliter (ng/mL) in urine samples. Some measurements have registered levels up to 800 ng/mL. Generally if a person has been a long-term smoker, it would take about 3 weeks before they wouldn't register on a test with a 50 ng/mL cutoff and another 3 weeks to be completely negative. In a few instances it has taken 10 weeks for the drug to clear completely. For someone who smoked a "joint" at a party but is not a long-time user, he or she usually tests negative 24–48 hours after use.

Generally marijuana

◇ impairs the ability to react properly to complex situations;

◇ induces drowsiness and impairs judgment (Mathias, 1996);

◇ and appears in the blood and urine three to five times more frequently in fatal drivers than in the general population (Gieringer, 1988).

The Medical Use of Marijuana

Controversy has always existed around marijuana. One major area of contention is whether it should be legalized, decriminalized, or kept illegal.

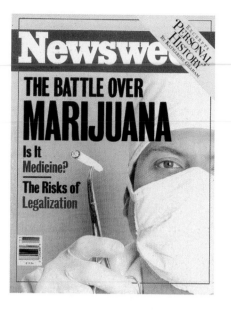

A second major area is whether it should be available for medical use.

Historically marijuana has been used

◇ to treat insomnia,

◇ to calm anxiety,

◇ to cure venereal disease,

◇ to relieve coughs (antitussive),

◇ to calm whooping cough,

◇ to control headaches,

◇ as a childbirth analgesic,

◇ as a topical anesthetic,

◇ to control asthma,

◇ to treat nerve pains (neuralgias) and migraine headaches,

◇ to treat withdrawal from opiates and alcohol,

◇ as an antibiotic,

◇ to control spasms and convulsions,

◇ and to induce childbirth.

(Mikuriya, 1973; Aldrich, 1997; Gurley, Aranow, & Katz, 1998)

Recently it has been recommended for some types of glaucoma, nausea control, and to help a patient who has lost too much weight (wasting disease) to gain it back by stimulating hunger.

There is evidence that marijuana does reduce intraocular pressure, does calm nausea, and does encourage people to eat, though there are other drugs that are as effective or in some cases better. Many people smoke marijuana therapeutically for their glaucoma, cancer, AIDS, or other illness even though it is

illegal. There are also people and places such as marijuana buyers clubs that procure marijuana for those who are ill. In addition, Marinol®, a synthesized form of THC, is theoretically available for treatment of these and other health problems but in practice is rarely prescribed. People say they prefer marijuana in its smokable form because it works faster than Marinol®. If they smoke, they can smoke just as much or as little as they need to relieve symptoms, whereas if they take a premeasured Marinol® capsule, it may not be enough or may be too much for their condition. A major obstacle with smoking or ingesting marijuana for medical purposes is the great variation in the amount of active ingredients in any given marijuana plant. Variations in Δ-9-THC potency, the relative concentration of other active cannabinoids, and the inconsistency of other botanical factors make it difficult to rely on this substance to treat medical problems. For example, some forms of marijuana have been shown to increase intraocular pressure, making someone's glaucoma worse, although normally most forms of marijuana will lower intraocular pressure.

But beyond the physiological effects, there are the mental effects of marijuana that are the real issue. Like opium cure-alls, such as theriac and laudanum, it is the mental effects of calming, anxiety relief, or mild euphoria that make people feel good and think they are getting better even if the drug isn't actually helping the illness.

There is however reluctance in the medical community to prescribe or even approve of marijuana for medical use for several reasons, including those already stated.

◇ There are a number of drugs on the market that physiologically have the same therapeutic effects or even better effects than marijuana or Marinol®.

◇ The THC content and even the potency of all the other chemicals vary from one "joint" to the next, so even if a few puffs worked a certain way one time, there's no guarantee the reaction would be the same the next time.

◇ Marijuana smoke contains a number of irritants, carcinogens, pathogens, and other chemicals, most of which have not been studied. If marijuana is baked in brownies or otherwise eaten, the respiratory effects are avoided but the 360 compounds contained in marijuana remain, along with all their side effects.

◇ Marijuana does somewhat impair the immune system, thus making the user more vulnerable to other illnesses.

◇ Marijuana is a psychoactive drug with abuse and addictive potential, which is particularly dangerous for those who are recovering from abuse or addiction.

Contrary to popular belief, medical research about marijuana continues in many countries. Since the 1970s there have been more than 12,500 scientific studies conducted on marijuana. Yet results continue to be conflicting, making it difficult to substantiate appropriate medical use of marijuana.

1999 REPORT FROM THE NATIONAL ACADEMY OF SCIENCES' INSTITUTE OF MEDICINE TO THE OFFICE OF NATIONAL DRUG CONTROL POLICY (ONDCP)

In 1999 a study entitled *Marijuana and Medicine: Assessing the Science Base* was released. It was commissioned in August 1996 by the White House Office of National Drug Control Policy. The Office asked the Institute of Medicine of the National Academy of Sciences to conduct a review of the scientific evidence and to do field research concerning the health benefits and risks of marijuana. We present, verbatim, their major conclusions and recommendations. We do this because when the report was originally released in 1999, both sides of the argument (pro- and antimarijuana forces) went in front of the media and translated the report colored by what they thought the report said. The result was that unless one read the original report, the public couldn't know what it really said.

Conclusions of the Report

Cannabinoid Biology

◇ Cannabinoids likely have a natural role in pain modulation, control of movement, and memory.

◇ The natural role of cannabinoids in immune systems is likely multifaceted and remains unclear.

◇ The brain develops a tolerance to cannabinoids.

◇ Animal research demonstrates the potential for dependence but this potential is observed under a narrower range of conditions than with benzodiazepines, opiates, cocaine, or nicotine.

◇ Withdrawal symptoms can be observed in animals but appear to be mild compared to opiates or benzodiazepines, such as diazepam (Valium®).

Efficacy of Cannabinoid Drugs

◇ Scientific data indicate the potential therapeutic value of cannabinoid drugs, primarily THC, for pain relief, control of nausea and vomiting, and appetite stimulation; smoked marijuana however is a crude THC delivery system that also delivers harmful substances.

Influence of Psychological Effects on Therapeutic Effects

◇ The psychological effects of cannabinoids, such as anxiety reduction, sedation, and euphoria, can influence their potential therapeutic value. Those effects are potentially undesirable for certain patients and situations and beneficial for others. In addition psychological effects can complicate the interpretation of other aspects of the drug effect.

Physiological Risks

◇ Numerous studies suggest that marijuana smoke is an important risk factor in the development of respiratory disease.

Marijuana Dependence and Withdrawal

◇ A distinctive marijuana withdrawal syndrome has been identified but it

Doonesbury

BY GARRY TRUDEAU

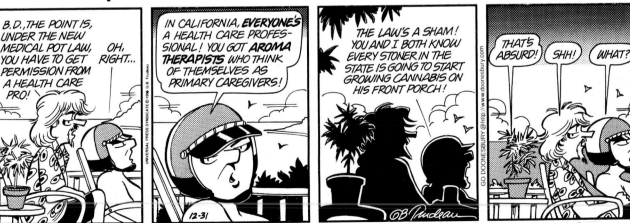

is mild and short-lived. The syndrome includes restlessness, irritability, mild agitation, insomnia, sleep EEG disturbance, nausea, and cramping.

Marijuana as a "Gateway" Drug

◇ Present data on drug use progression neither support nor refute the suggestion that medical availability would increase drug abuse. However, this question is beyond issues normally considered for medical uses of drugs and should not be a factor in evaluating the therapeutic potential of marijuana or cannabinoids.

Use of Smoked Marijuana

◇ Because of the health risks associated with smoking, smoked marijuana should generally not be rec-

'Marijuana Patch' May Aid Cancer Treatment

From Associated Press

ALBANY, N.Y.—A "marijuana patch" similar to the patches that help smokers kick the habit could help relieve the pain and side effects of cancer, researchers say.

The American Cancer Society is funding a three-year, $361,000 grant for research into a "marijuana patch" that announced today at

ommended for long-term medical use. Nonetheless for certain patients, such as the terminally ill or those with debilitating symptoms, the long-term risks are not of great concern. Further, despite the legal, social, and health problems associated with smoking marijuana, it is widely used by certain patient groups.

Recommendations of the Report

1. Research should continue into the physiological effects of synthetic and plant-derived cannabinoids and the natural function of cannabinoids found in the body. Because different cannabinoids appear to have different effects, cannabinoid research should include, but not be restricted to, effects attributable to THC alone.

2. Clinical trials of cannabinoid drugs for symptom management should be conducted with the goal of developing rapid-onset, reliable, and safe delivery systems.

3. Psychological effects of cannabinoids such as anxiety reduction and sedation, which can influence medical benefits, should be evaluated in clinical trials.

4. Studies to define the individual health risks of smoking marijuana should be conducted, particularly among populations in which marijuana use is prevalent.

5. Clinical trials of marijuana use for medical purposes should be conducted under the following limited circumstances: be conducted in patients with conditions for which there is reasonable expectation of efficacy; be approved by institutional review boards; and collect data about efficacy.

6. Short-term use of smoked marijuana (less than six months) for patients with debilitating symptoms (such as intractable pain or vomiting) must meet the following conditions:

   • failure of all approved medications to provide relief has been documented;

   • the symptoms can reasonably be expected to be relieved by rapid-onset cannabinoid drugs;

   • such treatment is administered under medical supervision in a manner that allows for assessment of treatment effectiveness;

   • and involves an oversight strategy comparable to an institutional review board process that could provide guidance within 24 hours of a submission by a physician to provide marijuana to a patient for a specified use.

(Institute of Medicine, 1999)

(The full report is available from the National Academy Press, Tel: (800) 624-6242.)

HEALTH-SCIENCE

The Mail Tribune, Friday, March 3, 2000   **9C**

Study: Pot makes heart attack more likely

By DANIEL Q. HANEY
The Associated Press

SAN DIEGO — Warning to middle-aged potheads: Smoking marijuana may be bad for your middle-aged hearts.

In the first study to find a link between pot and heart trouble, Harvard researchers reported Thursday that the risk of a heart attack is five times higher than usual in the hour after smoking a joint.

Until now, marijuana has not been much of an issue in heart disease, since older folks do not typically smoke pot. However, this could change as baby boomers take their pot-smoking habits beyond middle age.

The researchers said that for someone in shape, marijuana is about twice as risky as exercising or having sex.

The study was conducted by Dr. Murray Mittleman of the Harvard School of Public Health and Boston's Beth Israel Deaconess Medical Center. He presented the findings at a conference in San Diego of the American Heart Association.

The researchers questioned 3,882 heart attack victims — men and women — at 62 locations across the country about their habits and found that 124 were marijuana users. While pot was uncommon among the elderly heart patients, 13 percent of those under age 50 said they smoke it.

Among those questioned, 37 had their heart attacks within a day of using marijuana, including nine within an hour afterward.

The researchers calculated that someone's risk of a heart attack is five times higher during the hour after using marijuana. After an hour, the risk falls to twice normal. It soon returns to the usual level.

Whether a fivefold increase is a worry depends on whether someone has other risk factors, such as high blood pressure or diabetes. The increased risk is probably insignificant for a 20-year-old, whose chance of a heart attack is vanishingly small anyway.

"With baby boomers aging, more people in 40s and 50s are smoking marijuana than in prior generations," Mittleman said. "The risk of coronary artery disease increases with age. Whether this will emerge as a public health problem remains to be seen."

In any case, the risk of a heart attack from any single session of marijuana smoking is likely to be low. Mittleman said that for an otherwise healthy 50-year-old man, it is about 10 in 1 million.

Marijuana typically makes the heart speed up by about 40 beats a minute. Whether this is how it contributes to heart attacks is unclear. Mittleman noted that

while marijuana doesn't contain nicotine, the smoke is otherwise similar to cigarette smoke.

In general, the marijuana smokers in the study were more likely than other heart attack victims to be overweight and sedentary, but they were less apt to have diabetes, high blood pressure or badly clogged arteries.

"My advice on marijuana is, 'Don't,'" said Dr. Lynn Smaha of Sayre, Pa., president of the heart association. "If they have heart disease, I'd tell patients they are playing a dangerous game if they smoke marijuana."

CHAPTER SUMMARY

History

1. All arounders, also known as "psychedelics" and "hallucinogens," have been around since the origin of man. Virtually all of the early psychedelics were derived from plants including fungi. Recently the most popular psychedelics besides marijuana (e.g., LSD, MDMA) have been synthesized.

Classification

2. The most commonly used psychedelics are marijuana, LSD, PCP, peyote, psilocybin ("magic mushrooms"), and MDMA (or other variations of the amphetamine molecule).

General Effects

3. A major physical effect of psychedelics, other than marijuana, PCP, or anticholinergics, is stimulation.

4. The most frequent mental effects of psychedelics are intensified sensations (particularly visual ones, including illusions and delusions), mixed-up sensations (synesthesia), suppressed memory centers, and impaired judgment and reasoning.

5. The effects of all arounders are particularly dependent on the size of the dose, the emotional makeup of the user, the mood at the time of use, and the user's surroundings.

LSD, Psilocybin Mushrooms, & Other Indole Psychedelics

6. LSD is extremely potent. Doses as low as 25 micrograms (25-millionths of a gram) can cause some psychedelic effects.

7. Like many other psychedelics, LSD overloads the brainstem, the sensory switchboard for the mind, and creates illusions and delusions.

8. Psilocybin is the active ingredient in "magic mushrooms."

9. After initial nausea or vomiting, visual illusions and a certain altered state of consciousness are the most common effects of mushrooms.

10. Mushrooms and peyote buttons have been used in religious ceremonies by many Native American and Mexican Indian tribes.

Peyote, MDMA, & Other Phenylalkylamine Psychedelics

11. Mescaline is the active ingredient of the peyote cactus.

12. Eating peyote buttons or drinking them in a prepared tea causes color-filled visions and vivid hallucinations after an initial nausea and physical stimulation.

13. Club drugs abused at "raves," include MDMA, LSD, 2CB, GHB, and ketamine.

Belladonna & Other Anticholinergic Psychedelics

14. Belladonna and other nightshade plants contain scopolamine and atropine. In low doses these substances cause a mild stupor but as the dose increases, delirium, hallucinations, and a separation from reality are common.

Ketamine, PCP, & Other Psychedelics

15. PCP ("angel dust") is an anesthetic, now illegal, that besides deadening sensation, disassociates users from their surroundings and senses.

16. Effects of the drug PCP include amnesia, extremely high blood pressure, and combativeness. Higher doses can produce tremors, seizures, catatonia, coma, and even kidney failure.

17. Ketamine, another anesthetic, has become a popular drug in the "rave" club scene.

Marijuana & Other Cannabinols

18. Historically the *Cannabis* plant has been grown to produce fibers for rope and cloth, seeds for food, various chemicals for medicinal effects, and a psychoactive resin for psychedelic effects.

19. Marijuana is the most widely used illicit psychoactive drug. Use has increased, particularly in high school students since 1992 after a decade of decline.

20. Discoveries in the 1990s of a marijuana receptor site, a neurotransmitter (anandamide) that fits into that receptor site, and a marijuana antagonist, all have accelerated research into the effects of marijuana.

21. The two most widely used marijuana species are *Cannabis sativa* and *Cannabis indica*. *Cannabis sativa* can be used for hemp or psychedelic effects. *Cannabis indica* is used only for its psychedelic effects.

22. The sinsemilla technique of growing *Cannabis sativa* or *Cannabis indica* greatly increases the concentration of -9-THC, the main psychoactive ingredient in marijuana.

23. Street marijuana that is readily available in the 2000s is 5–14 times stronger than the marijuana of the 1960s and '70s. Much growing is done indoors to avoid detection.

24. Short-term effects of smoking marijuana include a dreamlike effect, sedation, and a mild self-hypnosis, making users more likely to exaggerate their mood and react to the surroundings.

25. Some of the negative effects of short-term marijuana use are lowered testosterone levels, a decrease in the ability to do complicated tasks, a temporary disruption of short-term memory, decreased tracking ability (an impairment of eye-hand coordination), a trailing phenomenon, and a loss of the sense of time.

26. Large amounts of marijuana or prolonged use can cause anxiety reactions, paranoia, and some illusions.

27. Respiratory effects include a decrease in the cilia lining the mucous membranes in the breathing passages that makes the smoker more susceptible to coughs, chronic bronchitis, emphysema, and possibly cancer. Smokers of both marijuana and cigarettes do much more damage to their air passages and lungs than a smoker of only one of the drugs.

28. Chronic marijuana use can make some smokers less likely to do anything they don't want to do, leading to a tendency to neglect life's problems or to think about problems rather than do something about them.

29. Tolerance develops fairly rapidly with chronic marijuana use.

30. When stopping chronic marijuana use, a person can suffer delayed withdrawal symptoms that include headache, anxiety, depression, irritability, aggression, restlessness, tremors, sleep disturbances, and continued craving for the drug.

31. Medical use of marijuana is the controversial new battleground. Although marijuana has been employed as a medicine for more than 5,000 years, it is very sparingly used today. Proponents say it should be available as a medicine whereas opponents say there are better medicines that are more reliable and don't have all the other chemicals with unresearched side effects. Several states have passed laws allowing the medical use of marijuana.

REFERENCES

Aceto, M. D, Scates, S. M., Lowe, J. A., & Martin, B. R. (1995). Cannabinoid-precipitated withdrawal by a selective antagonist: SR 141716A. *European Journal of Pharmacology, 282*(1–3), R1–R2.

Aldrich, M. R. (1997). History of therapeutic *Cannabis*. In M. L. Mathre (Ed.), Cannabis *in Medical Practice.* Jefferson, NC: McFarland & Company, Inc.

Atharva Veda. (1400 B.C.). *Atharva Veda*, 11.6.15.

Balster, R. L. (1995). Phencyclidine. In J. H. Jaffe (Ed.), *Encyclopedia of Drugs and Alcohol* (Vol. 2, pp. 809–818), New York: MacMillan Library Reference.

Bibra, B. E. (1855, reprint, 1995). *Plant Intoxicants.* Rochester, VT: Healing Arts Press.

Blum, K. (1984). Marijuana: Heaven or hell. In K. Blum (Ed.), *Handbook of Abusable Drugs.* New York: Garner Press, 447–534.

Brown, M. W., & Massaro, S. (1996). Attention and memory impairment in heavy users of marijuana. NIDA Notes, 2-20-99.

Carroll, M., & Comer, S. (1998). The pharmacology of phencyclidine and the hallucinogens. In A. W. Graham & T. K. Schultz (Eds.), *Principles of Addiction Medicine* (2nd ed., pp. 153–162). Chevy Chase, MD: American Society of Addiction Medicine, Inc.

Chilton, W. S., Bigwood, J., & Jensen, R. E. (1979). Psilocin, bufotenine and serotonin: Historical and biosynthetic observations. *Journal of Psychoactive Drugs, 11*(1–2), 61–69.

DEA (Drug Enforcement Administration). (1997). *Ketamine abuse increasing. http://www.usdoj.gov/dea/programs/diversion/divpub/substanc/ketamine.htm.*

DEA. (1998). The Supply of Illicit Drugs to the United States. DEA Publications. *http://www.usdoj.gov/dea/pubs/intel/nnicc97.htm.*

Devane, W. A., Hanus, L., Breuer, A., Pertwee, R. G., Stevenson, L. A., Griffin, G., Gibson, D., Mandelbaum, A., Etinger, A., & Mechoulam, R. (1992). Isolation and structure of a brain constituent that bonds to the cannabinoid receptor. *Science, 258*(5090), 1882–1884, 1946–1949.

Diaz, J. L. (1979). Ethnopharmacology and taxonomy of Mexican psychodysleptic plants. *Journal of Psychoactive Drugs, 11*(1–2), 71–101.

DuPont, R. L. (1997). *The Selfish Brain.* Washington, DC: American Psychiatric Press, Inc.

DuToit, B. M. (1980). *Cannabis in Africa.* Rotterdam: Balkema.

Efferink, J. G. R. (1988). Some little-known hallucinogenic plants of the Aztecs. *Journal of Psychoactive Drugs, 20*(4), 427–434.

Emboden, W. A. (1981). The genus *Cannabis* and the correct use of taxonomic categories. *Journal of Psychoactive Drugs, 13*(1), 15–22.

Fischer, C., Hatzidimitriou, G., Wlos, J., Katz, J., & Ricaurte, G. (1995). Reorganization of ascending 5-HT axon projections in animals previously exposed to recreational drug 3,4-methelenedioxymethamphetamine (MDMA, "ecstasy") *Journal of Neuroscience, 15*, 5476–5485.

Furst, P. T. (1976). *Hallucinogens and Culture.* San Francisco: Chandler & Sharp Publishers, Inc.

Gieringer, D. H. (1988). Marijuana, driving, and accident safety. *Journal of Psychoactive Drugs, 20*(1), 93–100.

Goldstein, A. (1994). *Addiction: From Biology to Drug Policy.* New York: W. H. Freeman and Company.

Gurley, R. J., Aranow, R., & Katz, M. (1998). Medicinal marijuana: A comprehensive review. *Journal of Psychoactive Drugs, 30*(2), 137–148.

Haney, M. et al. (1999). Abstinence symptoms following smoked marijuana in humans. *Psychopharmacology, 141*, 395–404.

Henderson, L., & Glass, W. (Eds.). (1994). *LSD Report.* Lexington, MA: Lexington Books.

Hollister, L. E. (1984). Effects of hallucinogens in humans. In B. L. Jacobs (Ed.), *Hallucinogens: Neurochemical, Behavioral, and Clinical Perspectives*, (pp.19–34). New York: The Raven Press.

Hollister, L. E. (1986). Health aspects of cannabis. *Pharmacological Revues, 38*(1), 1–20.

Hollister, L. E. (1992). Marijuana and immunity. *Journal of Psychoactive Drugs, 24*(2), 159–164.

Howlett, A. C., Evans, D. M., & Houston, D. B. (1992). The cannabinoid receptor. In L. Murphy & A. Bartke (Eds.), *Marijuana/Cannabinoids: Neurobiology and Neurophysiology* (pp. 35–72). Boca Raton, FL: CRC Press.

Institute of Medicine. (1999). *Marijuana and Medicine: Assessing the Science Base.* Washington, DC: National Academy Press.

Jaffe, J. H. (1989). Psychoactive substance abuse disorder. In H. Kaplan & B. J. Sadock (Eds.), *Comprehensive Textbook of Psychiatry* (5th ed., pp. 642–686). Baltimore: Williams & Wilkins.

Joy, J. E., Watson, S. J. Jr., & Benson, J. A. (Eds.). (1999). *Marijuana and Medicine: Assessing the Science Base.* Washington, DC: National Academy Press.

Kandel, D. B., & Yamaguchi, K. (1993). From beer to crack: Developmental patterns of drug involvement. *American Journal of Public Health, 83,* 851–855.

Kandel, D. B., Yamaguchi, K., & Chen, K. (1992). Stages of progression in drug involvement from adolescence to adulthood: Further evidence for the gateway theory. *Journal of Alcohol Studies, 53,* 447–457.

Kouri, E. M. et al. (1999). Changes in aggressive behavior during withdrawal from long-term marijuana use. *Psychopharmacology, 143,* 302–308.

Krupitsky, E. M., & Grinenko, A. Y. (1997). Ketamine psychedelic therapy (KPT). A review of the results of ten years of research. *Journal of Psychoactive Drugs, 29*(2), 165–183.

La Barre, J., & Weston, D. (1979). Peyotl and mescaline. *Journal of Psychoactive Drugs, 11*(1–2), 33–39.

Lerner, A. G., Oyffe, I., Isaacs, G., & Sigal, M. (1997). Naltrexone treatment of hallucinogen persisting perception disorder. *American Journal of Psychiatry, 154,* 437.

Longenecker, G. L. (1994). *How Drugs Work.* Emeryville, CA: Ziff-Davis Press.

Lyttle, T., Goldstein, D., & Gartz, J. (1996). Bufo toads and bufotenine: Fact and fiction surrounding an alleged psychedelic. *Journal of Psychoactive Drugs, 28*(3), 267–270.

Markert, L. E., & Roberts, D. C. (1991). 3,4 Methylenedioxyamphetamine (MDA) self-administration and neurotoxicity. *Pharmacology, Biochemistry and Behavior, 39,* 569–574.

Marnell, T. (Ed.). (1997). *Drug Identification Bible* (3rd ed.). Denver: Drug Identification Bible.

Mathias, R. (1996). Marijuana impairs driving-related skills and workplace performance. *NIDA Notes, 11*(3).

McMeens, R. R. (1860). Report to the Ohio State Medical Committee on *Cannabis indica.* In T. H. Mikuriya (Ed.), *Marijuana: Medical Papers 1839–1972.* Oakland, CA: Medi-Comp Press.

Mikuriya, T. H. (Ed.). (1973). *Marijuana: Medical Papers 1839–1972.* Oakland, CA: Medi-Comp Press.

Morgan, J. P. (1997). Designer drugs. In J. H. Lowinson, P. Ruiz, R. B. Millman, & J. G. Langrod, (Eds.), *Substance Abuse: A Comprehensive Textbook* (3rd ed., pp. 142–147). Baltimore: Williams & Wilkins.

National Institute of Justice. (1997). *Rise of hallucinogen use.* U.S. Department of Justice: Research in Brief. *http://www.ncjrs.org.*

NIDA (National Institute of Drug Abuse). (1995). Marijuana antagonist reveals evidence of THC dependence in rats. *NIDA Notes, 10*(6). *http://www.nida.nih.gov/.*

NIDA. (1998). Current trends in drug use worldwide. *NIDA Notes, 13*(2). *http://www.nida.nih.gov/.*

NIDA Advisory Council. (1999). Research Findings: Epidemiology, etiology, and prevention research. *Director's Report to the National Advisory Council on Drug Abuse. Information@lists.nida.nih.gov.*

NIDA INFOFAX. (1998). LSD (13550). *http://www.nida.nih.gov.*

NIH (National Institutes of Health). (1997). Workshop on the medical utility of marijuana (February 19–20). *Report to the Director, National Institutes of Health by the ad hoc group experts.* Bethesda, MD: NIH.

O'Brien, R., Cohen, S., Evans, G., & Fine, J. (1992). *The Encyclopedia of Drug Abuse* (2nd ed.). New York: Facts on File.

ONDCP (Office of National Drug Control Policy). (1999). *National Drug Control Strategy, 1999.* Office of National Drug Control Policy. Bethesda, MD: National Drug Clearinghouse.

Ott, J. (1976). *Hallucinogenic Plants of North America.* Berkeley. Wingbow Press.

Pechnick, R. N., & Ungerleider, J. T. (1997). Hallucinogens. In J. H. Lowinson, P. Ruiz, R. B. Millman, & J. G. Langrod, (Eds.), *Substance Abuse: A Comprehensive Textbook* (3rd ed., pp. 142–147). Baltimore: Williams & Wilkins.

Petersen, R. C. (1980). *Phencyclidine: a Review.* National Institute on Drug Abuse publication no. 1980-0-341-166/614. Washington, DC: U.S. Government Printing Office.

Reeve, V. C. et al. (1983). Hemolyzed blood and serum levels of delta-9-THC: Effects on the performance of roadside sobriety tests. *Journal of Forensic Sciences, 28*(4), 963–971.

Reynolds, J. R. (1890). Therapeutical uses and toxic effects of *Cannabis indica. Lancet, 1,* 637–638. In T. H. Mikuriya (Ed.), *Marijuana: Medical Papers 1839–1972.* Oakland, CA: Medi-Comp Press.

Rinaldi-Carmona, M. et al. (1994). SR141716, a potent and selective antagonist of the brain cannabinoid receptor. *Federation of European Biochemical Sciences Letters, 350*(2–3), 240–244.

SAMHSA (Substance Abuse and Mental Health Services Administration). (1999). *Summary of findings from the 1998 National Household Survey on Drug Abuse, H-9 & H-10.* Rockville, MD: National Clearinghouse for Alcohol and Drug Information.

Schultes, R. E., & Hofmann, A. (1980). *The Botany and Chemistry of Hallucinogens.* Springfield, IL: Charles C. Thomas.

Schultes, R. E., & Hofmann, A. (1992). *Plants of the Gods.* Rochester, VT: Healing Arts Press.

Siegel, R. K. (1985). LSD hallucinations: from ergot to electric Kool-Aid. *Journal of Psychoactive Drugs, 17*(4), 247–256.

Siegel, R. K., (1989). *Life in Pursuit of Artificial Paradise.* New York: E. P. Hutton.

Smiley, A. (1986). Marijuana: On-road and driving simulator studies. Alcohol, Drugs, and Driving: *Abstracts and Reviews, 2*(3–4), 121–134.

Smith, P. B. et al. (1994). The pharmacological activity of anandamide, a putative endogenous cannabinoid in mice. *Journal of Pharmacology and Experimental Therapeutics, 270,* 219–227.

Smith, M. V. (1981). *Psychedelic Chemistry.* Port Townsend, WA: Loompanics Unlimited.

Snyder, S. (1996). *Drugs and the Brain.* New York: W.H. Freeman and Company.

Stafford, P. (1992). *Psychedelics Encyclopedia* (Vol. 1, p. 157). Berkeley, CA: Ronin Publishing.

Stafford, P. (1985). Recreational uses of LSD. *Journal of Psychoactive Drugs, 17*(4), 219–228.

Tashkin, D P. et al. (1997). Respiratory symptoms and lung function in habitual heavy smokers of tobacco alone and nonsmokers. *American Review of Respiratory Disease, 135,* 209–216.

Tashkin, D. P., Simmons, M., & Clark, V.

(1988). Acute and chronic effects of marijuana smoking compared with tobacco smoking on blood carboxyhemoglobin levels. *Journal of Psychoactive Drugs, 20*(1), 27–32.

Tashkin, E. (1999). Effects of marijuana on the lung and its defenses against infection and cancer. *School Psychology International, 20,* 23–37.

Touw, M. (1981). The religious and medicinal uses of *Cannabis* in China, India, and Tibet. *Journal of Psychoactive Drugs, 13*(1), 23–33.

Tsou, K., Patrick, S., & Walker, M. J. (1995). Physical withdrawal in rats tolerant to delta-9-tetrahydrocannabinol precipitated by a cannabinoid receptor antagonist. *European Journal of Pharmacology, 280,* R13–R15.

University of Michigan. (1999). *Monitoring the Future Study.* Rockville, MD: SAMHSA. *www.MonitoringThe Future.org.*

Walton, R. P. (1938). *Marijuana: America's New Drug Problem.* Philadelphia: Lippincott.

Weil, A., & Rosen, W. (1993). *From Chocolate to Morphine.* Boston: Houghton Mifflin Company.

Wilkins, J. N., Conner, B. T., & Gorelick, D. A. (1998). Management of stimulant, hallucinogen, marijujana, and phencyclidine intoxication and withdrawal. In A. W. Graham & T. K. Schultz (Eds.), *Principles of Addiction Medicine* (2nd ed., pp. 583–592). Chevy Chase, MD: American Society of Addiction Medicine, Inc.

Wilkins, J. N., Gorelick, D. A., & Conner, B. T. (1998). Pharmacologic therapies for other drug and multiple drug addiction. In A. W. Graham & T. K. Schultz (Eds.), *Principles of Addiction Medicine* (2nd ed., pp. 465–485). Chevy Chase, MD: American Society of Addiction Medicine, Inc.

Young, C. R. (1997). Sertraline treatment of hallucinogen persisting perception disorder. *Journal of Clinical Psychiatry, 58,* 85.

Zukin, S. R., Sloboda, Z., & Javitt, D. C. (1997). Phencyclidine (PCP). In J. H. Lowinson, P. Ruiz, R. B. Millman, & J. G. Langrod, (Eds.), *Substance Abuse: A Comprehensive Textbook* (3rd ed., pp. 142–147). Baltimore: Williams & Wilkins.

CHAPTER 7

Other Drugs,
Other Addictions

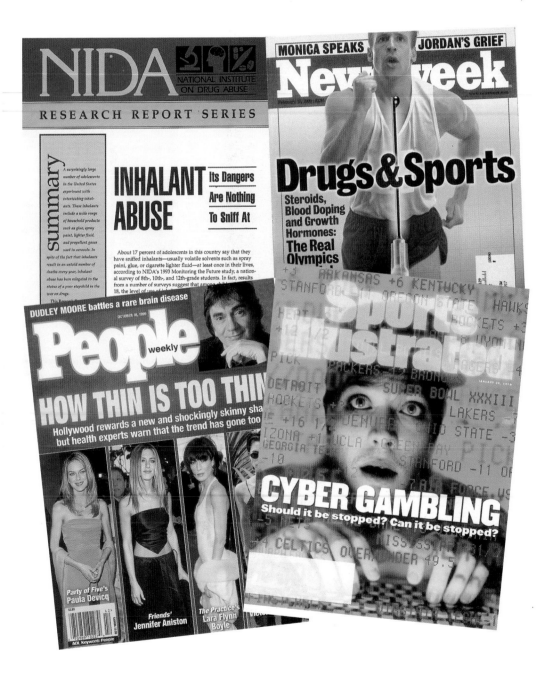

R esearchers, the media, and the general public have come to realize that addiction isn't limited just to hard drugs, alcohol and tobacco.

OTHER DRUGS

- **Inhalants:** The major inhalants (volatile solvents, volatile nitrites, and anesthetics) can cause CNS (central nervous system) depression, disorientation, and inebriation. Dangerous effects include nerve damage, learning disabilities, lack of coordination, and hypoxia (lack of oxygen leading to passing out or death).

- **Sports & Drugs:** Athletes have used therapeutic drugs, performance-enhancing (ergogenic) drugs, especially steroids and herbal supplements such as creatine, and recreational/mood-altering drugs (legal and illegal). Steroids can build muscles and increase weight but they can also cause aggression, physical problems, abuse, and addiction.

- **Miscellaneous Drugs:** Toad secretions, embalming fluid, hairspray, Bactine®, rubbing alcohol, cough medicine, hydrogen peroxide, and even C-4 explosives have been used to get high. Amino acids, herbal preparations, vitamins, and nutrients are used to improve health and brain power and slow aging.

OTHER ADDICTIONS

- **Compulsive Behaviors:** People get into compulsive behaviors to change their moods, forget problems, get a rush, or self-medicate in much the same way they begin to use psychoactive drugs. Compulsive behaviors include workaholism, shoplifting, hair pulling, and several other impulse control disorders.

- **Heredity, Environment, & Compulsive Behaviors:** These influences make compulsive behaviors progressive diseases just like substance addictions.

- **Compulsive Gambling:** Gambling has grown dramatically over the past 25 years. Almost eight million adults are problem or pathological gamblers.

- **Compulsive Shopping:** In an era of easy credit, shopping networks, and constant bombardment with advertisements, the debt load of the average American has exploded and a growing percentage of those are compulsive shoppers.

- **Eating Disorders:** There are three basic eating disorders.

  ◇ **Anorexia:** starving oneself by extreme measures including excessive exercise and laxatives but mostly by just not eating.

  ◇ **Bulimia:** uncontrolled overeating followed by techniques to avoid weight gain, such as vomiting, excess exercise, and laxatives.

  ◇ **Compulsive Overeating (including binge-eating disorder):** an uncontrolled desire to eat, often involving large weight gains—often a lifetime problem.

  All three eating disorders combine behavior and a substance (food) to create compulsive behaviors.

- **Sexual Addiction:** Sexual compulsivity, particularly pornography and masturbation, are often used to cope with personal problems and childhood trauma or stress.

- **Internet Addiction:** There are several kinds of compulsive use of the Internet that involve services such as chat rooms, list servers, and even e-mail.

  ◇ **Cybersexual Addiction:** This includes online pornography along with X-rated chat rooms, all a growing part of sexual addiction.

  ◇ **Computer Relationship Addiction:** This includes having relationships online in an obsessive manner.

  ◇ **Net Compulsions:** These include online gambling, shopping, auctions, and stock day trading.

  ◇ **Information Addiction:** This includes surfing the Net for information and data.

  ◇ **Computer Games Addiction:** Free computer games online are becoming as popular and as compulsive for some as the Sega® and Sony PlayStation® games.

- **Conclusions:** Because the roots of any compulsion are so similar, one has to treat the basic emotional causes of addiction as well as the specific substances or behaviors.

INTRODUCTION

One reason psychoactive drugs are used is to alter one's mood and state of consciousness. In fact, the definition of psychoactive drugs is "any substance that will alter one's nervous system." Users, whether through curiosity or desperation, have found many substances that alter their mood and perception in much the same way that psychoactive drugs do. When certain behaviors are practiced over a long period of time, they too can become compulsive and addictive in much the same way that cocaine or heroin use becomes compulsive and addictive.

"Addiction is a state of mind. I was thinking of what addictions I have or have had. Well eating, that's my addiction. Well, no, I gamble, I got that. I watch TV too much—four hours a day. Smoking, I smoked for 10 years—three packs a day. Drinking—I was drunk for six straight months in the Air Force and on a binge basis after that. It's not the substance. It's not the gambling. It's not the specific thing I do, it's all these behaviors. Instead of solving a problem to change how I feel, I take something or do something."
43-year-old male in recovery

OTHER DRUGS

In addition to stimulants, depressants, and psychedelics, many other drugs are used for their psychoactive effects. Inhalants have been around for millennia. Drugs used in sports to heal, increase performance, or to reward performance have also been around for several thousand years. Smart drugs and herbal preparations have been around since Neolithic times. Some herbal preparations have been discovered, forgotten, and discovered again. More recently, their active components have been synthesized in laboratories.

INHALANTS

"'Huffing'? I 'huffed' gas when I was like 9 years old. And then when I was 11 or 12, I 'huffed' for a year. I'd have 12 cans of air freshener a day. My mom would buy the big packs at Costco®— she didn't know I was 'huffing' them cause I'd throw them away and then when she found out, I had to stop. I'm surprised I'm not dead from it because I did it for a long time. I'd just sit there and use until I passed out."
17 year old in a therapeutic community

Inhalants, sometimes classified as deliriants, comprise a wide variety of volatile substances including certain gases, aerosol sprays, and liquids that give off fumes. The volatile substances are often present in commercial products. Inhalants are used for their stupefying, intoxicating, and, less often, slight psychedelic effects. Inhalants, which are inhaled through the nose and/or mouth and occasionally sprayed directly in the mouth or nose, are classified differently from those substances like tobacco and heroin that are heated or burned and then smoked, or powders like cocaine hydrochloride that are sniffed.

There is some disagreement as to how to classify inhalants. This chapter uses three groupings (Table 7-1):

◇ **volatile solvents and aerosols:** most of these substances are synthesized from petroleum and combined with other chemicals. Volatile solvents (hydrocarbons) are found

1894

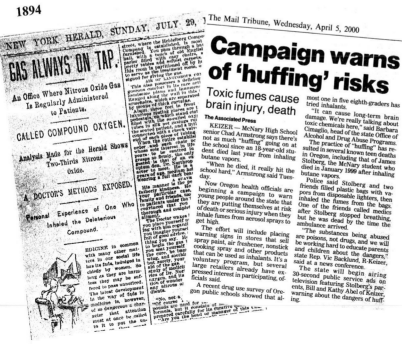

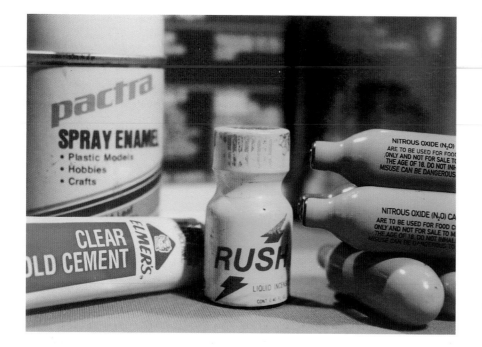

The three groups of inhalants are volatile solvents (including aerosols), volatile nitrites, and anesthetics.

TABLE 7–1 INHALANTS

Product	Chemicals
Volatile Solvents & Aerosols	
Airplane glue	Toluene, ethyl acetate
Rubber cement	Toluene, hexane, methyl chloride, acetone, methyl ethyl ketone, methyl butyl ketone
PVC cement	Trichloroethylene
Paint sprays (especially gold and silver metallic paints)	Toluene, butane, propane, fluorocarbons, hydrocarbons
Hairsprays and deodorants	Butane, propane, fluorocarbons
Lighter fluid	Butane, isopropane
Fuel gas	Butane
Dry cleaning fluid, spot removers, correction fluid, degreasers	Tetrachloroethylene, trichloroethane trichloroethylene
Nail polish remover	Acetone
Paint remover/thinners	Toluene, methylene chloride, methanol
Local anesthetic	Ethyl chloride
Analgesic/asthma sprays	Fluorocarbons
Volatile Nitrites	
Room odorizers, Locker Room®, Rush®, Climax® Quicksilver®, Bolt® Bullet® ("poppers")	(Iso)amyl nitrite, (iso)butyl nitrite, isopropyl nitrite
Anesthetics	
Nitrous oxide Whipped cream propellant (whippets, laughing gas, "blue nun," "nitrous")	Nitrous oxide
Chloroform	Chloroform
Ether	Ether

(Adapted from Sharp & Rosenberg, 1997)

in glues, gasoline, and nail polish remover. Some aerosols, which can be sprayed to produce a foggy mist, are inhaled for their gaseous propellants rather than for their primary contents. They can contain volatile hydrocarbons or, less often, other volatile organic compounds including esters, ketones (e.g., acetone), and glycols.

◇ **volatile nitrites:** these drugs, such as amyl and butyl nitrite, are used clinically as blood vessel dilators (vasodilators) for heart problems (amyl) and previously as over-the-counter room fresheners (butyl and isopropyl). They are also used recreationally, often in party or sexual situations.

◇ **anesthetics:** these were developed for anesthesia, however, their recreational use was discovered at the same time. Nitrous oxide (N_2O), also known as "laughing gas," is still used as an anesthetic and aerosol propellant as well as a party drug to make people giddy.

The *Diagnostic and Statistical Manual of Mental Disorders* (DSM-IV) classifies inhalant disorders as inhalant dependence and abuse, intoxication, induced delirium, dementia, psychotic disorder, mood disorder, and anxiety disorder. These are based on abuse of volatile solvents (hydrocarbon or other volatile compounds). DSM-IV classifies abuse of nitrites and anesthetics as psychoactive substance dependence not otherwise specified (APA, 1994).

Inhalants have some distinct differences from other psychoactive drugs.

◇ They are quick acting and have intense effects. They are absorbed through the lungs and into the bloodstream, which carries them rapidly to the brain. Their intoxicating effects occur within 7–10 seconds and last no more than 30 minutes to 1 hour after exposure has ceased. People who abuse inhalants can very quickly become intoxicated and with excess use can display strange, erratic, and unpredictable behavior and poor judgment. They can become violent, even suicidal.

◊ Inhalants are cheap, readily available, and widespread. More than 1,500 chemical products can be inhaled for their psychoactive effects.

◊ Because psychoactive gasses and liquids are present in a wide variety of substances in the home, garage, and workplace, they are readily accessible to children and adolescents. They have more direct effects on body tissues than most other psychoactive drugs.

◊ They get inadequate attention from parents, educators, the media, and law enforcement personnel because

of the low status of inhalant abuse as a drug problem. Derogatory and dismissive attitudes towards solvent abusers compound the difficulty of getting warnings and treatment to potential and existing users.

HISTORY (*also see Chapter 1*)

The practice of inhaling gaseous substances to get high goes back to ancient times. The Greek Oracle at Delphi was said to breathe in vapors from the earth (naturally occurring carbon dioxide) before uttering her prophecies. The carbon dioxide-induced lack of oxygen produced psychoactive effects (Giannini, 1991). In the Judaic world, burnt spices, gums, herbs, and incense were inhaled during religious ceremonies, a practice shared by other Mediterranean, African, and Native American peoples (Swan, 1995).

Our modern version of inhalant abuse began in the late 1700s with the

discovery of nitrous oxide (laughing gas), chloroform, and ether. The use of inhalants for anesthesia and recreation occurred together (Weil & Rosen, 1993). Nitrous oxide became popular and was reportedly used at parties and in bordellos in the United States, France, and the United Kingdom (Smith, 1974). Later, at the beginning of the twentieth century when petroleum began to be refined and manufactured into new products such as solvents, thinners, and glues, many more substances began to be inhaled for their intoxicating or euphoric effects. In the 1930s sniffing the carbon dioxide used to make seltzer bubbles had a brief fling with popularity as did gasoline sniffing (Giannini, 1991). Shortly after World War II, the abuse of glue and metallic paints rose dramatically, particularly in the midwestern United States and in Japan. The phrase "glue sniffing" is still used to include inhalation of many substances besides glue. The

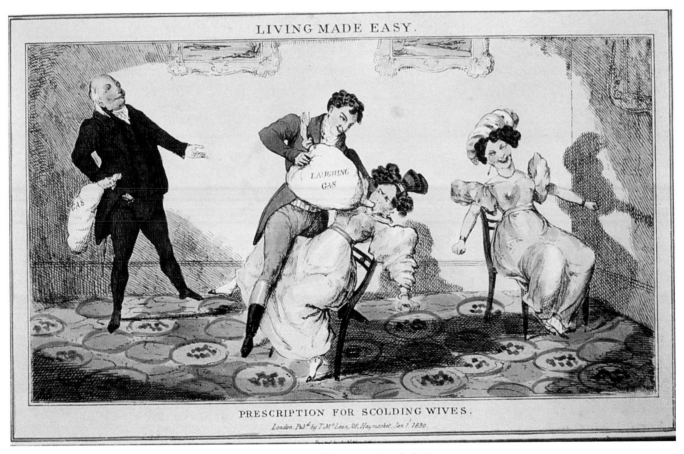

This 1830 print from England with its caption, "Living Made Easy," depicts a "gas frolic."

Courtesy of the National Library of Medicine, Bethesda

practice persists as a drug abuse problem into the twenty-first century; inhalants are responsible for about 1,200 deaths each year in the United States. The actual number of deaths is thought to be underreported since medical examiners probably mistake death from inhalant abuse for suicide, suffocation, or an accident.

EPIDEMIOLOGY

Since inhalants, especially volatile solvents, are readily available and inexpensive, they provide a cheap quick high, especially for those who are young and/or poor. Inhalant abuse often has an episodic pattern with brief outbreaks or "fads" in particular schools or regions. Abuse is most prevalent among young adolescents. However, adults also abuse inhalants, including painters, chemical company workers, health care professionals (especially in dentistry and anesthesiology), and others who have access to inhalants at work.

"In college we'd have whippet parties where someone would go and get six or seven of those small nitrous oxide cylinders and we'd pass them around. By the time it came around again, you'd be down from the giddy stupid feeling."
25-year-old ex-college student

In a survey in Texas some years ago, respondents were asked about inhalant use. The most frequently abused substances were typewriter correction fluid, glue, gasoline, and spray paints. When a mixture of substances were involved, the solvents toluene and trichloroethylene were the most frequently mentioned ingredients (Fredlund, Spence, Maxwell, & Kravinsky, 1990).

"We got a 911 call about a kid in a coma. It seems that three of them were inhaling a waterproofing spray and this one kid did too much. Basically he starved his head of oxygen because the spray temporarily replaced the oxygen. It took him three months to recover."
Emergency medical technician, Kansas City

TABLE 7–2   NUMBER OF AMERICANS WHO HAVE USED INHALANTS—1998

Age	Ever Used	Last Year	Last Month
12–17	1,387,000	664,000	253,000
18–25	3,023,000	895,000	308,000
26–34	3,151,000	173,000	37,000
35 & up	5,028,000	277,000	115,000
Total	12,589,000	2,009,000	713,000

Source: National Household Survey on Drugs (SAMHSA, 1999)

Inhalant abuse continues to be a worldwide problem, according to a World Health Organization Report. It afflicts primarily the young, the poor, street children, recent migrants to cities, and children exposed to chemicals daily, such as children of cleaners or shoemakers. The inhalant of choice in many countries is gasoline because of its wide availability, low price, and the rapid onset of psychoactive effects (WHO, 1998).

Use by Sex & Age

Generally more young people than adults abuse inhalants (Table 7-2) and among 12–17 year olds, more young men than young women. About 17% of the adolescents in the United States have sniffed inhalants at least once. In older populations, more men abuse inhalants than women but the numbers of overall abusers decline by 2/3 or more after the age of 25 (SAMHSA, 1998). The worrisome problem is that while inhalant use has decreased generally and leveled off among 12th graders, it has increased among 8th and 10th graders (University of Michigan, 1999).

Ethnically, earliest use is highest among Hispanics and lowest among Whites (SAMHSA, 1999; Padilla, Padilla, Morales, et al., 1979). The use of inhalants by Native American boys is also high.

METHODS OF INHALATION

Although there have been reports of people spraying aerosols onto bread and eating the bread or inserting small bottles of inhalants, such as typewriter correction fluid, into the nostrils, there are about seven common forms of inhalation.

1. "Sniffing" is breathing in the inhalant directly from the container. "Sniffing" puts the vapor into the lungs in contrast with snorting that puts solids, like cocaine, in contact with the mucosal lining of the nose.

2. "Huffing" is soaking a rag with a dissolved inhalant, putting the rag in one's mouth, and inhaling; also, inhaling from a solvent-soaked rag, sock, tissue, or glove through the nose. Generally "huffing" puts more vapors into the lungs.

3. "Bagging" is placing the inhalant or inhalant-soaked material in a plastic bag and inhaling by mouth or nose. Rebreathing the exhaled air intensifies the effect.

4. "Spraying" is spraying the inhalant directly into the nose or mouth.

5. Balloons and "crackers" is the use of a pin or other "cracking" device to puncture a can of nitrous oxide or other inhalant while a balloon is placed over the end of the can. The gas in the balloon is then inhaled.

Other methods include:

6. Putting a bag over one's head, spraying an aerosol into the bag, and inhaling is another form of use.

7. Pouring or spraying inhalants onto cuffs, sleeves, or collars and then sniffing over a period of time is occasionally used.

Some users heat the solvent to make it more volatile, a particularly dangerous practice that has resulted in explosions, burns, and deaths. (Blum, 1984; Marnell, 1997)

Directly breathing and spraying pressurized inhalants into the mouth or nose are particularly toxic methods. These techniques expose an abuser's fragile membranes to the caustic effects of these substances. They also put a harmful amount of pressure into the lungs and even cause a physical freezing effect as the substances vaporize quickly, taking heat from everything around them. "Bagging," because it limits oxygen, concentrates the effects. The choices of inhalant and method of inhalation allow great control over the intensity and duration of the effects.

"A Woodland boy died after he tried to get high by sniffing a common water repellent, Scotchguard®, and a 14-year-old friend who also was inhaling the aerosol was arrested on suspicion of involuntary manslaughter. The boys used a plastic bag to inhale the chemicals. They passed the bag back and forth. Suddenly the boy couldn't breathe."

Article from the Scripps-McClatchy News Service, 9-17-98

VOLATILE SOLVENTS

These solvents are often carbon- and hydrocarbon-based compounds that are volatile (turn to gas) at room temperature. Refined from petroleum, they are found in fuels, aerosols, and solvents. They include such common materials as gasoline and kerosene, paints (especially metallic paints), paint thinners, lacquers, nail polish remover, spot removers, glues and plastic cements, lighter fluid, and a variety of aerosols. Some are inhaled, not for the primary substance but for the effects of the solvents they are dissolved in or the propellant gasses used.

These volatile solvents are quick acting because they are absorbed into the blood almost immediately after inhalation and then they move to the heart, brain, liver, and other tissues. Solvents are exhaled by the lungs (in which case a telltale odor from the inhalant remains on the breath) or excreted by the kidneys (NIH, 1992).

Inhaling these substances produces a temporary stimulation, mood elevation, and reduced inhibitions before the central nervous system (CNS) depressive effects begin. Dizziness, slurred speech, unsteady gait, and drowsiness are seen early on. Impulsiveness, excitement, and irritability may also occur. Because judgment is impaired with abuse of these substances, there is danger of accident and injury.

High dosage or individual susceptibility has a greater effect on the central nervous system—illusions, hallucinations, and delusions may develop. The abuser may experience a dreamy stupor culminating in a short period of sleep. The effects resemble alcohol or sedative intoxication (inhalant abuse has been called a "quick drunk"). The intoxicated state may last from minutes to an hour or more, depending on the kind, quantity, and length of exposure to the substance inhaled. Headaches and nausea may follow as part of an inhalant hangover.

"I came to the conclusion that the headaches my son had been complaining about were due to 'huffing' because his cousin, whom he hung out with, was having the same headaches and the doctor could find nothing wrong with them. We found empty or depleted spray cans out in the woods near the house. Of course when I confronted him he said 'No way. Headaches must be from not having enough caffeine today.' There was a kid in school who finally confirmed that a number of the kids were doing it. They were doing bug spray, air freshener, Arid® deodorant, and whipped cream [the propellant]. When he was coming down, he would be real angry and violent. When loaded, they did stupid things."

Mother of 14-year-old "huffer"

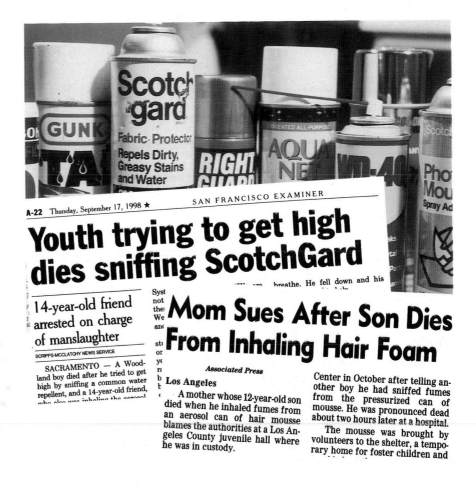

A-22   Thursday, September 17, 1998 ★   SAN FRANCISCO EXAMINER

Youth trying to get high dies sniffing ScotchGard

14-year-old friend arrested on charge of manslaughter

SCRIPPS-MCCLATCHY NEWS SERVICE

SACRAMENTO — A Woodland boy died after he tried to get high by sniffing a common water repellent, and a 14-year-old friend, who also was inhaling the aerosol

breathe. He fell down and his

Mom Sues After Son Dies From Inhaling Hair Foam

Associated Press

Los Angeles

A mother whose 12-year-old son died when he inhaled fumes from an aerosol can of hair mousse blames the authorities at a Los Angeles County juvenile hall where he was in custody.

Center in October after telling another boy he had sniffed fumes from the pressurized can of mousse. He was pronounced dead about two hours later at a hospital.

The mousse was brought by volunteers to the shelter, a temporary home for foster children and

After prolonged inhalation, delirium with confusion, psychomotor clumsiness, emotional instability, impaired thinking, and coma have been reported. Neurological effects from both low-level and high-level (acute) exposure to volatile solvents are usually reversible.

Chronic abuse (abuse that continues over a period of time) is characterized by lack of coordination, inability to concentrate, weakness, disorientation, and loss of weight. Because solvents have been shown to affect the hippocampus, a memory center, long-term use will affect memory (NCADI, 1999). Since chronic abuse can involve extremely high concentrations of fumes, sometimes thousands of times higher than industrial exposure, some mental and neurologic effects may be irreversible, though not usually progressive after abuse ceases. For example, chronic abuse of toluene can result in dementia, spasticity, and other CNS dysfunctions, whereas occupational exposure to toluene has not produced similar effects.

Complications may result from the effect of the solvent or other toxic ingredients, such as lead in gasoline. Injuries to the brain, liver, kidney, bone marrow, and particularly the lungs may result either from heavy exposure or from individual hypersensitivity. Blood irregularities and chromosome damage can result as well as cardiac arrhythmia, respiratory arrest, or asphyxia due to occlusion of the airway. With chronic abuse some of these solvents produce ulcers around the nose and mouth and cancerous growths. Body injuries result from falling, fainting, or other accidents experienced while under the influence of these substances (Dinwiddie, 1998; Sharp & Rosenberg, 1997; O'Brien, Cohen, Evans, & Fine, 1992).

Toluene (methyl benzene)

The most abused solvent is probably toluene, an aromatic hydrocarbon. It is a component of a myriad of substances—glues, drying agents, solvents, thinners, paints, inks, and cleaning agents. Several studies have suggested that toluene has an extremely high abuse potential (Sharp, Beauvais, & Spence, 1992). Chronic abuse can affect balance, hearing, eyesight, and, most often, neurological functions and cognitive abilities. In one study of chronic abusers of toluene in spray paint, 65% had neurologic damage (Hormes, Filley, & Rosenberg, 1986). Heavy abuse results in deafness, trembling, and dementia. Other severe abnormalities include midrange hearing loss and changes to the white matter of the central nervous system. "Texas shoeshine," spray paint containing toluene, is widely abused, often among painters. Kidney disorders are sometimes the result of toluene abuse.

Trichloroethylene (TCE)

This organic solvent is the most common solvent. It is used in typewriter correction fluids, paints, metal degreasers, and spot removers. Like two other volatile solvents, toluene and acetone, trichlorethylene (TCE) causes overall depression effects and moderate hallucinations. The toxic effects of TCE have been known for 50 years and are similar to those of toluene. It was once even used as an anesthetic despite dangerous side effects. The effects of low- to moderate-dose TCE is generally reversible but at higher doses, various neuropathies (any disorder affecting the nervous system) occur (Sharp & Rosenberg, 1997). Some of these neuropathies can be permanent.

N-Hexane & Methyl Butyl Ketone (MBK)

Used as a solvent for glues and adhesives, as a diluent for plastics and rubber, and in the production of laminated products, n-hexane has caused neurological damage. Similarly methyl butyl ketone, used as a paint thinner and solvent for dyes, causes some of the same damage. Both substances are metabolized to the same neurotoxin, 2,5-hexanedione. There are numerous reports of brain damage from occupational exposure as well as from deliberate recreational use. Recovery in severe cases can take three years after mild to moderate exposure (Sharp & Rosenberg, 1997).

Alkanes

The smaller molecules of this class of hydrocarbons are gases at room temperature. They include methane, ethane, butane, and propane. They are inhaled for their effects but unfortunately can also cause cardiac arrhythmias and sudden death (Siegal & Wason, 1990). The larger molecules of this class include hexane and pentane and as mentioned above are very neurotoxic (Wood, 1994).

Gasoline

Gasoline sniffing, especially common among solvent abusers on Native American reservations, introduces various components of gasoline into the system, including solvents, metals, and chemicals. Symptoms include insomnia, tremors, anorexia, and sometimes paralysis (Beauvais, Oetting, & Edwards, 1985). When leaded gas is inhaled, symptoms can also include hallucinations, convulsions, and the chronic, irreversible effects of lead poisoning. Internationally, gasoline is the substance of choice because even in remote areas, gasoline is used—it is cheap (especially if siphoned from a car or truck) and it is available in small quantities. For youngsters, especially in poorer countries, inhalants are often the first drug they use (WHO, 1992).

Alcohols

Ethanol, methanol, and isopropanol are the most commonly abused alcohol solvents. Remember the feeling when inhaling deeply from a brandy snifter? When inhaled too deeply and for too long a period of time rather than drunk, alcohols can cause nausea with vertigo, weakness, vomiting, headaches, and abdominal cramping. Formaldehyde is classified as an alcohol and can cause vision problems, dryness, and destruction of neurons in the central nervous system. Isopropanol, found in paints, rubbing alcohol, and perfumes, can induce severe CNS depression (Giannini, 1991).

Warning Signs of Solvent Abuse

Though inhalant abuse is difficult to spot, there are still various warning signs. They are

◇ headaches;

◇ chemical odor on body and clothes or in room;

◇ red, glassy or watery eyes and dilated pupils;

◇ inflamed nose, nosebleeds, and rashes around nose and mouth;

◇ slow, thick, or slurred speech;

◇ staggering gait, disorientation, and lack of coordination;

◇ pains in chest and stomach;

◇ fatigue;

◇ nausea;

◇ shortness of breath;

◇ loss of appetite;

◇ intoxication;

◇ irritability and aggression;

◇ seizure;

◇ coma.

VOLATILE NITRITES

These substances known as "aliphatic nitrites" include amyl nitrite as well as butyl and isobutyl nitrite. These inhalants dilate blood vessels, so the heart as well as other tissues receive more blood. Medically they are used for heart-related chest pains (angina pectoris) or for cyanide poisoning. Other effects include a rush of blood to the brain (cerebral arteries are also dilated) and the relaxation of smooth muscles in the body. Effects start in 7–10 seconds and last for about 30 seconds. Blood pressure reaches its lowest point in 30 seconds and returns to normal at 90 seconds. They are called "poppers" because amyl nitrite often comes in glass capsules wrapped in cotton that are broken open (with an audible pop) and sniffed (Weil & Rosen, 1993).

"My friend used to use 'poppers' at 'raves' because he thought it helped his dancing and made him more lively. It worked for him some of the time but a couple of times he got dizzy and fell over. The last time he fell over and broke his nose."

17-year-old "raver"

On inhalation, there is a feeling of a fullness in the head, a rush, and mild euphoria. (First-time abusers have reported feeling panic attacks.) This may be followed by severe headaches, dizziness, and giddiness. As the effects wear off, the user might experience headaches, nausea, vomiting, and a chill (because of dilation of blood vessels near the skin) (Wood, 1994). A tolerance develops rapidly to the gas, though excessive prolonged abuse may cause oxygen deprivation and possibly asphyxiation. An extreme increase in heart rate and palpitations can make nitrite inhalation unpleasant. First aid for the headaches includes abstinence. Overdose treatment requires removing the abuser from exposure and insuring that respiration and blood flow are maintained. Occasionally CPR is used.

Nitrites, thought to enhance sexual activity, are sought after especially by male homosexuals for both their euphoric and physiological effects that include relaxation of smooth muscles such as the sphincter muscle. Repeated abuse may alter blood cells and impair the immune system, thus increasing susceptibility to HIV infection. There is some evidence that nitrites inhibit the functioning of the white blood cells and

that the activity of these killer cells is suppressed. Nitrites are converted to nitrosamines in the body—nitrosamines are potent cancer-causing chemicals.

Recently warnings have been issued about using "poppers," Viagra®, and methamphetamine in combination (particularly at "rave" clubs and gay bathhouses) since the first two substances lower blood pressure and the combination of all three drugs can cause fainting or even death (AP, 1999).

Amyl nitrite, a volatile oily liquid with a wet dog or rotten banana odor is only available by prescription. Although butyl and propyl nitrites were banned, variants of these nitrites are still sold as room deodorizers, e.g., Rush®, Bolt®, and Locker Room®. Street supplies of the drug also come from diverted legal sources or are smuggled in from other countries.

ANESTHETICS

At the end of the eighteenth century, newly discovered volatile substances were found to have anesthetic as well as euphoric effects. Experimentation began in both directions with substances such as chloroform, ether, oxygen, and nitrous oxide. Abuse of ni-

Viagra, 'Poppers' Fatal Combination

Gay party scene hit hard by d

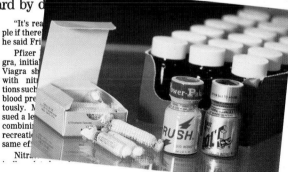

Associated Press

Los Angeles

The homosexual community, already coping with AIDS, has a new concern: Viagra.

The potency drug, when combined with inhaled stimulants known as "poppers" that long have been a fixture on the gay party scene, are a potentially deadly mix, doctors and the mayor of West Hollywood warn.

Unconfirmed reports that three gay men died after using

Isobutyl, butyl, or amyl nitrite, sold under various trade names from the 1970s, were some of the first successful designer drugs. For example, a prescription drug, butyl nitrite, was chemically rearranged to create a nonprescription derivative and sold as a room odorizer to circumvent drug laws. Presently amyl nitrite is only available by prescription while butyl nitrite and propyl nitrites were banned in 1991.

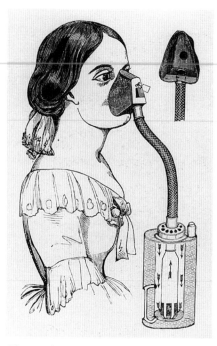

This mask was used not only by early day anesthesiologists but also by genteel inhalers at oxygen or nitrous oxide parties in the 1800s.

· ·

trous oxide was reported among Harvard medical students starting in the nineteenth century.

Abuse continues today by young experimenters as well as among middle class and affluent groups, including dentists, doctors, anesthesiologists, hospital workers and health-care professionals who abuse nitrous oxide, halothane, and other anesthetics like ether, ethylene, ethyl chloride, and cyclopropane.

Nitrous Oxide (N₂O)

Nitrous oxide, discovered by Dr. Joseph Priestly in 1776, was popularized by the physician Sir Humphrey Davy for its anesthetic and analgesic effects as well as for its euphoric effects. Davy talked about a pleasurable thrilling in the chest and extremities along with auditory and visual distortions. He also wrote about his recreational use of the gas. In 1869 the gas was first used to effervesce or aerate drinks (Lynn, Walter, Harris, et al., 1972).

Currently nitrous oxide (laughing

gas) is available in large blue-painted gas tanks for dental offices where it is used as an anesthetic and in bakeries where it is used as a propellant in whipped cream aerosol cans and small metal cylinders. Nitrous oxide is abused for its mood-altering effects. Within 8–10 seconds of inhalation, the gas produces giddiness and stimulation often accompanied by silly laughter. The maximum effect lasts only 2 or 3 minutes. There is a buzzing or ringing in the ears along with a sense that one is about to collapse or pass out. These feelings quickly cease when the gas leaves the body. Since the pain-numbing effects are also short acting, the gas is delivered continuously during oral surgery or other dental procedures.

Dangers from the abuse of nitrous oxide, especially if inhaled directly from a pressurized tank, include exploded or frozen lung tissue and frostbite of the tips of the nose and vocal cords. This risk is minimized when the gas is inhaled from a balloon inflated with the gas. Cognitive functioning is diminished during the peak of the high but returns to normal within 5 minutes. Experienced users seem to feel physical effects somewhat longer than novice users, possibly a form of reverse tolerance where less and less gas is needed to produce the same effects (Lynn et al., 1972).

Long-term exposure can cause central and peripheral nerve cell and brain cell damage due to lack of sufficient oxygen since nitrous oxide replaces oxygen in the blood. Symptoms of long-term exposure include numbness, loss of balance and dexterity, weakness and numbness in the arms and legs, and passing out (and occasionally getting hurt from the fall). Further, nitrous oxide abuse can lead to physical dependence in some users and has been a major addiction problem for dentists over the past few decades.

Halothane

Halothane is a prescription surgical anesthetic gas, sold under the trade name Fluothane®. Its effects are extremely rapid and powerful enough to

induce a coma for surgery. Because of its limited availability, it has been most often abused by anesthesiologists and hospital personnel.

DEPENDENCE

Though tolerance to volatile solvents will develop, the liability for physical and psychological dependence and addiction to these inhalants is less than for other depressants. Often younger children will get into long-term bouts with inhalants. Breaking the habit or treating the compulsion can be difficult because most users are young and immature and because the continued use can cause cognitive impairments. There have been isolated reports of withdrawal symptoms after cessation of long-term use (hallucinations, chills, cramps, and delirium tremens). A cross-tolerance to other depressants, including alcohol, will develop with long-term use (O'Brien et al., 1992). Interestingly, among drug addicts, inhalant abuse is looked down upon as low class and inferior to other highs. Although chronic dependence to nitrites is unusual, there has been some chronic addiction noted for nitrous oxide especially in dentists and in people who divert nitrous tanks from industrial gas suppliers.

PREVENTION

Inhalants present a special challenge to prevention efforts. The dangers of inhalant abuse have not been publicized as widely as the dangers of alcohol, tobacco, and other drugs. Young people may be unaware that they risk sudden death or brain damage from inhaling volatile substances. Inhalants are plentiful, cheap, and easily accessible even to young people. Law enforcement officers, health workers, and teachers may not be trained to recognize signs and symptoms of inhalant abuse and the youth that are particularly at risk are often far from the usual prevention resources. Further it is very difficult to control or monitor all of the potentially abusable substances that are used in industry and in common household products.

Drugs still haunt Strawberry

The Associated Press

TAMPA, Fla. — New York Yankees outfielder Darryl Strawberry tested positive for cocaine on Jan. 19 and might once again be suspended from baseball.

A high-ranking baseball official, speaking on the condition he not be identified, said Tuesday the commissioner's office is investigating and a ... take disciplinary ...

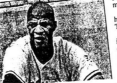

On Tuesday, Yankees manager Joe Torre gave a hint that something may have been up.

"I have a sense something will happen here that will stir the pot," Torre said.

Strawberry, who has been working out at the Yankees complex, could not be contacted after positive test became known. He already ha served two drug-related suspensior

The first, for 60 days, was in 1? after he tested positive for coca ...

Two Olympian track women test positive for drugs

The Associated Press

ATLANTA — In th... firmed drug cas... Games t...

McGwire taking hits over use of power pill

SOSA SWATS 2 – AT 51, 1,3,5,6C

By Dick Patrick
and Mel Antonen
USA TODAY

PITTSBURGH — Mark McGwire of the St. Louis Cardinals hit his 53rd home run Sunday then stepped up to defend his use of androstenedione, the controversial performance-enhancing substance.

"Is it legal? Yes," said McGwire.

McGwire said he has used the substance for a year and

that it is common in the majors. Toronto's Jose Canseco said Sunday he has used it for six months.

"Mark's supplementation is a non-concern," Cardinals trainer Barry Weinberg said.

The substance, which supporters say helps build muscle, can be purchased over the counter and is permitted in professional baseball.

But it is banned by the International Olympic Committee, the NFL and the NCAA. Randy Barnes, the Olympic shot put champion, faces a lifetime ban for using it.

McGwire has said he wouldn't use an unsafe product and is sure androstenedione is not harmful.

The Food and Drug Administration is aware of androsten-

edione's muscle-building capabilities but doesn't list it as a anabolic steroid.

Another authority disagrees. "It's a steroid," said Penn State professor and drug testing expert Chuck Yesalis. "It's a precursor to testosterone. It's a sex steroid. If you can buy androstenedione over the counter, you should be able to buy testosterone over the counter."

Said Don Catlin, head of the Olympic testing lab, "This can be debated at great length."

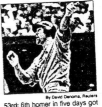

53rd: 6th homer in five days got him a curtain call — on the road.

By David Denoma, Reuters

... ting process. ... things," he said ... cases. "In one ... ly. In another ... ly what I feel ... it this later." ... ame on the ... the expul- ... s and two ... rmer So- ... se of the ... tan.

Athletes probably use drugs at the same rate as the general public but since they are in the spotlight, their problems get banner headlines.

SPORTS & DRUGS

"I was so wild about winning. Winning, winning, winning. I never thought about anything else."
Lyle Alzado, former NFL star

There are three main categories of drugs used in sports.

1. There are **therapeutic drugs** (e.g., analgesics, muscle relaxants, anti-inflammatories, and asthma medications) used for specific medical problems and only administered with proper medical supervision.

2. There are **performance-enhancing drugs (ergogenic drugs)** such as steroids, growth hormones and amphetamines, some legal and some illegal. Most are banned from competition.

3. And finally, there are **recreational** or **mood-altering drugs,** both legal and illegal (e.g., cocaine, marijuana, alcohol, and tobacco), used to induce euphoria, reduce pain or anxiety, lower inhibitions, escape boredom, or simply to enhance the senses.

It is the performance-enhancing drugs that are unique to athletics and that cause the most problems.

BACKGROUND

In an interview with Mark McGwire in 1998, a reporter asked about a bottle of medication on his locker shelf. The first baseman for the St. Louis Cardinals, on his way to smashing the 37-year-old home run record, identified it as androstenedione, a natural hormone that is a direct precursor in the biosynthesis of testosterone, the basic male hormone. At the time the so-called dietary supplement was legal in major league baseball but banned by the International Olympic Committee (IOC), the National Football League (NFL), the National Collegiate Athletic Association (NCAA), and professional tennis. McGwire said the supplement merely helped him train longer by energizing muscles but that the real work was the thousands of hours he spent training (Patrick, 1998). Possibly coincidentally, in 1999 steroid use increased in the 8th, 10th and, to a lesser extent, in the 12th grades (University of Michigan, 1999). In re-

sponse to his position as a role model, in 1999 McGwire announced he had stopped using the supplement. He still hit 65 home runs in 1999.

"I thought long and hard about it, and I don't like the way it was portrayed, like I was the endorser of the product, which I wasn't. [He stopped taking it 4 months before this interview]. But young kids take it because of me. I don't like that. I discourage young people from taking it. But if I have a message for kids, it's that you don't necessarily have to follow what somebody who's in the public eye does. If you're an adult, you elect to choose your own destiny."
Mark McGwire (AP, 1999)

Every two years Chicago physician Bob Goldman surveys several hundred superior athletes and asks, "You are offered a drug that will make you win every competition you enter for the next five years and then you will die from the side effects. Would you take it?" More than half the athletes said yes, meaning that they were willing to die just so they could be the best in their chosen sport.

Some athletes perceive drugs as the quick way to put on pounds, to increase stamina, to get up for a game, to relieve pain, or to keep up with other athletes suspected of using drugs. Since many drugs used in sports create feelings of confidence and excitement, drugs themselves can motivate athletes to abuse them.

"What you have to understand is that a young man doesn't think past tomorrow. All he is interested in is winning the neighborhood game and having the best-looking girl on his arm and looking the best that he possibly can. And these are technically the motivations for him taking the drug. And then he goes to college where peer pressure and the desire not to disappoint the hometown folks put further pressure on him. Then if he's lucky enough to make it to the pro ranks, it becomes a matter of money."
High school football coach giving testimony to congressional panel on drugs and sports

History

The use of drugs in sports is not new. Greek Olympic athletes in the third century B.C. ate mushrooms or meat to improve their performance. If they were caught, they were expelled from the games. About the same time, athletes in Macedonia prepared for their events by drinking ground donkey hooves boiled in oil and garnished with rose petals. Roman gladiators took stimulants (betel nuts or ephedra) to give them endurance (Hanley, 1983). In a native cactus, Aztec Indians found a stimulant that lasted up to three days that they used for running. By the 1800s, cyclists, swimmers, and other athletes used opium, morphine, cocaine, caffeine, nitroglycerin, sugar cubes soaked in ether (Dutch canal swimmers), and even strychnine (marathoners) (Mellion, 1985). Boxers drank water laced with cocaine between rounds. Long-distance runners were followed on bicycles by doctors who gave them a mixture of brandy and strychnine (Wooley, 1992).

Amphetamines, which were developed in the 1930s, increased alertness and energy for competition. In World War II, amphetamines were used by various countries to delay fatigue and increase the endurance of their troops. When veterans returned home to the playing fields, some continued to rely on the drugs to try to give themselves a competitive edge or increase their athletic endurance.

International Politics

The male hormone testosterone had been isolated in the 1930s and was used in its pure form or in compounds to help injury victims and survivors of World War II concentration camps gain weight. During the Cold War era, the Soviet weightlifting team used steroids in the 1952 Olympics to garner medals. When this information was revealed in 1954 to the U.S. weightlifting coach, the argument was soon made that the United States team should also have access to steroids if they wanted to have a chance of staying ahead of the Soviets and the rest of the Communist Bloc (Todd, 1987). The use of performance-enhancing drugs was thought to be the only way that Americans could maintain their competitiveness in international athletics. At the 1956 Olympics, the Soviets and many of the Communist Bloc countries, especially East Germany, were rumored to be using anabolic steroids not only in weightlifting and strength sports but in swimming as well. Use of ergogenic drugs continued in succeeding Olympics.

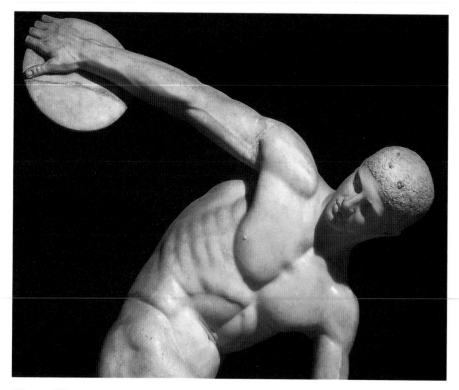

This marble copy of the classic bronze statue of the Discus Thrower by Myron (circa 450 B.C.) emphasizes the importance of sports in ancient Greece and the exalted position of the athlete. The five-foot-tall statue is on display at the Museo Nazionale delle Terme in Rome.
Reprinted, by permission, Gianni Dagli Orti/CORBIS.

"The athletes themselves came out and told that these coaches and scientists forced these drugs on them. And then they found the records of them. I've seen their health problems afterwards.

◇ analgesics (painkillers) and anesthetics,
◇ muscle relaxants,
◇ anti-inflammatories,
◇ and asthma medications.

Analgesics (painkillers)

These drugs are normally used to deaden pain. They include both topical analgesics that desensitize nerve endings on the skin (alcohol and menthol or local anesthetics, such as procaine and lidocaine), and systemic analgesics, such as aspirin, ibuprofen, and acetaminophen (Tylenol®), for mild to moderate pain, or narcotic (opioid) analgesics for moderate to severe pain. The most common opioids used in sports are hydrocodone (Vicodin®), the most prescribed, meperidine (Demerol®), morphine, codeine, and propoxyphene (Darvon®). These drugs are either ingested or injected. Besides the pain-killing effects, opioids can cause sedation, drowsiness, dulling of the senses, mood changes, nausea, and euphoria. Opioids allow users to play through the pain and perform at or near their previous levels.

"Pain is something you can play with and everybody experiences pain at one time in their life or another and your body's just telling you something. Injury is a totally different situation. Injury, you don't participate when you're injured."
Bob Visgar, strength coach, Sacramento State University

The biggest danger from these drugs results from their ability to block pain without repairing the damage. Normally pain is the body's warning signal that some muscle, organ, or tissue is damaged and that it should be protected. If those signals are constantly short-circuited, the user becomes confused about what the body is saying. In addition, since tolerance develops so rapidly with opioids, increasing amounts become necessary to achieve pain relief. The problem is that tissue dependence can develop, along with the analgesic effects, making it easier for the user to slip into compulsive use of the drug.

"I was on hydrocodone. You know it's kind of a super painkiller. And it felt good. I'd take one. The next hour and a half I'd be real sleepy and lightheaded, be dizzy. It's like being drugged. I developed a small addiction to it."
23-year-old weightlifter, ex-college football player

Muscle Relaxants

Muscle relaxants are drugs that depress neural activity within skeletal muscles. They are used to treat muscle strains, ligament sprains and the resultant severe spasms, and to control tremors or shaking. Some athletes also use them to control performance anxiety. The classes of muscle relaxants include skeletal muscle relaxants, such as carisoprodol (Soma®) and methocarbamol (Robaxin®), and benzodiazepines, such as diazepam (Valium®) or clonazepam (Klonopin®) (Arnheim & Prentice, 1993).

As with analgesics, the performance enhancement of these drugs is minimal because the drugs are depressants and can also cause sedation, blurred vision, decreased concentration, impaired memory, respiratory depression, and mild euphoria. Skeletal muscle relaxants are only occasionally abused for their mental effects. In recent years there has been an increase in the abuse of carisoprodol. Benzodiazepines and barbiturates have a higher dependence liability since accelerating use causes tolerance and tissue dependence. The benzodiazepines also stay in the body for a long period of time, causing delayed effects when they're not wanted.

"I couldn't imagine anyone performing under the influence of alcohol or a barbiturate. If they got to that point, they would probably hurt themselves. Occasionally some competed with a stimulant."
Former college diving champion

Anti-Inflammatory Drugs

These drugs control inflammation and lessen pain. Anti-inflammatory drugs come in two classes: **NSAIDs** or nonsteroidal anti-inflammatory drugs,

typically ibuprofen (Motrin® or Advil®), indomethacin (Indocin®), phenylbutazone (Butazoliden®), or sulindac (Clinoril®), and **corticosteroids,** such as cortisone and Prednisone® (corticosteroids are different than androgenic-anabolic steroids described below) (PDR, 1999).

But with the corticosteroids, side effects are a significant consideration. Prolonged use can cause water retention, bone thinning, muscle and tendon weakness, skin problems such as delayed wound healing, vertigo, headaches, and glaucoma. Psychoactive effects are minimal at low doses but severe psychosis results from excessive high-dose use (Arnheim & Prentice, 1993).

As with analgesics and skeletal muscle relaxants, when athletes are using anti-inflammatory drugs, a careful examination must be done to insure that the injury is not serious and that practice or play can continue without risk of aggravating the injury. There is the risk that these drugs will be used as a cure for the injury. They should not be used solely to enable the athlete to resume activity but should be part of the overall healing process. Ice, elevation, rest, physical therapy, and other treatment measures must accompany pharmacological relief of pain and inflammation.

Asthma Medications (beta$_2$ agonists)

Asthma affects 10% of the general population and is aggravated by heavy exercise in sports that requires continuous exertion, e.g., cycling, rowing, middle- to long-distance running. It is also aggravated by the excess stress that comes from preperformance anxiety. A lesser condition, exercise-induced asthma (EIA), has been found. The incidence of EIA is 11% to 23% in athletes (Fuentes & DiMeo, 1996; Rupp et al., 1993). Because asthma is so widespread in athletics, permission to use certain asthma medications is given. Medications used to control asthma include beta$_2$ agonists like clenbuterol (banned) and albuterol (limited use). Beta$_2$ stimulation also increases muscle energy and growth but to a lesser extent (about 10% to 25%) than steroids. (Beta$_2$ agonists are widely used

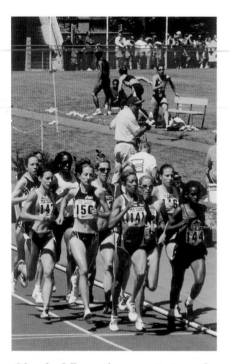

Often the difference between winning and coming in fifth is a fraction of a second. Athletes look for any edge, occasionally an illegal one.

on cattle to promote growth and have therefore been banned. Other asthma medications like ephedrine cause too much stimulation to the brain and are also banned.) These drugs can slightly increase oxygen intake by bronchodilation that is helpful to the asthmatic. Tolerance to the muscle-building effects seems to develop, so the benefits to muscle growth become less and less with continued use. Other medications such as theophylline and cromolyn are freely allowed by both the IOC and NCAA (Rosenberg, Fuentes, Wooley, et al., 1996).

ANABOLIC STEROIDS & OTHER PERFORMANCE-ENHANCING (ergogenic) OR APPEARANCE-ENHANCING DRUGS

To this very broad general category of drugs we will add other substances and even techniques used to enhance performance. Most of the drugs, substances, and techniques are banned by various sports-governing bodies such as the IOC and the NCAA.

The goals that motivate users make these drugs different from alcohol and other psychoactive drugs. These ergogenic or energy-producing drugs, substances, and techniques are thought to possess various capabilities for boosting an athlete's performance by giving a physical competitive edge (e.g., muscle building, fatigue delay). They are also abused to enhance self-image by adding muscle mass (bulking up) and shaping physique. Young adolescents might want them to hasten maturity or to develop the look of others using them. Unfortunately one of the side effects in young adolescents is to limit growth. Steroid use in junior high and high school will limit increases in height. The final reason performance-enhancing drugs are used is to increase aggression (Brower, 1995).

Anabolic-Androgenic Steroids (AAS or "roids")

"It's a performance-enhancing drug. I mean, that's what it did. It enhanced my performance. There were a few side effects but for the most part, I had pretty good results from them as far as gaining strength and power."
24-year-old weightlifter

The most abused performance-enhancing drugs today, anabolic-androgenic steroids are derived from the male hormone testosterone or are synthesized versions of it. Anabolic means "muscle building," androgenic means "producing masculine characteristics"; and steroid is the chemical classification of the natural and synthetic compounds resembling hormones like testosterone. Anabolic steroids are used by physicians to treat testosterone insufficiency, osteoporosis, certain types of anemia, some breast cancers, endometriosis, and a few other conditions (Lukas, 1998).

For the athlete these drugs have marked benefits that include increases in body weight, lean muscle mass, and increased muscular strength. The drugs can also increase aggressiveness and confidence, traits that are of value in many sports (Brower, 1992).

"I don't think Lyle thought of steroids as a drug. He thought of them as some kind of magic potion that was going to allow him to play football better and he also took a human growth hormone

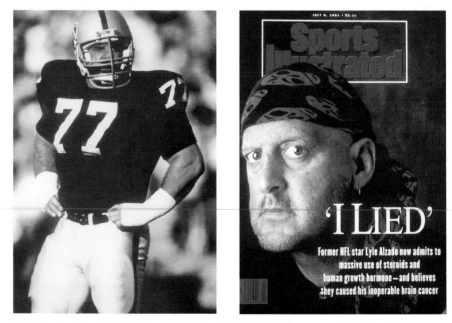

Lyle Alzado played football for the Raiders in the 1980s. He was one of the few players to speak out publicly about his use of performance-enhancing drugs. He blamed his use of human growth hormone and steroids for the brain cancer that eventually killed him. He said, "If I had known I would be this sick now, I would have tried to make it in football on my own, naturally." He died in 1992 at the age of 42.

that they got out of a cadaver. And I mean, that's how ferocious his need was to fill whatever he felt his insecurities were."

Peter Alzado, brother of NFL football star Lyle Alzado now deceased probably due to steroid and growth hormone use

Many students use AASs strictly to enhance personal appearance. As with any drug that's misused, less desirable side effects occur such as bone weakness, tendon injury, cancer, sexual problems, and even feminization in males or masculinization of women. So far no pharmacological process has been able to separate the desirable muscle-building properties of AAS from their undesirable or dangerous hormonal side effects.

"The men I knew who used steroids the most were 5'8" and under and they talked about how they were the runts of the class and the 98-pound weakling at the beach. Steroid use is one way they felt they could overcome that."

Ex-weightlifter

Patterns of Use: Cycling & Stacking. Anabolic steroid users may take from 20–200 times the usually prescribed daily dosage. Instead of a normal prescribed dose of 75–100 mg per week, weightlifters, bodybuilders, and other illicit users have taken 1,000 mg to 2,100 mg per week (Yesalis, Herrick, Buckley, et al., 1988). Some athletes practice steroid stacking by using three or more kinds of oral or injectable steroids and by alternating between cycles of use and nonuse.

"Basically I go on about 10 weeks, then I'll go off for a little while. So I would kind of cycle it to where it would peak me out at a certain time in the season."

24-year-old weightlifter

Cycling means taking the drugs for a 4- to 18-week period during intensive training and then stopping the drugs for a period of several weeks to several months to give the body a pharmacological rest and then beginning another cycle. Some athletes cycle to escape detection. Studies have reported that 82% of those using "roids" during a training cycle combined three or more different anabolic steroids in that time and 30% used seven or more. Of special concern is the fact that up to 99% of "roid" users have injected the drug and most increase their dosage during the course of their training (Kashkin, 1992).

Physical Side Effects. In men the initial masculinization effect includes an increase in muscle mass and muscle tone. Most users also report an initial bloated appearance. However, long-term use results in suppression of the body's own natural production of testosterone. As a consequence, men who are long-term steroid users develop more feminine characteristics (e.g., swelling breasts, nipple changes), decreased size of sexual organs, and an impairment of sexual functioning (Pope & Katz, 1994).

In women similar gains in muscular development may be considered beautiful to some but long-term use results in masculinizing effects such as increased facial hair, decreased breast size, lowered voice, and clitoral enlargement (Strauss, Liggett, & Lanese, 1985).

"Outwardly you have people experience the bad acne. With women, I've seen a change in the facial jaw line—their voices too. There are definitely things that, as a woman, are not in your favor. And the lasting results, too, are something that I often wonder why a person chooses to go that route."

Female bodybuilder

If injections of steroids are taken to supplement oral doses and the large gauge reusable needles purchased on the black market are shared, users are liable to contract or transmit the HIV infection that can lead to AIDS. They are also at risk for other blood-borne pathogens like hepatitis B and C.

Mental & Emotional Effects. Anabolic steroids can make users feel more confident and aggressive while using these substances. Some researchers think that the confidence that "roids" can induce is as sought after as the physical effects. As use continues, emotional balance starts to swing from confidence to aggressiveness, to emotional instability, to rage, and back to depression or to psychosis. This "roid rage" can lead to irrational behavior (Pope & Katz, 1994).

"After a dinner date, this one guy attacked me in my apartment. He was in the middle of a 'roid' cycle. I put up a great fight and he gave up, but if he was determined, there was no way I could have overpowered him. I don't know if it was the drugs or he was just crazy."

Female college student

The "roid rage" is more likely to occur in people who already have a tendency to anger or who take excessive amounts of steroids. One study of 12 bodybuilders compared to a control group found much higher tendencies towards paranoid, schizoid, antisocial, borderline, histrionic, and passive-aggressive personality profiles due to use. Before use the two groups were about equal in regards to abnormal personality traits (Cooper, Noakes, Dunne, et al., 1996).

Compulsive Use & Addiction. About 1/3 of the users experience a sense of euphoria or well-being (at least initially) that contributes to their continued and compulsive abuse of "roids." In a survey of hard-core AAS users in their senior year in high school, 38% said they wouldn't stop using even if it were proven beyond a doubt that AASs cause permanent sterility, liver cancer, or heart attacks (Kusserow, 1990).

Various surveys of weightlifters found distinct withdrawal symptoms, which are strong signs of dependence and abuse. Withdrawal symptoms include craving, fatigue, dissatisfaction with body image, depressed mood, restlessness, insomnia, lack of appetite, headaches, and lack of sexual desire (Brower, Blow, Young, & Hill, 1991). Even between cycles, users will continue with low doses to avoid withdrawal. As with other drug use, compulsive use of steroids makes the user more likely to use other psychoactive drugs to enhance performance, as a reward, or in social situations.

"It was addicting, mentally addicting. I just didn't feel strong unless I was taking something. When I retired, I kept taking the stuff. I couldn't stand the thought of being weak."

Lyle Alzado, former NFL star

Do Steroids Work?   In 1984 the American College of Sports Medicine stated that steroids could increase mass and muscle strength when combined with diet and exercise. A 1996 study by Dr. Shalender Bhasin of Charles R. Drew University in Los Angeles showed large measurable increases in strength and weight due to steroids in a double blind study involving 43 male volunteers. When steroid use was combined with exercise, the gains in muscle size and strength were significantly greater (Bhasin, Storer, Berman, et al., 1996). What the study didn't cover was the use of multiple steroids and the use of excessive amounts of steroids over long periods of time.

"I took steroids from 1976 to 1983. In the middle of 1979, my body began turning a yellowish color. I was very aggressive and combative, had high blood pressure and testicular atrophy. I was hospitalized twice with near kidney failure, liver tumors, and severe personality disorders. During my second hospital stay, the doctors found I had become sterile. Two years after I quit using and started training without drugs, I set six new world records in power lifting, something I thought was impossible without the steroids."

Richard L. Sandlin, Former Assistant Coach, University of Alabama (U.S. Congress, 1990)

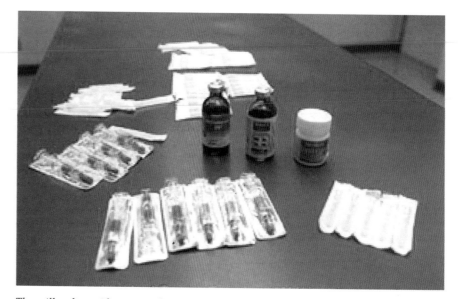

These illegal steroids were confiscated at the Mexican/U. S. border when a young teenage American boy tried to smuggle them in.
Courtesy of the U.S. Customs Service (James R. Tourtellotte and Todd Reeves, photographers)

Supply & Cost.   Athletes obtain steroids in different ways: from the black market (at gyms, from mail order companies, or friends) or from unscrupulous doctors, veterinarians, or pharmacists. Serious users spend $200 to $400 per week on anabolic steroids and other strength drugs, so a single cycle can cost thousands of dollars. Some professional athletes spend $20,000 to $30,000 a year. At a conservative estimate, the black market for steroids grosses up to $300–500 million a year (Brower, 1992; NIDA, 1997). Most of the product comes from approximately 20 underground laboratories in the United States and foreign countries.

"We all knew who was using. We exchanged information on any new drugs that were on the market. We got our steroids through the gym owner. In fact he would inject them for us in the rear."

28-year-old weightlifter

STIMULANTS

Central nervous system stimulants often start out as performance boosters but the basic pharmacology of most stimulants often makes use self-defeating. The IOC and all other sports organizations have banned the use of any kind of amphetamine and most other strong stimulants in competition. Stimulants used in sports include methamphetamines, diet pills, methylphenidate, ephedrine, caffeine, nicotine, occasionally cocaine, and some herbal or dietary supplements.

Amphetamines

Amphetamines are referred to as "sympathomimetics" because they mimic and stimulate the effects of the sympathetic nervous system, that part of the nervous system that controls involuntary body functions, including blood circulation, respiration, and digestion. Some use amphetamines ("crank," "whites," "black beauties") as a way of getting up for competition. Initially many users feel energetic and alert. Athletes also take (or are given) amphetamines to make themselves more aggressive and confident. Some take them after an event to sustain the competitive high. Studies have shown that amphetamines will increase strength by about 3% to 4% and endurance by 1.5% in low doses (Rosenberg et al., 1996). Other studies have shown

TABLE 7–4 ANABOLIC-ANDROGENIC STEROIDS

Chemical Name (DEA schedule)	Trade Name
U.S. Approved	
Adanazol (N/S)	Danocrin®
Fluoxymesterone (III)	Halotestin®
Methyltestosterone (III)	Android®, Metandren®, Testred®, Virilon®
Nandrolone phenpropionate (III)	Durabolin®
Nandrolone decanoate (III)	Deca-Durabolin®
Oxandrolone (III)	Oxandrin®
Oxymetholon (III)	Anadrol-50®
Stanozolol (III)	Winstrol®
Testolactone (III)	Teslac®
Testosterone cypionate (III)	Depo-Testosterone®, Virilon IM®
Testosterone enanthate (III)	Delatestryl®
Testosterone propionate (III)	Testex®, Oreton Propionate®
Not U.S. Approved	
Bolasterone	Finiject 30®
Ethylestrenol	Maxibolan®
Mesterolone	—
Methandrostenolone	Dianabol®
Methenolone	Primobolan®
Methenolone enanthate	Primobolan Depot®
Norethandrolone	Nilexor®
Oxandrolone	Anavar®
Oxymesterone	Oranabol®
Oxymethalone	Anadrol-50®
Testosterone proponiate	Testex®, Oreton Propionate®
Veterinary	
Boldenone	Equipoise®
Mibolerone	Cheque® Drops
Stanozolol	Winstrol®-V
Zeranol	Ralgro®

that much of the increase in performance comes from the focusing effects of amphetamines and the increase in aggressiveness rather than specific muscular changes as are seen with anabolic steroids. Improvement seems to be in complex tasks that require concentration (Laties & Weiss, 1981).

"When you have played before 70,000 people and come off the field, you're back down to normal so to speak. You want to get back up there with cocaine. It replaces that high with an artificial stimulation. But the comedown from cocaine is very, very draining, emotionally, physically, and nutritionally. It's totally different than coming down from the natural high."
Delvin Williams, former NFL rushing back, recovering cocaine user

Tolerance to amphetamines develops quite rapidly and as it develops, the beneficial effects diminish. Negative effects include anxiety, restlessness, and impaired judgment. In some cases amphetamine users (e.g., football players) can overreact to plays and literally overrun the action. The increase in aggressiveness caused by amphetamines can get out of hand causing injury to the users and their opponents. Physically, heavy use can bring on heart and blood pressure problems, exhaustion, and malnutrition. There have been reports of fatal heat stroke among athletes since these strong stimulants redistribute blood away from the skin thereby impairing the body's cooling system (Fischman, 1995). Mentally they can bring on paranoia and even amphetamine psychosis.

Caffeine

This mild stimulant is found in coffee, tea, cola-flavored beverages, and cocoa. It also comes in liquid form and can be very toxic. It can increase wakefulness and mental alertness at blood levels of 10 mg/ml by stimulating the cerebral cortex and medullar centers. It also increases endurance slightly during extended exercise and supposedly increases muscle contraction (Spriet, 1995). The Olympic Committee puts a limit on caffeine of 12 mg/ml, about three strong cups of coffee just before competition (Bell & Doege, 1987). Some athletes have been using a combination of caffeine, ephedrine, and aspirin to try and increase endurance even though the cardiovascular effects can be risky. Caffeine also acts as a mild diuretic, increasing urine flow and dehydration (Partin, 1988).

Ephedrine (ma huang)

This mild stimulant, extracted from the ephedra bush or synthesized in laboratories, is found in hundreds of legal, over-the-counter cold and asthma medications as well as in some herbal teas and sports energy bars (NCAA, 1999). It is used by itself or in combination with other mild stimulants (e.g., pseudoephedrine and phenylpropanolamine) to supposedly increase strength and endurance and/or promote weight loss. Excess use can cause jitteriness, anxiety, headaches, high blood pressure, and overheating. A study of 36 female weightlifters that used ephedrine showed that many had used the drug for years, mostly in high doses, and about 20% exhibited signs of dependence. Eating disorders appeared to be especially prevalent among them (Gruber & Pope, 1998).

Tobacco

Initially the nicotine in cigarettes is a mild stimulant but does little for performance and in fact, reduces lung capacity. Like other stimulants, it also constricts blood vessels, thus raising blood pressure. After the mild stimulation, it often acts as a relaxant probably due to suppression of withdrawal symptoms. Smokeless tobacco (spit tobacco) has many of the same effects as cigarettes except for a reduction in lung capacity. Chewing tobacco was a mainstay of baseball dugouts and the image of the baseball player with a large wad of chewing tobacco in his cheek, spitting in the dugout was common. Fortunately it is becoming less popular partly due to an increasing number of players who speak out about their developing health problems due to their habit, e.g., Brett Butler, the ex-Dodger leadoff man, underwent surgery for throat cancer that he feels was caused by chewing tobacco.

"You know the first time you try chewing tobacco, it is absolutely disgusting. You get dizzy because of all the nicotine rushing into your bloodstream. I saw some baseball player from the '50s—he had to have a big old chew in his mouth, so now, like half of his face is gone."
28-year-old weightlifter

In 1994, the NCAA banned the use of all tobacco products during NCAA-sanctioned events.

HUMAN GROWTH HORMONE (HGH)

HGH is a polypeptide hormone produced by the pituitary gland that stimulates growth in children. It is used by athletes to increase muscle strength and growth. It was thought that the side effects of HGH were less damaging than steroids. Studies have found that HGH reduces fat by altering lipolytic effects. It also increases muscle mass, skin thickness, and connective tissues in muscles (Terney & McLain, 1990). Some studies have found that it has little effect on muscle development in those with normal HGH production. Gigantism and acromegaly, along with metabolic and endocrine disorders, have been widely reported. Abuse is also associated with cardiovascular disease, goiter, menstrual disorders, decreased sexual desire, and impotence. It decreases the life span by up to 20 years (Jacobson, 1990). HGH used to be harvested from human cadavers but techniques for synthesis were developed in 1986. Cadaver HGH usually contains contaminants, unlike synthetic HGH that is pure.

HGH is banned by both the USOC and NCAA although it is difficult to detect because it is found naturally in the body.

OTHER PERFORMANCE-ENHANCING DRUGS

Androstenedione & DHEA (dehydroepiandrosterone)

Androstenedione made headlines when Mark McGwire said he used it to help his stamina during baseball training. Androstenedione is not a steroid but

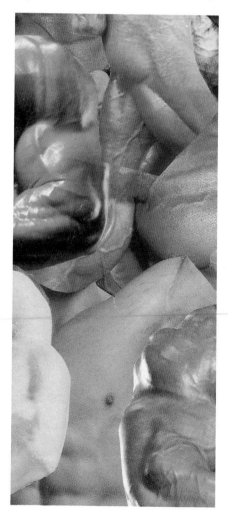

rather a precursor (one step removed) to testosterone synthesis in the body. It is produced in all mammals by the gonads and adrenal glands and metabolized in the liver into testosterone. An eight-week study of healthy men with normal testosterone levels was done. Half of 20 subjects used androstendione and half used a placebo but they all did resistance training for the eight weeks. They found no change in testosterone levels between the two groups but there was a higher level of estradiol, a female hormone, in the group that used the drug. There was also no difference in strength between the two groups. Unfortunately there was an increase in high-density cholesterol in the group that got the hormone (King, Sharp, Vukovich, et al., 1999). In women, according to an older study, there was a four- to seven-fold increase in their testosterone level (Mahesh & Greenblatt, 1962). The logical conclusion of both studies would be that in people with low normal testosterone levels, the substance would increase levels of the male hormone and increase endurance and muscle size but in those with normal levels, it probably will not. So unless further studies take into account the normal production of testosterone in its subjects, then the tests will not be accurate. The drug is banned by the IOC and by the NFL among others. Major League Baseball (MLB) is reevaluating its policy of allowing use of the hormone.

A somewhat similar hormone, DHEA (dehydroepiandrosterone), has been tried in an attempt to increase gonadal and peripheral testosterone as well as estrogen production since it is a precursor for these hormones. Over-the-counter sales were banned in 1985. Studies have found little effect from the substance but it has shown some unwanted side effects such as reduced natural testosterone production and liver damage (DiPasquale, 1994).

Beta Blockers (propranolol [Inderol®] & atenolol [Tenormin®])

Beta blockers are normally prescribed by physicians to lower blood pressure, decrease heart rate, prevent arrhythmias, and reduce eye pressure.

Beta blockers are also banned by the IOC and most athletic organizations for specific events. Because they are therapeutic drugs, permission to use them is often given. They work by blocking nerve cell activity at the brain, heart, kidney, and blood vessels. They keep adrenaline from binding onto beta receptors on the heart. Their ability to block nerve cell activity in the brain calms and steadies the body (Gordon et al., 1991). Beta blockers are also used to control the symptoms of a panic attack or performance fright. Because of their ability to calm the brain and tremors, they are sought by some athletes involved in riflery, archery, diving, ski jumping, biathlon, and pentathlon (Fuentes, Rosenberg, & Davis, 1996).

Beta blockers can cause fatigue, lethargy, dreams, occasional nausea, vomiting, and temporary impotence. Another negative effect of these drugs is interference with production of the liver enzyme needed to eliminate wastes. A great danger in the use of these drugs is their potential to intensify some forms of asthma and heart problems that can be fatal to the user.

Blood Doping

While not involving a drug, the practice of injecting extra blood, either one's own or someone else's, is used to increase endurance by increasing the number of red blood cells available to carry oxygen. Normally about two units of the athlete's own blood are withdrawn, frozen to minimize deterioration, and then reinfused five or six weeks later (about one to seven days before competition) after the athlete's blood volume has returned to normal (Williams, Wesseldine, Somma, & Schuster, 1981). Blood doping is used by athletes in such sports as cycling, long-distance running, cross-country skiing, and other events that require endurance. Tests have shown that performance times for a five-mile race drop an average of 45 seconds (Williams et al., 1981) and a three-mile run about 24 seconds (Goforth, Cambell, Hodgdon, & Sucec, 1982).

Because doping involves blood transfusion, dangers include poor storage, viral or bacterial infections, and even fatal reactions due to mislabeling. No test yet exists to accurately detect blood doping, so athletes have a clear-cut decision to make: to cheat or not to cheat.

Creatine

Creatine, an amino acid, is a nutritional supplement, synthesized naturally in the body and also found in fish and meat. It is used by athletes to delay muscle fatigue, store energy that can be used in short bursts, extend workout time, and help muscles recover faster. Three pounds of meat contain five grams of creatine. Sales have exploded in recent years. The use of creatine in muscle energy metabolism has been researched for the past 100 years (Rosenberg et al., 1996). A recent study in which athletes were given 20 grams of creatine suggests the supplement helps the body store energy and helps muscles to recover faster. Cyclists increased their endurance from 30 minutes to 37 minutes (Becque, Lochmann, & Melrose, 2000). The creatine was coupled with 6 weeks of resistance training.

"It gives you energy so your muscles don't get tired and just takes away some of the soreness that enables you to work out longer and harder."
College football player

Creatine supplementation also seems to benefit sprint disciplines of running, swimming, cycling, and other power exercises.

"The greatest danger that I see with nutritional supplements is that there's the tendency of athletes to try to overuse them to compensate for other things. For example, if a certain supplement supposedly works at one dosage, a lot of times an athlete will take two or three times that because they think that will give them more of an effect."
Lawrence Magee, M.D., team physician, University of Kansas

Since it is classified as a nutritional supplement, creatine is sold over the counter and is not banned by any sports agency.

Diuretics

Diuretics (e.g., furosemide, ethracrynic acid, and toresemide) are drugs that increase the rate of urine formation, thus speeding the elimination of water from the body. Athletes use these drugs

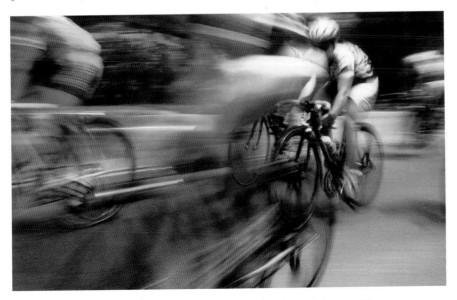

Because endurance is critical in bicycle racing, some racers try to increase the oxygen-carrying capacity of their blood either by blood doping (transfusing stored blood) or the use of EPO, a drug that increases the oxygen-carrying red blood cells.

◇ to lose weight rapidly which is important in sports where people compete in certain weight classes;

◇ to avoid detection of illegal drugs during testing by increasing urination.

(Arnheim & Prentice, 1993)

"I was given a diuretic a week before I was to compete with instructions not to drink more than 1/2 cup of water per day. I probably lost 12 pounds of water that week. I left the dorm the morning of my competition and my neighbor across the hall didn't recognize me because my face was so drawn. I wouldn't have placed second if the gym owner hadn't given me the diuretic."

Competitive wrestler

Erythropoietin (EPO)

In the 1998 Tour de France bicycle race, several competitors were expelled from competition when drugs, including EPO, were found in their rooms and team trucks (AP, 1998). EPO is a synthetic version of the human peptide hormone that stimulates bone marrow to produce more red blood cells that carry oxygen to muscles. It is used as a substitute for blood doping and there is evidence that it increases performance in endurance sports such as bicycle racing. It takes two to three weeks after beginning injections for full manifestation of the effects.

The dangers from unsupervised EPO administration result from the thickening of the blood that can lead to clots that might cause stroke or heart attack. Sweating and the accompanying increase in blood viscosity magnify this potential danger of blood clots. A number of deaths among European cyclists from this kind of blood doping have been reported over the last 15 years. EPO is banned by the NCAA, the United States Olympic Committee (USOC), and most every other sport.

GHB (gamma-hydroxybutyrate)

This supplement is sold as a fat burner, anabolic agent, sleep aid, mus-cle definer, and psychedelic. It is touted as an amino acid that acts like a diuretic to reduce anabolic steroid water weight gain and raise levels of HGH (human growth hormone). It is now illegal in the United States.

Soda Doping

Some athletes believe that ingesting alkaline salts (sodium bicarbonate) about 30 minutes prior to exercise delays fatigue by decreasing the development of acidosis. It seems somewhat effective for shorter events, 30 seconds to 10 minutes, rather than endurance activities (Rosenberg et al., 1996).

Weight Loss

Getting to a specific weight is necessary or strongly desired in a number of sports, especially wrestling, gymnastics, and horse racing (jockeys usually weigh under 125 pounds). Athletes trying to make their weight will use diuretics, laxatives, exercise, fasting, self-induced vomiting, and excess sweating in a sauna. This is done in spite of the evidence that dehydration significantly diminishes performance. Some athletes will lose three to five percent of their weight in a couple of days.

"We can definitely see that gymnasts are worried about their weight. I mean we walk around in leotards and we still say we're fat and there's probably not an ounce of fat on any of our bodies."

19-year-old college female gymnast

Besides dieting and exercise, stimulants are used to control weight. Diet pills (prescription and over-the-counter), illegal amphetamines, tobacco, and caffeine are used. In addition laxatives, diuretics, excessive exercise, and even self-induced vomiting are tried when the need to lose weight becomes a compulsion. After a few months of continuous use, most diet pills and amphetamines don't work as well and the rising tolerance and development of tissue dependence can trigger abuse and addiction. In fact a major cause of amphetamine addiction stems from their overuse in trying to control weight. Bulimia (eating and purging) and anorexia (starvation eating) can also be the result of the desire to stay thin or make a weight. The NCAA recently changed training rules for wrestlers as a result of an increasing number of injuries and deaths due to dehydration and excess weight loss.

Weight-loss deaths jar wrestling

The Associated Press

Two days before his season-opening wrestling match, high school sophomore Frank Angelone needed to shed 5 pounds to com

and I think we'll see it," says Iowa State coach Bobby Douglas. "We don't want to put a Band-Aid on a gaping wound

the school and throughout the NCAA.
The NCAA

class offers an advan-

■ SPORTS DIGEST

U.S. Gymnast Henrich, 22, Dies of Eating Disorders

Associated Press

Christy Henrich, a gymnast who missed qualifying for the 1988 U.S. Olympic team by 0.118 points, died Tuesday as a result of eating disorders. She was 22.

A victim of anorexia nervosa and bulimia, Henrich died of multiple-organ-system failure after more than two weeks in Research Medical Center in Kansas City, Mo., near her hometown of Independence. Hospital officials wouldn't say how much she weighed at her death, but she had wasted away to 60 pounds a year ago.

was throwing herself into the equipment because she couldn't do the routines. I set up all these appointments with the nutritionists, and then I found out she wasn't attending those sessions."

and riding an exercise bike he died while trying to shed pounds. He was 22.

Nov. 9, 19-year-old Billy Saylat North Carolina's Campbell versity died trying to drop 6 nds for a match.

nce Reese's death, Michigan suspended its wrestling pron until after Christmas while it ws how the sport operates at

his 21 years as coach, will study the findings and report to the NCAA Wrestling Rules Committee.

"We've got to have some regulation to prevent any dangerous situation," Gabie told the Chicago Tribune. "I want to find out what happened so it won't happen again."

The U.S. Food and Drug Administration said it will investigate the effects of creatine, a synthetic muscle-building supplement widely used by athletes. The agency wants to know whether the wrestlers' deaths were linked to dietary supplements.

Among wrestlers, there is a prevailing belief that regardless of risks, losing pounds swiftly to compete in the lowest possible weight

at Fraser High School in suburban Detroit.

wrestling coach

"Wrestlers consider themselves the best-conditioned athletes that exist, and they like the fact that they can go where no one's gone before. The instilled attitude among these kids is that if they push and push, it'll pay off with a victory."

Angelone, the 16-year-old in North Carolina, agreed.

"Most wrestlers can be stubborn, hard-headed and think that can't happen to them," he said. "I really didn't think what happened to that Campbell dude would happen to me."

The NCAA bars college wrestlers from participating in more than three weight classes in a season. But there are no rules on how much weight one can lose in a season.

Although deaths from weight loss are rare, deaths from excessive exercise due to dehydration and overheating caused by sweat suits, diuretics, and drugs are somewhat more common.

Wrestlers are not allowed to use any mechanism for shedding weight during training. The NCAA also allowed greater flexibility in weight, permitting up to a seven-pound variance in the listed weight categories.

The flip side of anorexia is a newly defined disorder called "muscle dysmorphia" that is a preoccupation with body development—no matter how sculptured their body is, they look in a mirror and still see the 98-pound weakling, so they continue to lift weights and often take supplements and steroids.

Miscellaneous Drugs Used in Sports

◇ **Bee pollen:** This supplement is sold in pellets that consist of plant pollens, nectar, and bee saliva that contain 30% protein, 55% carbohydrates, some fat, and minerals. The anecdotal reports claim that it increases energy level and performance, boosts immunity, relieves stress, and improves digestion. Most scientific studies do not show any performance or energy benefits and for someone allergic to bee stings, an inadvertent stinger or other contaminant could be dangerous. However it is not banned by the IOC or NCAA (USOC, 1996).

◇ **Calcium pangamat:** This nonvitamin (its deficiency is not linked to any disease), also called "vitamin B_{15}" or "pengamic acid") supposedly keeps muscle tissue better oxidated but these desired effects are testimonials rather than scientific research. It is reportedly a carcinogen.

◇ **Cyproheptadine (Periactin®):** Used for colds and allergic reactions, this antihistamine (serotonin and histamine antagonist) is believed to cause weight gain and increase strength. Some users believe that this prescription drug acts like steroids but in fact the increase in muscle size comes from excess caloric intake caused by serotonin's effect on appetite control. Side effects include decreased performance, sweating, and sedation.

◇ **HCG (human chorionic gonadotropin):** This drug and clomiphene or tamoxifen is occasionally used after anabolic steroid treatment to restart the body's own testosterone production. Toxic effects on the liver and reproductive system have been reported.

◇ **Ornithine & arginine:** These amino acids are taken to try and increase muscle mass because these substances supposedly release growth hormone used in sports to increase growth and performance. High doses can lead to kidney damage.

◇ **Primagen:** This drug increases steroid production in the body and is mainly used by European athletes.

◇ **Vitamin B-12:** This vitamin is injected supposedly to ward off illness and provide extra energy. It's also used to mitigate the effects of heavy drinking.

◇ **Adrenaline & amyl or isobutyl nitrite:** This combination is taken by weightlifters just prior to their performance to increase strength. The downside includes dizziness (a dangerous side effect with a 400-pound barbell over one's head), rapid heart beat, and hypertension.

THE RECREATIONAL/ MOOD-ALTERING USE OF DRUGS BY ATHLETES

Many of the more common psychoactive drugs, legal and illegal, are used to enhance performance but also to adjust moods, to help the user fit into social situations, to comply with peer pressure, to imitate the behavior of older role models, or to conform to their image of an athlete. Athletes may also turn to drugs to help cope with the demands of a heavy schedule (practice, travel time, course work), to reduce stress, to compensate for loneliness, or to fill up time on long road trips.

"I don't think you could find too many college programs—basketball programs, football, track, any sport—

that their athletes don't drink. And I'm sure that there are a lot of people who smoke weed too."
21-year-old college basketball player

Stimulants

Many stimulants, such as amphetamines, caffeine, and tobacco, are used to enhance performance but are also used recreationally. The advantages and problems with these drugs are the same as with use by nonathletes as discussed elsewhere in this book.

Cocaine, one of the strongest stimulants, isn't often used as a performance enhancer for two reasons. First it is short acting, 30 minutes to 1 hour, so one would have to reuse during the game for a consistent effect and second, the spike of energy and euphoria is too intense for the sustained effort needed in a game.

Sedative-Hypnotics

Some athletes will use drugs such as alprazolam (Xanax®), barbiturates, and even opioids, as self-rewards for enduring the stress they experience while performing before so many people. They also use these drugs as a tranquilizer to calm down after the excitement of competition or to counteract the effects of stimulants used to enhance their performance. Regarding performance-enhancing effects, depressants are counter-productive, although their painkilling effects can benefit recovery.

Alcohol

"We were 16 and 17 years old and our club coach told us, 'If you can go get hammered the night before the game and still come out and play awesome and play to your maximum performance, go ahead. But if you can't, and you know your body, and you know you won't be able to play well enough if you get drunk the night before, don't do it.'"
20-year-old college soccer player

In general, alcohol consumption negatively affects reaction time, coordination, and balance, although studies suggest that low-dose alcohol consumption does not produce impaired performance in all people. The NFL Drug Policy statement calls alcohol "without question the most abused drug in our sport." The problem is how to alert athletes to the health and performance consequences of a drug that has general social, legal, and moral acceptance in society.

"When you have a problem with alcohol or marijuana, things of that nature, you'll see a decline in their academics. You'll see a decline in athletics. You just see a decline in everything. And we see it as coaches and the players see it, so we try to address it right away."

Patti Phillips, college women's soccer coach

The NCAA specifically bans alcohol for riflery competition. It is however not banned by the USOC since it does not enhance performance. The problem with alcohol in sports is its excess use as a reward for performance (or nonperformance), as a way to unwind, or to prove that one can drink to excess. Excess use causes the same problems that are found in the general population. A survey by the NCAA found similar levels of drinking among student-athletes as among the general population but one study found a five times greater incidence of acquaintance rape, about five percent of athletes, and alcohol is involved in most cases of date rape (Bausell, Bausell, & Siegel, 1994).

"Women are more vulnerable sexually when they've had too much to drink. They're more likely to be raped, date-raped, or otherwise. Study after study has shown that. Male athletes, when they've had too much to drink, tend to become extraordinarily aggressive."

Judith Davidson, Ph.D., athletic director, Sacramento State University

Because of the money involved in professional athletics, alcohol becomes a problem when it interferes with the athletes performance. Alcohol is generally not tested for unless the athlete exhibits abuse and addiction problems, such as occurred with Bob Welch, the ex-Dodger pitcher who was in and out of alcohol rehabilitation half-a-dozen times before he left baseball permanently.

Unfortunately athletes are less likely than other college students to turn to professionals in their university or community for help with substance abuse problems, especially alcohol (Grossman & Gieck, 1992).

Marijuana

Marijuana can either stimulate or depresses the user depending on the strength of the drug and the mood of the smoker. The most consistent effect of marijuana use is an increase in pulse rate of about 20% during exercise (Arnheim & Prentice, 1993). Marijuana also

◇ lowers blood pressure, which has caused fainting spells in football linemen who have to go quickly from a down position to a standing one many times during a game;

◇ inhibits sweating, which has caused heat prostration and strokes in athletes;

◇ impairs the ability of users to follow a moving object like a ball in play (decreased tracking ability);

◇ hinders the ability to do complex tasks, such as hitting a golf ball;

◇ diminishes hand-eye coordination;

◇ decreases oxygen intake since it is smoked;

◇ is a banned substance that will result in a one-year loss of eligibility from any NCAA sport;

◇ is illegal and can destroy an athlete's career.

Since marijuana is extremely fat-soluble and lasts so long in the body, impairment can persist for a day or two after casual use and longer after cessation of chronic use.

In a study at a major university, athletes admitted who was using marijuana and who wasn't. All of the athletes thought they were doing well and performing well but when an objective study was made of their performance, those that smoked marijuana did much worse—they dropped more passes, committed more errors, and suffered more injuries during their college career.

Currently the NCAA bans all marijuana use more for ethical and moral reasons than because of performance reasons while the IOC bans it for certain sports, although there has been much controversy within the Committee about recreational use.

TESTING

In an effort to reduce the use of illicit drugs in sports, various drug-testing programs have been instituted by sports organizations and even individual colleges. For example, the NCAA has two drug-testing programs. The first, started in 1986, tests at all NCAA championships and at the post-season football bowl games. The second program is a year-round anabolic steroid testing program that started in 1990. Banned drugs can be therapeutic, performance enhancing, and recreational, including anabolic steroids, diuretics, beta blockers, alcohol, methamphetamines, most street drugs, and even high levels of caffeine. The first positive test causes the student to lose eligibility for one year and a second positive test to lose college eligibility permanently. In a survey of NCAA schools, only 56% of all respondents had a drug/alcohol education program for student-athletes. Three-fourths of the respondents said they refer student-athletes with problems to community agencies (NCAA, 1998).

Testing for the Olympics over the years has generated much controversy. In 1999, the IOC reached agreement on the creation of a world antidrug agency to coordinate drug-testing programs, intensify research, create educational programs, and publish an annual list of banned substances.

ETHICAL ISSUES

Using illegal drugs and using drugs illegally to improve athletic performance is against the rules in all sports and is illegal in most states. Drugs undermine the assumption of fair competition on which all sports rest. It is a kind of cheating that goes on before a game as well as during a game. Drugs violate the very nature of sport, which since the time of the Greeks, was a measure of personal excellence, the result of a sound mind in a healthy body. The outcome of athletic contests should be determined by discipline, training, and effort.

There is a real threat today that the public will walk away from sports if they perceive that winning is based on access to the latest pharmacology and schemes to evade drug testing. Drugs also rob the athlete of feelings of self-accomplishment and tarnish the pride of winning. Because our society treats sports figures as heroes and role models, drug-abusing athletes diminish all of us.

"If I could take a drug and set the world record out of reach for everybody and the tradeoff would be I would be dead in five years, I definitely wouldn't do it. I mean because to me, why is it so important? I want to have a chance to grow old and play with my grand kids and my great grand kids."

Allen Johnson, 1996 Olympic Gold Medallist, 110-meter hurdle

MISCELLANEOUS DRUGS

UNUSUAL SUBSTANCES

Besides the dozens of obscure psychedelic plants that are used mostly in Africa and South America, it's amazing what substances and methods some people will use to get high. They include inhaling typewriter correction fluid, chewing dandelion root, smoking camomile tea leaves, drinking rubbing alcohol, ingesting C-4 (a plastic explosive), smoking aspirin, drinking hydrogen peroxide, putting Ambusol® in the eye, and smoking toad secretions. Cough suppressants, ginseng root, and

even other people's heart medications are also abused.

Other psychoactive substances are provided by street chemists who either synthesize drugs that were once legally available, such as Quaaludes®, PCP, and fentanyl, or produce illegal drugs, including MDMA, MDE, and methcathinone (synthetic khat). The danger is that street drugs have not been tested and are not made under any kind of control. Irregular doses, unexpected effects, or contaminants in the manufacturing process can have disastrous effects on an unsuspecting user.

For example, in the 1980s a group of heroin users who had been sold a supposedly synthetic Demerol® derivative, MPPP, were later found to have an 80% incidence of Parkinson's disease symptoms (rigid muscles, loss of voluntary body control) caused by contamination of the drug during the chemical process. Street drugs can also be dozens of times stronger than the expected dose. Ultrapotent street fentanyl killed 30 users in Baltimore in 1993.

Camel Dung

Some Arab countries produce hashish by force feeding ripe marijuana plants to camels. Their four-chambered stomachs convert the marijuana into hashish camel dung.

C-4 Explosive

Modern veterans have been known to ingest C-4 or cyclonite plastic explosives for their psychedelic effects. Tremors and seizure activity can result but usually not an explosion since it takes a blasting cap to set off the chemical.

Toad Secretions (bufotenine)

The *Bufo* genus of toads (Colorado River, Sonoran Desert, Cane, and others) secrete a psychedelic substance from pores located on the back of their necks. This substance, bufotenine, is milked and harvested onto cigarettes that are then smoked to induce a psychedelic experience.

Embalming Fluid (formaldehyde)

Mortuaries have been broken into and robbed of their embalming fluid. It can either be directly abused (inhaled for its depressant and psychedelic effects) or it can be used in the manufacture of other illicit drugs. Some abusers soak marijuana "joints" or cigarettes in the fluid and smoke them. Called "clickers," "clickems," or "Sherms," the mixture gives a PCP-like effect. Formaldehyde, the main ingredient of embalming fluid, is a known carcinogen. Recently formaldehyde has also been used in the illicit manufacture of "crank" or "crystal" methamphetamine.

Gasoline

In spite of the toxicity of leaded or unleaded gasoline, a few people have been known to mix it with orange juice and drink it. They call it "Montana Gin," a particularly lethal beverage. Most often gasoline fumes are inhaled for their effects.

Ginseng Root

Ginseng has been used for thousands of years as an herbal tonic or health aid. Today the plant extract is

SPIDER COCKTAIL: Doctors at a California emergency department report they successfully treated a 37-year-old woman who had crushed a black widow spider, mixed it with distilled water and injected it to get high. "One hour later she (complained) of severe cramping ... headache and anxiety," say Drs. Sean Bush, John Naftel and David Farstad in the April *Annals of Emergency Medicine*. She had an extremely fast heart rate and trouble breathing, but three days of hospital treatment returned her to normal. The heart and lung problems could have been from an allergy to the spider protein or a direct result of the spider venom. The woman was referred to a psychiatrist.

It's amazing what some people do to get high.

. . . .

also used to help develop muscles rapidly. The root does contain small amounts of anabolic steroids and can cause blood problems in massive doses.

Kava Kava

The roots of the South American *Piper methysticum* plant are chewed or crushed into a soapy liquid and drunk. This milky exudate of the root, kava kava, contains at least six chemicals that produce a drunken state, similar to that of alcohol. Users claim that the effects are more pleasurable, relaxing, and psychic than the effects of alcohol, without the hangover. Since human saliva is an important ingredient in the preparation of this drug, its use has not found popularity.

Raid®, Hairspray, & Lysol®

Abusers puncture the aerosol cans, draining out the liquid that they swallow mainly for its alcohol content. These items are rarely abused in the general population but find more use in rural isolated areas where access to alcohol is limited.

M-99®

M-99®, a powerful injectable opioid that is 400–1,000 times stronger than morphine, is sold under the trade names of M-99® or Immobilion®. This drug is used in veterinary practices to immobilize large animals. Its abuse seems limited to the veterinary professionals since it is highly toxic. In fact when it is abused, the user will also have a needle into a vein, ready to administer the antidote Narcan®.

Dextromethorphan (Robitussin D.M.®, Romilar®, & other cough syrups)

This chemical has been known to be a psychedelic compound for 25 years. A full six ounces of the liquid is ingested to get a proper dose of dextromethorphan. This also provides the abuser with six ounces of up to 20% alcohol, so the effects are that of a drunken deliriant.

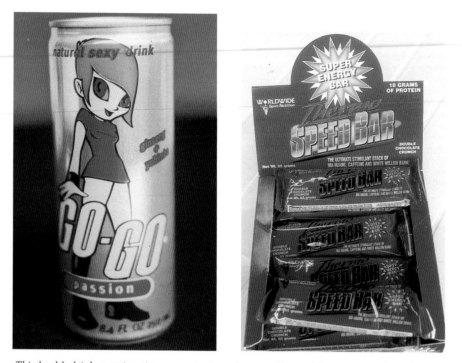

This health drink contains ginseng root extract (supposedly good for energy and muscles) and yohimbe (a mild stimulant and supposed aphrodisiac). The energy bar contains ma huang (ephedra), caffeine, and willow bark (source of aspirin).

Coricidin®, Benadryl®, & Sudafed®

Decongestants and antihistamine tablets or capsules, sold over the counter to relieve cold symptoms, are taken in excessive doses (6–10 pills at-a-time) to produce sedation or psychic effects.

SMART DRUGS

Smart drugs ("SDs") are the drugs, nutrients, drinks, vitamins, extracts, and herbal potions that manufacturers, distributors, and proponents think will boost intelligence, improve memory, sharpen attention, increase concentration, detoxify the body, especially after alcohol or other drug abuse, and energize the user. Popular drugs have included Cloud 9®, Herbal Ecstasy®, Brain Tonix®, Brain Booster®, Nirvana®, SAMe® (S-adenosylmethione), and many others. Proponents range from AIDS activists to health faddists, New Agers, antiaging questors, and members of the technoculture who feel they are on the edge of a new field of mental development.

For some consumers, smart drinks are nonalcoholic, usually a mixture of vitamins or powdered nutrients and amino acids in fruit drink, purchased in a smart bar for $4 to $6 or at a health foods store. More recently smart drinks and drugs have contained combinations of medications usually prescribed for Parkinsonism, Alzheimer's disease, or dementia. It is felt that these drugs more effectively rebalance the brain after abusing drugs, for instance, MDMA during a "rave." It is also claimed that they will slow or reverse the aging process. The consumers are typically young (17–25) urban students or professionals looking for an intellectual edge or more stamina to work or party harder.

Vitamin supplements and nutrient products, once purchased through ads in New Age magazines, are sold through health food stores. Critics of these supplements and products attribute their success to either a placebo effect (only the expectation, not the product, produces the effect) or to the caffeine and sugar that are part of the ingredients. Smart drugs containing stimulants could lead to problems if someone with high blood pressure, for example, were to take too high a dose.

Investigation of New Age smart drugs like hydergine, vasopressin, ginkgo biloba, piracetam, ginseng, and acetyl-L-carnitine has led to the proposal for a new classification of these drugs as **nootropics** (acting on the mind). Substances in this new psychotropic drug class would be those that improved learning, memory consolidation, and memory retrieval without other central nervous system effects and with low toxicity, even at extremely high doses (Dean & Morgenthaler, 1991).

Americans import nootropic drugs from Europe where many can be purchased that are not yet approved by the Food and Drug Administration (FDA) for sale in the United States. Critics of these and other prescription drugs, including researchers, doctors, and the FDA, point out that, at the very least, claims for the efficacy of the drugs have not been substantiated. Advocates argue that these and other smart drugs improve mental ability for people suffering from debilitating mental disorders and that they can enhance mental capacity in normal people too. Nootro-

pic drugs include those prescribed for debilitating mental disorders (but not FDA approved for other uses). These substances include ergoloid mesylates, selegiline hydrochloride, phenytoin (Dilantin®), and vasopressin. Other nootropics are prescription drugs not approved in the United States for any use such as piracetam, aniracetam, hydergine, fipexide, metformin, tacrine, vinpocetine, and oxiracetam (Dean & Morgenthaler, 1991).

OTHER ADDICTIONS

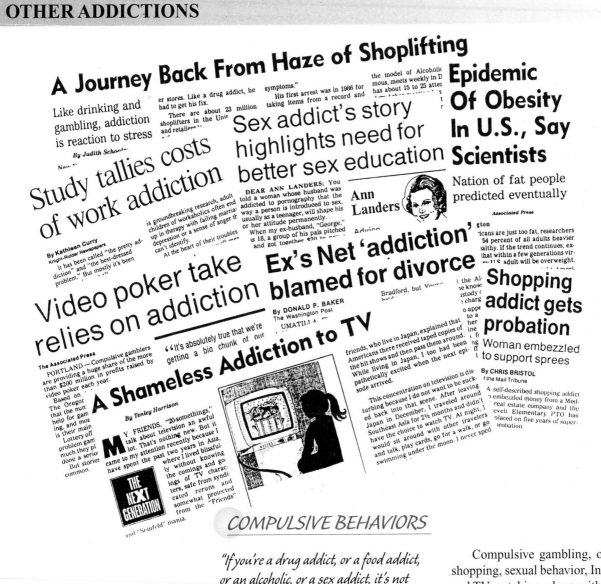

COMPULSIVE BEHAVIORS

"If you're a drug addict, or a food addict, or an alcoholic, or a sex addict, it's not about the addiction, it's about all the other things in your life that you're doing."
36-year-old recovering compulsive overeater

Compulsive gambling, overeating, shopping, sexual behavior, Internet use, and TV watching, along with pathological lying, shoplifting, hair pulling, and fire setting, all offer opportunities for repetitive, compulsive behaviors. Some of these disorders are classified as impulse control disorders (e.g., compulsive gambling, hair pulling) while some have their own classification (eating disorders). Some people confuse impulse control disorders with obsessive-compulsive disorder. The hallmark of impulse control disorders as listed in the DSM-IV is a failure to resist an impulse that is harmful to the individual or others but often starts out as pleasurable. The other major hallmark is an increasing sense of tension or arousal before actually committing the act, often followed by gratification, pleasure, and relief and then remorse and guilt over the consequences of that act (McElroy, Soutullo, & Goldsmith, 1998). The hallmark of obsessive-compulsive disorders, including hand washing, checking things, ordering, counting, and praying, are repetitive activities whose goal is to reduce anxiety or distress, not to provide pleasure or gratification (APA, 1994).

A growing number of researchers believe that vulnerability to all addictions (substance and behavioral) can be genetically transmitted, aggravated by environmental factors, and set into motion with the use of drugs or acting out of the behavior (Blum, Braverman, Cull, et al., 2000). In fact substance abuse disorders were classified as impulse control disorders until recently when they received their own classifications. A number of studies of compulsive buyers, about 37%, had substance use disorders at some time in their lives (Christenson, Faber, De Zween, et al., 1994; McElroy, Keck, Pope, et al., 1994).

Vulnerability to addictive behavior varies widely among people, as does its effect on brain chemistry.

"Every thought we have, every single thought we have, every action we do has an impact on the brain. I mean the brain in some ways causes it but then the thought or the behavior actually loops back and impacts the brain, so you can actually get a high from a sexual act, you can get a high from the excitement that comes from stealing things, you can get a high from being

in a gambling environment, which is likely related to dopamine and people then start to chase the high."
Dr. Daniel Amen, Director, Amen Clinic for Behavioral Medicine

The reasons that people engage in compulsive behavior are the same reasons that they engage in compulsive drug use: to get an instant rush, to forget problems, to control anxiety, to oblige friends, to alter consciousness, to self-medicate, and so forth. Above all, they desire to change their mood—alter their state of consciousness (Nakken, 1996).

But to understand how similar they are, it is instructive to look at the major hallmarks of addiction to psychoactive substances and compare them to compulsive behaviors. These hallmarks are

◇ using and thinking about using most of the time;

◇ the development of tolerance with continued use;

◇ the onset of withdrawal symptoms when abstinence begins;

◇ continued use despite adverse medical, social, family, and legal consequences;

◇ denial that use is a problem;

◇ a strong tendency to relapse after stopping use.

If one takes these elements of drug addiction and replaces the word using with the words eating, gambling, surfing the Internet, shopping, watching TV, or having sex, then it is easier to see that compulsion isn't limited to psychoactive substances (although many regard certain foods as psychoactive substances).

Compulsive gamblers

◇ are always playing a poker machine, buying lottery or keno tickets, trying to raise money, or thinking about where they are going to gamble;

◇ gradually increase the amount bet whether it's a machine or a high-stakes poker table;

◇ feel intensely restless and discontent when not gambling (Rosenthal & Leseur, 1992);

◇ though they lose most of their pay check each month through slot/poker machines, lotteries, or table games, they continue gambling;

◇ think they can control their gambling and their only problem is a cash flow problem;

◇ when they can't gamble or are forced to quit, they become restless, irritable, and discontent (withdrawal) and have to find some action.

Compulsive eaters

◇ wake up in the morning thinking about what and where they are going to eat that day and then they eat many times during the day (anorexics figure out how they are going to avoid eating);

◇ gain greater amounts of weight as the disease progresses and they eat larger amounts of food;

◇ experience agitation and restlessness when they begin a diet;

◇ continue overeating despite diabetes, increased risk of heart disease, impaired relationships, isolation, and a decreased ability to function physically;

◇ say they could stop eating compulsively but their metabolism makes it impossible to lose weight even if they hardly eat anything while anorexics still think they are too fat and bulimics see nothing wrong with vomiting to avoid weight gain—why give up something that gives instant pleasure, blocks out worries, and is as easy to find as the next fast-food restaurant.

◇ even when they lose large amounts of weight by dieting, almost always gain all that back and more.

"Well food does for me what alcohol and drugs and other things do for other people. If I'm feeling angry and I eat, it takes the anger away. If I'm feeling lonely or sad and I eat, it takes care of the feelings. If I feel inadequate or empty, I fill myself with food, or I used to. I don't do it any more. It's just a drug to me."
36-year-old recovering compulsive overeater

Another example of the relationship between compulsive drug use and compulsive behaviors is that in 12-step groups that help people with compulsive behaviors such as gambling, overeating, or obsessions with sex, the members use literature taken directly from Alcoholics Anonymous. Even the structure of the meetings is similar, as is the philosophy that tries to get people to understand that addiction involves lack of control over the behavior and tries to make them see the necessity of changing their lifestyle and beliefs (Nakken, 1996).

"I have to work on my behavior. How do I act with my husband? How do I act with my children? How do I act in relationships? My addiction carries over to all that—carries over to my whole life. So, I had to change the way I treat people, the way I treat myself."
36-year-old recovering compulsive overeater

HEREDITY, ENVIRONMENT, & COMPULSIVE BEHAVIORS

Apparently, like substance abuse, these behaviors can be triggered by genetic predisposition, by environmental stresses, and by the comfort, reassurance, or escape provided by the repetitive behavior itself. Increased dopamine levels in those involved in the behaviors suggest a common biochemical thread.

HEREDITY

Twin studies have already identified a genetic connection to alcoholism or other drug addictions. Other twin studies have shown a connection between heredity and other compulsive behaviors that don't involve psychoactive drugs.

"I never was a very good alcoholic, though my dad and granddad were quite good at it. Now eating—that I

excelled in. I could put down five or six meals a day without a second thought. I got pretty good at cards and slots. I can play poker for 20 hours straight without a thought for going home. And work—I can get lost in that too. In truth, I don't do anything halfway. Check that, I can't do anything halfway."
58-year-old recovering compulsive overeater, compulsive gambler, etc.

Compulsive overeating was the first addiction shown to be partly hereditary. A recent study by the National Institutes of Health of 400 twins over a period of 43 years found that "cumulative genetic effects explain most of the tracking in obesity over time." This means that a much higher than normal percentage of twins born to obese parents but subsequently raised in totally different households ended up obese. The researchers also found that "shared environmental effects were not significant" in affecting the twins' weight gain (Rosenbaum & Leibel, 1988; Bouchard, 1994). Five studies of adopted children bolstered this finding by discovering that the family environment, such as size and frequency of meals, the amount of food in the house, and the level of exercise of the family, plays very little or no role in determining the obesity of children. They found that only dramatic environmental differences could mitigate the influence of a genetic profile that made one susceptible to obesity.

Twin studies of risk takers have also found a genetic component that resulted in a higher percentage of children of risk takers being risk takers themselves.

By the mid-1990s, genetic connections between alcohol abuse, compulsive drug use, and other compulsive behaviors were starting to be confirmed by research efforts. Kenneth Blum, John Cull, Eric Braverman, David Comings, researchers at various universities, and others have postulated a genetic basis not only for alcoholism but for people with other addictive, com-

pulsive, and impulsive disorders, such as compulsive overeating, pathological gambling, attention deficit disorder, and Tourette's syndrome (compulsive verbal outbursts or strong tics). They call this genetic predisposition the "reward deficiency syndrome" (Blum, Cull, Braverman, & Comings, 1996; Blum et al., 2000).

Specifically their studies indicate that a marker gene associated with the most severe forms of alcoholism also has a strong association with several addictive compulsive behaviors. This is only one of several yet-to-be discovered marker genes that indicate a deficiency of certain neurotransmitters in the reward/pleasure center. They found that, whereas this marker gene (DRD_2 A_1 allele gene) appears in only 19% to 21% of nonalcoholic, nonaddicted, and noncompulsive subjects, it exists in

◇ 69% of alcoholic subjects with severe alcoholism;

◇ 45% of compulsive overeaters;

◇ 48% of smokers;

◇ 52% of cocaine addicts;

◇ 51% of pathological gamblers;

◇ 76% of pathological gamblers with drug problems;

◇ and in 45% of the people with Tourette's syndrome.

In addition a study of children with attention deficit disorder found that 49% had the marker gene compared to only 27% of the control group (Blum et al., 2000).

These findings suggest that a biochemical deficiency or anomaly draws some people to compulsive behaviors. The researchers postulate that carriers of this A_1 allele gene have a deficiency of dopamine receptors in the reward/pleasure center. What the dopamine receptor site deficiency means is that activities that will normally give people a surge of satisfaction, pleasure, and satiation by releasing dopamine do not give that same level of satisfaction in people with a lack of dopamine receptor sites. Such people are more likely to seek out substances and activities that release additional dopamine (e.g., alcohol, drugs, and repetitive compulsive behaviors). The release of extra amounts of dopamine caused by compulsive, repetitive behaviors stimulates the reward/pleasure center to a greater degree than normal. People with this lack of receptors all of a sudden feel pleasure that they normally don't experience.

It is important to note that there isn't just one marker gene for compulsive drug use and behaviors. This is because there are several neurotransmitters involved in the reward cascade chain and several that can alter the reward reinforcement sites in the brain (*see Chapter 2*). For example, in the urine and spinal fluid of pathological gamblers, researchers have discovered higher than normal levels of norepinephrine, the neurotransmitter that produces stimulation, alertness, and confidence. Scientists funded by the National Institute of Mental Health discovered abnormal functioning in serotonin and norepinephrine in acutely ill bulimic and anorexic patients, further suggesting a link between these disorders at the level of neurotransmitters.

ENVIRONMENT

It is fairly easy to understand how environment could intensify compulsive behaviors.

◊ Compulsive gambling is influenced environmentally by the abundance of state lotteries, slot and poker machines, the growth of gambling casinos and gambling riverboats in states outside of New Jersey and Nevada, along with the growth of Internet betting and legal off-track betting.

◊ Compulsive overeating is magnified by all the fast-food restaurants; by the abundance of fat and refined carbohydrates that can induce a certain euphoria; by parents who overfeed their children; by the endless ads for mostly high-fat high-sugar foods such as ice cream; by chaotic childhoods that make people search for an instant escape; by the lack of daily physical activity that allows fat rather than muscle to form; and

by the endless media examples of how important it is to look thin.

◊ Compulsive sexual activity is abetted by the abundance of sexual activity on television, in the movies, in music, and most of the media. Practice is encouraged by an abundance of latch key kids without supervision or without close emotional family connections. It is encouraged by an overabundance of easily accessible erotic material and pornography on the Internet.

◊ Internet addiction is encouraged by a rapidly expanding network of games, gambling, pornography, and chat rooms. Since isolation is a hallmark of many addictions, the very anonymity of doing one's thing while sitting alone feeds into that compulsion.

◊ Compulsive shopping is spurred on by the ease of obtaining credit, the endless barrage of advertisements and catalogues, shopping networks urging people to buy, accessibility to Internet shopping and auction sites, and a materialistic view of how life should be lived.

The presence of physical and sexual abuse and other childhood traumas in many that practice these compulsive behaviors also suggests the importance of environmental conditioning and reinforcement.

COMPULSIVE BEHAVIORS

It is also easy to understand how engaging in the activity itself could lead to compulsive acting out. Having a big win while gambling imprints the brain in much the same way a potent dose of cocaine would (Shaffer, 1998).

◊ Straining the digestive system with excessive food, particularly fats and sugars, or eating too many reward foods rather than life-enhancing foods changes the body's chemistry, so the person eats to change mood rather than sustain life (Carr & Papadouka, 1994).

◊ The compulsive shopper walking through the mall or phoning The Home Shopping Network® imprints

the brain, so it can anticipate buying a coveted item, thereby kindling a surge of pleasure with no regard for financial responsibility or even the need for such an item.

◊ The repeated use of pornography and participation in other compulsive sexual behaviors can make the participant avoid normal relationships.

It is instructive to look at specific compulsive behaviors to better appreciate the similarities among most addictions.

COMPULSIVE GAMBLING

"You go over it and over it and over it in your mind and say, 'How could you be this stupid? How could you not have any inkling of what was happening to you? How could you be so bright in academia and so stupid in your everyday life.'"
53-year-old recovering poker player - table and machines

Gamblers Anonymous defines gambling as "any betting or wagering, for self or others, whether for money or not, no matter how slight or insignificant, where the outcome is uncertain or depends upon chance or skill (GA, 1998). This includes

◊ poker, blackjack, craps, roulette wheels, and pai gow;

◊ standard slot machines and poker machines;

◊ horse and dog races;

◊ jai alai;

◊ bingo and raffles;

◊ state run lotteries and keno games;

◊ sports betting, both legal and illegal;

◊ office pools and bets on the golf course;

◊ school ground games: lag pennies, flip coins;

◊ bar games, e.g., liar's dice;

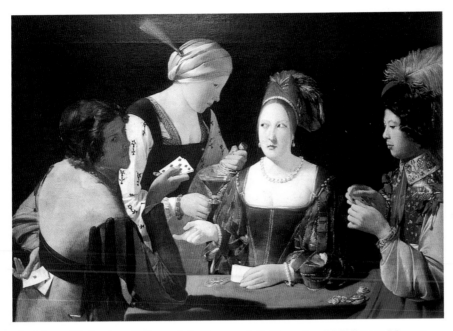

The Cheat with the Ace of Diamonds *by Georges de La Tour, circa 1647, Louvre Museum, Paris.*

Courtesy of Simone Garlaund

◇ stock speculation such as day trading, commodities, and options;

◇ and most recently, online gambling.

In the present day, there are more opportunities for gambling than ever before and the sheer availability of all these outlets, mostly legal now, are triggering problem and pathological gambling in greater and greater numbers of people. The problems that result from pathological and problem gambling are as severe as any drug-based addiction.

HISTORY

Gambling in Ancient Civilizations

The record of human gambling predates recorded history. Archeologists have unearthed prehistoric gambling bones from 40,000 B.C. called "astragali," small four-sided rolling bones from the ankles of small animals. They were used to make decisions on matters believed to be in the gods' hands, e.g., rain or drought. Six-sided dice made from pottery, wood, and ivory were used as early as 1400 B.C. in Iraq and India. Other gaming artifacts, such as throwing sticks, have been found in ancient Britain, Greece, Rome, and in

Mayan ruins in pre-Columbian America. The casting of lots is recorded in the *Bible* as a means of ending disputes or distributing property. It also records that Roman soldiers cast lots for the robes Jesus wore at the Crucifixion. Centuries later, crusading knights gambled at dice (Herman, 1984).

Along with the desire to gamble came prohibitions against gambling. Originally many of the upper classes kept gambling from the lower classes, e.g., Roman emperors kept "dicing" to themselves. Churchmen sermonized against gambling in the Middle Ages and Louis IX of France made dice illegal in 1255. Henry VIII made public gaming houses unlawful in England because he thought they distracted young men from the arts of war. That prohibition lasted until the 1960s when private gambling clubs became very popular in Great Britain (Fleming, 1992).

Gambling in America

Three waves of gambling have swept the United States. The first wave was in revolutionary times. Lotteries, popular for centuries in both Asia and Europe, were imported to the American

colonies in the 1700s where, among other things, their proceeds were used to support roads, build schools (e.g., Harvard University), hospitals, and other public works. Betting on horse races, cockfights, and dogs fights was popular. Gambling financed some of the Revolutionary War, though certain antigambling laws were later passed by the original 13 states. Corruption and scandal brought lotteries to an end in the 1820s and 1830s (Clotfelter, Cook, Edell, et al., 1999).

The second wave began at the end of the Civil War in 1865 with the expansion of the western frontier. Riverboat gambling on the Mississippi, saloon card games, roulette wheels, and dice games became part of the lore of the Wild West. But again, scandals and Victorian morality caused their demise around 1910.

The third wave began in the 1930s with the legalization of gambling in Nevada and the opening of racetracks in 21 states. New Hampshire rediscovered the state lottery in 1964 but it wasn't until the late 1970s that gambling really took off with the opening of casinos in Atlantic City, the expansion of lotteries to 38 states, off-track betting, riverboat casinos, and finally, the legalization of gambling casinos on Native American lands.

For much of the nineteenth and twentieth centuries, gambling continued to be popular, though it was considered immoral and preyed on human weakness. Gamblers have also been considered decadent, irresponsible, or insane. But in the last 40 years, gambling has become a respectable pastime and its legalization has vastly increased. By the mid-1990s, all states except Hawaii and Utah had established some kind of gambling. In addition the Indian Gaming Regulatory Act that had been approved in 1988 had caused a construction explosion of Indian-run casinos. By 1998, 146 of the 554 Native American tribes in the United States had 298 gambling facilities in 31 states. Revenues from 1988 to 1997 went from $220 million to $6.7 billion (Bureau of Indian Affairs, 1999).

State-supported lotteries were es-

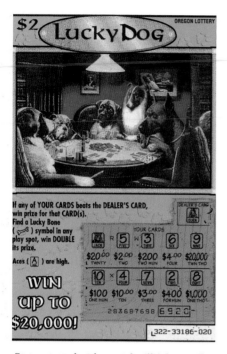

States started with scratch-off tickets and lotteries as a way to raise money for education and other state services. They have expanded the action to Keno, sports betting, and poker machines.

⋅ ⋅

tablished through the 1980s and '90s to supplement tax dollars and generate jobs. From 1974 to 1997, the public increased its wagers on legal gambling from $17 billion to over $400 billion per year, generating profits in 1997 of over $36 billion. Some argue that legalized gambling imposes a very regressive tax on low-income gamblers. The poor devote two and a half times more of their income on gambling than the middle class (NORC, 1999).

"I could be behind on bills for my electric, my rent, whatever . . . telephone, and I'll be like, 'Well I don't have the money but if I get the urge to go gamble I'll find a way that day to come up with a couple of hundred dollars. Amazing what you can do."
23-year-old compulsive sports gambler

With the increasing accessibility of the Internet in the 1990s, online gambling is exploding. Revenues from a variety of games plus the software to operate them, including poker, roulette,

dice, and even online poker machines went from $445 million in 1997, to $919 million in 1998, and an estimated $2.3 billion by 2001 (Sinclair, 1999). In Congress, the House Justice Subcommittee is trying to put limits on Internet gambling—Congress has yet to decide. Even credit card companies are refusing to act as a conduit for offshore companies because of lawsuits and the fact that pathological gamblers run up a lot of credit debt, whether online or in regular gambling venues, that often can't be paid.

"Well I certainly started to realize when I went into such debt on credit cards that I was running to the mailbox so that my husband wouldn't see 22 credit cards with $10,000 and $20,000 limits maxed out."
53-year-old recovering poker player—table and machines

Unfortunately most states have not adequately studied compulsive gambling nor have they established prevention or treatment programs. Critics contend that government encourages gambling and legitimizes it but does not address the problem of gambling addiction. The gambling industry often sees excess concern over compulsive gambling as an impediment to its growth, since the majority of their income derives from problem gamblers.

"I worked in a dozen casinos over the years and was a compulsive gambler. And I tell you, in every place I worked, a healthy percentage of the employees were compulsive gamblers. At one place, at the end of the day, the casino would pay us half our salary in cash and of course those of us who got paid usually gambled—and lost. We were cheap employees and the casino knew it."
55-year-old compulsive gambler

The media directly or indirectly supports gambling by publishing odds, sports' scores, players' injury reports,

winning lottery numbers, stories of big winners, and ads for gambling excursions. CNN Headline News offers a sports ticker listing running scores across the bottom of the screen. There is also simultaneous picture-in-picture coverage of multiple games. It is possible to gamble in airports, gas stations, bars, and supermarkets.

National Gambling Impact Study Commission Report

The proliferation of gambling forced the creation of the National Gambling Impact Study Commission. After two years they delivered their report to the President and Congress on the effect of gambling on the United States. Their studies found that in 1998 Americans lost $50 billion gambling, the equivalent of $200 for every man, woman, and child in the United States. The amount of money bet was $500 billion and even though that figure is 10 times the amount lost, that ratio is deceiving because a gambler recycles almost all winnings, so the same amount of money is counted many times (NORC, 1999; NRC, 1999).

EPIDEMIOLOGY

There is controversy as to estimates of the number of gamblers and the number of gamblers with problems. The three categories generally used are pathological gamblers (the most serious), problem gamblers, and at-risk gamblers (Rosenthal, 1989). A meta-analysis study at the Harvard Medical School estimated that 125 million adult Americans gamble and of those, 2.2 million are pathological gamblers and 5.3 million are problem gamblers (Shaffer, Hall, & Bilt, 1997). In addition there are about 1.1 million pathological adolescent gamblers (NRC, 1999). Another study by the University of Chicago estimated the total number of adult gamblers at 148 million, pathological gamblers at 2.5 million, problem gamblers at 3 million, and at-risk for problem gambling at 15 million (NORC, 1999). For most people who gamble, gambling is an occasional recreational pastime but for growing numbers of Americans,

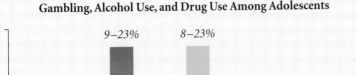

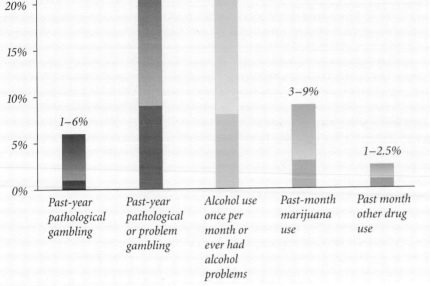

Gambling, Alcohol Use, and Drug Use Among Adolescents

Figure 7-1 •

This graph gives the range of gambling, alcohol, and marijuana use among adolescents. One can see that adolescent gambling rivals alcohol and overshadows marijuana as a problem among adolescents.

gambling is compulsive and pathological. Male compulsive gamblers outnumber female compulsive gamblers 2 to 1. Women more than men seem to use gambling as a means of escape from depression, traumas, or relationship problems.

College students have a higher rate of pathological gambling than the general population—5 1/2%, with 15% reporting at least some problems associated with gambling. College male pathological gamblers outnumbered their female counterparts approximately 4 to 1, suggesting that problem gambling surfaces at an older age for women. Among college students, pathological gamblers were more often absent and got lower grades than other students (Lesieur, Cross, Frank, et al., 1991).

CHARACTERISTICS

There are four kinds of gamblers.

1. There are the **recreational/social gamblers** who are able to separate gambling from the rest of their lives. Those are the majority of gamblers.

2. There are **professional gamblers** and they are able to take losses as part of the game. It's a business for them and they are able to make a living at it. They are few and far between.

3. There is the **antisocial gambler** who will steal to gamble and has no conscience.

4. Finally there are **pathological gamblers** who are obsessed with gambling, getting the money to gamble, and figuring out ways to stay in action. There are two types of pathological gamblers, the action-seeking gamblers and the gamblers. The **action-seeking compulsive gambler** is the stereotype of the gambler—always in action, frenetic, excited (Hunter, 1997). The other type that is growing in numbers, the **escape-seeking compulsive gambler**, is often drawn to slot machines, especially poker machines.

"There were no feelings. That's why I played it. There were no feelings.

Blocked all the feelings. Blocked all the stress. Blocked all the anxiety. There were no feelings."
42-year-old recovering escape-seeking compulsive slot machine player

Like other addictions, pathological gambling seems to be a progressive disorder requiring more episodes and larger amounts of money bet to relieve anxiety and tension. The similarity to substance addictions is emphasized by the fact that there is a high rate of other addictions among pathological gamblers—other behavioral and substance addictions occur in 25% to 63% of pathological gamblers (NORC, 1999).

"I didn't see that one was just making the other worse. The more drugs and alcohol I did, it seemed that I wanted to gamble more. The more I gambled, if I lost, especially, then I wanted to do more drugs."
24-year-old recovering compulsive gambler

Symptoms of persistent recurrent pathological gambling (positive diagnosis with five or more of the following) are:

1. preoccupation with gambling (reliving past experiences, planning future ones);

2. gambling with increased amounts of money;

3. repeated unsuccessful efforts to control, cut back, or stop gambling;

4. restlessness and irritability when attempting to control, cut back, or stop;

5. gambling as an escape;

6. attempts to recoup previous losses;

7. lying to others to conceal gambling;

8. illegal acts to finance gambling;

9. jeopardization or loss of job, relationship, or educational or career opportunity;

10. reliance on others to bail gambler out of pressing debts.

(Adapted from the *Diagnostic and Statistical Manual of Mental Disorders*) (APA, 1994)

A pathological male gambler often begins gambling as an early adolescent. Female pathological gamblers typically begin in later life. They both are more likely than the general population to have a parent who was a problem gambler. One study found the risk of heavy or compulsive gambling was 65% if the father gambled, 30% if the mother gambled, and 40% if a sibling gambled (Lesieur, Blume, & Zoppa, 1986).

Dr. Robert Custer, a clinician at the Brecksville, Ohio VA Hospital treatment unit, the first unit for compulsive gamblers, described three phases of gambling—winning phase, losing phase, and desperation phase. To these three, researchers Henry Lesieur and Robert Rosenthal added a giving-up phase (Custer & Milt, 1985; Lesieur & Rosenthal, 1991).

Winning Phase

Initially gambling is recreative and pleasurable for the action-seeking gambler. Bets are small and consequences negligible. The feelings that come from playing and winning or breaking even seem to satisfy the gambler.

"For me it was a rush, you know—nothing like alcohol, nothing like anything I've ever experienced. It was nervousness yet excitement and if you won, you know, the excitement turned into happiness. If you lost, you didn't feel too good unless there was another race and you had more money."
23-year-old recovering sports gambler

Skills improve and the gambler becomes more confident and even overconfident of his/her abilities. The winning phase can last 1 year or 10 years. Early on, in 70% to 80% of compulsive gamblers, there is a big win (from a few hundred to tens of thousands of dollars) that fuels the craving to gamble. The big win to the gambler is like the first intense rush to the cocaine user—never forgotten and forever chased.

"I had a winning phase that lasted me for probably 12 to 15 years and I actually lived on my gambling. I thought I was a semi-professional but I still did it in the closet."
42-year-old recovering male compulsive gambler

A gambler with a susceptibility to compulsion begins to devote more time and wager more money. Stakes increase from a nickel and dime poker to $5–$10 and table-stake games while blackjack goes from $2 a hand to $20 on two different hands; sports bets escalate from $5 on the Super Bowl to $100 on 10 different football games on the weekend. A $2 bet on the favorite at the racetrack ends up with $20 on the trifecta and $100 on every other race. Day traders start by depositing $500 to cover their trades and soon up it to tens of thousands if they have a run of luck good or bad. The player comes to rely more and more on the high to deal with undesired moods and relationships or other problems.

"The longer you could stay in action, the more you could—for me anyways—the more I could escape from the reality of what my life really had become."
43-year-old recovering action-seeking gambler

They begin to believe in luck and magic to solve their problems. They remember their wins and minimize their loses. Their self-esteem is boosted by their gambling ability and the camaraderie of other gamblers.

"More than anything, I just wanted to be a big shot. I didn't care if I was winning or losing or if you saw me go back to the same place day after day after day, somebody was going to think, 'God, this kid is a high roller or something because he's here every single day.'"
23-year-old recovering action-seeking compulsive gambler

A winning phase doesn't really exist for escape gamblers, such as poker machine, slot machine, keno, bingo, and lottery players, if they play on a regular basis. They will have days where they win but overall they will lose. For them, a good day is breaking even while staying in action for hours at a time.

"It gave me power. I didn't have to think about, 'Well, I'm a mother. Somebody needs me at home. I'm a wife. I'm somebody's daughter.'"
48-year-old recovering gambler

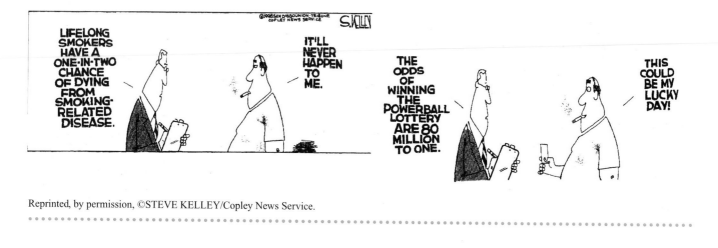

Losing Phase

"The losses were getting bigger and bigger and I realized I was in trouble the last one and a half years or so and didn't really know what to do about it. I just thought I better start winning to pay some of these credit card bills off."

45-year-old recovering horse racing compulsive gambler

Since intense emotional needs and self-esteem are satisfied by playing and winning, losing is particularly devastating to compulsive gamblers. A losing phase often starts with a losing streak that is inevitable due simply to the laws of chance but if the gambler's tolerance has increased and they are betting large sums, the suddenness of heavy indebtedness can be startling. They begin to try to recoup their loses—they begin chasing. A sports gambler may listen to three or four games simultaneously while a compulsive stock or commodities speculator may call for quotes frequently or be glued to a quote screen. Social, job, and family tensions multiply. Gamblers may deny there is a problem or lie to conceal the amount of money involved or the frequency of the gambling. Now emotional satisfaction, ego, self-esteem, and money are involved. The magic is gone and the emotional anguish of appearing to be a loser can be overwhelming. Chasing brings other changes in the gambler: depression, lying, isolation, and irritability. But even when losing, gamblers still rely on gambling for their emotional satisfaction.

"At our GA meetings, I asked which is more exciting, to go into a casino and get $400 ahead early on and stay there for the evening and walk out a couple of hundred ahead or be down $400 and battle and struggle and get back to only $50 down? And in every case they preferred being down and coming back. Said it gave them more of an adrenaline rush."

58-year-old recovering compulsive gambler

As losses multiply, the gambler tries to recover them by gambling more, tries unsuccessfully to cut back, swears he or she will never gamble again (but always does) and even seeks a bailout to get out of trouble.

Desperation Phase

In the end stages, which may take decades to develop or might just take a year, especially with machine players, compulsive gamblers often lose jobs because of absenteeism or poor work performance. They max out credit cards, borrow from friends and family, and even turn to illegal activities like theft, embezzlement, and drug dealing. Law enforcement officials point to problems associated with gambling such as illegal loans, extortion, threats, and beatings to collect debts. Their desperation causes them to play badly because they lose patience and common sense. They play too many hands in poker, they get mad at the poker or slot machines and swear they won't let a machine beat them, and their sense of being lucky and good turns into a lament that they are the unluckiest people in the world. What they fail to acknowledge at this stage is that they keep playing and keep making bad decisions.

"After the 15 years, it got really bad in dollars, hundreds of thousands of dollars lost, loss of my marriage, my self-esteem of course, my vehicles, my homes. At one other point in time, I lost my mother's home. I don't even know how I got them [my parents] to sign on the dotted line."

43-year-old recovering gambler

The gambler often bankrupts his or her family and often suffers divorce or separation because of deteriorating family relations, long absences from home, arguments over money, and indifference to the welfare of family members and others.

Giving-Up Phase

At this stage, pathological gamblers stop thinking they will win it all back and just want to stay in action. Gamblers can experience insomnia attacks, health problems, and elated moods when they win and mania, depression, panic attacks, and suicidal thoughts or actual attempts when they lose. One study of Gamblers Anonymous members found severe depression in 72% of those who say they have hit bottom and suicide attempts in 17–24% of them (Linden, 1985). In Gulfport, Mississippi, suicide attempts went from 24 in 1992 before casinos came in, to 85 in 1995 after casinos opened and 137 in 1996.

"Every time I get out from the casino I want to kill myself. Then it's going to be over. Then it's going to end. I tried to kill myself twice. I took my car to the mountain. I just wanted to—I decided I didn't want the pain anymore."

38-year-old recovering compulsive gambler (casino games and scratch-off tickets)

Often the problems become so overwhelming that they can precipitate the final crisis that hopefully leads the compulsive gambler into treatment rather than to suicide.

VIDEO POKER MACHINES (the "crack" cocaine of gambling)

"I preferred that the bell didn't go off. I mean, winning was only temporary. I was sitting there till it was all gone anyway, so why draw attention to myself. . . . Toward the end, when I would ask for a rack at a $25 video poker machine, they bring you a small rack—well that's $2,500."

42-year-old recovering escape-seeking compulsive slot machine player

There are some things that make some games more potent and more powerful than others according to Robert Hunter, an expert in the field of pathological gambling. For the average gambler, it means the game is more exciting or more interesting. For the 5% who are pathological gamblers, what makes a game exciting for the average person makes it deadly for them:

◇ immediacy, finding out right now if you're winning or losing;

◇ an ability to increase both the time and money to play longer as well as higher amounts of bets;

◇ the ability to lose yourself in the game; to block out external stimuli; to get lost and focus solely on what's in front of you;

◇ the perception of a skill component; it's only perception of the skill component because how do you outwit a microchip?

"The illusion of control? Yeah, you have some say so in this. You are so smart. You are smarter than this computer chip that has already randomly done this. Yeah, you are so smart. It gives you the illusion of control. It's a lot better than just pulling a handle. Any idiot can pull the handle but boy to pick out those cards and decide which ones to hold, that takes smarts, doesn't it?"

43-year-old recovering compulsive video poker player

If you think of those four qualities (immediacy, ability to increase, perception of skill or control, and the ability to get lost), then there's not a form of gambling in the world that maxes out all four of those except video poker. What's probably tied for second place in this addictive hierarchy is cards and dice and traditional casino table gambling. In states with video poker machines, 70% to 80% of people entering treatment listed video poker as their game of choice.

"Women, I have noticed, get hooked on the video poker machines because it is the isolation. They don't have to worry. They can escape. No one's going to judge them. They don't have to feel stupid because they don't know how to play blackjack, or they don't know the point spread, or they don't know the crap table."

42-year-old recovering video poker player

GAMBLERS ANONYMOUS

Gamblers Anonymous was formed in 1967 on the model of Alcoholics Anonymous as an organization that would let problem/compulsive/pathological gamblers help themselves by not only refraining from gambling but by developing spirituality and ultimately changing the way they live. At present it is almost the only stopgap and hope between compulsive gamblers and their addiction.

Gamblers Anonymous lists several characteristics of the compulsive gambler including inability and unwillingness to accept reality, emotional insecurity, and immaturity. These traits lead the compulsive gambler into a dream world that can lead to destruction.

"A lot of time is spent creating images of the great and wonderful things they are going to do as soon as they make the big win . . . . When compulsive gamblers succeed, they gamble to dream still greater dreams. When failing, they gamble in reckless desperation and the depths of their misery are fathomless as their dream world comes crashing down. Sadly they will struggle back, dream more dreams, and of course suffer more misery. No one can convince them that their great schemes will not someday come true. They believe they will for without this dream world, life for them would not be tolerable."

Gamblers Anonymous Combo Book (GA, 1998)

The above statement is read as part of each meeting. Members also read and answer the 20 questions in the little

TABLE 7–5   THE 20 QUESTIONS OF GAMBLERS ANONYMOUS

1. Did you ever lose time from work or school due to gambling?
2. Has gambling ever made your home life unhappy?
3. Did gambling affect your reputation?
4. Have you ever felt remorse after gambling?
5. Did you ever gamble to get money with which to pay debts or otherwise solve financial difficulties?
6. Did gambling cause a decrease in your ambition or efficiency?
7. After losing did you feel you must return as soon as possible and win back your losses?
8. After a win did you have a strong urge to return and win more?
9. Did you often gamble until your last dollar was gone?
10. Did you ever borrow to finance your gambling?
11. Have you ever sold anything to finance gambling?
12. Were you reluctant to use "gambling money" for normal expenditures?
13. Did gambling make you careless of the welfare of yourself and your family?
14. Did you ever gamble longer than you had planned?
15. Have you ever gambled to escape worry or trouble?
16. Have you ever committed, or considered committing, an illegal act to finance gambling?
17. Did gambling cause you to have difficulty in sleeping?
18. Do arguments, disappointments, or frustrations create within you an urge to gamble?
19. Did you ever have an urge to celebrate any good fortune by a few hours of gambling?
20. Have you ever considered self-destruction or suicide as a result of your gambling?

Most compulsive gamblers will answer yes to at least seven of these questions.

(GA, 1998)

yellow meeting booklet that reminds gamblers of the havoc their addiction can have on themselves and their families. It is also a good self-test for those who are not sure if they are problem or pathological gamblers.

TREATMENT

(See Chapter 9 for information about treatment of compulsive gambling.)

COMPULSIVE SHOPPING

The inability to handle money in a responsible manner is the hallmark of almost any addict. To the addict, money is a means to buy drugs, gamble with, sit at a bar longer, buy as much binge food as needed, or purchase things that stimulate, sedate, or alter one's mood as much as possible. The craving can overwhelm common sense. The addict does what feels good at the time—immediate gratification or immediate relief from anxiety and pain. For this reason, budgets, layaway shopping, avoiding debt and/or borrowing from friends are generally not in the addict's vocabulary. Compulsive shopping (oniomania) is often a manifestation of the personality factors that are present in most addicts. The DSM-IV puts compulsive shopping under Impulse Control Disorders Not Otherwise Specified. These also include sexual addictions and even repetitive self-mutilation (APA, 1994). Compulsive shoppers have described the relief from depression and subsequent high when buying as being similar to the high from cocaine and both result in a subsequent crash accompanied by more depression and guilt than felt before buying (McElroy, Satlin, Pope, et al., 1991).

Americans are more than $1.2 trillion ($1,200,000,000,000) in debt. That works out to about $5,000 for every man woman and child. Studies in the United States, Germany, Canada, and the United Kingdom put the number of compulsive shoppers somewhere between 2% and 10% (University of Sussex, 1997). Some put the number of Amer-

icans who are extreme impulse or compulsive buyers at 5% to 10% of the population, people whose debts are measured in the tens of thousands or even hundreds of thousands (Mjoseth, 1999). Clearly, poor countries generally do not have this problem except in the middle or wealthy classes.

The roots of compulsive shopping are similar to many aspects of compulsive gambling. Compulsive gamblers come to feel their worth and self-esteem come from gambling because they believe they have control—the house brings them free drinks at casinos and if they lose a lot, they are treated like kings and queens. Casinos and clubs issue membership cards to frequent gamblers and they are treated, if not with respect, at least they are not put down.

"Almost every addict, and I've talked to thousands of addicts in groups and individually, has said that they have a background in which they felt inferior, inadequate, guilty, ashamed, rejected, unwanted, all of that captured in this point phrase, 'No matter what I did, it was never enough.'"
Dewey Jacobs, psychologist, addictions specialist and lecturer

With shopping, if they have money, they are treated well, and if they can spend a lot, they are graciously waited upon. That's just good business. For most shoppers, shopping is a pleasant outing, a chance to buy needed or desired items but to some, it's one of the few places they can get respect or get lost in fantasy, much like the action-seeking and escape-seeking gamblers. All they need is a charge card or some checks. A study of 25 compulsive shoppers found a number of commonalties. Buying urges occur from a few times a week to once a week and although they try to fight the urges, they give in 74% of the time. However when they enter the shopping area or mall, they often don't know what they want to buy and frequently purchase on impulse. About 50% of household income goes toward paying debts (Christenson et al., 1994).

In preliminary studies by the Eco-

nomic and Social Research Council in the United Kingdom, researchers found a large discrepancy between the way shopping addicts see themselves (their actual self) and the way they wish to be (the ideal self). They believe that buying and acquiring things will bring them closer to their ideal selves. Others with the same problem might turn to drugs or compulsive eating. Women tend to buy things that enhance their uniqueness, including jewelry, clothes, and cosmetics, while men prefer high-tech, electronic, and sports equipment (Dittmar, 1997). Debt counseling, much like a temporary bailout for compulsive gamblers, is only a stopgap measure because the roots of the condition have not been addressed.

Winter time is when consumers incur 40% of their actual debt, often because the holidays can bring up old resentments and magnify feelings of loneliness and depression (Mellan, 1995). Depression seems a major part of compulsive shopping. In one study 10 of 13 compulsive shoppers who received antidepressants reported a complete or at least partial reduction in their compulsive buying behavior (McElroy et al., 1998). Dr. Eric Hollander of the Compulsive, Impulsive and Anxiety Disorders Program at Mt. Sinai School of Medicine in New York believes that low serotonin levels (which cause depression) lead women more to compulsive shopping and eating disorders while it leads men to risk taking and violence (Mjoseth, 1999).

Weekly therapy that helps interrupt the cycle of compulsive buying, making out a budget and sticking to it, plus working on the inner issues regarding self-image and self-esteem are steps towards recovery. As with other addictions, attending a self-help group for support is an alternative to going out shopping. There are more than 400 Debtors Anonymous groups in the United States.

EATING DISORDERS

"I went to this eating disorder clinic for my bulimia. There were also

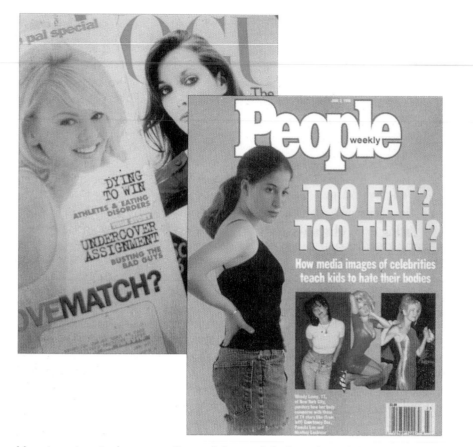

Magazines give mixed messages. One week they extol the "most beautiful people" and the next week they write about eating disorders.

by fashion magazines, television, ads featuring painfully thin models, and films featuring slender stars with large bosoms.

The paradox of body image in modern society is that while the ideal splashed in the media is thinness associated with youth and beauty, the advertisements promote pizza, cookies, milk, and candy bars; the supermarket shelves are loaded with high-calorie foods side by side with low-calorie versions and diet aids to further imprint the emaciated ideal. Being greatly overweight may also subject a person to social isolation, job discrimination, and ridicule that create feelings of inferiority and guilt. A common compliment in our society is, "You've lost weight, you look good." People are given mixed messages—look thin, stay slim, but eat up.

The average height and weight of women in the United States is 5'4" and 142 lbs. The average height and weight of fashion models is 5'9" and 110 lbs. (Wolf, 1992). Diet and exercise industries capitalize on this disparity and persistently urge us to achieve a slim look. A few years ago, Americans spent $30 billion on diet programs and diet products, Kellogg's Frosted Flakes® alone spent $32 million just on advertising while the government spent $34 million on obesity research (Grunwald, 1995). That a number of chronic eating disorders have sprung from these conflicting messages is no great surprise.

The three main eating disorders are anorexia nervosa, bulimia nervosa, and compulsive overeating.

◇ **Anorexia nervosa** is an addiction to weight loss, fasting, and control of body size.

◇ **Bulimia nervosa** is an addiction to binge eating of large amounts of food often followed by purges using self-induced vomiting, laxatives, or fasting.

◇ **Compulsive overeating (including binge-eating disorder)** is an obsessive consumption of food to regulate mood and feelings of anxiety, depression, and emptiness. Binge-eating disorder is basically defined as "bu-

anorexics and overeaters there. At the meal table, the staff kept an eye on everyone. They made sure the anorexics ate something and didn't give it to the overeaters or bulimics, or go to the bathroom immediately after to throw up, or start exercising to incredible excess. They also checked under the table for thrown away food. We bulimics, they just had to keep away from the bathroom, so everyone had to stay in the meal room for at least a half hour after eating. A year after I stopped throwing up because of health reasons, I ballooned up to 360 pounds. Now I'm just a plain old compulsive overeater."

35-year-old recovering bulimic (male, ex-college wrestler)

Since ancient times, the concept of beauty has changed from generation to generation and from culture to culture. Usually thinness used to be a sign of poverty and being from a lower class while plumpness was a sign of wealth and upper class membership. For example, in the United States at the beginning of the twentieth century, the ideal of the upper-class, buxom, bustle-supported full-figured grand dame of the Victorian era gave way to the svelte fun-loving flappers of the 1920s promoted in books, magazines, and films. Following the Depression and World War II, the "voluptuous female" that had become popular, typified in the '50s by Marilyn Monroe and Jane Russell, gave way in the '60s to the very boyish figures of Audrey Hepburn and the British model Twiggy. That ideal has remained and been reinforced

limia without vomiting, laxatives, or other compensatory activities."

Like other addictions, eating disorders involve a sense of powerlessness when dealing with food or eating even though it is a desire to have control over something in one's life that often leads to eating disorders. Eating disorders also involve obsession with thoughts of food, use of food to escape from undesirable feelings, secretive behavior, guilt, denial, dysfunctional reliance on eating (or not eating), and continued overeating regardless of the harm done.

Some regard eating disorders as learned behaviors that can be unlearned with treatment. Others believe they are physiological and psychological addictions. Many believe the causes of these behaviors arise during infancy and early childhood. Evidence suggests that eating disorders are a combination of genetic, neurochemical, psychodevelopmental, and sociocultural factors (Becker, Grinspoon, Klibanski, & Herzog, 1999). There is also a high incidence of comorbid disorders, especially depression, anxiety disorders, substance abuse, and personality disorders (Herzog, Nussbaum, & Marmor, 1996).

Recent research on genetic and biochemical factors have been particularly suggestive. Some bulimics, for instance, report feeling a rush while purging or a peacefulness afterwards. Anorexic women describe feelings of powerfulness, blissfulness, and even a floating sensation because starving oneself releases endorphins that in turn release dopamine in the reward/pleasure center, similar to an endorphin or opioid high (Kaye, Pickar, Naber, & Eben, 1982). Overeaters say that when they load up on carbohydrates, they feel like they're loaded on alcohol. High levels of sugar have been found to lower stress hormones by reducing the levels of corticosteroids, the body's stress hormones (Bell, 1999). Preliminary studies indicate that there is an addiction to the neurotransmitters produced during both bingeing and purging. Clearly, eating often involves control of moods through compulsive eating and the process can be addicting (Gold, Johnson, & Stennie, 1997). Eating disorders are complex syndromes with multiple causes.

EPIDEMIOLOGY

Most eating disorders begin in adolescence, are chronic, and they affect women disproportionately (Herzog, Dorer, Keel, et al., 1999). About three percent of young women have one of the three main DSM-IV eating disorders: anorexia nervosa, bulimia nervosa, and the newest, binge-eating disorder (Becker et al., 1999). With a national obesity rate approaching 18%, the number of women and men who are compulsive overeaters, a diagnosis not listed in the DSM-IV, is much greater.

Anorexia & Bulimia

Anorexia and bulimia are overwhelmingly female disorders. An estimated 90–95% of anorexics and bulimics are women (Kaplan & Garfinkel, 1995). Women have been socialized to regard their self-worth as closely tied up with their physical appearance, especially their size and weight. In *The Beauty Myth,* Naomi Wolf points out that, whereas a generation ago models weighed 8% less than average, today they weigh 23% less (Wolf, 1992). Secondly, both bulimia and anorexia involve collateral elements of low self-esteem, depression, and secrecy. Often practice of the illness is triggered by a stressful event like the break-up of a relationship, social rejection, or going off to college.

Today anorexia and bulimia seem more common in developed nations with an abundance of food and media promotion of thin-body beauty ideals for women. But recent studies of school girls in Cairo, Egypt found rates for anorexia and bulimia about the same as those in England. At the Hospital for Anorexia and Bulimia in Buenos Aires, Argentina, hundreds of emaciated teenage girls are patients. More than 70 new ones arrive each week. Almost 1 in every 10 Argentine teenage girls suffers from clinical anorexia or bulimia (Washington Post, 1997). The globalization of pop culture seems to have spread these disorders.

Certainly in the United States, anorexia and bulimia are quickly increasing. From the mid-1950s to the mid-'70s, cases of anorexia grew by 300% (NOAH, 1996; Fairburn & Beglin, 1990). Currently, according to one survey of the health care professionals at 490 colleges and universities, it is estimated that anywhere from 10% to 20% of college women have an eating disorder. The same survey asked coeds if they ever had an eating disorder, 11% answered yes. The disparity in self-reporting vs. objective reporting is probably due to denial or unawareness that there is a problem (People, 1999).

Anorexia nervosa is most frequent in young women from 14–18 years old. It afflicts an estimated 0.5–1.0% of women in their late teens and early adulthood. Women over 40 seldom develop anorexia (APA, 1994). The illnesses do, however, strike all age groups from children to the elderly. A high incidence of anorexia in males is found in high school and college wrestlers who must maintain a certain weight to stay in a category. There is also a high incidence among rowers.

"It was our coach who taught us how to throw up to maintain our weight in high school on the wrestling team. We'd go to smorgasbords, eat a bunch, throw up in the bathroom, eat again, throw up again. Most of the team did it. Of course we weren't supposed to tell anybody but about a year and a half later, word got out and he was fired."

College wrestler, senior

Females involved in sports who are at risk include gymnasts, runners, swimmers, dancers, cheerleaders, and figure skaters, many of whom are prodded or compelled by teachers, coaches, and trainers to maintain a certain weight, no matter what.

A complex of disorders afflicting women athletes has been called the "female athlete triad." It consists of

◇ an eating disorder such as anorexia and bulimia but also includes elim-

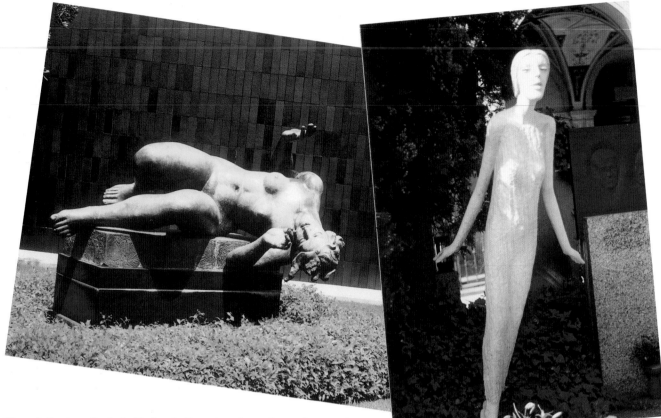

The artistic view of a desirable female figure has changed over the centuries.

ination of certain food groups and abuse of weight control methods such as dieting, fasting, and use of diet aids and laxatives;

◇ irregular menstruation, i.e., missing more than one period;

◇ osteoporosis or irreversible loss of bone density, which can result in pain or fractures.

It is not clear whether eating disorders precede or follow women's participation in sports.

ANOREXIA NERVOSA

Historically anorexia appeared in the Middle Ages as the "holy anorexia" during which monks and nuns piously starved themselves to achieve a control over the desires of the flesh and an ideal of holiness. Over the last three centuries, starting in 1694, there have been numerous descriptions of anorexia that were quite similar to the modern day definition (Bell, 1985; Morton, 1694).

Definition

Although anorexia means "without appetite," the condition has less to do with loss of appetite than with what one expert calls "weight phobia." Some anorexics, the so-called anorexia restrictors, will maintain weight by limiting their food intake through dieting, fasting, the use of amphetamines and other diet pills, and excessive exercise. Binge-eating/purging types limit weight by purging through the use of diuretics, laxatives, or enemas (APA, 1994). Some people even control weight through liposuction (surgical removal of fat). Sometimes the line between anorexia and bulimia becomes blurred. Bulimic symptoms appear in 30% to 80% of all anorexics.

"Bingeing and purging is the choice of my best friend and it's easy to see the signs: the skin on a finger eaten away and yellow from the acids in the vomit. You feel guilt for eating even a salad

with no dressing. If you eat only once a day, your mind screams at you to not eat, to say no. The guilt of eating anything almost consumes you. I used to do it too."

19-year-old female college student

People afflicted with anorexia nervosa are afraid of weight gain and eventually may lose from 15–60% of their weight. They will not maintain a normal body weight and they have a distorted perception of their body's shape and size, often feeling, even when emaciated, that their body or parts of it are overweight. Their emotional state is tied to their weight. They let the scale dictate how they feel about themselves. Often there is ignorance or denial of the seriousness of low body weight. Peer approval may aggravate the condition by praising the anorexic and encouraging "the look," which confers high status among adolescents (Aronson, 1993).

"Our whole culture promotes a thin look. I never realized how bad I looked. I wore baggy clothes so no one could tell. Even when I wore a bathing suit, my friends told me how good I looked, not how sick I was."

Recovering anorexic

Causes

Some psychologists see anorexia as a compensatory behavior for people who are too concerned with following directions and pleasing others. Young females may be considered good girls and be model students, academically talented, good athletes, and may have a tendency to perfectionism, but they may lack self-esteem and a sense of self. A refusal to eat gives them a measure of control in their lives and continuous loss of weight can be an index of their discipline, achievement, self-esteem, and status among their peers.

"I didn't have a sense of myself or my body growing up but I tried to be so perfect. But whenever I do anything, I feel I'm going to be criticized for it, especially by my mother. I mean, even when she's not around, I still hear her. And she's not a bad person. So the only thing I could control was my eating. And the more they tried to get me to eat, the more I could say no. I thought that if I could control my eating, I could control the rest of my life."

19-year-old recovering from anorexia

Additional characteristics of anorexia include delusions (persistent, unshakable ideas that one is unattractive or overweight) and compulsions (rigid, self-imposed rituals, such as weighing food, dividing it into small pieces, or eating in a prescribed order). There is also a growing belief that the early use of amphetamines and other strong stimulants to control weight will disrupt normal functioning of the body's weight control mechanisms.

Family studies, including twin studies, indicate a higher prevalence of anorexia if one has an immediate relative who is anorexic (Treasure & Cambell, 1994). A current theory suggests that what initially may begin as a strict diet, in about three months begins to change brain chemistry, so that more of the body's natural opiates (endorphins) are produced and the person becomes addicted to those brain chemicals (Marazzi & Luby, 1989). The act of eating something precipitates a kind of opiate withdrawal encouraging further refusal to eat.

Effects

The results of semistarvation can put strains on all the body systems, including the heart, liver, and brain. Dehydration from vomiting depletes electrolytes, a dangerous condition that can lead to cardiac arrest. In addition, mild anemia, swollen joints, constipation, and light-headedness can also occur. Females can decrease their estrogen levels, and males, their testosterone levels. Amenorrhea (absence or abnormal cessation of the menses) often occurs in women practicing anorexia. It can take several months into treatment before a normal menstrual cycle is reestablished. Other disturbances include stomach cramps, dry skin, and lanugo (a downy body hair that develops on the trunk).

With anorexia nervosa, osteoporosis, sterility, miscarriage, and birth defects are additional dangers. Death rates among anorexic patients have been estimated at 4–20% over the life of the disease, with risks increasing as weight loss approaches 60% of normal. The most frequent cause of death is heart disease, especially congestive heart failure. The other most frequent cause of death is suicide (APA, 1994).

Treatment

Most severely ill anorexic patients have to be admitted to a hospital because of the extreme weight loss, disturbed heart rhythms, extreme depression, and often suicidal ideation. It usually takes 10–12 weeks for full nutritional recovery. Many hospitals and clinics treat this eating disorder and the rate for full recovery is about 40%. A first priority in treatment is to prevent death by starvation. Severely ill patients are monitored for body weight, serum electrolytes, and diet as the patient is returned to normal nutrition. Fluoxetine (Prozac®), other SSRIs, antidepressants, and MAO inhibitors have been tried to help patients improve eating behavior by treating the underlying depression. Generally though, antidepressants and antipsychotic drugs have had marginal effects in aiding recovery (Jacobi, Dahme, & Rustenbach, 1997; Jimerson, Herzog, & Botman, 1993).

For an adolescent, a weight gain of 4 oz. (0.1 kg) per day is aimed for. The patient is generally monitored by staff for 2–3 hours after eating to prevent self-induced vomiting. The recovery rate among 84 anorexic women after 12 years in one study was 54% based on the restarting of menstruation (41% based on the criterion of general well-being). The mortality rate was 11% (Psychology Today, 1995).

One of the first problems in treatment is convincing the patient that anorexia is a potentially fatal problem. Often it is a parent who brings a young woman to treatment. She herself will think that her body weight is normal or that she is overweight. Programs involve stabilizing the patient and psychological counseling to alert the anorexic to the problem and its causes; to devalue an overemphasis on thinness, weight, dieting, and food; to build self-esteem; and to promote healthy behaviors. They also involve family therapy to provide the family with understanding, support, and the ability to cope.

BULIMIA NERVOSA

Definition

"I just remember saying, 'Hey, I can eat,' but feeling so full after bingeing, feeling so full and wanting to get rid of it, and then purging. It's kind of like you want to have your cake and eat it too. No pun intended but it's an awful disease. And I was grateful because I

only did it for a year. I kept eating but I stopped the purging and eventually I got into recovery from a 12-step program."
Recovering bulimic

Although bulimia means "ox hunger" ("I'm so hungry I could eat an ox"), the term generally is used to designate the eating disorder characterized by eating large amounts of food in one sitting, bingeing, followed by inappropriate methods of ridding oneself of the food. These methods may include self-induced vomiting (used by 80–90% of those with this disorder), use of diuretics or laxatives, fasting, and excessive exercise. These methods of eliminating food are used primarily to keep from gaining weight (APA, 1994).

"I discovered I was practicing bulimia when I realized I lost weight by eating high levels of sugar. I activated my diabetes to disrupt my body's ability to process food and I drank huge amounts of water which acted as a diuretic, so I was able to indulge my binge eating and still lose weight. I was in essence damaging myself to lose weight, a perfect definition of abuse."
58-year-old recovering bulimic

People with bulimia often are ashamed of their behavior, do it secretly, and consume food rapidly. Although a slightly overweight condition may precede bulimia, those suffering from the disorder often are within normal weight ranges. People with bulimia may feel loss of control during binges and guilt after them. Bulimia was first described in 1979 (Russell, 1979).

Generally a binge means "an abnormally large amount of food on the order of a holiday meal, eaten in two hours or less but definitely more than other people would eat in the same time." Continuous snacking during the day does not constitute a binge. Diagnosis of bulimia requires that bingeing and purging average at least twice a week for three months. Although many binge eaters prefer sweet high-caloric foods like ice cream, soft drinks, and cookies, bulimia has more to do with the large amount of food consumed than the types of food. During binge episodes, there may be a feeling of frenzy, of not being in control, and a sense of being disconnected from one's surroundings. Between binges, typically low-calorie foods and drinks are consumed.

Causes

As with anorexia, the causes of bulimia are multiple. Because bulimia spans different races and classes, it is clear that all American women are subject to the social pressures to be slim. Except for a few notable exceptions, most television personalities are slender, a look promoted by fashion and other entertainment industries. When television was widely introduced in 1995 in the Pacific Island nation of Fiji, only 3% of girls reported they vomited to control their weight. Three years later the number had grown to 15%. In addition Anne Becker, a Harvard researcher, found that 74% of the Fijian girls reported feeling "too big or fat" while almost 2/3 reported dieting in the past month. In the past, before the slender bodies of Melrose Place and Xena, Warrior Princess were on television, losing weight was a sign of illness. About 84% of women were overweight or obese but there was an acceptance of that condition (Becker et al., 1999).

Some claim that the socialization of women to an ideal of excessive thinness begins with the Barbie® dolls young girls receive; dolls, which, if extrapolated into an adult female's measurements, would produce a woman with a 36-inch bust, an emaciated 18-inch waist, and 33-inch hips. The average model's measurements are 36-23-33. The contemporary "starved" look popularized by the 92-pound, 5'6" inch Twiggy has given way to the "heroin chic" emaciated look of current models such as Kate Moss. One study that examined *Playboy*® centerfold models and Miss America contestants found average weights declined from 1959 to 1978. Another study found that between 1979 and 1988, weights of the models and contestants averaged 13–19% below the average weights of women in relevant age groups (Wiseman et al., 1992).

The biochemical changes involved with bulimia can make the disorder self-perpetuating. A severe diet can precipitate a bulimic cycle. Like other addictions, the process of bingeing and purging may encourage and continue the condition. There is evidence that metabolism adapts to the cycle and slows down, so that more weight is gained with the same intake of food. This increased weight gain is then seen as even more reason to continue to binge and purge. There is also evidence that purging through vomiting or laxatives produces higher levels of natural opioids (endorphins), so that people suffering from bulimia become addicted to the body's own natural drugs (Gold et al., 1997).

"It was like depression, you know. I'd just keep eating all day, and so I got to the point where I was gaining weight too fast, and I spoke with a friend about it and she said, 'Do like I do, throw it up.' I went into this mad trip of eating everything I could shove down my throat and then if I felt bad about it or if I felt any guilt at all, I could throw it back up and all the guilt would go away, and so to me, it was like stuffing down all my problems— the drinking, the smoking, and all of that stuff was replaced with the food and then throwing it back up."
28-year-old recovering bulimic

Effects

Effects and health consequences are less severe with bulimia that does not progress into anorexia. Problems include dental complications and a greater liability for alcohol and drug abuse than other people including those suffering from anorexia. Dependency on laxatives for normal bowel movements can result. There is a high rate of depression associated with bulimia as well as a greater risk of suicide.

Because of the frequency of vomiting, bulimia puts people at risk for stomach acid burns to the esophagus and throat resulting in chronic sore throat and greater risk of cancer. When vomiting is practiced with either bulimia or anorexia, the tooth enamel can be permanently eaten away by acid, high incidence of cavities can occur, and front teeth can appear ragged, chipped, and mottled. Dental professionals often are the first to spot bulimic activities. The back of the fingers and hands can become scarred from abrading the skin on the teeth while pushing the hand down the throat to induce vomiting. As with anorexia, heart problems, such as arrhythmias, can develop as can electrolyte imbalances and irregular menstrual periods or no periods at all.

Psychological effects include loneliness and self-imposed isolation, difficulty in dealing with any activities involved with food, irritability, mood changes, and depression.

Treatment

Bulimia presents special problems. As with other eating disorders, bulimia is best treated in its early stages. But because people with bulimia often are in a normal weight range, their problem may escape detection for years. After diagnosis is made, a decision is made to treat an individual in a hospital or on an outpatient basis.

Because of the multiple problems involved, a multidiscipline integrated treatment is generally used. An internist advises on medical problems. A nutritionist provides help with diet and eating patterns. A psychopharmacologist may counsel on which psychoactive medications might be effective (NOAH, 1996). In recent years antidepressants have been used, especially selective serotonin reuptake inhibitors, along with monamine oxidase inhibitors. One scientist combined naltrexone, usually prescribed to help people get off heroin or alcohol, in combination with psychotherapy for 19 women

with bulimia or anorexia with good effects (Jonas & Gold, 1988; Goldbloom, 1997). A psychotherapist provides emotional support and counseling and may begin therapy that involves changing attitudes and behaviors.

Family and group therapies also are useful to provide understanding and emotional support to the patient. Group therapy may provide great relief for a person who doesn't need to keep the disorder secret any longer. Family, friends, and colleagues can help an ill person start and complete treatment and then provide the encouragement to make sure the disorder does not reoccur. There are also self-help and peer-support groups organized specifically for bulimia but these are currently less effective than groups for compulsive overeating.

"During your life, my child, see what suits your constitution,
do not give it what you find disagrees with it;
for not everything is good for everybody,
nor does everybody like everything.
Do not be insatiable for any delicacy;
do not be greedy for food,
for over-eating leads to illness and excess leads to liver attacks.
Many people have died from over-eating;
control yourself, and so prolong your life."
Sirach, 37, 27, Bible

COMPULSIVE OVEREATING (including binge-eating disorder)

"If I say, 'I'm an alcoholic,' people say, 'Oh, you're an alcoholic,' or, 'I'm a drug addict,' 'Oh, that must be tough.' But when you tell people you're a food addict, some people laugh, like, 'What's a food addict? How can you be a food addict?'"
36-year-old recovering compulsive overeater

The prevalence of obesity in the United States is increasing. Obesity is

defined as greater than 30 kg/m². For example, if a 6-ft. (1.83 m) tall person weighs more than 100 kg or 220 lbs., they are classified as obese. One major study found that obesity increased from 12.0% in 1991 to 17.9% in 1998. The greatest increase was found in 18–29 year olds, in those with some college education, those of Hispanic ethnicity, and those from the South Atlantic states (Mokdad, Serdula, Dietz, et al., 1999). Internationally, for the first time in history, there are as many people overweight as underweight, about 1.1 billion of each out of a worldwide population of 6 billion. In Europe, overweight outnumbers underweight by a ratio of 9 to 1, North America, 12 to 1, and Latin America, 5 to 1, while in Africa they are about equal and in Southeast Asia there are 5 times as many underfed as overfed people (Halwell & Gardner, 2000).

Definition

There is much debate concerning obesity. Some of the questions are, "Is obesity a specific syndrome or is it a symptom of a number of conditions such as metabolic disorders, psychological disorders, or simply situational factors (there are too many fast-food restaurants and people don't get enough exercise)?" "Is obesity an outcome of the metabolic changes wrought by excessive eating and overuse of refined carbohydrates or is it the result of childhood traumas and damaged self-image that occurred in infancy?" In addition to a diagnosis of "eating disorder not otherwise classified," the current *Diagnostic and Statistical Manual of Mental Disorders* (DSM-IV) is examining a condition called "binge-eating disorder" that they say affects 4.6% of the community at large and 28.7% of those in a weight-loss program (Spitzer, Yanovski, Wadden, et al., 1993). Binge-eating disorder is marked by recurrent episodes of binge eating without use of vomiting, laxatives, or other compensatory activities. A pattern of frequent eating and snacking over a period of several hours is also a symptom of compulsive overeating.

Certain foods and excessive intake activate the mesolimbic dopaminergic

Researchers find another fat gene

But don't expect a wonder pill

The Associated Press

Two research groups identified the first gene kn~~ suppress obesity and re~~ the burning of calories — that could lead the way to~~ drug that keeps people tr~~

But don't reach for that ~~jelly doughnut just yet.

The gene, known as ~~gany, or the MG gene, was ~~ered in mice. It is the sixth~~ found to be implicated in o~~ But researchers said it is t~~ discovered to regulate me~~ism and the expenditure ~~ergy.

In one of two studies put~~ in today's issue of the jour~~ture, scientists at Mille~~ Pharmaceuticals in Caml~~ Mass., tested groups of mi~~ normal and mutated MG ~~ They fed the mice diet~~ varying percentages of fa~~

Mice with a mutated M(~~ did not gain weight regar~~ whether they ate a high-f~~ or a low-fat one. Mice wi~~ normal gene gained wei~~ the high-fat diet.

Researchers said they

optimistic that the gene would

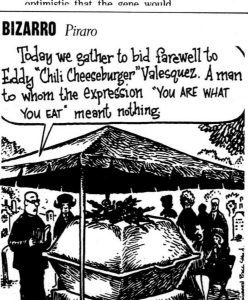

BIZARRO *Piraro*

Today we gather to bid farewell to Eddy "Chili Cheeseburger" Valesquez. A man to whom the expression "YOU ARE WHAT YOU EAT" meant nothing.

reward system during ingestion of food and not only give pleasure but block out unwanted emotions (Blum et al., 2000). This chapter will use the phrase "compulsive overeater" and acknowledge that there are several causes of obesity but the main ones are remarkably similar. Many of the diagnostic criteria for binge-eating disorder can be applied to compulsive overeating. With compulsive overeating or binge-eating disorder, people eat in response to emotional states rather than to hunger signals. Symptoms of compulsive overeating and binge-eating disorder include the following:

◇ frequent episodes of eating what other people consider large quantities;

◇ a feeling of lack of control while overeating or bingeing;

◇ eating rapidly and swallowing food without chewing;

◇ eating when uncomfortably full;

◇ eating large amounts when not feeling physically hungry;

◇ eating alone because of being embarrassed by how much one is eating;

◇ feeling disgusted and distressed when one is overeating;

◇ a preference for refined carbohydrates including high-sugar junk food as well as high-fat foods.

(Adapted from APA, 1994)

"Eating at 3 o'clock in the morning. Sneaking food when my husband was asleep and my kids were in bed. Hiding food so my kids wouldn't know I had it because I didn't want to share it with them. And it would be junk. It would be cakes and cookies and sweet stuff... sugars. That was probably the height of it and feeling so lousy about myself because of the weight."
Recovering binge eater

People with a binge-eating disorder feel that they cannot control the amount eaten, the pace of eating, or the kind of food eaten. They will only stop when it becomes painfully uncomfortable. Most who suffer from this disorder are obese but those with normal weight suffer this disorder as well.

Causes

Food is used to modify emotions, especially anxiety, solitude, and stress. Depression is found in about half of those with the disorder, though it is not clear whether depression is in fact a contributing cause. Food has a calming and sedating effect on some. Dieting may trigger binge-eating disorder in some cases but in one study nearly 50% of all cases had the disorder before starting to diet. Some report that solitude, boredom, anger, or other negative feelings can initiate binge eating. Unfortunately, weight gain may increase stress, guilt, and depression, perpetuating the overeating cycle.

"I was molested, sexually abused at 12, and I remember feeling really uncomfortable about my body after that and using food to just feel comfortable and maybe as a layer of protection, to keep people away. Not wanting to look good because then I might have to interact with the opposite sex and maybe have some kind of altercation. I was just afraid of men after that."
36-year-old recovering compulsive overeater

Effects

People who compulsively overeat are generally overweight and may suffer from those conditions associated with obesity, including high cholesterol, diabetes, high blood pressure, gall bladder disease, and heart disease. They are at greater risk for cancer, stroke, gout, and arthritis. They also have higher rates of depression than the population at large. Psychological problems often develop. People who binge eat become distressed, develop a negative body image, and avoid going out in public or gathering socially.

Treatment

Many people with this disorder have unsuccessfully attempted to control it. Professional treatment generally recognizes that either physiological or psychological causes underlie the disorder and address those issues before initiating a weight-loss program. Treatment often concentrates on resolving childhood issues, accomplishing positive lifestyle changes, and not just focusing on the narrower issues of eating behavior or the emotional states associated with the disorder itself. Common treatment methods include:

◇ psychotherapy that focuses on changing attitudes and ideals;

◇ psychiatric counseling that addresses underlying traumas;

◇ behavioral therapy to help monitor and control responses to stress and to change eating habits;

◇ pharmacological treatment with antidepressants (e.g., Zoloft® or Paxil®) or with the opioid blocker naltrexone;

◇ self-help groups, such as Overeaters Anonymous (OA), to reassure people who overeat that they are not alone and to provide the examples and support for positive changes.

As with all eating disorders, because people must eat to live, abstinence from all food is impossible, unlike alcohol and other drug dependencies where total abstinence is possible. A current saying among those recovering from eating disorders is, "You must walk the tiger three times a day and hope it doesn't eat you." The treatment goal is to learn to manage one's intake and to avoid foods that trigger binges, such as refined sugars, chocolate, or carbohydrates. Binge foods are substances that give a much greater emotional reaction than other foods and they vary from person to person. The goal in treating eating disorders is to teach people to solve underlying problems without resorting to destructive eating behaviors.

"Addiction for me is a state of mind. It's not the food, it's not the gambling, it's not the procrastination, it's not the alcohol and smoking. I had five or six really good addictions. It's a state of mind, and so if I am going to recover fully, I have to give them all up."
58-year-old recovering overeater, gambler, alcohol abuser, smoker

SEXUAL ADDICTION

"A patient had just fallen in love and he had just spent the day at the beach with a girlfriend. And when I saw him, he just looked like he was intoxicated . . . and so we [SPECT] scanned him on love and what we found, it worked right in the basal ganglia, which are the structures in the brain that produce dopamine. And he looked like someone had just injected him with cocaine. And it was just amazing. So love is a drug and if you get that feeling, you want it again."
Dr. Daniel Amen, Director, Amen Clinic for Behavioral Medicine

DEFINITION

"Early on we came to feel disconnected from parents, from peers, from ourselves. We tuned out with fantasy and masturbation. We plugged in by drinking in the pictures, the images, and pursuing the objects of our fantasies. We lusted and wanted to be lusted after. We became true addicts:

TABLE 7–6   COMPULSIVE OVEREATING SELF-DIAGNOSTIC TEST

The following questions are used by Overeaters Anonymous to help someone determine whether he or she is involved in compulsive overeating. Members of OA typically answer "yes" to many of the questions.

1. Do you eat when you're not hungry?
2. Do you go on eating binges for no apparent reason?
3. Do you have feelings of guilt and remorse after overeating?
4. Do you give too much time and thought to food?
5. Do you look forward with pleasure and anticipation to the time when you can eat alone?
6. Do you plan these secret binges ahead of time?
7. Do you eat sensibly before others and make up for it alone?
8. Is your weight affecting the way you live your life?
9. Have you tried to diet for a week (or longer) only to fall short of your goal?
10. Do you resent others telling you to "use a little willpower" to stop overeating?
11. Despite evidence to the contrary, have you continued to assert that you can diet on your own whenever you wish?
12. Do you crave to eat at a definite time, day or night, other than mealtimes?
13. Do you eat to escape from worries or troubles?
14. Have you ever been treated for obesity or a food-related condition?
15. Does your eating behavior make you or others unhappy?

sex with self, promiscuity, adultery, dependency relationships, and more fantasy. We got it through the eyes; we bought it, we sold it, we traded it, we gave it away. We were addicted to the intrigue, the tease, the forbidden. The only way we knew to be free of it was to do it."

Sexaholics Anonymous Big Book (SA, 1989)

Sexual addiction is marked by sexual behavior over which the addict has no control and no choice. Compulsive sexual behavior is practiced by males and females, young and old, gay and straight. It can include masturbation, pornography, serial affairs, phone sex, or visits to topless bars and strip shows. Some sexual activity that can be compulsive has legal penalties, such as prostitution, sexual harassment, sexual abuse, voyeurism, exhibitionism or flashing, child molestation, rape, and incest. Pornography and masturbation are the most frequent combination (Goodman, 1997). The incidence of sexual addiction in some studies is 3–6% (Carnes, 1997; Coleman, 1992). The DSM-IV diagnostic manual lists some separate sexual disorders under the heading of paraphilias (including exhibitionism, fetishism, frotteurism (clandestine rubbing against another person), pedophilia, sexual masochism, sexual sadism, transvestic fetishism, voyeurism). These are different from sexual compulsivity.

"Once I got married, the first time, I wanted it all the time. And I masturbated quite a bit, you know. I mean, we had sex all the time but that wasn't enough. And it got to the point where I masturbated, four, five, six times a day and wanted to go home and have sex with my wife."

34-year-old recovering sex addict

Collateral addictions include love addictions, such as romance addiction, the compulsion to fall in love and be in love, and relationship addiction, either a compulsive relationship with one person or with relationships in general.

"I'll pursue somebody and then a lot of times, once the relationship gets started, after a few months or a couple of years or whatever, depending on what the situation is with that individual, then the steam tends to go out of it, or once I know she's been caught, it's like the excitement's over."

33-year-old recovering sex addict

EFFECTS & SIDE EFFECTS

Compulsive sexual behavior is practiced as a way to cope with anxiety, stress, solitude, or low self-worth. The body becomes conditioned to the release of pleasure-giving neurotransmitters, especially dopamine, enkephalins and endorphins, with the repetitive practice of the sexual activity (Goodman, 1997). But compulsive sex is not an effective way of solving problems. Often, progressively more time must be spent in the sexual activity to reduce the stressor. Damage is done to careers, relationships, self-image, and peace of mind but the activity continues despite all negative consequences.

"Even though sex was on my mind a lot, in my teenage years, early teenage years, all through my teenage years, pornography was always an issue."

34-year-old recovering sex addict

With sexual addiction, sex becomes the person's most important all-consuming activity. Part of the elevated mood generated by the activity may involve risk. The pursuit of the addiction has been described as trance-like. A special routine or pattern may be followed that increases the excitement. Usually there is a culminating sexual event (orgasm, exposure, rape, molestation) over which the addict has no control. It is often followed by remorse, guilt, fear of being discovered, and resolutions to stop the behavior. Throughout, the sexual behavior is pursued with a sense of desperation and the person is demoralized and may suffer from low self-image, self-hatred, and despair over the time and money wasted or the

danger of injury involved. Sexaholics Anonymous (SA) and other affiliated groups see compulsive sex as a progressive disease that can be treated.

"I think it was compulsive sexuality because I used to love just a man being with me. I liked the money, for one. I like the money that men would give me for sex. So I think that anytime I would see someone that I knew personally, not as a prostitute, I would always have that temptation that I wanted to have sex with this person and I would always do it. I would always have sex with men who would be friends of mine or so-called friends."

38-year-old female recovering polydrug abuser and sex addict

It is postulated that the activity of the neurotransmitter serotonin is involved in stimulating or inhibiting sexual activity and that drugs that act to inhibit or stimulate serotonergic activity can be used to treat sexual addiction or other sexual dysfunctions (Meston & Gorzalka, 1992).

INTERNET ADDICTION

"I would wait until my wife was asleep, about one or two in the morning, and I would go into the dining room where the computer was, and I would go to the thumbnail porno pictures or play Texas hold-em online. I'd play for a couple of hours, lose a few hundred dollars, try to go back to bed, and wake up tired for the office. It wasn't until I blew $1,700 at online poker and I got a lousy job evaluation that I tried to get help. Unfortunately only Gamblers Anonymous was available but that did help."

28-year-old compulsive gambler/Internet addict

DESCRIPTION

The predecessor to the Internet was the Advanced Research Projects

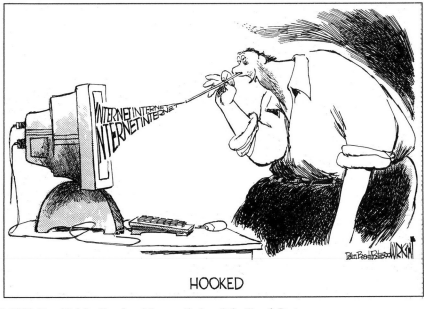

HOOKED

Agency Network (ARPA), a military network started in 1969 that was eventually opened to defense researchers at universities and other companies. In the late 1980s, most universities and many companies had come online. In 1989 a British-born computer scientist, Tim Berners-Lee, proposed the World Wide Web project. When commercial providers were allowed to sell online connections to individuals in 1991, the explosion of the Internet began. Ten thousand new subscribers come online everyday in the United States alone (Greenfield, 1999).

The electronic media, like any business, offered services that users wanted. Of course what many wanted were games, erotic material, and gambling, all pleasurable activities to many but which also had the potential for compulsive/impulsive use, abuse, and addiction. In addition the ease and anonymity of the Net enabled people to start relationships and do things that they might have avoided in the past. A survey by ABC News of 18,000 Internet users worldwide found that almost 6% of participants met the criteria for a serious compulsive addictive problem with another 4% having mild to moderate problems (Greenfield, 1999).

America Online established a chat group (room) for those suffering from cyberaddiction, an AOL-Anon group that deals with the addictive relationship with the Internet. Also called "Internet compulsion disorder" or "Internet addiction disorder," cyberaddiction is marked by compulsive involvement in chat groups, game playing, stocks or commodities market watching, sexual relationships, and other aspects of the Internet. Symptoms of Internet addiction include

◇ logging on every chance one gets at home, work, or school;

◇ thinking about the Internet constantly;

◇ needing progressively more time online to get the same satisfaction;

◇ losing track of time while logged on, so that hours go by like minutes;

◇ neglecting responsibilities while online;

◇ allowing your relationships with spouse, family, co-workers, and friends to deteriorate;

◇ increasing the time you spend online;

◇ posting more and more messages, downloading more and more data;

◇ eating in front of your monitor;

◇ checking your e-mail as soon as you get up in the morning and before you go to bed at night; getting up in the middle of the night to check it just in case.

Some people experience a stimulant-like rush when online while others speak of being tranquilized by their quiet, isolated online time. Repetitive compulsive use of the Net induces tolerance and changes in mental states. Other symptoms of Internet (and computer game) addiction include blurred vision, lack of sleep, twitching mouse fingers, and relationship problems. People who spend hours of free time every day on the Internet or log on during work or school despite negative consequences may have a compulsive dependency problem.

According to the Center for Online Addiction, there are a number of areas on the Internet where problems occur.

Cybersexual Addiction

The use of the Internet to view an incredible amount of pornography that is free on the Internet, along with development of anonymous sexual relationships that can start out with the person masturbating while chatting online or viewing pornography and escalate into phone sex and even meetings in person, is often tied to sexual addiction. According to estimates by the industry, in 1998 there were about 70,000 sex-related Web sites with 200 more being added every day. Over 10 million Web users logged onto the 10 most popular sex sites in one month (Netaddiction, 1998). The difference is that the sheer availability of the medium, along with the anonymity inherent in the Net, feeds into traits found in many people bothered by sexual compulsivity and addiction. The availability also encourages the idea that it's okay and accepted by society.

Many of those with cybersexual addiction use the chat rooms and message boards to find sexual partners. Unfortunately sexual predators are sometimes involved, preying mostly on children and women. The problem has caused many police departments to create Internet crimes units.

As the compulsion increases, compulsive cybersexual "surfers" will become more secretive, hiding their activities from their partner. They can now avoid expensive 900 sex phone lines, visits to X-rated bookstores, and visits to prostitutes. They often will exclude other forms of normal sexual activity.

Computer Relationship Addiction

If the connections made on the Internet don't particularly aim towards sexual activity but become compulsive, then they could be called "cyberrelationships." The problems begin when the online relationships draw the Net surfer from his or her real-life relationships. The online friendships can lead to "cyberaffairs" often to the devastation of the forgotten partner. As with so many behavioral addictions, when use increases, it squeezes out other parts of the user's life.

Net Compulsions

The biggest problem with Net compulsions is that of accessibility. There are hundreds of virtual casinos, online trading companies and auction houses. People can lose fortunes, or at least their mortgage payments, from the comfort of their own home, day or night. While there isn't quite the excitement of going to a casino, the element of control is also important: "I can do it when and where I want." Online traders don't have to rely on brokers to buy stocks. They don't need these so-called experts. The promise of large winnings and profits is a spur to activity. For some these elements of accessibility and control can lead to compulsive gambling as described earlier in the chapter. The online gambler or trader goes through the same stages as compulsive gamblers: winning, losing, desperation, and don't care phases (*see compulsive gambling*).

Information Addiction

The ability to access any libraries of information from the comfort of one's home is attractive to a wide variety of Internet surfers. The number of Web sites seems to be growing geometrically. The problem with surfing the Net is that it requires little direct human contact. So if Net surfers start young and find the cyber activity less threatening than dealing with people, they will be less likely to learn how to deal with people, which will then cause them to rely more and more on the electronic communication. Like other addictions, only a small percentage of users will have a problem.

Computer Games Addiction

Nintendo®, Sony PlayStation®, and other computer game systems are receiving stiff competition from all the games available online or as part of operating programs. The early game of choice was solitaire, played for hours at a time by new computer users. It is still popular but dozens of other games such as Minesweeper have been added along with hundreds of online games which can be played for fun or money. Game playing is more common among men, teenagers, and children.

CONCLUSIONS

As useful as seeing the similarities among substance abuse and other all-consuming behaviors, the danger in generalizing the concept of addiction is obscuring the distinctive characteristics of a specific addiction that need to be addressed in treatment. For example, in eating disorders and sex addiction, returning to normal levels of behavior is the preferred option, unlike alcohol and other drug abuse that stress abstinence. Fortunately pharmacology, psychotherapy, and behavioral therapies tailored to specific compulsive disorders offer hope for treatment and recovery.

CHAPTER SUMMARY

OTHER DRUGS

Inhalants

1. The three main types of inhalants are volatile solvents and aerosols, volatile nitrites, and anesthetics.

2. Inhalants are popular because they are quick acting, cheap, readily available at work and in the home, and problems with them are ignored.

3. Volatile solvents and aerosols consist of hydrocarbon gases and liquids refined from oil, including gasoline, kerosene, airplane glue, nail polish remover, lighter fluid, carbon tetrachloride, and even embalming fluid.

4. The effects of volatile solvents, mostly depressant effects, include dreaminess, dizziness, stupor, and slurred speech. Impulsiveness and irritability occasionally give way to hallucinations. Eventually, delirium, clumsiness, and impaired thinking occur.

5. Prolonged use of volatile solvents, especially leaded gasoline, can cause brain, liver, kidney, bone marrow, and especially lung damage. Death can occur from respiratory arrest, asphyxiation, or cardiac irregularities.

6. Volatile nitrites ("poppers"), such as butyl or isobutyl nitrite, are sold as Bolt®, Rush®, and Locker Room®. The major effects are muscle relaxation, blood vessel dilation, and increased heart rate causing a blood rush to the head. Dizziness and giddiness also occur. Too much can lead to vomiting, shock, unconsciousness, and blood problems.

7. Nitrous oxide, usually used as an anesthetic in the dentist's office, produces a temporary giddiness that lasts for just a couple of minutes. If not done very carefully, inhaling directly from the tank can cause frozen and exploded lung tissue.

Sports & Drugs

8. Athletes use drugs to lessen pain, improve performance, socialize, increase confidence, and as a reward.

9. Drug use among athletes dates from the time of the early Greeks. Drug use continues through the present because of increased availability of drugs, synthesis of new drugs, a "win at any cost" attitude, and increased financial incentives to succeed.

10. Although use among collegiate and professional athletes is decreasing (possibly because of increased testing), use continues, especially among high school athletes.

11. Three classes of drugs available to athletes are therapeutic drugs, performance- or appearance-enhancing drugs, and recreational drugs.

12. A danger of various pain-killing drugs is that athletes will aggravate injuries while playing injured. Other undesirable effects of analgesics, such as opioids, include mood changes, nausea, and tissue dependence.

13. The two kinds of anti-inflammatory drugs are NSAIDs and corticosteroids. Side effects of the latter are more serious than those of the former.

14. Androgenic-anabolic steroids are derived from or imitate the male hormone testosterone. Athletes use them to increase weight, strength, muscle mass, and definition. Some use them to boost aggressiveness or confidence.

15. The side effects of anabolic steroid abuse are acne, lowered sex drive, shrinking of testicles in men, breast reduction in women, bloated appearance, anger, and aggressiveness.

16. Amphetamines, including methamphetamines, are used to boost the athlete's confidence and to increase energy, alertness, aggression, and reaction time. The negative effects from occasional use of amphetamines include irritability, restlessness, anxiety, and heart or blood pressure problems.

17. Blood doping involves injecting extra blood into an athlete to increase the oxygen content of the blood. Because of the risk of infection, it is considered dangerous.

18. Marijuana acts either as a stimulant or depressant and it is the most widely abused illegal drug. Athletes turn to marijuana to relax or calm down.

19. Cocaine may be used by athletes for its stimulant effects and as a recreational drug.

20. Drug use in sports risks loss of fan support. It imperils the notion of fair competition and it robs athletes who abuse drugs of a sense of self-worth and personal achievement.

Miscellaneous Drugs

21. Other substances used to get high have included embalming fluid, gasoline, hairspray, C-4 explosive, and even camel dung.

22. Smart drugs are a mixture of vitamins, powdered nutrients, and amino acids. Some prescription drugs used to treat diseases of aging, such as Parkinson's disease or Alzheimer's disease, are also used as smart drugs.

OTHER ADDICTIONS

Compulsive Behaviors

23. Compulsive behaviors are practiced for the same reasons that compulsive drug use occurs.

24. Many of the symptoms of compulsive behavior are the same as the symptoms of compulsive drug use, such as doing the behavior or thinking about doing it most of the time and continuing the behavior despite adverse consequences.

Heredity, Environment, & Compulsive Behaviors

25. Besides emotional needs created by chaotic childhoods, environmental influences that make users more susceptible to compulsive behaviors include bad diets, a glut of fast-food restaurants, state-sponsored lotteries, and easy-to-get credit cards.

26. Heredity plays a role in compulsive behaviors making some people more susceptible.

27. A hereditary susceptibility to compulsive behavior involves many of the same areas of the brain and neurotransmitters that are involved in drug abuse.

28. A number of researchers postulate that a lack of arousal in the reward/pleasure centers causes people to engage in compulsive and repetitive behaviors to raise their level of arousal.

Compulsive Gambling

29. Historically gambling has been used by governments to raise funds, although at times, it was looked on as a vice.

30. Compulsive gambling includes commodities, stock, and day trading.

31. One to 3% of American adults are compulsive gamblers. Male compulsive gamblers outnumber female compulsive gamblers two to one but only a fraction of women, compared to men, seek help.

32. More than 5% of college students are compulsive gamblers with an-

other 10% experiencing some problems.

33. Other behavioral and substance addictions, such as alcoholism, occur in 30% to 50% of compulsive gamblers.

34. Some characteristics include preoccupation with gambling, betting progressive amounts of money, risky attempts to recoup losses, restlessness and irritability when trying to stop, and jeopardization of family, relationships, and job.

35. Compulsive gambling is treatable through Gamblers Anonymous, individual therapy, and abstinence from all gambling.

Compulsive Shopping

36. The inability to handle money is a hallmark of almost any addict.

37. Compulsive shopping (buying) is an impulse control disorder. This means that the behavior relieves tension and gives pleasure unlike obsessive compulsive disorders that only relieve tension and discomfort and are not pleasurable.

38. The control a compulsive shopper feels adds to a feeling of self-worth.

Eating Disorders

39. Society's promotion of underweight models has set up a false ideal of how we should look.

40. The three main eating disorders are bulimia, anorexia, and compulsive overeating.

41. Up to 95% of anorexics and bulimics are female.

Anorexia Nervosa

42. Anorexia is similar to a weight phobia. It occurs mostly in women who are too concerned with pleasing others. They lack self-esteem and a sense of self.

43. Anorexic individuals lose up to 60% of their body weight. The health risks are enormous.

44. Treatment is difficult because anorexics think their weight is normal or even too high even though to others, they look emaciated.

Bulimia Nervosa

45. Bulimics usually look normal but they stay that way by bingeing and then purging (throwing up) the large amounts of food they eat. The also use excessive exercise, laxatives, and fasting to control their weight.

46. One to three percent of adolescent females have bulimia.

47. Low self-esteem, pursuit of thinness, and biochemical changes induced by constant dieting trigger and perpetuate bulimia.

48. Bulimia is best treated in its early stages through psychotherapy, emotional support by family and friends, and self-help groups.

Compulsive Overeating (including binge-eating disorder)

49. With compulsive overeating, the desire to eat is triggered more by emotional states than by true hunger, e.g., to calm, to satisfy, to control pain, and to combat depression.

50. About 300,000 people die prematurely due to eating disorders:

heart disease, diabetes, stroke, gout, cancer, and arthritis.

51. Treatment includes psychotherapy, self-help groups such as Overeaters Anonymous, pharmacological treatment with antidepressants or amphetamine congeners, and behavioral therapy to change eating habits and lifestyle.

Sexual Addiction

52. Compulsive sexual behavior such as pornography, masturbation, phone sex, voyeurism, and flashing, is practiced as a way to control anxiety, stress, solitude, and low self-esteem.

53. The sexual activity is usually followed by guilt, remorse, fear of being caught, and resolutions to stop the behavior.

Internet Addiction

54. Internet addictions include cybersexual addiction, cyber-relationship addiction, Net compulsions, information overload, and computer games addiction.

55. Cyberaddiction means "using the Internet or the computer to the exclusion of a socially interactive lifestyle."

56. Cyberaddiction can be stimulating or sedating while online.

Conclusions

57. Because the roots of any compulsion are so similar, one has to treat the basic emotional causes of addiction as well as the specific substance or behavior.

REFERENCES

AP (Associated Press). (1999). Viagra, 'poppers' fatal combination. *San Francisco Chronicle*, 6-22-99.

AP. (1998). Another two teams quit. *San Francisco Chronicle*, 7-31-98.

AP. (1999). Why stop at 500?: Others laud slugger for axing Andro. *Associated Press*, 8-6-99.

APA (American Psychiatric Association). (1994). *Diagnostic and Statistical Manual of Mental Disorders* (4th ed.). Washington, DC: Author.

Arnheim, D. D., & Prentice, W. E. (1993). *Principles of Athletic Training* (8th ed.). St. Louis, MO: Mosby-Year Book, Inc.

Aronson, J. K. (1993). *Insights in the Dynamic Psychotherapy of Anorexia and Bulimia: An Introduction to the Literature*. Northvale, NJ: Jason Aronson, Inc.

Bausell, R. B., Bausell, C. R., & Siegel, D. G. (1994). *The links among alcohol, drugs and crime on American college campuses: A national follow-up study*.

Unpublished report. Towson, MD: Towson State University Campus Violence Prevention Center.

Beauvais, F., Oetting, E. R., & Edwards, R. W. (1985). Trends in the use of inhalants among American Indian adolescents. *White Cloud Journal, 3*, 3–11.

Becker, A., Grinspoon, S. K., Klibanski, A., & Herzog, D. (1999). Eating disorders. *New England Journal of Medicine, 340,* 1092–1098.

Becque, M. D., Lochmann, J. D., & Melrose, D. R. (2000). Effects of oral creatine supplementation on muscular strength and body composition. *Medicine and Science in Sports and Exercise, 32*(3), 654–658.

Bell, E. (1999). *Presentation at a symposium sponsored by the National Alliance for Research on Schizophrenia and Depression.* Great Neck, NY. *Newsday, 10-29-99.*

Bell, J. A., & Doege, T. C. (1987). Athletes' use and abuse of drugs. *The Physician and Sportsmedicine, 15*(3), 99–108.

Bell, R. M. (1985). *Holy Anorexia.* Chicago: University of Chicago Press.

Bhasin, S., Storer, T. W., Berman, N., et al. (1996). The effects of supraphysiologic doses of testosterone on muscle size and strength in normal men. *New England Journal of Medicine, 335,* 1–7.

Blum, K. (1984). *Abusable Drugs* (pp. 211–236). New York: Gardner Press, Inc.

Blum, K., Cull, J. G., Braverman, E. R., & Comings, D. E. (1996). Reward Deficiency Syndrome. *American Scientist, 84,* 132–135.

Blum, K., Braverman, E. R., Cull, J. G., Holder, J. M., Luck, R., Lubar, J., Miller, D., & Comings, D. E. (2000). "Reward deficiency syndrome" (RDS): A biogenetic model for the diagnosis and treatment of impulsive addictive, and compulsive behaviors. *Journal of Psychoactive Drugs, 32*(1).

Bouchard, C. (Ed.). (1994). *Genetics of Obesity.* Boca Raton, FL: CRC Press.

Brower, K. J. (1992). Anabolic steroids: Addictive, psychiatric, and medical consequences. *American Journal on Addictions, 1,* 100–114.

Brower, K. J. (1995). Anabolic steroids. In J. H. Jaffe (Ed.), *Encyclopedia of Drugs and Alcohol* (Vol. I, pp. 117–122). New York: Simon & Schuster MacMillan.

Brower, K. J., Blow, F. C., Young, J. P., & Hill, E. M. (1991). Symptoms and correlates of anabolic-androgenic steroid dependence. *British Journal of Addiction, 86*(6), 759–768.

Bureau of Indian Affairs. (1999). Oral communication with Bureau. In National Gambling Impact Study Commission, *National Gambling Impact Study Commission Final Report.* Washington, DC: Author.

Carnes, P. (1992). *Out of the Shadows: Understanding Sexual Addiction* (2nd ed.) Minneapolis: CompCare Pubishers.

Carr, K. D., & Papadouka, V. (1994). The role of multiple opioid receptors in the potentiation of reward by food restriction. *Brain Research, 639*(2), 253–260.

Christenson, G. A., Faber, R. J., DeZwaan, M., et al. (1994). Compulsive buying: Descriptive characteristics and psychiatric comorbidity. *Journal of Clinical Psychiatry, 55,* 5–11.

Clotfelter, C. T., Cook, P. J., Edell, J. A., & Moore, M. (1999). *State Lotteries at the Turn of the Century: Report to the National Gambling Impact Study Commission.* Chapel Hill, NC: Duke University.

Coleman, E. (1992). Is your patient suffering from compulsive sexual behavior? *Psychiatric Annual, 22,* 320–325.

Cooper, C. J., Noakes, T. D., Dunne, T., Lambert, M. I., & Rochford, K. (1996). A high prevalence of abnormal personality traits in chronic users of anabolic-androgenic steroids. *British Journal of Sports Medicine, 30*(3), 246–250.

Custer, R., & Milt, H. (1985). *When luck runs out: help for compulsive gamblers and their families.* New York: Facts On File Publications.

Dean, W., & Morgenthaler, J. (1991). *Smart Drugs & Nutrients.* Santa Cruz, CA: B&J Publications.

Dinwiddie, S. H. (1998). The Pharmacology of Inhalants. In A. W. Graham & T. K. Schultz (Eds.), *Principles of Addiction Medicine* (2nd ed., pp. 187–194). Chevy Chase, MD: American Society of Addiction Medicine, Inc.

DiPasquale, M. G. (1994). DHEA. *Drugs in Sports, 2*(4), 2–3.

Dittmar, H. (1997). Compulsive shopping. *http://www.sussex.ac.uk.*

Fairburn, C. G., & Beglin, S. J. (1990). Studies of the epidemiology of bulimia nervosa. *American Journal of Psychiatry, 147,* 495–502.

Fischman, M. W. (1995). Amphetamine. In J. H. Jaffe (Ed.), *Encyclopedia of Drugs and Alcohol* (Vol. I, pp. 105–109). New York: Simon & Schuster MacMillan.

Fleming, A. M. (1992). *Something for Nothing: A History of Gambling.* New York: Delacorte Press.

Fredlund, E. V., Spence, R. T., Maxwell, J. C., & Kavinsky, J. A. (1990). *Substance use among Texas Department of Corrections inmates.* Austin: Texas Commission on Alcohol and Drug Abuse.

Fuentes, R. J., & DiMeo, M. (1996). Exercise-induced asthma and the athlete. In R. J. Fuentes, J. M. Rosenberg, & A. Davis (Eds.), *Athletic Drug Reference '96* (pp. 217–234). Durham, NC: Clean Data, Inc.

Fuentes, R. J., Rosenberg, J. M., & Davis, A. (1996). *Athletic Drug Reference, '96.* Glaxco Wellcome. Durham, NC: Clean Data, Inc.

GA (Gamblers Anonymous). (1998). *Gamblers Anonymous Combo Book.* Los Angeles: Gamblers Anonymous.

Gerstein, D, Volberg, R., Harwood, H., et al. (1999). *Gambling Impact and Behavior Study: Report to the National Gambling Impact Study Commission.* Chicago: National Opinion Research Center at the University of Chicago *http://www.norc.uchicago.edu.*

Giannini, A. J. (1991). The volatile agents. In N. S. Miller (Ed.), *Comprehensive Handbook of Drug and Alcohol Addiction* (pp. 395–403). New York: Marcel Dekker, Inc.

Goforth, H. W. Jr., Cambell, N. L., Hodgdon, J. A., & Sucec, A. A. (1982). Hematological parameters of trained distance runners following induced erythrocythemia. *Medicine and Science in Sports and Exercise, 14,* 174.

Gold, M. S., Johnson, C. R., & Stennie, K. (1997). Eating disorders. In J. H. Lowinson, P. Ruiz, R. B. Millman, & J. G. Langrod (Eds.), *Substance Abuse: A Comprehensive Textbook* (3rd ed., pp.319–329). Baltimore: Williams & Wilkins.

Goldbloom, D. S. (1997). Pharmacotherapy of bulimia nervosa. *Medscape Women's Health, 2*(1).

Goodman, A. (1997). Sexual addiction. In J. H. Lowinson, P. Ruiz, R. B. Millman, & J. G. Langrod (Eds.), *Substance Abuse: A Comprehensive Textbook* (3rd ed., pp. 340–354). Baltimore: Williams & Wilkins.

Gordon, N. F. et al. (1991). Effect of beta-blockers on exercise physiology: implication for exercise training. *Medical Science Sports Exercise, 23*(6), 668.

Greenfield, D. N. (1999). *Virtual Addiction.* Oakland, CA: New Harbinger Publications.

Grossman, S. J., & Gieck, J. (1992). A model alcohol and other drug peer education program for student athletes. *Journal of Sport Rehabilitation, 1*, 337–349.

Gruber, A. J., & Pope, H. G. (1998). Ephedrine abuse among 36 female weightlifters. *American Journal on Addictions, 7*(4), 256–261.

Grunwald, L. (1995). Do I look fat to you? *Life Magazine, February, 1995*.

Halwell, B., & Gardner, G. (2000). *Underfed & Overfed: The Global Epidemic of Malnutrition*. Worldwatch Institute Report 150. *http://www.world-watch.org/pubs/paper/150.html*.

Hanley, D. F. (1983). Drug and sex testing: Regulations for international competition. *Clinical Sports Medicine, 2*, 13–17.

Herman, R. D. 1984. Gambling. *Encyclopaedia Britannica* (Vol. 7, pp. 866–867). Chicago: Encyclopaedia Britannica.

Herzog, D. B., Dorer, D. J., Keel, P. K., et al. (1999). Recovery and relapse in anorexia and bulimia nervosa. A 7.5 year follow-up study. *Journal of the American Academy of Child and Adolescent Psychiatry, 38*, 829–837.

Herzog, D. B., Nussbaum, K. M., & Marmor, A. K. (1996). Comorbidity and outcome in eating disorders. *Psychiatric Clinics of North America, 19*, 843–859.

Hormes, J. T., Filley, C. M., & Rosenberg, N. L. (1986). Neurologic sequelae of chronic solvent vapor abuse. *Neurology, 36*, 698–702.

Hunter, R. (1997). Interview with Rob Hunter, Gambling Counselor. Author's files.

Jacobi, C., Dahme, B., & Rustenbach, S. (1997). Comparison of controlled psycho- and pharmacotherapy studies in bulimia and anorexia nervosa. *Psychotherapiek Psychosomatik, Medizinische Psychologie, 47*, 346–364.

Jacobson, B. H. (1990). Effect of amino acids on growth hormone release. *Physical Sportsmedicine, 18*(1), 63.

Jimerson, D. C., Herzog, D. B., & Botman, A. W. (1993). Pharmacologic approaches in the treatment of eating disorders. *Harvard Review of Psychiatry, 1*, 82–93.

Jonas, J. M., & Gold, M. S. (1988). The use of opiate antagonists in treating bulimia: A study of low-dose versus high-dose naltrexone. *Psychiatry Research, 24*(2), 195–199.

Kaplan, A. S., & Garfinkel, P. R. (1995). General principles of outpatient treatment—eating disorders. In G. O. Gabbard (Ed.), *Treatments of Psychiatric Disorders* (Vol. 2). Washington, DC: American Psychiatric Press.

Kashkin, K. B. (1992). Anabolic steroids. In J. H. Lowinson, P. Ruiz, R. B. Millman, & J. G. Langrod (Eds.), *Substance Abuse: A Comprehensive Textbook* (2nd ed., pp. 380–395). Baltimore: Williams & Wilkins.

Kaye, W. H., Pickar, D. M., Naber, D., & Eben, M. H. (1982). Cerebrospinal fluid opioid activity in anorexia nervosa. *American Journal of Psychiatry, 139*, 643–645.

King, D. S., Sharp, R. L., Vukovich, M. D., et al. (1999). Effect of oral androstenedione on serum testosterone and adaptations to resistance training in young men. *Journal of the American Medical Association, 281*(21).

Kusserow, R. P. (1990). *Adolescents and Steroids: A User's Perspective*. Washington, DC: Office of Inspector General, Office of Evaluations and Inspections, Department of Health and Human Services.

Laties, V. G., & Weiss, B. (1981). Amphetamines and sports. *Federation proceedings, 40*, 2689–2692.

Lesieur, H. R., Blume, S. B., & Zoppa, R. M. (1986). Alcoholism, drug abuse and gambling. *Alcohol Clinical Experimental Research, 10*(1), 33–38.

Lesieur, H. R., Cross, J., Frank, M., et al. (1991). Gambling and pathological gambling among university students. *Addictive Behaviors, 16*, 515–527.

Lesieur, H. R., & Rosenthal, R. J. (1991). Pathological gambling: a review of the literature (prepared for the American Psychiatric Association Task Force on DSM-IV. *Journal of Gambling Studies, 7*(1), 5–39.

Linden, R. D. (1985). Pathological gambling and major affective disorder: preliminary findings. *Journal of Clinical Psychiatry, 47*, 201–203.

Lukas, S. E. (1998). The pharmacology of steroids. In A. W. Graham & T. K. Schultz (Eds.), *Principles of Addiction Medicine* (2nd ed., pp. 173–186). Chevy Chase, MD: American Society of Addiction Medicine, Inc.

Lynn, E. J., Walter, R. G., Harris, L. A., Dendy, R., & James, M. (1972). Nitrous oxide: It's a gas. *Journal of Psychoactive Drugs, 5*(1), 1–7.

Mahesh, V. B., & Greenblatt, R. B. (1962). The in vivo conversion of dehydroepiandosterone and androstenedione to testosterone in the human. *Acta Endocrinology, 41*, 400–406.

Marazzi, M. A., & Luby, E. D. (1989). Anorexia nervosa as an auto-addiction. *Annual of the New York Academy of Science, 575*, 545–547.

Marnell, T. (Ed.). (1997). *Drug Identification Bible*. Denver: (800) 772-2539.

McElroy, S. L., Keck, P. E. Jr., Pope, J. F. Jr., et al. (1994). Compulsive buying: A report of 20 cases. *Journal of Clinical Psychiatry, 55*, 242–248.

McElroy, S. L., Satlin, A., Pope, H. G. Jr., Hudson, J. I., & Keck, P. E. Jr. (1991). Treatment of compulsive shopping and antidepressants. A report of three cases. *Annals of Clinical Psychiatry, 3*, 199–204.

McElroy, S. L., Soutullo, C. A., & Goldsmith, R. J. (1998). Other impulse control disorders. In A. W. Graham & T. K. Schultz (Eds.), *Principles of Addiction Medicine* (2nd ed., pp. 1047–1062). Chevy Chase, MD: American Society of Addiction Medicine, Inc.

Mellan, O. (1995). *Overcoming Overspending*. Walker and Company.

Mellion, M. B. (1985). Drugs and doping in athletes. *Resident & Staff Physician: Problems in Primary Care*.

Meston, C. M., & Gorzalka, B. B. (1992). Psychoactive drugs and human sexual behavior: The role of serotonergic activity. *Journal of Psychoactive Drugs, 24*(1), 1–40.

Mjoseth, J. (1999). Overzealous shopping: A higher prevalence of compulsive shopping among women may be attributable to their response to low levels of serotonin. *APA (American Psychological Association) Monitor*.

Mokdad, A. H., Serdula, M. K., Dietz, W. H., et al. (1999). The spread of the obesity epidemic in the United States, 1991–1998. *Journal of the American Medical Association, 282*(16), 1519–1522.

Morton, R. (1694). *Phthisiological; or a treatise of consumptions*. London: Smith and Walford.

Nakken, C. (1996). *The Addictive Personality*. Center City, MN: Hazelden.

NCAA (National Collegiate Athletic Association). (1997). *Survey of college student-athletes*.

NCAA. (1998). Drug testing shows state of drug education programs at member schools. *NCAA News. http://www.ncaa.org/news/*.

NCAA. (1999). Latest drug-testing results indicate concern for ephedrine use. *NCAA News. http://www.ncaa.org/news/*.

NCADI (National Clearinghouse for Alcohol and Drug Information). (1999).

Inhalant abuse. *http://www.health. org/kidsarea/funstuf/brain/inhal.htm.*

Netaddiction. (1998). Center for On-Line Addiction. *Netaddiction.com.*

NIDA (National Institute of Drug Abuse). (1997). Questions and answers about anabolic steroids. *NIDA Notes, 12*(4).

NIH (National Institutes of Health). (1992). *Inhalant Abuse: A Volatile Research Agenda. NIH Publication no. 93-3475.* Rockville, MD.

NOAH (New York Online Access to Health). (1996). Eating disorders: anorexia and bulimia nervosa. *http://www. NOAH.cuny.edu/wellconn/eatdisorders.html.*

NORC (National Opinion Research Center). (1999). *Gambling Impact and Behavior Study, Report to the National Gambling Impact Study Commission. http://www.norc.uchicago.edu.*

NRC. (1999). National Research Council, Pathological Gambling: A Critical Review. *Committee on the Social and Economic Impact of Pathological Gambling.* Washington, DC: National Academy Press.

O'Brien, R., Cohen, S., Evans, G., & Fine, J. (1992). *The Encyclopedia of Drug Abuse* (2nd ed., pp. 149–150). New York: Facts on File.

Padilla, E. R., Padilla, A. M., Morales, A., Olmedo, E. L., & Ramirez, R. (1979). Inhalant, marijuana, and alcohol abuse among barrio children and adolescents. *International Journal of Addiction, 14,* 945–964.

Partin, P. (1988). Effects of caffeine on athletes. *Athletic Trainer, 23.*

Patrick, D. (8-24-98). McGwire taking hits over use of power pill. *USA Today.*

PDR. (1999). *Physicians' Desk Reference.* Montvale, NJ: Medical Economics Company.

People. (4-12-99). Wasting away: Eating disorders on campus. *People Magazine Survey.*

Pope, H. J., & Katz, D. L. (1994). Psychiatric and medical effects of anabolic-androgenic steroid use. A controlled study of 160 athletes. *Archives of General Psychiatry, 51*(5), 375–382.

Psychology Today. (Mar/Apr 1995).

Rosenbaum, M., & Leibel, R. L. (1988). Pathophysiology of childhood obesity. *Advanced Pediatrics, 35,* 73–137.

Rosenberg, Fuentes, R. J., Woolley, B. H., Reese, T., & Podraza, J. (1996). Questions and answers–What athletes commonly ask. In R. J. Fuentes, J. M. Rosenberg, & A. Davis (Eds.), *Athletic*

Drug Reference '96. Durham, NC: Clean Data, Inc.

Rosenthal, R. J. (1989). Pathological gambling and problem gambling: Problems in definition and diagnosis. In H. J. Shaffer, S. A. Stein, B. Gambino, et al. (Eds.), *Compulsive Gambling: Theory, Research, and Practice* (pp. 101–125). Lexington, MA: Lexington Books.

Rosenthal, R. J., & Lesieur, H. R. (1992). Self-reported withdrawal symptoms and pathological gambling. *American Journal of Addictions, 1,* 150–154.

Rupp, N. T. et al. (1993). The value of screening for risk of exercise-induced asthma in high school athletes. *Annual Allergy, 70, 33–39.*

Russell, G. (1979). Bulimia nervosa: an ominous variant of anorexia nervosa. *Psychological Medicine,* 429–448.

SAMHSA (Substance Abuse and Mental Health Services Administration). (1999). *Summary of findings from the 1998 National Household Survey on Drug Abuse.* Rockville, MD: Substance Abuse and Mental Health Services, Office of Applied Studies.

SA (Sexaholics Anonymous). (1989). *Sexaholics Anonymous.* New York: SA Literature.

Shaffer, H. J., Hall, M. N., & Bilt, J. V. (1997). *Estimating the prevalence of disordered gambling behavior in the United States and Canada: A meta-analysis.* Boston: President and Fellows of Harvard College.

Shaffer, H. Lecture to casino executives, Las Vegas gaming convention. *Medford Mail Tribune,* 2-28-98. Medford, OR .

Sharp, C. W., Beauvais, F., & Spence, R. (1992). Inhalant abuse: a volatile research agenda. *NIDA Research Monograph Series No. 129, NIH publication no. 93-3480.* Rockville, MD: National Institutes of Health.

Sharp, C. W., & Rosenberg, N. L. (1997). Inhalants. In J. H. Lowinson, P. Ruiz, R. B. Millman, & J. G. Langrod (Eds.), *Substance Abuse: A Comprehensive Textbook* (3rd ed., pp. 246–263). Baltimore: Williams & Wilkins.

Siegal, E., & Wason, S. (1990). Sudden death caused by inhalation of butane and propane. *New England Journal of Medicine, 323*(23), 1638.

Sinclair, S. (1999). *The Birth of an Industry: Gambling and the Internet.* Gambling Report III.

Smith, G. (1974). *When the Cheering Stopped.* Toronto: MacLeod.

Spitzer, R. L., Yanovski, S., Wadden, T., et

al. (1993). Binge-eating disorder: its further validation in a multi site study. *International Journal of Eating Disorders, 13,* 137–153.

Spriet, L. L. (1995). Caffeine and sports. *International Journal of Sports Nutrition, 5,* S84–S99.

Strauss, R., Liggett, M., & Lanese, R. (1985). Anabolic steroid use and perceived effects in ten weight-trained woman athletes. *Journal of the American Medical Association, 253,* 2871–2873.

Swan, N. (1995). Inhalants. In J. H. Jaffe (Ed.), *Encyclopedia of Drugs and Alcohol* (Vol. 2, pp. 590–600). New York: Simon & Schuster MacMillan.

Terney, R., & McLain, L. G. (1990). The use of anabolic steroids in high school students. *American Journal of the Disabled Child, 144,* 99–103.

Thomason, H. (1982). Science and sporting performance: Management or manipulation. In B. Davies & G. Thomas (Eds.), *Drugs and the Athlete.* Oxford: Clarendon Press.

Todd, T. (1987). Anabolic steroids: The gremlins of sport. *Journal of Sports History, 14,* 87–107.

Treasure, J, & Campbell, I. (1994). Editorial: A biological hypothesis for anorexia nervosa. *Psychiatric Medicine, 24,* 3–8.

U.S. Congress. House. (1990). Hearing before the Subcommittee on Crime of the Committee on the Judiciary, House of Representatives, March 22, 1990. *Abuse of Steroids in Amateur and Professional Athletics.*

University of Michigan. (1999). *Monitoring the Future Study.* Rockville, MD: SAMHSA. *http://www.MonitoringThe Future.org.*

University of Sussex. (1997). Shopping addicts need help. Bulletin in the University of Sussex Newsletter. *http://www.sussex.ac.uk.*

USOC (United States Olympic Committee). (1996). *USOC Drug Education Handbook 1993–1996,* (pamphlet).

Washington Post. Argentina struggles with record anorexia. *Washington Post,* 7-6-97.

Weil, A., & Rosen, W. (1993). *From Chocolate to Morphine.* Boston: Houghton Mifflin Company.

WHO (World Health Organization). (1992). *Programme on Substance Abuse: Solvent Abuse.* Geneva: World Health Organization. WHO/PSA/93.8.

WHO. (1998). *Volatile Solvent Use: A Global Overview.* Geneva: Substance

Abuse Department, World Health Organization. WHO/HSC/SAB/99.7.

Williams, M. H., Wesseldine, S., Somma, T., & Schuster, R. (1981). The effects of induced erythrocythemia upon 5-mile treadmill run time. *Medicine and Science in Sports and Exercise, 13,* 169–175.

Wiseman, C. V. et al. (1992). Cultural expectations of thinness in women: An update. *International Journal of Eating Disorders, 11*(1).

Wolf, N. (1992). *The Beauty Myth: How Images of Beauty Are Used Against Women.* New York: Anchor Books/ Doubleday.

Wood, R. W. (1994). Inhalants. In J. H. Jaffe (Ed.), *Encyclopedia of Drugs and Alcohol* (Vol. 2, pp. 590–595). New York: Simon & Schuster MacMillan.

Wooley, B. H. (1992). Drugs of abuse in sport. In R. Banks, Jr. (Ed.), *Substance Abuse in Sport: The Realities* (2nd ed., pp. 3–12). Dubuque, IA: Kendall/Hunt Publishing Company.

Yesalis, C. E., Herrick, R. T., Buckley, W. E., et al. (1988). Self-reported use of anabolic-androgenic steroids by elite powerlifters. *Physiology of Sportsmedicine, 16,* 91–100.

Drug Use & Prevention:
From Cradle to Grave

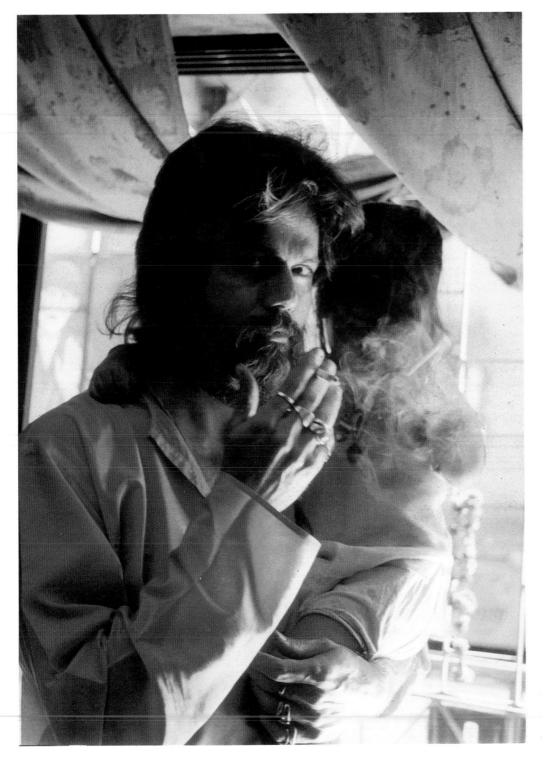

M any new prevention
strategies focus on secondhand smoke.

Courtesy of Shyam Sharma

◇ **Introduction:** Drug use affects people from cradle to grave, so prevention should be taught from cradle to grave.

PREVENTION

◇ **Concepts of Prevention:** Historically substance abuse prevention has included a vast array of interventions from total prohibition to temperance to harm reduction. Scare tactics, drug information programs, skill-building programs, and resiliency programs have been some of the methods used over the years.

◇ **Prevention Methods:** The three main prevention methods are supply reduction (enforce legal penalties and interdict drugs), demand reduction (reduce craving for drugs), and harm reduction (minimize harm without requiring abstinence).

◇ **Challenges to Prevention:** The impediments to prevention efforts include the abundance of legal drugs and the availability of illegal drugs, the relatively slow rate of success of prevention programs, the difficulty of properly evaluating these efforts, and the lack of adequate funding.

FROM CRADLE TO GRAVE

◇ **Patterns of Use:** A pattern of earlier age of first use and high levels of overall use are worrisome. Drug abuse is not restricted to any age, race, intelligence, or sex.

◇ **Pregnancy & Birth:** Drugs cross the placental barrier and affect the fetus more strongly than the mother. Drug effects continue after birth. The infant can be born addicted and must go through withdrawal.

◇ **Youth & School:** Alcohol is still the number one drug problem in schools. Tobacco is second and marijuana third. Increased alcohol abuse is being countered by recognizing risk factors, bolstering resiliency, and using normative assessment. Prevention efforts are required throughout all grades.

◇ **Love, Sex, & Drugs:** Psychoactive drugs are used to lower inhibitions in order to enhance sexual activity. Initially some drugs may increase sensation but with continued use they can diminish sexual performance and pleasure. Sexual violence, such as date rape, is strongly associated with drug use. High-risk sex practices, aggravated by lowered inhibitions and contaminated needles, spread sexually transmitted diseases (STDs), HIV/AIDS, hepatitis C, and other infections.

◇ **Drugs at Work:** Employee assistance programs (EAPs) help control substance abuse in the workplace that costs businesses and society more than $110 billion a year in lost productivity, lost earnings, and increased health care.

◇ **Drug Testing:** Preemployment testing, testing of people in treatment, military testing, sports testing, and random testing of workers responsible for public safety (e.g., pilots, nuclear technicians) are the most widely used kinds of drug testing.

◇ **Drugs & the Elderly:** The elderly are more susceptible to the pharmacological effects of drugs. Alcohol abuse and prescription drug abuse are the biggest problems.

◇ **Conclusions:** To be successful, prevention programs must be specific to age, ethnic, and cultural group and the message must be consistent. It must also be continued through one's lifetime.

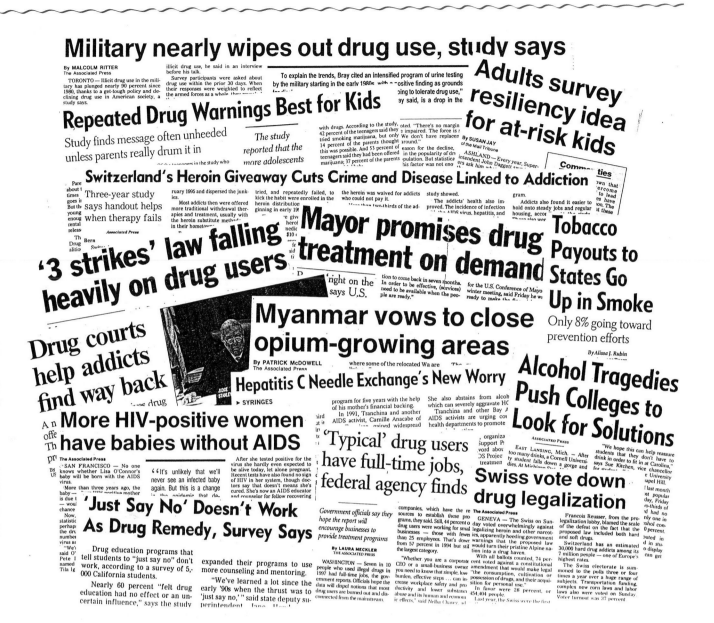

Military nearly wipes out drug use, study says

By MALCOLM RITTER
The Associated Press

TORONTO — Illicit drug use in the military has plunged nearly 90 percent since 1980, thanks to a get-tough policy and declining drug use in American society, a study says.

illicit drug use, he said in an interview before his talk.

Survey participants were asked about drug use within the prior 30 days. When their responses were weighted to reflect the armed forces as a whole, they...

To explain the trends, Bray cited an intensified program of urine testing by the military starting in the early 1980s, with a positive finding as grounds ...going to tolerate drug use," ...ay said, is a drop in the

Repeated Drug Warnings Best for Kids

Study finds message often unheeded unless parents really drum it in

The study reported that the more adolescents

with drugs. According to the study, 42 percent of the teenagers said they tried smoking marijuana, but only 14 percent of the parents thought this was possible. And 53 percent of teenagers said they had been offered marijuana; 37 percent of the parents

Adults survey resiliency idea for at-risk kids

By SUSAN JAY
of the Mail Tribune

ASHLAND — Every year, Superintendent John Daggett... ers ask him an...

Switzerland's Heroin Giveaway Cuts Crime and Disease Linked to Addiction

Three-year study says handout helps when therapy fails

'3 strikes' law falling heavily on drug users

Mayor promises drug treatment on demand

Tobacco Payouts to States Go Up in Smoke

Only 8% going toward prevention efforts

Drug courts help addicts find way back

Myanmar vows to close opium-growing areas

By PATRICK McDOWELL
The Associated Press

Hepatitis C Needle Exchange's New Worry

Alcohol Tragedies Push Colleges to Look for Solutions

More HIV-positive women have babies without AIDS

'Typical' drug users have full-time jobs, federal agency finds

Swiss vote down drug legalization

'Just Say No' Doesn't Work As Drug Remedy, Survey Says

INTRODUCTION

"Preventing addiction should be easy but it's been a difficult process. It's been difficult because moral issues become involved with the medical issues. We should have the ability to prevent this condition as well as to treat this condition. Unfortunately many of the things that people look at from an addictive standpoint seem to concentrate on the illegality, on the

police scene, on interdiction, and on stopping drugs at the border. The more we try to stop drugs from coming into the United States, the more drugs it seems are available."

Dr. Darryl Inaba, CEO, Haight-Ashbury Free Clinics

Psychoactive drugs and addictive behaviors affect people's lives from conception to death. For example:

◊ a fetus absorbs heroin through the umbilical cord when an addicted mother injects the drug;

◊ an 8 year old drinks a beer that's been kept cold in the refrigerator;

◊ a 14 year old is offered MDMA at a "rave" party so she can get "rolling";

◊ a college student smokes marijuana on the weekend to unwind from a tough week of exams;

◊ a college coed troubled by bulimia makes herself throw up five times a week;

◊ a young mother with three children hides in her room to smoke "crack";

◊ while having sex, a 28-year-old IV methamphetamine user infects his girlfriend with the HIV virus he got through a contaminated needle;

◊ an office worker takes alprazolam (Xanax®) to cope with job stress and anxiety while a coworker with major depression is prescribed Prozac®, an antidepressant, to help him function;

◊ a mother, whose children have grown, battles boredom by compulsively playing poker machines;

◊ a 50-year-old salesman on the road smokes and drinks to cope with boredom;

◊ a 74 year old borrows a prescription painkiller from a neighbor to relieve arthritic pain.

Since drug use and abuse affects all ages, prevention and treatment programs should also be continued throughout people's lifetimes. Some strategies include

◊ encouraging pregnant mothers to attend prenatal care programs to teach them how drugs affect their fetuses;

◊ limiting the use of club drugs at parties through greater parental involvement;

◊ offering counseling on eating disorders in high schools and colleges;

◊ keeping the doctor aware of a patient's excess use of Xanax® and educating the patients about the possibility of delayed withdrawal convulsions;

◊ using outreach workers to encourage drug users to practice safe sex and use clean needles in order to prevent HIV or hepatitis C infection and to get them to consider treatment;

◊ coercing a heavy-drinking salesman into an employee assistance program;

◊ holding seminars to enlighten senior citizens about the dangers of borrowing medications;

◊ teaching all ages about resiliency, support services, and healthy alternatives to using psychoactive drugs.

If the basic premise of practicing prevention at every age is accepted, then the questions that need to be answered are, "What are the different theories and methods of prevention?" "Which prevention methods work?" and "How should they be implemented throughout people's lives?"

PREVENTION

CONCEPTS OF PREVENTION

PREVENTION GOALS

Each society has to decide exactly what they are trying to prevent and since there is such a diversity of cultures from country to country and within each country, that decision can be difficult. Are they trying to prevent any use of any psychoactive drug, are they just trying to ban illicit drugs or are they just trying to limit the damage caused by use, abuse, and addiction? In the United States and most countries, a combination of the two concepts is employed. Thus prevention needs to have several goals. They include

◊ keeping the disease of addiction from ever having a chance to develop by teaching skills that will help the individual to resist drug use, make wise decisions, and resolve inner pain and conflict—all aimed at instilling resiliency and creating alternatives to drug use;

◊ stopping inappropriate or potentially destructive use as soon as possible where it has begun;

◊ in more advanced stages of abuse and addiction, reversing the progression, restoring people to health, and helping them find an alternative way of thinking and living.

"And so I set out on a mission to rebuild myself. So I said, 'Okay, now what would you do if you had to rebuild a car?' Well you would take everything apart and you'd start all over. So what I had to do was shed all the negativity and step down naked so to speak and just build myself up all over again. And this time, not making mistakes and not making choices that I made before."

48-year-old recovering addict—currently a counselor at the Haight-Ashbury BASN treatment unit

Traditionally there have been three methods used to achieve the above goals:

1. **reduce the supply** of illegal drugs available in society. This is usually done through interdiction of drugs supplies, legislation against use, and legal penalties for possession, distribution, and use;

2. **reduce the demand** for all psychoactive drugs, legal and illegal. This is done through treatment of drug abuse/addiction, education, emotional development, moral growth, and individual and community activities;

3. **reduce the harm** that drugs do to users, relatives and friends of users, and society as a whole. This more controversial alternative is done through such methods as promoting temperance, instituting needle exchanges with outreach components, using drug substitution programs (e.g., methadone), providing resources to lessen the consequences

of abuse (e.g., designated drivers), and decriminalizing drug use.

Historically, supply reduction and harm reduction (temperance) have been the most widely used methods. In the twentieth century, with the recognition of addiction as a disease process, demand reduction has become a viable method of prevention. In 2001 about 1/3 of the projected $19.2 billion in federal funds requested for drug control is allocated for demand reduction (ONDCP, 2000). In comparison, the total drug control budget for 1991 was approximately $11 billion.

"A common fault in drug policy has been anticipating or promising dramatic results within an unrealistically brief period. Reducing and stopping drug use requires fundamental changes in the attitudes of millions of Americans and that shift in attitude is more gradual than we would wish. The National Drug Control Strategy promotes a steady pressure against drug use and underscores why drug control must be lifted out of partisan conflict."

Barry R. McCaffrey, Director, Office of National Drug Control Policy (ONDCP, 1999)

HISTORY & DESCRIPTION OF PREVENTION TECHNIQUES

Temperance vs. Prohibition

Attempts to regulate drugs, particularly alcohol, have wavered between moderation of use and prohibition. In the United States, eighteenth- and early nineteenth-century attempts to regulate alcohol consumption initially focused on the ideal of "temperance." The guiding assumptions were that heavy drinking and especially drunkenness were destructive, sinful, and immoral but moderate use could improve health and mood. Initial efforts consisted of convincing drinkers to switch from distilled spirits (hard liquor) to beer, wine, and fermented cider (White, 1998).

By the 1850s, the ideal of total abstinence had replaced that of temperance. These efforts eventually led to passage of the Eighteenth Amendment to the Constitution, forbidding the manufacture, sale, and transportation of alcohol. People's desire to drink again and the increase of criminal activity involved in illegal trafficking led to the repeal of Prohibition 13 years later (Jaffe, 1995).

This conflict between moderate use of psychoactive drugs and moral/legal abhorrence of any use of any amount persists to the present day.

Historically with alcohol, the concept of complete prohibition or lately, zero tolerance, seems to run on a 70-year cycle: 1780, 1850, 1920, 1990. Over the last 15 years, all states raised their drinking age to 21 while some states decreased the allowable blood alcohol concentration (BAC) from 0.10 down to .08. In 1995 Louisiana became the first state to lower the drinking age back to 18 years. Currently several states have enacted zero tolerance laws that suspend driver licenses of youths under 21 convicted of driving with a BAC of just .01, the equivalent of about half a beer.

Did Prohibition Really Fail?

Popular belief over the decades has been that Prohibition, enacted into law in 1917 (and enforced starting in 1919) by the Eighteenth Amendment and repealed in 1933, was ineffective. An examination of medical records concerning diseases caused by excess alcohol consumption as well as criminal justice records show the truth to be different.

◇ Admissions to mental hospitals for alcoholic psychosis in Massachusetts fell from a rate of 14.6 per 100,000 in 1910, to 6.4 in 1922, and 7.7 in 1929. In New York, the rate fell from 11.5 in 1910, to 3.0 in

TABLE 8–1   NATIONAL DRUG CONTROL BUDGET, 1991–2001 (Total budget is $19.2 billion)

FUNCTIONAL AREAS	1991	1993	1995	1997	1999	2001
Demand Reduction			(in millions)			
Drug abuse treatment	$1,877.3	$2,251.6	$2,692.0	$2,756.2	$2,949.0	$3,382.0
Drug abuse prevention	1,479.2	1,556.4	1,559.1	1,643.3	1,953.5	2,122.3
Prevention research	150.6	164.3	179.6	230.7	285.6	340.0
Treatment research	187.9	242.0	261.2	312.7	382.5	439.6
Total Demand Reduction	**$3,695.0**	**$4,214.3**	**$4,691.9**	**$4,942.9**	**$5,570.6**	**$6,283.9**
Supply Reduction						
Criminal justice system	$4,385.6	$5,692.4	$6,757.0	$7,446.4	$8,557.6	$9,385.5
Other research	111.6	91.9	101.4	111.8	113.2	118.6
Intelligence	104.1	138.1	125.0	142.3	277.3	305.3
International	633.4	523.4	295.8	424.1	774.7	907.7
Interdiction	2,027.9	1,511.1	1,311.6	1,723.3	2,417.9	2,213.4
Total Supply Reduction	**$7,262.6**	**$7,956.0**	**$8,590.8**	**$9,847.9**	**$12,140.7**	**$12,930.5**

(ONDCP, 2000)

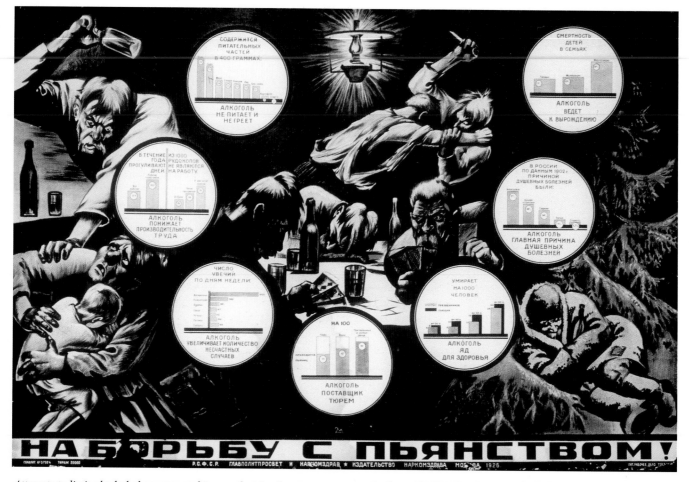

Attempts to limit alcohol abuse was and is prevalent in almost every country in the world. This Russian anti-alcohol poster from 1926 coincided with Prohibition in the United States.

Courtesy of the National Library of Medicine, Bethesda

1920, and up to 6.5 in 1931 (Aaron & Musto, 1981).

◊ Nationally death rates from cirrhosis of the liver went from 14.8 per 100,000 in 1907, to 7.1 in 1920, and stayed below 7.5 through the rest of the 1920s (Jaffe, 1995).

◊ In addition there were decreased legal costs of jailing drunks, less domestic violence, and less crime in general.

◊ Per capita alcohol consumption dropped in half and did not climb back to pre-Prohibition levels until 20–30 years after Prohibition was repealed.

As bootlegging increased the supply of alcohol in the late 1920s, medical problems increased again but still stayed way below pre-Prohibition levels.

The myth that Prohibition created organized crime wasn't really true. Criminal organizations existed long before Prohibition, although organizational techniques were refined during Prohibition and prepared the mobs to step into smuggling and distribution of illicit drugs.

Even though Prohibition did reduce illness and crime, or possibly because it did, concern for and treatment of the alcoholic decreased. Prohibitionists thought that all they needed to do was ban alcohol and the problems would be solved (Lender & Martin, 1987). The Prohibitionists also tried to criminalize drinking itself even though Prohibition only banned the "manufacture, sale, and transportation of intoxicating liquors." There was support for Prohibition from President Hoover and most

state governors in 1928 and if the Great Depression hadn't occurred in the 1930s, the Eighteenth Amendment might have lasted years longer. The need for increased tax revenue, the activities of the anti-Prohibition forces called the "Wets," and the desire to drink again on the part of the general public caused the repeal of the Prohibition amendment.

Scare Tactics & Drug Information Programs

Concerted attempts to lessen substance abuse didn't begin in earnest until the 1960s when recreational drugs came out of the ghettos and barrios and began to affect middle-class kids. A number of grassroots prevention movements began in the 1960s and '70s as the percentage of Americans who had used any illicit drug went from 2% in 1962 to 31% in 1979 (Rusche, 1995; SAMHSA, 1999).

Early prevention programs in the '60s and '70 assumed that young people lacked knowledge about the dangerous effects of psychoactive drugs. Knowledge-based programs were established to teach students about pharmacological effects, causes of addiction, health effects of drug use, and legal penalties. Providing factual information with a heavy dose of scare tactics was considered enough to reduce drug use. Often the scare tactics overwhelmed the information or made even correct information suspect to students. Unfortunately, early scare tactics also presented nonfactual or distorted information about drugs, destroying the credibility of the message.

"In the early 1970s, the government asked a group of treatment professionals, including myself, to review 297 drug education films that were available. We found that we could only recommend 1 or 2 of the films because most of them had bad information, relied only on scare tactics, or were just poorly made."

Dr. Darryl Inaba, CEO, Haight-Ashbury Free Clinics

Although factual information produced documentable increases in knowledge and changes in attitude and is still thought to persuade some young people into rational abstention, there is little evidence that drug information alone causes changes in behavior.

"I received only one drug education lesson in my ninth grade health class. They talked a lot about all the different types of drugs and drug use. The class actually made me quite aware that I was missing out on a whole lot of drugs. By the time I ended up in therapeutic boarding school, I knew a lot about drug use and abuse but only because of the extensive drug history I had."

Recovering 21-year-old college student

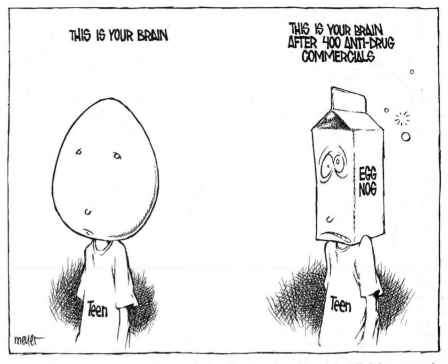

THIS IS YOUR BRAIN

THIS IS YOUR BRAIN AFTER 400 ANTI-DRUG COMMERCIALS

EGG NOG

Teen

Teen

The role of knowledge in comprehensive prevention programs is still unknown. Some studies indicate that among certain adolescent audiences, factual information actually stimulates experimentation (Moskowitz, 1989). It has been suggested that adolescents' feelings of immortality and invulnerability, a limited view of the future, and an indifference to long-term health consequences all frustrate information-only approaches. School-centered knowledge-based programs may also miss those who skip school frequently and are most at risk for health and crime problems associated with drug abuse. However, prevention efforts greatly lessen drug problems at a fraction of the cost of supply reduction efforts. These programs often suffer from underskilled teachers and trainers or they are not appropriate to the developmental level of targeted students.

Skill-Building & Resiliency Programs

Prevention efforts then expanded to address the psychological and developmental factors that might predispose individuals to turn to drugs and the social skills that might protect them from experimentation and abuse. The more risk factors that youths have, the more likely they are to abuse drugs (Hird, Khuri, Dusenbury, & Millman, 1997; Bry, McKeon, & Pandina, 1982). Thus increasing skills that effectively address these risks may result in a solid prevention strategy.

Areas included are as follows,

◇ **general competency building:** The aim is to teach people how to adjust to life through training in self-esteem, in socially acceptable behavior, and in decision making, self-assertion, problem solving, and vocational skills. Programs employing these prevention strategies continue to report positive results but once training ceases, the gains are soon lost. Periodic booster shots throughout a student's educational career improve the effectiveness of this kind of prevention education;

◇ **special coping skills:** Coping skills, like parenting classes, stress management, and even breathing classes, are taught to help people face stressful situations. Coping skills are seen as ways of developing the self-reliance, confidence, and inner resources needed to resist drug use;

◇ **reinforcing protective factors and resiliency:** These are ways to build on natural strengths that people already have available. The factors that seem to increase resiliency are optimism, empathy, insight, intellectual competence, self-esteem, direction or purpose in life, and determination (Kumpfer, 1994). These factors, along with supportive friends and family and opportunities to belong to meaningful groups in their own communities, all emphasize that the coping resources available to people are close at hand;

◇ **support system development:** The purpose of this method is to provide easy access to sympathetic resources, such as telephone reassurance for elderly who are living alone or homework hotlines for students struggling with the stress of school.

Changing the Environment

Gradually prevention programs began to look beyond individuals to the social and environmental influences on drug use, such as family and peer-group values and practices as well as media influences. Community organization was stressed as a way to ensure cultural sensitivity and to provide local control over prevention efforts, like billboard and advertising distribution controls. Some community programs focused on societal and organizational change, such as altering practices in schools, work situations, organizations, cultures, and society at large. These community-based systems-oriented programs have been effective in getting entire neighborhoods to take responsibility for preventing substance abuse.

Typical community coalition activities include

◇ assessing the needs of the community and the patterns of drug abuse;

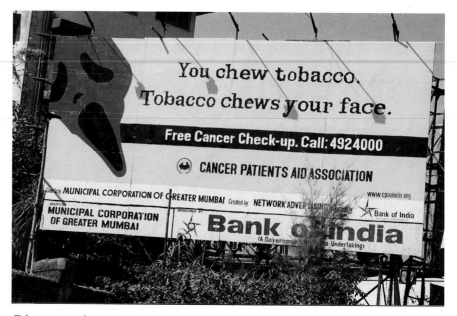

Tobacco use, along with its attendant health consequences, is a greater problem in many countries outside the United States. This modern anti-chewing tobacco advertisement in Bombay, India is in response to a high rate of precancerous oral lesions caused by chewing tobacco, either by itself or with minced betel nut in a mixture called "gutkha."
Courtesy of Shyam Sharma

◇ coordinating existing services to avoid costly redundancy and fill in the service gaps;

◇ changing laws and public policy to reduce availability of alcohol and tobacco;

◇ increasing funding for family, school, and community prevention services;

◇ community-wide training and planning.

(Kumpfer, Goplerud, & Alvarado, 1998)

Public Health Model

As the complexity of prevention efforts increased, a model was needed to better understand the relationships between all elements in society. The result was the public health approach to prevention.

The public health model holds that addiction is a disease in a genetically predisposed host (the actual user) who lives in a contributory environment (the actual location and the social network of the host) in which an agent (the drug or drugs) introduces the disease. Prevention is designed to affect the re-

lationship of these three factors to control addiction (Hoffman, 1998).

For example, programs to regulate cigarette advertising are designed to limit the pervasiveness of the agent in the environment. Programs to raise the drinking age or to have drug-free zones around schools are designed to limit the host's access to the agent. National antismoking, drunk driver, and HIV risk-reduction campaigns, which constitute the bulk of the highly visible programs, seek to limit the influence of the environment on the host.

Other prevention activities aimed at the environment-host relationship are designed to reinforce the emotional strengths and protective elements already existing in people's lives or to improve the economic and emotional environment of those most at risk.

Family Approach

Recently a family-focused approach has been embraced by treatment and prevention specialists. The family approach makes sense since susceptibility to addiction often stems from family dynamics. Family support, skills training, and therapy, along with parenting programs, seem to reduce the risk factors that lead to drug abuse and addiction (Kumpfer et al., 1998). Certainly any process that reduces abuse, decreases parental use of drugs, and helps the family members improve their relationships with each other must be of benefit to a potential abuser. Unfortunately much of the focus is on the potential addict rather than the total environment and relationships that have the greatest effect on susceptibility to addiction.

PREVENTION METHODS

Whatever model is used, a good way to understand the effectiveness of the various approaches to prevent drug abuse and addiction is to examine supply, demand, and harm reduction in more detail.

SUPPLY REDUCTION

Supply reduction seeks to decrease drug abuse by reducing the availability of drugs through regulation, restriction, interdiction, and law enforcement. Supply reduction is the responsibility of

◇ state and local police departments;

◇ the Department of Justice (including the Federal Bureau of Investigation [FBI], the Bureau of Prisons, the Immigration and Naturalization Service [INS], and the Drug Enforcement Administration [DEA]);

◇ the Treasury Department (including the Bureau of Alcohol, Tobacco, and Firearms [ATF], the Internal Revenue Services [IRS], and the Customs Service);

◇ the Department of Transportation (including the U.S. Coast Guard and the Federal Aviation Administration [FAA]);

◇ the Department of Defense.

This complex network of agencies is coordinated by the Office of National Drug Control Policy (ONDCP) and headed by Barry McCaffrey.

Some of the supply reduction activities include

◇ interdicting drug smugglers by air, sea, and highway;

◇ increasing law enforcement activities at border crossings;

◇ interdicting and limiting the supply of precursor chemicals used in the manufacture of illicit drugs (e.g., ephedrine, a precursor of methamphetamines);

◇ funding the addition of 100,000 community police officers;

◇ supporting local and state police in high-intensity drug-trafficking areas (HIDTA) as well as coordinating intelligence information and activities;

◇ identifying, disrupting, and dismantling criminal gangs and organized crime;

◇ supporting and passing more severe laws while trying to make sentencing policies fair;

◇ disrupting money laundering activities and seizing assets of drug dealers to limit the profits from illegal drug activities;

◇ breaking up domestic and foreign sources of supply by supporting eradication and the antidrug efforts of countries like Colombia, Pakistan, and Mexico;

◇ enacting treaties and other international agreements to work conjointly towards supply reduction goals.

(ONDCP, 2000)

Legislation & Legal Penalties

Historically laws to control the use of opium and other drugs did not exist in America prior to the nineteenth century. It wasn't until 1860 that the first antimorphine law was passed and not until 1906 that the Pure Food and Drug Act was passed. In 1914 the Harrison Narcotics Act was passed, enacting the first major drug controls. Since then laws such as the Comprehensive Drug Abuse and Control Act of 1970, the Sentencing Reform Act of 1984, and the Anti-Drug Abuse Acts of 1986 and 1988 established federal guidelines for mandatory minimum sentences including a minimum five-year sentence for possession of five grams of cocaine base.

To curtail drug availability, stiffer penalties that include long prison terms and asset forfeiture, are given to suppliers (those who manufacture, smuggle, and distribute). On the other hand, in the past 15 years, increased jail time just for use has dramatically increased. Legal penalties increase for each conviction for possession. In most states, laws also make it illegal just to possess syringes (Carlson, 1998). Such laws, however, increase the possibility that injection drug users will share needles and increase exposure to blood-borne viruses.

The other aspect of legal approaches to supply reduction is the fact that more than 51% of inmates reported drug use while committing the offense that put them in jail or prison (Mumola, 1998).

Women have been prosecuted because they used dangerous substances during their pregnancy (USA Today, 1998). Prosecution, however, can be counterproductive in that pregnant drug abusers might be less likely to present themselves for prenatal treatment of drug abuse and even normal prenatal care if they fear that they will be jailed or lose their babies. Lack of prenatal care seems to have greater long-term adverse effects on the baby than use of cocaine (Klein & Goldenberg, 1990). Pilot programs in New York City and in Michigan have tied welfare payments to drug testing as a way of routing clients into treatment (Alcoholism & Drug Abuse Weekly, 1999).

The so-called three strikes and you're out law requires a life sentence for three convictions (originally to get habitual violent criminals off the street but later expanded to other crimes). As a result of this and other laws, the prison population (federal, state, and local) has more than tripled between 1980 and

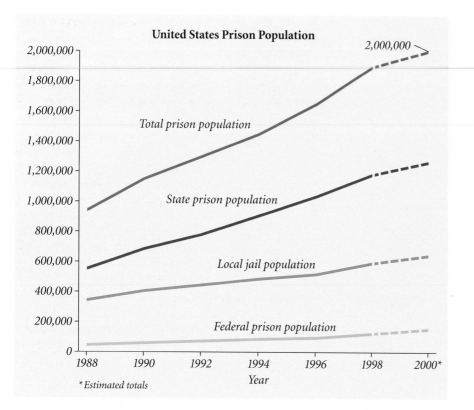

United States Prison Population

Figure 8-1 •

Nearly one in four inmates in state and local prisons or jails is incarcerated for violating a specific drug law. In federal prisons, that figure is close to 60%.

1999 Bureau of Justice Statistics Bulletin

2000 to approximately 2 million (DOJ, 2000). Nearly 60% of the inmates in federal prisons in 1998 were sentenced for drug offenses, up from 53% in 1990 (Beck & Mumola, 1999). Today between 60–80% of those in all prisons are there for drug-related crimes, such as use and possession, for crimes committed under the influence of alcohol or other drugs, and for crimes committed to raise money for a drug habit (ONDCP, 2000; DOJ, 2000).

Sales to minors or sales near schools may earn a perpetrator up to twice the usual sentence. Supply reduction legislation sometimes extends to laws against products made from hemp and to advertising or sales of drug paraphernalia, the devices used to prepare or consume drugs, such as roach clips and bongs sold in so-called "head shops" (Sher, 1999). Governments also promulgate laws that regulate the sale of legal prescription drugs and the availability of alcohol and nicotine. Recent propos-

als target even more precursor chemicals used to manufacture drugs illegally (e.g., ephedrine, ether, sulfuric acid).

Outcomes of Supply Reduction

The successes of supply reduction approaches to the drug problem are debatable. Clearly the estimated 10–15% of drugs that are kept off the market means that a significant amount of illegal drugs never reach the streets (DEA, 1998; ONDCP, 2000). The number of people imprisoned for drug crimes cuts down on the use and distribution of drugs and an unknown number of people are dissuaded from becoming involved with drugs by the threat of imprisonment. Strict policies and strong penalties delay the impulse to use, get people to treatment, and keep people in treatment say the advocates of supply reduction.

Some, however, argue that increased law enforcement, court costs, and implementation of international

drug-policing agreements make this an extremely costly approach with relatively minor impact on the supply. In fact, despite a five-fold increase in federal expenditures for supply reduction efforts since 1986, cocaine is about 25% cheaper today than a decade ago (ONDCP, 2000).

One of the bright spots in law enforcement is the increased use of drug courts to avoid clogging the justice system with thousands of minor drug-use arrests. First-time offenders are diverted to treatment, thus shifting a supply reduction technique to a demand reduction strategy. Further, treatment outcome studies suggest that mandated treatment of drug abuse by law enforcement results in better outcomes than those achieved through voluntary treatment (Anglin, 1988; Nurco, Hanlon, Bateman, & Kinlock, 1995)

DEMAND REDUCTION

The second major area of current prevention strategy has focused on reducing the demand for drugs. Those pursuing demand reduction believe that the health and crime problems associated with drug abuse could be greatly lessened at a fraction of the cost of supply reduction efforts if any of three conditions were met:

1. if individuals never develop an interest in using psychoactive drugs,

2. if those using never progress to abuse or addiction,

3. or if those who abuse drugs or are addicted to them can get treatment and stop their continued use of drugs.

"Drug use is preventable. If children reach adulthood without using illegal drugs, alcohol, or tobacco, they are unlikely to develop a chemical dependency problem later in life. To this end, the strategy seeks to involve parents, coaches, mentors, teachers, clergy, and other role models in a broad prevention campaign."

Barry McCaffrey, Chief, Office of National Drug Control Policy (ONDCP, 2000)

There are three levels of demand reduction (prevention) programs that have been developed to decrease drug abuse. They are primary, secondary, and tertiary prevention.

Primary Prevention

Primary prevention tries to anticipate and prevent initial drug use. It is intended mainly for young people who have little or no experience with alcohol, tobacco, or other drugs, especially those who are most at risk. Its goals are generally to

◇ promote nonuse or abstinence;

◇ help young people refuse drugs;

◇ delay the age of first use, especially of the legal drugs alcohol and tobacco;

◇ encourage healthy nondrug alternatives to achieving altered states of consciousness (for example, Friday night, nonalcoholic dance parties).

Primary prevention involves education about harmful consequences of psychoactive substance use, along with personal skill-building exercises designed to prevent or delay experimentation with abusable drugs. It attempts to instill resistance by teaching skills in coping, decision making, conflict resolution, and other abilities that assist young people from ever using psychoactive substances (Hazelden, 1993). It also undertakes to build self-esteem by examining the roots of susceptibility to addiction and helping children handle the confusion, anger, or pain of growing up. In a broad sense, primary prevention also includes nonpersonal strategies such as legislation, policy formulation, and school curriculum design meant to prevent or delay first use.

Though the importance of primary prevention is universally accepted, outcome evaluation of its effectiveness gives mixed reviews of program results. Controversy also exists over the best way to accomplish this important level of prevention (Kumpfer et al., 1998).

Recently the Office of National Drug Control Policy designed a set of principles upon which good prevention programming can be based.

Secondary Prevention

Secondary prevention seeks to halt use once it has begun. It strives to keep experimental, social/recreational, and habitual use, along with limited abuse, from turning into prolonged abuse and addiction by taking action when symptoms are first recognized. It educates people about specific health effects, legal consequences, and effects on a family. It can also provide counseling.

Secondary prevention adds intervention strategies to education and skill building. Once drug use is recognized, a number of different intervention techniques are employed to engage the user in educational and counseling processes that encourage abstinence and provide skills to avoid further use or abuse.

Drug diversion programs (e.g., drug courts) used at this level of prevention for first-time drug offenders have been proven to be useful and cost-effective. Drug diversion programs route those arrested for possession or use to education and rehabilitation programs instead of jail.

Secondary prevention is somewhat handicapped by two actions typical of drug abusers and even casual users: concealment that makes use more difficult to detect, and denial that prevents the user from acknowledging that there is a problem. On the average, it takes two years for parents to recognize drug use and abuse in their children.

Also complicating secondary prevention is the **lag phase,** the time between first use of a drug and the development of problematic use. The lag phase is particularly long for tobacco since it may take decades for severe

---

TABLE 8–2   EVIDENCE-BASED PRINCIPLES FOR SUBSTANCE ABUSE PREVENTION

A. Address appropriate risk and protective factors for substance abuse in a defined population.

   1. Define a population (e.g., by age, sex, race, and neighborhood).

   2. Assess levels of risk, protection, and substance abuse for that population.

   3. Focus on all levels of risk with special attention to those exposed to high risk and low protection.

B. Use approaches that have been shown to be effective.

   4. Reduce the availability of illicit drugs and of alcohol and tobacco for the underaged.

   5. Strengthen antidrug use attitudes and norms.

   6. Strengthen life skills and drug refusal techniques.

   7. Reduce risk and enhance protection in families by strengthening family skills.

   8. Strengthen social bonding and caring relationships.

   9. Ensure that interventions are appropriate for the populations being addressed.

C. Intervene early at important stages and transitions.

   10. Intervene at developmental stages and life transitions that predict later substance abuse.

   11. Reinforce interventions over time with repeated exposure to accurate and age-appropriate information.

D. Intervene in appropriate settings and domains.

   12. Intervene in appropriate settings that most affect risk, including homes, schools, and peer groups.

E. Manage programs effectively.

   13. Ensure consistency and coverage of programs and policies.

   14. Train staff and volunteers to communicate messages.

   15. Monitor and evaluate programs to verify that goals and objectives are being achieved.

(ONDCP/Prevention, 2000)

health problems to develop after initial smoking begins. Because most drug users describe their initial use of drugs to be enjoyable and problem free, denial and a sense of personal invulnerability to adverse consequences, along with the lag phase, make them less likely to believe that information about harmful effects applies to them.

"I didn't have a clue. Why couldn't I handle this? I never really attributed all the problems that I had to the drinking because I was a periodic drinker, so I could go for periods of abstaining. But once I started, there was always going to be repercussions. So it was hard for me to identify the problems in the beginning."

42-year-old recovering alcoholic

Tertiary Prevention

Tertiary prevention seeks to stop further damage from problematic relationships (especially addiction) with drugs and to restore drug abusers to health. It joins drug abuse treatment with strategies employed in primary and secondary prevention, such as intervention and drug diversion programs. Tertiary prevention seeks to end compulsive drug use with such strategies as

◇ group intervention to engage a person in a treatment program focused on detoxification, abstinence, and recovery;

◇ cue extinction therapy that desensitizes clients to people, places, or things that trigger use;

◇ family therapy (especially for younger users), group psychotherapy, or residential treatment in therapeutic communities;

◇ psychopharmacological strategies like methadone maintenance and drugs that reduce craving;

◇ promotion of a healthy lifestyle;

◇ development of support and aftercare systems, often 12-step programs.

Advocates of demand reduction, while admitting that interdiction decreases the availability of drugs, point out that young people reported alcohol and other drugs to be more available in 1999 than students did in 1980 (University of Michigan, 1999).

"In our experience over the past 30 years, the best and most cost-effective prevention & harm reduction strategy is treatment on demand."

Dr. Darryl Inaba, CEO, Haight-Ashbury Free Clinics

Treatment of alcoholism and drug addiction has been extensively researched and has consistently been documented to be effective. Treatment results in abstinence or decreased drug use in 40–50% of cases, a great reduction in crime (74%), and a savings of $7–$20 for every $1 spent by a community (Gerstein, Johnson, Harwood et al., 1994). Despite these results, funding for treatment programs consistently falls short of meeting the needs of those seeking treatment. (The Haight-Ashbury Detox Clinic in San Francisco alone has over 400 people on their waiting list every month. Only 20–30% of those on its waiting list ever come into treatment at the Clinic, possibly because they initially came for help at their most vulnerable and treatable moment.)

Drug courts have further increased treatment demand without providing more treatment resources. Drug courts are collaborations of the court, prosecution, public defenders, probation officers, treatment providers, and sheriff's department to coordinate treatment and facilitate processing of convicted drug offenders. As of 1998, there were 500 drug courts operating in the United States (Belenko, 1998).

HARM REDUCTION

Harm reduction is a prevention strategy that recognizes the difficulty of getting and keeping people in recovery. It focuses on techniques to minimize the personal and social problems associated with drug use rather than making abstinence the primary goal.

One example of a harm reduction tactic is providing clean syringes to addicts. A panel jointly convened by the National Research Council (NRC) and the National Institute of Medicine (NIM) found that bleach distribution and needle exchange efforts can reduce the spread of the AIDS virus without increasing illegal drug use. It is interesting to note that the study did not say "does reduce" or "has reduced," only that it "can reduce" the spread of AIDS (NRC & NIM, 1995). As of 1999, 47 U.S. states had laws that make it illegal for injection drug users to possess syringes (Blumenthal, Kral, Erringer, & Edlin, 1999). The controversy continues as to whether needle exchange itself actually works. More than 55 needle exchange programs provide approximately 8 million syringes to IV drug users in the United States. In Australia with a population 1/10 that of the United States, 10 million syringes are exchanged from 4,000 outlets. Less than 5% of Australian drug users are HIV positive compared to an estimated 14% in the United States (Wodak & Lurie, 1997). The estimated smaller number of HIV infections in Australia saved about $220 million at a cost of $8 million for the 10 million needles and syringes (Feacham, 1995).

"The reason why we are so intent on needle use is because it's the route to the heterosexual population and to babies. If you can stop the needle from infecting heterosexual men, then you stop most of the cause of the spread to heterosexual women and to babies."

John Newmeyer, Ph.D., drug epidemiologist, Haight-Ashbury Clinic

Another example of harm reduction involves replacing a legal drug addiction for an illegal one as in methadone maintenance programs. These programs have been shown to decrease crime and health problems in the user. In 1999 about 115,000 patients were enrolled in methadone programs, about 15% to 20% of all heroin addicts in the United States. A study by the University of Pennsylvania found that comprehensive methadone treatment combined with intensive counseling reduced illicit drug use by 79%. Clients were also five times less likely to get AIDS (Metzger, Woody, McLellan, et al., 1993). Additionally criminal activity was reduced by 57% while full-time employment increased by 24% (Hubbard, Craddock, Flynn, Anderson, & Etheridge, 1997).

In the broad sense of reducing the harm of use without promoting abstinence, some harm reduction tactics for alcohol and tobacco have already been used. Examples include designated driver programs, encouraging eating when drinking, prohibiting smoking in all public places, regulating alcohol and tobacco advertising, and providing users with information on less harmful ways to use drugs.

These legal drug prevention tactics receive some criticism because they may be misapplied. For example, someone gets even drunker when there is a designated driver, or someone uses moderation as an excuse to break abstinence, or someone augments methadone with alcohol and other drugs to try to get a rush. Harm reduction practices and proposals that are very controversial include

◇ responsible use education that accepts some level of experimental or social use and seeks to inform people of ways of using drugs that minimize dangers;

◇ treatment of addicts merely to reduce their habits to manageable levels;

◇ behavioral management to minimize the amount of drugs used;

◇ permitting addicts to totally design and manage their intervention and treatment processes;

◇ decriminalization or even legalization of all abused drugs.

Some harm reduction tactics also seem to be in conflict with federal drug policy based on zero tolerance (no use of illegal drugs). Changes in laws and policies will probably not be forthcoming soon since many elected officials are afraid of appearing soft on crime and drugs. War on drugs advocates fear that any attempt at decriminalization or legalization would introduce the kind of ambiguity about drugs that prevailed in the 1970s, creating confusion about whether drug use is undesirable and leading inevitably to more drug problems. (*See Chapter 9 for further discussion of harm reduction.*)

"I had a parole officer who told me to leave those other drugs alone. Drinking is O.K. or smoking a little 'pot' now and then but I have come to believe that I can't take any mood-altering chemical into my body today and still remain in recovery. That is still what I stick to and believe in."
Recovering heroin addict

CHALLENGES TO PREVENTION

LEGAL DRUGS IN SOCIETY

For all the effort put into prevention of illicit drug use, we are still primarily an alcohol-drinking, tobacco-smoking, prescription and over-the-counter drug-using society. The social and health problems from alcohol abuse, along with the health problems from tobacco abuse, are far greater than those of illicit drugs. Wisely, drug abuse prevention efforts over the last decade have increased the emphasis on alcohol and tobacco abuse and most recently on behavioral addictions, such as gambling, eating disorders, and sexual addiction that also have devastating effects on society.

Legal drugs, such as tobacco and alcohol, are widely available and actively marketed by sophisticated advertising campaigns that attempt to show the fun to be found in psychoactive drugs and that try to establish brand recognition and brand loyalty at an early age. Joe Camel® and the Budweiser® frogs were examples of familiar cartoonlike characters that targeted young potential smokers and drinkers. The frogs are still around but Joe Camel® is gone. Each year alcohol companies spend over $2 billion and tobacco companies over $6 billion on advertising and promoting their products. This is not surprising since alcohol sales are about $100 billion per year and tobacco sales over $46 billion per year in 1998 (U. S. Department of Agriculture, 1999). (There is something to be learned here. If advertising was successful by targeting age-specific and culture-specific populations, prevention groups can do the same by customizing their messages.)

Billions more are spent advertising over-the-counter drugs, thus promoting the concept that there is a chemical solution for any ailment or discomfort. This two-tiered approach, acceptable and unacceptable drugs, breeds cynicism and disbelief of prevention messages in adolescents and young adults. If prevention messages aren't consistent, they are usually ineffective.

One of the realities of prevention is that there is no quick fix. If modern attempts to reduce smoking began with the first health warnings issued in the mid-1950s, then the success of the anti-smoking efforts have taken almost a half a century and are still developing so as to be more effective. First knowledge must change, then attitudes, and finally practices. These changes can take a generation or more. When change comes, it can be profound—no smoking in public buildings, restaurants, offices, etc. was unheard of a few decades ago.

A second reality of prevention is that the job is never complete. Each year there is a new group entering grammar school, middle school, high school, and college who need to learn or at least be reminded of the potential dangers of smoking, drinking, or using illicit drugs. The rise in adolescent smoking in the last decade is due in part to a diminished antismoking campaign, compared with relatively strenuous efforts conducted in the late '60s through the '70s, such things as public service ads on TV, limitations on tobacco broadcast advertising, and increased cigarette taxes.

Third, any prevention campaign becomes progressively more difficult. Prevention techniques succeed better with people ready to listen—those already predisposed to heed warnings. After initial successes, it becomes harder to penetrate deeper into any particular generation to change attitudes and behaviors.

Another challenge to prevention is that no single approach has been shown to work consistently, probably because there are so many variables that contribute to substance abuse and addiction. There is no doubt that if and when prevention efforts become consistently and documentably successful, they will be cost effective. The difficulty is find-

ing undeniably effective prevention programs.

FUNDING

As previously mentioned, prevention (demand reduction) gets a small share of the total federal expenditure in the war on drugs. It generally receives about 1/3 of the total budget that in 2001 will be $19.1 billion (ONDCP, 2000). Prevention is vastly underfunded especially when compared to the cost of the consequences of alcohol and drug abuse and the moneys committed

to tobacco and alcohol advertising. Cocaine-exposed babies alone are estimated to cost the United States $352 million annually (NIDA Media Advisory, 1998). In 1995 the economic cost of drug and alcohol abuse to the United States was an estimated $276 billion (e.g., lost earnings, health care, and crime control). Another $63.2 billion was diverted from the economy by users to purchase the drugs while the total national expenditure for primary prevention in the same year was just $8 billion (ONDCP, 1999, 2000).

FROM CRADLE TO GRAVE

PATTERNS OF USE

Since drug use affects us directly or indirectly from cradle to grave, by examining the patterns of use of different age groups in our society, it is possible to design prevention programs that have a better chance of success.

AGE OF FIRST USE

Over the past 35 years, one of the most important changes in drug abuse has been the gradual lowering of the age of drug users. This is of particular concern since one of the most reliable indicators of future addiction problems is early-onset drug use. The younger a person starts drugs, the more likely they are to develop addiction problems. A 1999 survey by the University of Michigan found that from 1991–1999, the use of marijuana by 8th graders tripled and the use by 10th graders doubled while the use by 12th graders went up 50%, although use in the past 3 years has leveled off (University of Michigan, 1999). Another measure of increased use (and possible increased law enforcement) is that the percentage of male juvenile arrestees testing positive for any drug except alcohol went from 22% in 1990 to 55% in 1998 (ADAM, 1999).

USE BY RACE & CLASS

Addicts are often portrayed in the media as weak, bad, stupid, crazy, immoral, poor, inner-city dwellers, or as the disenfranchised who have nothing else to turn to except drugs. When drug use is studied on a regional basis, the facts show that rural and small urban areas use as many and in some cases more drugs than large urban areas (SAMHSA/CSAT, 1999). Even in large cities, less than five percent of alcoholics live on skid row in the poor sections of cities. When ethnicity was used as a measure, the differences in overall

drug use were minimal, although the use of some specific drugs is higher in certain ethnic, cultural, economic, or social communities (Joseph & Paone, 1997).

The group least likely to have a substance problem was African Americans. Contrary to common beliefs, urban African Americans who are under 16 years of age and are in school have relatively low rates of use of alcohol and other drugs (SAMHSA, 1999). The relatively high rate of African Americans in prisons suggests that this ethnic group tends to fall prey more readily to the negative aspects of addiction, including the lure of the drug trade. They may also

TABLE 8–3   AVERAGE AGE OF INITIATION OF DIFFERENT SUBSTANCES: 1965–1998

(These figures show the average age of first use among those who have used various drugs.)

Drug	1965	1975	1985	1990	1994	1998
Cigarettes (first use)	16.0 yrs.	15.3 yrs.	15.6 yrs.	15.4 yrs.	15.9 yrs.	15.5 yrs.
Inhalants	14.9	17.4	16.6	16.6	16.2	16.7
Alcohol	17.6	17.1	16.6	16.6	17.3	17.4
Hallucinogens	18.8	19.1	19.3	18.4	17.9	18.7
Marijuana/hashish	18.9	18.5	17.9	17.7	16.9	18.2
Heroin	N/A	19.3	23.8	26.4	21.2	22.3
Cocaine	N/A	21.4	22.4	22.4	21.4	21.7

(SAMHSA, 1999)

be the target of greater enforcement efforts. African Americans with drug problems tend to be incarcerated at a greater rate and receive treatment through the criminal justice system whereas others are more likely to get probation and receive treatment from medical and social service programs.

"They come to Black neighborhoods to cop dope. It's like a pretty regular thing to see wealthy White people go slipping around through there at night. Now 'crack' cocaine is not Black or White. 'Crack' cocaine is dope. It doesn't care who it gets. And it has no inhibitions at all. That dope doesn't have a name on it. I have sat down with people up here and I have sat down with people from down there and when we do dope, it is all the same."
Recovering cocaine addict

Alcoholics and addicts include not only residents in the inner city but also the most skilled, talented, intelligent, and sensitive individuals in our society. For example, physicians are as likely to be as addicted or possibly slightly more so than members of the general population possibly due to accessibility to drugs and a higher income level to make drugs more affordable (Anthony & Hetzer, 1991; Centrella, 1994). Intelligence is not a guaranteed protection against addiction. Members of MENSA, a high-IQ society, also have a relatively high rate of addiction, as do gifted high school students. Members of the American clergy also have a relatively high rate of alcoholism. Even nuns had a higher-than-average incidence of prescription drug abuse. One predictor of cocaine addiction in New York was a high annual income. If people use psychoactive substances, they are liable to addictive disease no matter what race, class, or region of the country they live in. Addiction is a nonbiased equal opportunity disease.

USE BY AGE

The absolute numbers of Americans who used illicit drugs in the past month (13.6 million in a population of

TABLE 8–4   DRUG USE BY AGE GROUP, 1998

Age Group	Ever Ever Used	Used Past Year	Used Past Month
12–17 (23 million)			
Any illicit drug	21.3%	16.4%	9.9%
Cigarettes	35.8%	23.8%	18.2%
Alcohol	37.3%	31.8%	19.1%
18–25 (28 million)			
Any illicit drug	48.1%	27.4%	16.1%
Cigarettes	68.8%	47.1%	41.6%
Alcohol	83.2%	74.2%	60.0%
26–34 (35 million)			
Any illicit drug	50.6%	12.7%	7.0%
Cigarettes	71.8%	36.6%	32.5%
Alcohol	88.2%	74.5%	60.9%
35 & up (132 million)			
Any illicit drug	31.8%	5.5%	3.3%
Cigarettes	75.2%	26.7%	25.1%
Alcohol	86.6%	64.6%	53.1%
Total, 12 & up (218 million)			
Any illicit drug	35.8%	10.6%	6.2%
Cigarettes	68.8%	47.1%	28.8%
Alcohol	81.3%	64.0%	51.7%

National Household Survey on Drug Abuse: Population Estimates 1998 (SAMHSA, 1999)

218 million, 12 and older) may seem small, however, they have an exaggerated effect on all levels of society, especially in regard to economic loss, accidents, assaults, suicides, crime, and domestic or other violence (SAMHSA, 1999; ONDCP, 2000).

In the rest of this chapter, we will examine the consequences of drug use during pregnancy, in school, on the job (including a section on drug testing), by the elderly, and some of the most dangerous consequences of drug use—sexually transmitted diseases, hepatitis C, and AIDS. We will then examine some of the prevention and early intervention programs designed for those groups.

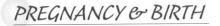

PREGNANCY & BIRTH

OVERVIEW

Drug and alcohol use during pregnancy continues to be a national prob-

lem that results in many infants born with alcohol-related birth defects. Drug abuse during pregnancy occurs in women of all ethnic and socioeconomic backgrounds. According to NIDA (National Institute of Drug Abuse), 18.6% of infants were exposed to alcohol during gestation, 4.5% were exposed to cocaine, 17.4% to marijuana, and 37.6% to tobacco (NIDA, 1994; Young, 1997). Fetal alcohol syndrome (FAS) is the third most common birth defect and the leading cause of mental retardation in the United States. Most psychoactive substances may be harmful to the developing fetus. Problems associated with substance abuse during pregnancy are now beginning to be understood.

In the California Perinatal Substance Exposure Study in 1991–1993, the California Department of Alcohol and Drug Programs tried to determine the prevalence of drug-exposed newborns (Table 8-5). While these rates are high, the actual exposure is probably

TABLE 8–5   PERCENTAGE OF INFANTS BORN EXPOSED TO DRUGS

Substance	Asian & Pacific Islander	African American	Hispanic	White	Other	All
Alcohol	5.07	11.58	6.87	6.05	4.03	6.72%
Tobacco	1.73	20.12	3.29	14.82	4.81	8.82%
Prescription drugs	1.49	2.38	1.26	1.96	1.31	1.71%
All illicit drugs	0.39	11.90	1.51	4.92	1.57	3.49%
Marijuana	0.21	4.59	0.61	3.25	1.21	1.88%
Cocaine	0.06	7.79	0.55	0.60	0.20	1.11%
Opioids	0.34	2.54	1.06	1.59	1.11	1.47%
Amphetamines (illicit & legal)	0.06	0.19	0.35	1.32	0.24	0.66%
Total Positives (excluding tobacco)	14.22%	24.02%	9.37%	12.28%	6.76%	11.35%

Source: California Perinatal Substance Exposure Study, 1993 (Noble, Vega, Kolody, Porter, Hwang, Merk, & Bole, 1997)

even higher since most drugs are nondetectable three days after exposure. If one looks at drug use at various times during pregnancy, the use of alcohol is higher (Fig. 8–2).

Maternal Risks

Historically the effects of drugs and alcohol on women, including periods of pregnancy when drug use also affects the fetus, have been poorly researched. Even when female opium and morphine addicts outnumbered male addicts at the beginning of the twentieth century, most treatment facilities were aimed at men (Worth, 1991; Young, 1997). In fact, although damage to the fetus due to drinking has been recognized since ancient times, the identification of a specific clinical syndrome, fetal alcohol syndrome (FAS), was not identified until 1973 (Jones & Smith, 1973). Starting in the 1980s interest and research on perinatal effects of drugs increased, as did funding by the National Institute of Drug Abuse (NIDA), the National Institutes of Health (NIH), and other governmental agencies.

When added to the normal stresses and medical complications of pregnancy, drug and alcohol abuse during this period puts women at even higher risk for medical and obstetrical compli-

cations. Some conditions aggravated in a pregnant woman include anemia, sexually transmitted diseases, diabetes, high blood pressure, and poor nutrition. Intravenous use of heroin, cocaine, amphetamines, and other drugs increases risk for additional complications, such as hepatitis, endocarditis (a heart infection), or even fetal death (Miller, 1998; Briggs et al., 1986). Contaminated needles further increase the risk of a woman becoming infected with the HIV or he-

patitis C viruses and passing the disease to her fetus. Eighty percent of children with the HIV virus in the United States were born to mothers who were or are IV drug abusers or sexual partners of IV drug abusers. That figure jumps to 90% worldwide in infants and children. The life expectancy of an infant born with HIV is less than two years. Surprisingly, in the United States, if AZT (an AIDS drug) therapy is used, only 8% of the newborns will be infected with the virus. If AZT is not used, there is a 25% infection rate (NIAID, 1995). In underdeveloped countries, that rate jumps to 35–40% (JAMA, 1999; Quinn, 1996; UN-AIDS, 1998; CDC, 1998).

Multiple drug use is now commonplace and can further complicate a pregnancy. A typical pregnant drug addict is often in poor health and presents herself for treatment late in pregnancy. She often has had no prenatal care or medical intervention and often lives a chaotic lifestyle. A further complication of drug use is adolescents who become pregnant. Of the more than 1 million adolescent females who become pregnant annually, about 10% use psychoactive drugs besides alcohol (Marques & McKnight, 1991). Even without the complicating factors of drug use, the infants of adolescent mothers are at higher risk than those born to women

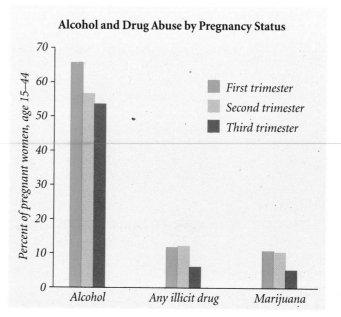

Alcohol and Drug Abuse by Pregnancy Status

Figure 8-2•

Notice that in the first and second trimesters when the fetus is most vulnerable, drug use, particularly alcohol use, is much higher than just before birth.

Office of Applied Studies, National Household Survey on Drug Abuse, 1998. Unpublished Data (SAMHSA, 1998, 1999)

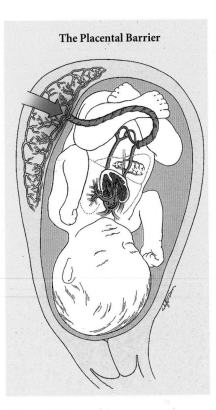

The Placental Barrier

Figure 8-3•

The developing baby and its circulation are protected by the placental barrier that screens out substances that would affect the fetus. All psychoactive drugs breach this protective barrier and affect the baby, usually much more than the mother.

over 18. All areas of functioning are affected since the adolescent herself has not yet developed physically, emotionally, or behaviorally (Hechtman, 1989; Kaminer, 1994).

Fetal & Neonatal Complications

Psychoactive drugs can easily cross the multiple cell layers of the membrane separating the baby's and the mother's blood, the placental barrier (Fig. 8-3). So a fetus is exposed to the same chemicals that a mother uses. After birth, many drugs can pass into a nursing mother's breast milk and expose a nursing infant to dangerous chemicals.

Because of the fetus's and subsequently infant's metabolic immaturity, each surge of effects from the psychoactive drug that the mother injects, ingests, snorts, or smokes may be pro-

longed in the fetus, causing greater problems for the fetus than for the mother.

The period of maximum fetal vulnerability is the first 12 weeks. During this first trimester, development and differentiation of cells into fetal limbs and organs occur. This is when drugs pose the greatest risk to organ development. Because the central and peripheral nervous systems develop throughout the entire pregnancy, the fetus is vulnerable to neurological damage no matter when a woman uses drugs. The second trimester involves further maturation of the already developed body parts. Drug exposure at this stage creates a risk of abnormal bleeding or spontaneous abortion. The third trimester includes maturation of the fetus and preparation for birth. Dangerous drugs such as heroin or cocaine can cause severe withdrawal in the newborn and perhaps premature birth. Since drugs can have such a magnified effect on the fetus throughout pregnancy, it is crucial that a pregnant woman abstain from all unnecessary drug exposure.

The immaturity of the fetus's metabolic system also causes drugs to remain in the fetus for a longer period and in higher concentrations than in the mother. Diazepam (Valium®) or cocaine and their metabolites may remain in the fetus's or newborn's system for days, even weeks longer than in the mother. Because of the persistence of the drug in the neonate's system, intoxication or withdrawal in a baby born exposed to PCP may last for days, weeks, or even months after birth. The problems of fetal drug exposure extend beyond the period of pregnancy. Many babies are born with compromised immune systems due to drug use. Definite syndromes of neonatal withdrawal, intoxication, and developmental or learning delays have been attributed to a variety of drugs, including alcohol (Finnegan & Kandall, 1997). In a Florida study, the cost of newborn care of those affected by drugs was more than double the normal cost of care for newborns, $11,188 vs. $4,741 (AHCA, 1999).

Long-Term Effects

Research is still being done on the long-term effects in drug-exposed children when they enter school. Symptoms range from convulsive disorders in the most extreme cases, to poor muscular control and cognitive skills, hyperactivity, difficulty concentrating or remembering, violence, apathy, and lack of emotion. The good news is that recent research indicates that the majority of drug-exposed babies who receive prenatal, perinatal, and postnatal care, along with continued pediatric services, manage to catch up in their development to other non-drug-exposed children after a slow start (Kaltenbach & Finnegan, 1989). Even without care, some of the effects are reversible. In a study in Ottawa, Canada, children of moderate-drinking mothers showed lower cognitive scores at 36 months but not at 48, 60, or 72 months (Fried, O'Connel, & Watkinson, 1992). Though many of the effects not only of alcohol but of other drugs are reversible, the cost of necessary intensive care is high.

SPECIFIC DRUG EFFECTS

Despite difficulties with scientific research on fetal effects of drug use during pregnancy, medical scientists have identified prenatal and postnatal symptoms and conditions due to specific psychoactive drugs.

Alcohol (*see Chapter 5 for complete coverage of alcohol's neonatal effects*)

Alcohol's effect on the developing fetus is the most widely researched drug in relation to pregnancy. Fetal alcohol syndrome (FAS) is a definite pattern of physical, mental, and behavioral abnormalities in children born to mothers who drank heavily during pregnancy. Symptoms include retarded growth (reduced height, weight, head circumference, brain growth, and brain size) facial deformities (specifically shortened eyelids, thin upper lip, flattened midface, groove in the upper lip), occasional problems with heart and limbs, delayed intellectual development, neurological abnormalities, behavioral problems, visual problems, hearing loss, and balance or gait problems (Sokol & Clarren, 1989).

The incidence of fetal alcohol syndrome (FAS), fetal alcohol effects (FAE), and other abnormalities is well documented. Statistics show that anywhere from 0.33 to 2.9 cases per 1,000 live births have FAS. In the United States, African Americans have an incidence of 6 FAS births per 1,000; Asians, Hispanics, and Whites about 1–2; and Native Americans about 10–30 (May, 1996; Hans, 1998).

Dr. Sterling K. Clarren and his associates at Children's Hospital in Seattle located and interviewed 80 mothers of children with FAS. They asked them about 2,000 questions to get a profile of the patients.

"What we learned was really startling—100% of them had been severely physically and sexually abused. About 60% of it occurring before they were adults and the rest as adults. About 80% of them had major mental health diagnoses and not just one but many. The average patient had 6 distinct mental health diagnoses made through the DSM-IV system. Some of them had more than 10. Schizophrenia, manic depression, phobias, posttraumatic stress disorder, and on and on."

Dr. Sterling K. Clarren (Clarren, 1999)

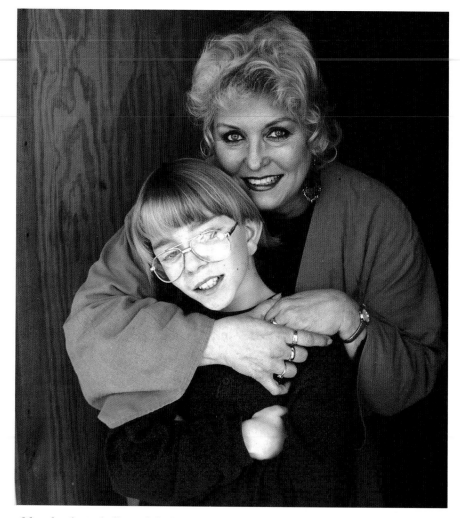

Often the physical effects of alcohol are not obvious as one can see on this child diagnosed with FAS (fetal alcohol syndrome).

Courtesy of Sterling K. Clarren, M.D., Children's Hospital, Seattle

Cocaine & Amphetamines

Currently in the United States, about 200,000 regular heavy cocaine and "crack" abusers are women (the number is growing yearly) with an average age in the early 20s, the most fertile childbearing years (SAMHSA, 1999). A percentage of these women use cocaine during pregnancy, although the rates vary widely from hospital to hospital and among different ethnic groups. In the 1980s when cocaine use was at its highest levels, it was estimated that about 4.5% of infants were exposed to cocaine in utero (Gomby & Shiono, 1991). Other studies show that from 15–25% of babies born in some inner-city hospitals are born cocaine affected (Bateman & Heagarty, 1989). The recent increase of amphetamine abuse will certainly result in increased numbers of pregnancies affected by this stimulant.

"My one year old was born toxic. She had 'crack' in her system, and the hospital called CPS (Child Protective Services), and they kept her, and then I figured it was time for me to stop this. I went into recovery a month after that."

24-year-old recovering "crack" user

The stimulants cocaine and amphetamines increase heart rates and constrict blood vessels, causing dramatic elevations in blood pressure in both mother and fetus. Constriction of blood vessels reduces the flow of blood, nutrients, and oxygen to the placenta and fetus, sometimes resulting in retarded fetal development, especially when the mother is a habitual user or addicted. Increased maternal and placental blood pressure can, in rare cases, cause the placenta to separate prematurely from the wall of the uterus (abruptio placenta), usually resulting in spontaneous abortion or premature delivery, life threatening for both mother and fetus.

Acutely elevated blood pressure in

the fetus can also cause a stroke in the brain of the fetus. Fetal blood vessels in the brain are very fragile and may be easily damaged by exposure to cocaine and particularly amphetamines. Third trimester use of cocaine can induce sudden fetal activity, uterine contractions, and premature labor within minutes after a mother's ingesting cocaine (Plessinger & Woods, 1998).

Although there is no specific set of physical abnormalities connected to cocaine or amphetamine use during pregnancy, exposed babies can be growth retarded with smaller heads, genito-urinary tract abnormalities, severe intestinal disease, and abnormal sleep and breathing patterns (Cherukuri, Minkoff, Feldman, Parekh, & Glass, 1989).

Infants exposed to cocaine during pregnancy often go through a withdrawal syndrome characterized by extreme agitation, increased respiratory rates, hyperactivity, and occasional seizures. Because these babies are in withdrawal, intoxicated, or both, they are highly irritable, difficult to console, tremulous, and deficient in their ability to interact with their environment. Many of these initial effects disappear within a few weeks after birth, assuming the mother is not nursing with cocaine-contaminated milk.

Infants exposed to cocaine, when studied at 3, 12, 18, and 24 months, seemed to require more stimulation to increase arousal and attention but were less able to control higher states of arousal than unexposed children (Mayes, Grillon, Granger, & Schottenfeld, 1998). A study of 150 cocaine-exposed infants also found that the amount of alertness and attentiveness was directly related to the amount of cocaine used during pregnancy (Eyler, Behnke, Conlon, Woos, & Wobie, 1998). Many of these infants show some patterns of neurobehavioral disorganization, irritability, and poorer language development. These infants may also have a slightly higher incidence of sudden infant death syndrome (SIDS), although it is often hard to separate environmental and nutritional factors from the direct effects of drugs (Finnegan & Kandall, 1997).

A study of 69 amphetamine-using pregnant women showed a high perinatal mortality rate, high incidence of health complications, low birthweight, several congenital malformations, and neurological abnormalities (Eriksson, Larsson, & Zetterstrom, 1981). A later study also found a connection between increased amphetamine use and poor psychometric testing (aggressive behavior and problems with adjustment) (Billing, Eriksson, Jonsson, Steneroth, & Zetterstrom, 1994). As with cocaine, many of the problems resolved themselves within a few years, although more longitudinal studies are needed that search for more subtle and long-term problems.

There is hope for parents, educators, and others involved with the education and care of these children. Many abnormal neurobehavioral effects improve over the first three years of life. Recent studies suggest that earlier predictions of severely impaired cocaine babies have been exaggerated. Cocaine does harm the fetus, especially when the mother is a heavy user but most children prenatally exposed to cocaine will have more normal behavior by the age of three than was feared. However, reports of attention deficit disorder and low frustration levels are related by teachers and parents (Harvard, 1998).

Opioids

Physical dependence on opioids leads to more long-term use, so the effects on the fetus seem greater than with binge drugs such as cocaine. People addicted to heroin, morphine, codeine, meperidine (Demerol®), hydrocodone (Vicodin®), oxycodone (Percodan®) and other opioids have a greater risk for fetal growth retardation, miscarriages, stillbirths, abruptio placenta as well as severe infections from intravenous use, e.g., endocarditis, septicemia, hepatitis, and, of course, AIDS.

For pregnant heroin users, the periods of daily withdrawal that alternate with the rushes following each drug injection cause dramatic fluctuations in autonomic functions in the fetus, believed to harm the fetus and contribute to maternal/fetal complications. Babies born to heroin-addicted mothers are often premature, smaller, and weaker than normal (Fulroth, Phillips, & Durand, 1989). Prenatal exposure to heroin has also been associated with abnormal neurobehavioral development. These infants have abnormal sleep patterns and are at greater risk for crib death, sudden infant death syndrome (SIDS). A 600% increase in SIDS deaths was found in a study of 16,409 drug-exposed infants in New York City (Kandall, Gaines, Habel, Davidson, & Jessop, 1993).

If a mother becomes truly addicted to opioids, so does the fetus. Depending on the mother's daily dose of shorter-acting opioids, such as heroin, a majority (60% to 80%) of opioid-exposed infants exhibit the neonatal abstinence syndrome (withdrawal) 48–72 hours after birth (Finnegan & Ehrlich, 1990). With longer-acting opioids, such as methadone, it can take 1–2 weeks. Symptoms include hyperactivity, irritability, incessant high-pitched crying, increased muscle tone, hyperactive reflexes, sweating, tremors, irregular sleep patterns, increased respiration, uncoordinated and ineffectual sucking and swallowing, sneezing, vomiting, and diarrhea. In severe cases, failure to thrive, seizures, or even death may occur. These withdrawal effects may be mild or severe and may last from days to months (Kandall, 1998).

Since the onset of symptoms varies, close observation of the opioid-exposed neonate is necessary. Most cases of neonatal narcotic withdrawal can be treated with good nursing care, loose swaddling in a side-lying position, quiet and dimly lit surroundings, good nutrition, and normal maternal/ infant bonding behaviors. Opioids have been found in breast milk in sufficient concentration to expose newborns. Only in severe cases is medication required for the infant and then it should be a milder opioid such as tincture of opium (Kandall, 1993).

Marijuana

Marijuana is used by 5% to 10% of pregnant women during their pregnancy. Recent research has found high levels of anandamide in the uterus of mice and suggests that this neurotransmitter, mimicked by marijuana, helps regulate the early stages of pregnancy. They found that high levels of anandamide inhibit the progression of the fertilized egg from blastocyst stage to embryo (Paria, Das, & Dey, 1995; Paria et al., 1999; Schmid et al., 1997). These discoveries might give a better understanding of the process of gestation but they also suggest that the use of marijuana (that slots into anandamide receptors) might disrupt the development process.

Most marijuana exposure in newborns goes undetected or is masked by the use of other drugs that can also cause problems. Some studies have reported reduced fetal weight gain, shorter gestations, and some congenital anomalies, however, most studies have found minimal developmental effects in regards to motor skills and mental functioning (Richardson, Day, & Goldschmidt, 1995). However, long-term development studies (Ottawa Prospective Prenatal Study) showed that intrauterine exposure to marijuana led to poorer short-term memory and verbal reasoning at age three (Day, Richardson, Goldschmidt, et al., 1994; Richardson, 1998). Between the ages of 5–6 and 9–12 years, according to the Ottawa study, marijuana-exposed children scored somewhat lower on verbal and memory performance tests, impulsive/hyperactive behavior, conduct problems, and distractibility. They also scored lower on tasks associated with executive function—the individual's ability to plan ahead, anticipate, and suppress behaviors that are incompatible with a current goal (Fried et al., 1992; Fried & Watkinson, 1997; Fried, Watkinson, & Gray, 1998).

Many of the problems with marijuana have to do with the delivery system—marijuana is smoked and therefore limits oxygen to the body and fetus, irritates alveoli and bronchii, and causes babies to weigh about 3.4 ounces less on average (Zuckerman, Frank, Hingson, et al., 1989; Fried, 1995).

"Smoking marijuana, that was the big one. It has caused behavioral problems for my children. I think that it has affected their ability to learn and remember, based on what I deal with today with them."
35-year-old mother of three

Since there are withdrawal symptoms after ceasing heavy or long-term use of marijuana and since the fetus is also exposed, it is logical to assume that neonates would exhibit withdrawal symptoms. Anecdotal reports relate that these marijuana-exposed babies had abnormal responses to light and visual stimuli, increased tremulousness, "startles," and a high-pitched cry associated with drug withdrawal. Unlike infants undergoing narcotic withdrawal, marijuana babies were not excessively irritable. New research is needed to reevaluate the risk of current higher-potency marijuana on pregnancy and the fetus.

Prescription & Over-the-Counter Drugs

Over-the-counter and prescribed medications are the most common drugs used by pregnant women. About 2/3 of all pregnant women take at least one drug during pregnancy, usually vitamins or simple analgesics, such as aspirin. Medications to treat maternal discomfort, anxiety, pain, or infection must be prescribed carefully, for a variety of prescription drugs are harmful to the human fetus. Sedative-hypnotics are among the most studied of these drugs.

Benzodiazepines such as diazepam (Valium®) or alprazolam (Xanax®) accumulate in the fetal blood at more dangerous levels than in maternal blood at dosages normally safe for the mother alone. Besides high fetal drug concentrations, excretion is also slower. The drugs and their metabolites remain in fetal and newborn systems days or even weeks longer than in the mother, resulting in dangerously high concentrations of the drug, leading to fetal depression, abnormal heart patterns, or rarely, death.

In the Physician's Desk Reference (PDR) under alprazolam, the warnings read:

"Because of experience with other members of the benzodiazepine class, Xanax® is assumed to be capable of causing an increased risk of congenital abnormalities when administered to a pregnant woman during the first trimester. Because use of these drugs is rarely a matter of urgency, their use during the first trimester should almost always be avoided. The possibility that a woman of childbearing potential may be pregnant at the time of institution of therapy should be considered."
(PDR, 2000)

A newborn addicted to benzodiazepines may exhibit a variety of neonatal complications. Infants may be floppy, have poor muscle tone, be lethargic, and have sucking difficulties. A withdrawal syndrome, similar to narcotic withdrawal, may also result and may persist for weeks.

Studies have indicated an increased risk of cleft lip and/or cleft palate when diazepam was used in the first six months of pregnancy. Because diazepam and its active metabolites are excreted into breast milk, it has been thought to cause lethargy, mental sedation/depression, and weight loss in nursing infants. Because diazepam and other benzodiazepines can accumulate in breast-fed babies, its use in lactating women is ill advised.

Barbiturates are also to be avoided during pregnancy.

"Barbiturates can cause fetal damage when administered to a pregnant woman. Retrospective case-controlled studies have suggested a connection between the maternal consumption of barbiturates and a higher-than-expected incidence of fetal abnormalities."
(PDR, 2000)

Withdrawal symptoms occur in infants born to mothers who receive barbiturates throughout the last trimester of pregnancy. Withdrawal symptoms include hyperactivity, disturbed sleep, tremors, and hyperreflexia. Prolonged withdrawal can be treated through tapering the infant with phenobarbital over a period of two weeks.

Anticonvulsants such as phenytoin (Dilantin®) increase a pregnant woman's chances of delivering a child with congenital defects such as cleft lip, cleft palate, and heart malformation. Consequently, the physician must carefully weigh the dangers of seizures vs. the chances of congenital defects in the neonate. Pregnancy also alters the absorption of the drug, so there is a chance of more frequent seizures (PDR, 2000).

Even antibiotics such as tetracycline can cause a variety of adverse effects. For example, the PDR says:

"The use of drugs of the tetracycline class during tooth development in the last half of pregnancy, infancy, and childhood to the age of eight years may cause permanent discoloration of the teeth (yellow-gray-brown)."
(PDR, 2000)

Many over-the-counter medications contain stimulants such as caffeine and ephedrine and their use should also be carefully monitored by the pregnant woman and the physician.

Nicotine

In the overall population, the percentage of women who smoked in the past month has steadily increased from 5% in the 1920s to 28.2% in 1997 but finally dropped to 25.7% in 1998. In comparison, smoking by males decreased from 50% to about 29.7% during the same period (SAMHSA, 1999). In an earlier study, the percentage of pregnant women who were using tobacco at the time they gave birth was 8.82%. The highest rates were among African Americans (20.12%) and Whites (14.2%) (Noble et al., 1997).

Smoking during pregnancy is particularly dangerous because tobacco smoke contains more than 2,000 different compounds including nicotine and carbon monoxide. Both have been shown to cross the placental barrier and reduce the fetal supply of oxygen. In addition smoking is a continual activity—one, two, or three packs-a-day—so the impact on the fetus is constant.

Recent studies now indicate that women smokers with a heavy habit are about twice as likely to miscarry and have spontaneous abortions as nonsmokers. Nicotine damages the placenta and has adverse effects on the developing fetus. Stillbirth rates are also higher among smoking mothers (Cook, Petersen, & Moore, 1994).

As with many other psychoactive substances, smoking decreases newborn birthweights. Babies born to mothers who smoke heavily weigh on the average 200 grams (7 ounces) less, are 1.4 centimeters shorter, and have a smaller head circumference compared to babies from nonsmoking or non-drug-abusing mothers (Martin, 1992). Although the incidence of physical birth defects is very low in babies born to smoking mothers, there is still a significant increase in cleft palate and congenital heart defects. Smoking leads to potential minor brain and nerve defects that may be hard to detect. Because nicotine is toxic and creates lesions in that part of animal brains that controls breathing, it is given as one possible reason for the increase in SIDS (sudden infant death syndrome or crib death) seen in babies born to mothers who smoke heavily (Jaffe & Shopland, 1995).

Babies born to heavy smokers have been shown to have increased nervous nursing (weaker sucking reflex) and possibly a depressed immune system at birth, resulting in more pneumonia and bronchitis, sleep problems, and less alertness than other infants.

Long-lasting effects of smoking exposure before birth can include lower IQ and cognitive ability, along with lower verbal, reading, and mathematical skills (Rush & Callahan, 1989). There is even some association with smoking

during pregnancy and the incidence of attention deficit/hyperactivity disorder (Milberger, Biederman, Faraone, & Jones, 1998).

Caffeine

Neonates, newborns, and infants have less tolerance for caffeine than adults do. In addition pregnant women have decreased ability to metabolize methylxanthines, so the stimulatory effects of caffeine last longer in the fetus. No long-lasting effects have been found but physicians recommend avoiding caffeine during pregnancy.

Prevention

Since drugs can have such a magnified effect on the fetus throughout pregnancy, it is crucial that a pregnant woman abstain from all unnecessary drug exposure.

It is estimated that only 55% of women of childbearing age know about fetal alcohol syndrome, although as many as 375,000 children every year may be impacted by their mother's drug use. Reaching pregnant women with appropriate prevention messages, through OB/GYN health professionals, prenatal and well-baby clinics, and public service messages, is essential to reducing the effects of alcohol and drug use on babies (NIDA, 1994).

Many professionals feel that if a drug-abusing pregnant woman can be gotten off drugs in the third trimester, the baby will not be born addicted and will not have to go through detoxification. Most prevention professionals agree that because the effects of alcohol on a developing fetus are not yet fully known, clear multiple warnings to women not to drink or use drugs if they are pregnant or planning pregnancy should be given. Complete abstinence is the safest choice.

A challenge to prevention exists in some states where mothers have been convicted of drugging babies or have lost custody of their children. Some experts fear that such measures encourage pregnant addicts to avoid prenatal clinics and doctors and to give birth outside hospitals to avoid imprisonment or loss of their children. Other ju-

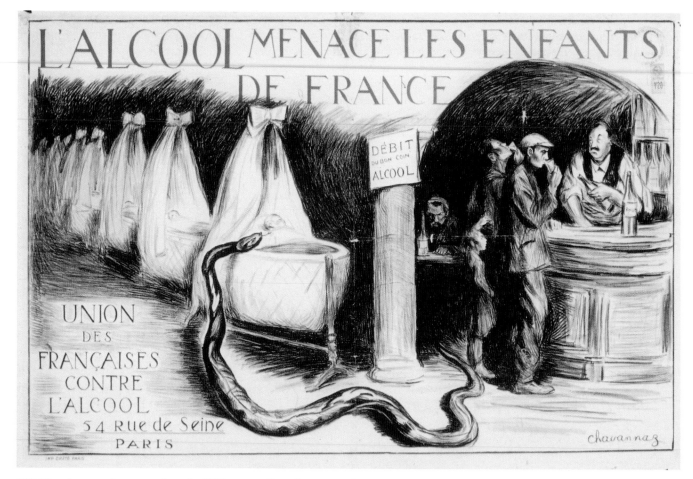

This French prevention poster from the 1920s warns about the impact of parental alcohol use on infants.
Courtesy of the National Library of Medicine, Bethesda

risdiction use a treatment alternative to jail. It has been suggested that if women do not have to give up their babies when they enter treatment, the treatment option will be more acceptable.

YOUTH & SCHOOL

In spite of all the headlines about "crack," MDMA, and methamphetamine use among adolescents and college students, the <u>most serious drug problem by far is still alcohol. Tobacco is a close second and marijuana third.</u>

"In high school we'd have 'keggers.' We found out whose parents wouldn't be home, have a keg delivered, and have the party there. In college the drug

scene was a little different; besides the alcohol, you could get a better selection of drugs: opium, hashish, mescaline, peyote, LSD, but mostly just marijuana. We were too poor in high school for those."
19-year-old college sophomore

A problem with high school, college, and other drug surveys is that many users lie about or minimize their use of drugs even when assured that the survey is confidential. This is part of the denial process. What has been found is that most figures on current or frequent use of illicit drugs in high schools and colleges are underreported (Comerci, 1998).

"We were supposed to put on a skit about drugs and the minute we sat

down we said, 'Now what do the parents want to hear about that?' That's the general attitude all my friends have in dealing with these programs, 'What do the parents want to hear from us?' And a lot of the people teaching these drug programs are also telling us what they think the parents want us to hear. It's all very stereotypical."
15-year-old high school student

The other problem with doing surveys is that problematical use means different things for different people and for different drugs. For example, if a college freshman gets drunk only on Friday and Saturday nights, usually leading to a fight or unprotected sex, the student would probably swear that he or she doesn't have a drinking problem. But by the definition of abuse, that kind of drinking is a problem.

With cocaine, if a student goes on a three-day binge just once a month, spends all available money on the drug, and has nothing left for food or textbooks, that also could be defined as abuse. The true value of youth surveys is that they show trends in drug use, so it is possible to see changes from year to year in order to have a sense of where our society is headed. Surveys also give us a rough benchmark for measuring the effectiveness of the prevention efforts we as a society are expending.

ADOLESCENTS & HIGH SCHOOL

How Serious Is the Problem?

Several ideas present themselves when we look at the figures about drug use in adolescents (Fig. 8-4). Besides the high prevalence of the legal drugs, alcohol and tobacco, with all their at-

tendant health consequences, the use of marijuana has continued to rise since 1990 after dropping almost in half, in the 1980s. Next the recent increases in legal and illegal drug use by young people show that effective prevention efforts are needed more than ever.

Much of the alcohol and other drug use in high schools is experimental, social, or habitual with bouts of abuse. However, most students haven't had enough time for addiction to occur. Unfortunately they also don't have much experience and maturity in their drinking and drug taking habits, so inappropriate use, including intoxication, drunk driving, and unsafe sex is more likely. Another factor that can lead to inappropriate use is when young people drink or take drugs to control emotional turmoil and they don't look on it as dangerous. Part of the reason is society's contradictory attitudes toward legal psychoactive drugs.

"There is no way that you are going to get a majority of teenagers to say

alcohol is an evil substance. That's because it's legal to buy. And how can you say that cigarettes are evil or awful things when everyone over 18 can buy them?"
17-year-old high school student

Finally, because many adolescents think of themselves as invulnerable to the consequences of use, their level of concern is lower than that of older users. Whereas the majority of teenagers who experiment with drugs will not become addicted, some will and for them the legal, psychological, and physical effects of psychoactive drugs will cause problems (they can also cause problems for social and habitual users). Some of the problems are

◇ 70% of teen suicides involve alcohol or drugs;

◇ 50% of date rapes involve alcohol (victim and/or rapist);

◇ 40% of drownings involve alcohol.

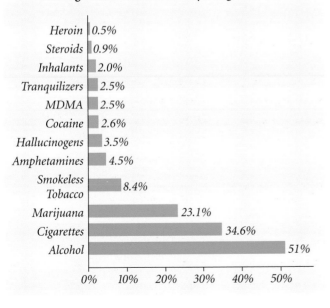

U.S. High School Seniors 30-Day Drug Use – 1999

Drug	Percentage
Heroin	0.5%
Steroids	0.9%
Inhalants	2.0%
Tranquilizers	2.5%
MDMA	2.5%
Cocaine	2.6%
Hallucinogens	3.5%
Amphetamines	4.5%
Smokeless Tobacco	8.4%
Marijuana	23.1%
Cigarettes	34.6%
Alcohol	51%

Figure 8-4•
Since 1992, decreased funding, greater availability of drugs, and a tolerance to drug use have led to sharp increases in drug use among high school seniors as well as 8th and 10th graders.
University of Michigan, 1999

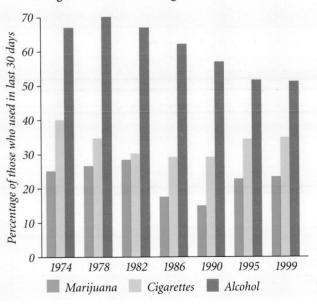

U.S. High School Seniors Drug Use Trend – 1974–1999

Figure 8-5•
This graph compares the change in the 30-day use of alcohol, marijuana, and tobacco over the last 20 years by high school seniors.
University of Michigan, 1999

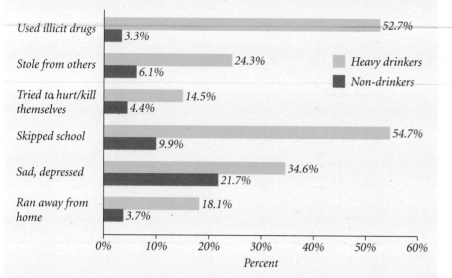

Past Month Adolescent Heavy Drinking and Emotional/Behavioral Problems

Used illicit drugs — 52.7% / 3.3%
Stole from others — 24.3% / 6.1%
Tried to hurt/kill themselves — 14.5% / 4.4%
Skipped school — 54.7% / 9.9%
Sad, depressed — 34.6% / 21.7%
Ran away from home — 18.1% / 3.7%

Heavy drinkers
Non-drinkers

0% 10% 20% 30% 40% 50% 60%
Percent

Figure 8-6•
A survey of 12–17 year olds showed that heavy drinkers were more likely to have emotional and behavioral problems. Some of the problems led to experimentation and eventually heavy use of alcohol while others were caused by the heavy use itself.
SAMHSA, 2000

Crime

The biggest effect of alcohol and drug use is on crime. In some cities, the youth guidance centers or juvenile halls are clogged because of crimes related to drugs. Nationally, according to the Arrestee Drug Abuse Monitoring Program, in 1998 more than half of juvenile male arrestees tested positive for one or more illegal drugs, with marijuana being by far the most frequent (ADAM, 1999). If the authorities had also tested for alcohol, the figures would be much higher. It has been estimated that the cost of youth alcohol abuse is more than $58 billion (e.g., $36 billion in violent crime, $18 billion in traffic accidents).

"We're not immortal. We know that we can die but life for us is not as meaningful as for adults who have kids and responsibilities. If I die, only my friends and my family would be sad but it's not like I'm skipping out on anyone as if I were a parent or had a big position in a company."
16-year-old high school student

The Effects of Drugs on Maturation

In the United States, levels of legal and illegal substance abuse among teenagers are estimated to be the highest found in any developed country in the world. If true, this trend is particularly alarming from two perspectives: first, drug use among our youth gives us a preview of future levels of drug abuse in our society and second, since teenagers are still maturing and developing physically, drugs are generally more toxic and cause disruption of psychological and emotional growth.

"When you begin to use drugs around 12, 13, or 14, you never have rites of passage. You never get indoctrinated into the adulthood of society. Many people that we talk to who come into treatment actually began using substances at that age, so their rites of passage haven't yet occurred when we see them at 30 or 35. And essentially, we're talking to a 14—15 year old in a

30- to 35-year-old body, and that's where we have to begin."
Counselor, Haight-Ashbury Detox Clinic

When drugs or alcohol are commonly used in adolescence to avoid feelings, drown out problems, or as a shortcut to feeling good, then young people will not fully learn how to deal with their emotions and life's problems without psychoactive substances. They will not learn patience, they will not learn that emotional pain can be accepted and used to grow on, and they will learn that doing things they don't like to do, such as studying or chores, are part of the maturation process.

Risk-Focused & Resiliency-Focused Prevention for Adolescents

Recent studies indicate that a number of conditions put adolescents more at risk for substance abuse and other behavioral addictions. These risks include

◊ getting pregnant;

◊ dropping out of school;

◊ living in poverty;

◊ having emotional and mental disturbances;

◊ getting caught in the juvenile justice system;

◊ lacking self-esteem;

◊ being exposed to peer group tolerance or encouragement of drug use;

◊ lacking alternative activities;

◊ being in a school that has no policies, detection procedures, or referral services for users;

◊ being in a family that tolerates use, has no consistent rules, lacks consistent discipline, and has absent and uninvolved parents or especially parents that use drugs.

(ONDCP, 2000; Juliana & Goodman, 1997)

"I believe both my parents were alcoholics. My brother's an addict and alcoholic. It runs in the family. So I basically followed in my father's

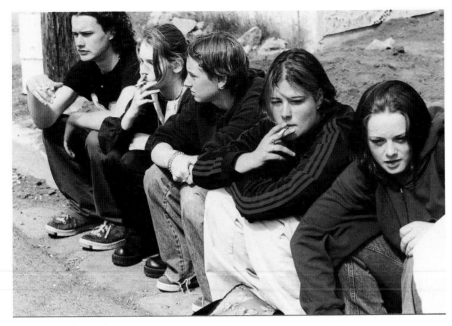

The teenage years are a period of invulnerability, romanticism, and adventure.
Courtesy of Simone Garlaund

. . . .

you can make yourself happy. When I'm with friends doing something that's fun or even important, then I don't even think about drugs."
16-year-old student

Primary, Secondary, & Tertiary Prevention for Grades K through 12

When prevention programs are planned, they need to keep the risk and resiliency factors in mind and tailor programs not only for the age groups but also for ethnicity, sex, culture, and any other factors that will get the message across.

Primary Prevention.   Since the purpose of primary prevention is to prevent or at least minimize drug experimentation and use, it needs to start as early as kindergarten. Coordinated efforts among parents, teachers, and other community members are of great value. Parent-teacher sessions and the incorporation of drug prevention lesson plans within the school's overall curriculum are the first steps. School-based prevention programs can teach life skills, resistance education, and/or normative education (Bates & Wigtil, 1994).

A **life-skills program,** Life Skills Training (LST), being taught in grades 7 to 10, focuses on increasing social skills and reducing peer pressure to drink. An evaluation of this program showed a decrease in the frequency of drinking and excessive drinking (Botvin, Baker, Dusenbury, Tortu, & Borzin, 1990).

One of the most widely used resistance education programs is the **DARE (Drug Abuse Resistance Education)** that consists of 16 or 17 weekly one-hour sessions conducted by uniformed police officers and presented to 5th or 6th graders. The program teaches self-esteem, decision-making skills, and peer-resistance training. Several studies have shown that the program has modest short-term (one year) effects on reducing drug use although it improved self-assertiveness and increased knowledge about the dangers of alcohol and

footsteps—the drinking, the running around."
Recovering alcoholic

The challenge for prevention specialists is to develop programs that clearly identify the above risks and teach adolescents to deal with them while enhancing the protective elements that promote healthy lifestyles and personal accomplishments. Researchers Steven Glenn, Ph.D. and Richard Jessor, Ph.D. present four antecedents or predictors of future drug use in children by age 12 that often differentiate future drug abusers from future nondrug abusers.

1. Strong sense of family participation and involvement: By age 12, those children who feel that they are significant participants in and valued by their families seem to be less prone towards substance abuse in the future.

2. Established personal position about drugs, alcohol, and sex by age 12: Children who have a position on these issues and who can articulate how they arrived at their position, how they would act on it, and what

effect their position would have on their lives seem less likely to develop drug or alcohol problems.

3. Strong spiritual sense and community involvement by age 12: Young people who feel that they matter and contribute to their community and that they are individuals with a role and purpose in society also seem less likely to develop significant drug or alcohol problems.

4. Attachment to a clean and sober adult role model other than one's parents by age 12: Children who can list one or more nondrug-using adults for whom they have esteem and to whom they can turn for information or advice seem less prone to develop drug abuse problems. These positive role models, often persons like a coach, a teacher, activities leader, minister, relative, neighbor, or family friend play a critical role in the formative years of a child's development.

"There is stuff around you in your life, including if you are just bored, that makes you want to experience the effect of a drug. You can change that if

other drugs (Ennet, Tobler, Ringwalt, & Flewelling, 1994).

Another resistance education program similar to DARE is **AMPS (Alcohol Misuse Prevention Study)** that consists of a four-session curriculum for 5th and 6th graders. It educates as well as develops peer resistance skills. Studies of high-risk students who had taken the course found a 50% reduction in use after 26 months and through grade 12 (Dielman, 1995).

Normative education is a strategy that aims to correct erroneous beliefs about the prevalence and acceptability of alcohol use and drug use among peers. This strategy was found to be a strong adjunct to resistance education, causing substantial drops in alcohol use among high school students (Hansen & Graham, 1993).

The most pertinent point about primary prevention is that it needs to be continued, not just limited to a one-year attempt at inoculating students against drug and alcohol use. Education and skills-training booster sessions need to continue through high school and into college (CSAT, 1994). The most effective prevention programs seem to be those in which the students are taught self-esteem and confidence and in which they learn not be afraid of their feelings.

Since the roots of most addiction come from the family, **family-focused primary prevention** is a necessary adjunct to any school-based program. Programs such as parental-skills training through the school, reduction in parental use of drugs or alcohol in front of the children, and greater positive participation of parents in their children's lives have a great influence on children's behavior. Results from a study by the Partnership for a Drug-Free America indicate that parents who have repeated discussions with their children about the risks of illicit drugs do make a difference in adolescent drug use. About 45% of teenagers who heard nothing at home about drug risks used marijuana in the last year. That figure drops to 33% for those who learned a little at home and 26% for those who learned a lot (Partnership, 1998).

Secondary Prevention. Once experimentation, social use, habituation, and occasional abuse have begun, usually starting in the 7th and 8th grades, school-based prevention programs need to continue primary prevention but also need to add a number of new lesson plans and definitive drug policies. Teachers and staff should be trained in recognizing drug use and dealing with the consequences. Training to enable parents to recognize problems due to drug use in their children, supporting their children, and seeking counseling should also be included. Additional services should include crisis intervention and referral. Other essential (but sometimes neglected) services include follow-up aftercare, support to make sure use does not reoccur, and continuing care to insure that emotional, social, and physical problems leading to substance use are being corrected. Often these services are available through utilization of existing community services rather than hiring new and expensive staff.

At this level, some other programs found to be effective in minimizing experimentation with drugs include peer educator programs, prevention curricula, Students Against Drunk Driving (SADD), positive role models, health fairs, and Friday Night Live alternative activities.

"When I was going through my wild stage, I think what changed my mind about drugs was seeing someone who went through their wild days and never stopped. So I think that there is a point when you cross over from experimentation and go on to abusing."
22-year-old former college student

Tertiary Prevention. This program (for students who have had a problem with drugs) uses student assistance programs, teenage Narcotics/Cocaine/Alcohol/Addictions Anonymous meetings, peer intervention teams, and other activities geared at getting drug abusers into early treatment to limit abuse. The honesty of peers seems most effective in reaching students who are in trouble.

Home drug tests provide one way parents monitor drug abuse. They use these drug tests when behavior suggests that family rules have been violated. Teenagers, however, may resent the tests as a breach of trust and an invasion of privacy.

Children of Alcoholics & Drug Abusers. Whether it's primary, secondary, or even tertiary prevention, teachers, counselors, and health professionals have to recognize that children are affected by drugs and alcohol even when they don't use and have to be able to identify and deal with the different roles a child will take in a family since many of these roles will affect future drug use. These roles include

◇ the hero, a hard-working student who tries to bring pride to the family but is still affected by the intense stress of having an addict or alcoholic in the family;

◇ the lost child who is extremely shy and deals with problems by avoiding family and social activities;

◇ the problem child who exhibits disruptive behaviors at an early age;

◇ and the mascot who tries to ease tension in a dysfunctional family by being funny or cute and has trouble maturing.

(Adger, 1998; Sher, 1997)

COLLEGES

Although illegal drugs appear on college campuses, alcohol is the drug that predominates. In a Carnegie Foundation survey, college presidents ranked alcohol abuse as the "quality of campus life" issue that was their greatest concern. Drinking is embedded in college traditions and norms. College students are particular targets for advertising by the alcoholic beverage industry since a freshman who prefers a particular brand is expected to generate $20,000–$50,000 in sales over his or her lifetime.

Prevalence

Various reports confirm that from 80–90% of students on most college

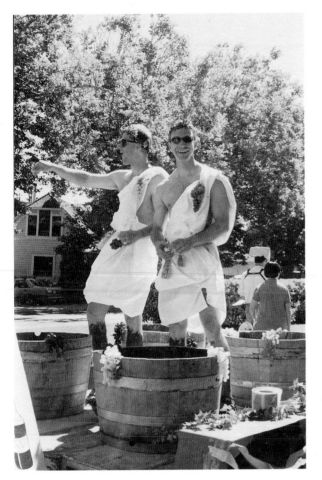

Alcohol is still the number one problem in colleges despite the continued use of marijuana, MDMA, and methamphetamines.

. . . .

campuses drink at least some alcohol. Research by Harvard University Professor Henry Wechsler and his colleagues indicates that

◇ 44% of the students surveyed on college campuses binge drink (five or more drinks in a session for men, four or more for women at least once every two weeks);

◇ about 1/2 of binge drinkers are frequent binge drinkers (five or more drinks at one sitting three or more times in the past two weeks);

◇ men bingers outnumber women bingers 50% to 39% but the number of women binge drinkers has been increasing in recent years;

◇ the rate of binge drinking is even higher for members of fraternities and sororities: almost 65%. If they live in a fraternity or sorority house, the rate jumps to 79%;

◇ fraternity men lag behind nonfraternity men in cognitive develop-ment, especially critical thinking skills after the freshman year;

◇ on the positive side, the number of abstainers increased from 15.4% to 19.2%.

(Wechsler, Lee, Kuo, & Lee, 2000)

Secondhand Drinking

Many problems that occur on campuses are related to **secondhand drinking,** that is, the effect binge drinkers and heavy drinkers have on other students. On campuses where more than 50% of students binge, 86% of nonbinge-drinking students reported being victims of assault or unwanted sexual advances, having sleep and study time interrupted, suffering property damage, having to care for or clean up after a drunken student, or suffering from the general impairment of the quality of life on campus (Wechsler et al., 2000). Recently on many campuses, efforts have been made to protect students from the damage that other people's drinking does to them.

Prevention in Colleges

College drinking games and songs date back centuries, as do attempts to control the damage students do to themselves and to one another. A sheriff still leads the commencement parade at Harvard graduation ceremonies, a centuries-old tradition to prevent drunken rowdy behavior.

Contemporary college prevention efforts date from the Federal Anti-Drug Abuse Act of 1986 that set aside funds for higher education and designated the Fund for the Improvement of Post-Secondary Education (FIPSE) as the granting agency that reviewed prevention grant proposals and dispersed funds. Many current drug courses and campus prevention programs derive from that legislation. Newer programs include counter-advertising campaigns of the National Association of State Universities and Land Grant Colleges as well as programs by individual colleges.

Normative Assessment. One prevention approach that has had success is a program that aims to change common misperceptions that drug and alcohol use among peers is higher than it really is. This process, called "normative assessment," recognizes that if students think that heavy drinking or drug use is the normal thing to do, they will be more likely to do it themselves. If they recognize that heavy drinking or illicit drug use is not normal, then they are more likely not to use. At Hobart and William Smith Colleges in Geneva, New York, studies found that 68% of the students believed that their peers found frequent intoxication acceptable when in fact only 14% found it acceptable (Perkins, Meilman, Leichliter, Cashin, & Presley, 1999).

Instead of talking about drug and alcohol use, normative assessment emphasizes that prevention efforts should talk about **not using**. The key is to let students know what constitutes normal use on a particular campus rather than letting their perceptions be formed by sensational stories in the media or the exaggerations of their friends and classmates.

Perception Versus Reality

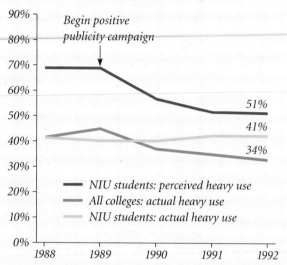

Heavy drinkers are those who have had 5 or more drinks at 1 sitting at least once every 2 weeks.

Figure 8-7•

This study from Northern Illinois University advertised the results of a campus survey that assessed students' perception of the amount of heavy drinking on campus. Students believed that 70% of their fellow students were heavy drinkers when in fact the real figure (and the national average) was about 43%. When the school advertised this fact and showed that heavy drinking wasn't as prevalent as the students thought, heavy drinking dropped even lower, down to 34%.

an eye on and help but if I'm too strict, they just drink off campus and come back and make noise and throw up. As dorm supervisor I turn a partial blind eye to the older students who have learned how to drink and close their doors and have a few beers or wine. I can't burst into their rooms and I don't want to lurk behind doors but I do have to protect the other students. I do know that when the university instituted alcohol-free dorms they were instantly popular."

Resident assistant at university dormitory

It is crucial to recruit peer counselors who are themselves clean and sober and will model the kind of attitudes and behavior desirable in a prevention program.

Other Programs. The following is a list of different campus programs directed at controlling alcohol use and abuse:

◇ campus regulation of drinking (25% of campuses ban beer, 32% prohibit liquor on campus, and 98% prohibit kegs in dorms) (Wechsler, Kelley, Weitzman, Giovanni, & Seibring, 2000);

◇ no alcohol at campus events;

◇ alcohol-, tobacco-, and drug-free dorms (wellness halls) (2/3 of campuses offer such dorms);

◇ requirement that food and nonalcoholic beverages be served when alcohol is available;

◇ server training for bartenders at college-sponsored functions;

◇ banning or regulating alcoholic beverage advertising in campus newspapers (50% ban such advertising);

◇ curricular infusion (substance abuse education incorporated into many courses);

◇ prohibition of alcohol at fraternity and sorority rush parties;

◇ having a substance abuse officer and a task force to deal with on-campus use and abuse;

◇ programs to work with the neighborhood and community;

◇ announcement and enforcement of campus alcohol and other drug policies;

◇ higher education prevention consortia in which several campuses pool their knowledge and effort; about 90 such consortia exist;

◇ early detection, intervention, enforcement, and referral by residence hall assistants, peer counselors, the health and counseling centers.

At the college level, primary prevention also includes well-publicized alcohol-free parties, weeklong "red ribbon" alcohol and drug-free celebrations, and active outreach activities, especially those promoting safe sex.

In an effective college prevention program, the three levels of drug abuse prevention (primary, secondary, and tertiary) need to be tailored mostly for 17, 18, 19, and 20 year olds. Experience has shown that as most students mature, their alcohol and drug use becomes more sensible.

"It's the freshman that are the biggest pain—not all of them. They are free from their parents' supervision for the first time, they are in an exciting but lonely place, and they try out their wings. Those are the ones I try to keep

LOVE, SEX, & DRUGS

"The deepest human need is the need to overcome the prison of our aloneness."
Erich Fromm

Over the last few years, the appearance of Viagra® (sildenafil citrate) to treat erectile dysfunction has been the biggest change in the use of drugs to enhance human sexuality. It releases nitric oxide that eventually relaxes smooth muscles in the corpus cavernosum erectile tissue allowing greater blood flow. After years of searching, a so-called aphrodisiac that works has been discovered. The rush to find more medications to enhance sexuality continues. However it is important to remember that Viagra® has no effect in the absence of sexual stimulation (PDR, 2000). This limited effect of Viagra® emphasizes the complexity of human sexuality.

Our desire for friendship, affection, love, intimacy, and sex is a primary driving force in men and women. That primary force is affected by drugs in many different and complicated ways. For example, some psychoactive drugs, such as alcohol, marijuana, and "ecstasy,"

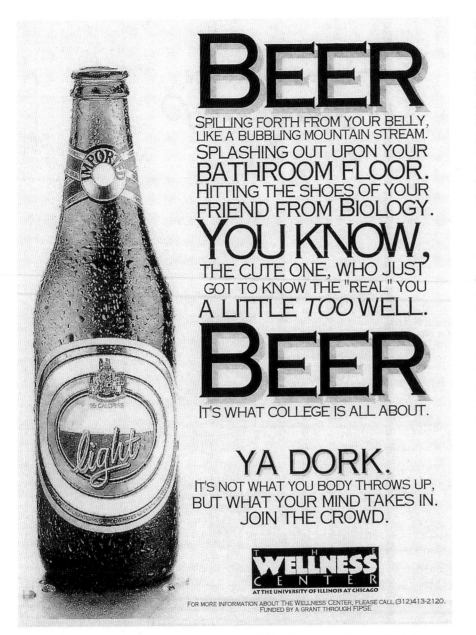

BEER
SPILLING FORTH FROM YOUR BELLY,
LIKE A BUBBLING MOUNTAIN STREAM.
SPLASHING OUT UPON YOUR
BATHROOM FLOOR.
HITTING THE SHOES OF YOUR
FRIEND FROM BIOLOGY.
YOU KNOW,
THE CUTE ONE, WHO JUST
GOT TO KNOW THE "REAL" YOU
A LITTLE *TOO* WELL.
BEER
IT'S WHAT COLLEGE IS ALL ABOUT.

YA DORK.
IT'S NOT WHAT YOU BODY THROWS UP,
BUT WHAT YOUR MIND TAKES IN.
JOIN THE CROWD.

THE **WELLNESS** CENTER
AT THE UNIVERSITY OF ILLINOIS AT CHICAGO

FOR MORE INFORMATION ABOUT THE WELLNESS CENTER, PLEASE CALL (312)413-2120.
FUNDED BY A GRANT THROUGH FIPSE

Many colleges have campaigns to control excess drinking. This campaign was funded by a FIPSE grant from the federal government.
Courtesy of the University of Illinois, Chicago

lower inhibitions. Others, including cocaine, amphetamines, marijuana, and some inhalants, are used to intensify and otherwise alter the physical sensations of sexuality and to counter low self-esteem or shyness. Often, psychoactive drugs substitute a simple physical sensation, or the illusion of one, for more complex (and yet more rewarding) true emotions, such as desire for intimacy and comfort, love of children, or release from anxiety. What

many psychoactive drugs do is artificially manipulate natural biochemicals, thereby stimulating, counterfeiting, blocking, or confusing physical sensations and true emotions and sensations about romance, love, and sex.

Drugs are used to have an impact on all phases of sexual behavior from puberty, through dating, to marital relations. Unfortunately drugs can also trigger sexual aggression, sexual harassment, rape (including date rape),

and child molestation. Sexual violence occurs because certain psychoactive drugs decrease inhibitions, increase aggressiveness, and disrupt judgment, particularly in those already prone to such behavior. Drugs also encourage high-risk sexual behavior like multiple partners, anonymous sex, unprotected sex, anal sex, and even prostitution, all of which can spread sexually transmitted diseases, like syphilis, gonorrhea, hepatitis B and C, and HIV disease.

"I'm monogamous. I'm with just one boyfriend at a time. I've been with him for two months now. The one before, I was with for four months."
Teenage high school junior

The 1960s and '70s signaled an increase in the use and availability of marijuana, amphetamines, and several other psychoactive drugs, all of which could affect sexual activity. This increased availability of drugs, along with less severe attitudes towards sexual activity, increased sexual contacts and drug experimentation. In addition the onset of the cocaine and "crack" epidemic in the '80s and methamphetamine surge in the '90s increased high-risk sexual activity. The mood-altering effects of the drugs, along with the need to make money to buy the drugs, added to the problem.

"These were women that otherwise I would never even have the nerve to approach. Once I've got 'crack,' then I'm someone who's desirable and I can do with these women anything that I want to. And that's what got me involved with 'crack' cocaine."
"Crack" user

GENERAL EFFECTS

The three main effects of psychoactive drugs on sexual behavior are on desire, excitation, and orgasm. Physically, psychoactive drugs affect hormonal release (testosterone, estrogen, adrenaline, etc.), blood flow, blood pressure, nerve sensitivity, and muscle tension that in turn affect excitation (erectile ability) and orgasm. For example,

◊ heroin desensitizes penal and vaginal nerve endings;

◊ alcohol dilates blood vessels, making it harder for excess blood to stay in the genital area, thereby making it difficult to maintain an erection;

◊ steroids increase testosterone that stimulates the fight center of the brain, making a user more sexually aggressive;

◊ cocaine and amphetamines release dopamine that stimulates our pleasure center in the limbic system, the same system stimulated during excitation and orgasm;

◊ many psychoactive drugs affect the hypothalamus that can trigger hormonal changes.

"It's a very euphoric satisfying kind of effect and it's similar to sex—but different. If I have heroin, I don't want or need real sex."
Heroin user

The actual effect of drugs in contrast with their expected effect can vary radically. In a survey we conducted at the Haight-Ashbury Detox Clinic, regular drug users said they combined sex and drugs in order to

◊ lower their inhibitions;

◊ try to make themselves perform better;

◊ increase their fantasies.

"As a teenager, I was sort of shy and the 'meth' made me feel I was super smart, super pretty, a super person. At that age, I felt very awkward and uncomfortable without the drug."
Recovering "meth" user

SIDE EFFECTS

People combine sex and drugs, searching for a shortcut to complex emotions but the reaction to psychoactive drugs is so variable, often escalating into compulsive and addictive behavior, that many of the initial, desired effects on desire and performance change with time. Diminished sexual performance, even to the point of impotence, is experienced by males who are heavy users of a number of drugs, including heroin and alcohol, as is diminished interest in physical and emotional contact.

Sex and love are such complicated processes and so tied in with our mental state that people use drugs not only to enhance their sexuality but also to shield themselves from their sexuality and even from any emotional involvement.

THE DRUGS

Drug-using behavior takes on a life of its own as tolerance, withdrawal, and side effects overwhelm the original intentions of the user.

Uppers (cocaine & amphetamines)

Amphetamines and cocaine are popular with heterosexuals and particularly some male homosexuals because for some, use increases confidence, prolongs an erection, increases endurance, and intensifies an orgasm during initial low-dose use. Cocaine and amphetamines increase the supply of dopamine in the nervous system that induces a rush of pleasure by affecting centers in the brain involved with sexual activity, mostly in the limbic system (Gold & Miller, 1997). This extra rush is often associated with sex that occurred under the influence. However, the myth of stimulant effectiveness often outweighs the reality of controlled studies (which are limited). Also, as with all drug use, preexisting sexual proclivities are directly related to the effect and effectiveness of a drug (Meston & Gorzalka, 1992). For example, someone who is shy or sexually inhibited will often get a larger boost of confidence from cocaine or methamphetamines while someone who has unusual sexual practices normally will be more likely to intensify those practices under the influence.

"The kind of feeling you get when you inject it—it's sort of like the feeling when you're making love with your wife. After a while, when you keep doing it, you're impotent and it doesn't have any effect. The opposite sex can do anything they want to you and you won't react."
Recovering cocaine addict

The effects of high-dose and prolonged use have quite the opposite effect on sexuality. In men, heavy or prolonged use often causes delayed ejaculation, decrease in sexual desire, and especially with cocaine, difficulty achieving an erection. In women, abuse can disrupt the menstrual cycle, cause difficulty in achieving orgasm, and decrease desire (Buffum, 1982; Smith, Wesson, & Apter-Marsh, 1984).

Then too there is a higher incidence of antisocial and other personality disorders as well as a number preexisting social and emotional problems. It is often difficult to measure just the effects of the stimulants.

"I was so loaded in the beginning that I would just blank my mind. I didn't want to think he was on top of me or anything because it would bring back [memories of] my stepfather. It would bring back what he was doing. He used his hands all over me."
Recovering 42-year-old polydrug abuser

Tobacco

From Humphrey Bogart puffing on cigarette after cigarette in *Casablanca* to Brad Pitt smoking in *The Fight Club*, the use of cigarettes in romantic and sexual situations has been encouraged by the movie industry and particularly by the tobacco industry. The image of a cigarette after sexual activity was so common that now it is used satirically to denote sex. Physically nicotine can both stimulate and relax depending on the set and setting. In social situations it is a great distracter, something to do while figuring out what to do. How-

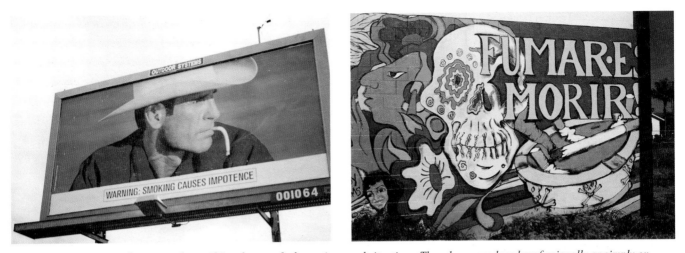

Antitobacco advertising focuses on demystifying the use of tobacco in sexual situations. The ads are produced professionally or simply on community walls.

ever, long-term tobacco use has been associated with impotence in men and reduced fertility in women, although not nearly to the degree caused by excessive cocaine or alcohol use (USD-HHS, 1988).

Opioids

Downers are often used to lower inhibitions, though the physiological depressive effects often decrease desire and performance. Some "nod out" when using, some feel "up." These differences can be explained by selective tolerance of different functions of the body to the effects of opioids. In a study at the Haight-Ashbury Clinic in 1982 of men and women who had come in for heroin treatment, the majority of those who had some sexual dysfunction before using reported an initial improvement in sexual activity functioning when they first began to use the drug. Men reported an increased delay in ejaculation while women reported an increase in relaxation and lowered inhibitions, however, with continued use, some users became disinterested in sex while others wanted to repeat the experience. Long-term users reported a decrease in sexual drive and impaired performance. Reduced testosterone in men led to impotence in some while long-term female users reported menstrual irregularities, reduced fertility, and frigidity (O'Brien, Cohen, Evans, & Fine, 1992).

"You start to look more masculine. You feel out of your skin. You can't really feel yourself anymore. The same sort of people you really loved aren't attracted to you anymore."
Female heroin user

In the study, 60% of heroin addicts reported an overall decrease in desire (impaired sexual desire or libido). While they were high on heroin, that figure jumped to 90%. In another study, 70% reported delayed ejaculation when using, which is why some premature ejaculators self-medicate. Further, the overall rate of impotence (inability to become aroused) in one study of male addicts was 39%, jumping to 53% when they were actually high (Shen & Sata, 1983; Buffum, 1982).

Sedative-Hypnotics

Many sedative-hypnotics, such as the benzodiazepines, barbiturates, and street Quaaludes®, have been called "alcohol in pill form" and touted as sexual enhancers. As with alcohol, it is a case of lowered inhibitions and relaxation vs. physical depression that makes one unable to perform or respond sexually.

"Sexually and mentally, everything is so down. If I were a man, I couldn't have an erection. As a woman, I don't

have an orgasm. Your mind is just mush but you don't care. The last thing you worry about is sex."
37-year-old benzodiazepine addict

Along with the disinhibition, sedative-hypnotics also impair judgment, making the user more susceptible to sexual advances. As the dose increases, the sedative effects take over, making the user less able to ward off unwanted sexual advances. The user becomes lethargic and sleepy and experiences extensive muscle relaxation. With abuse comes sexual dysfunction and total apathy towards sexual stimulation (Buffum, 1982).

Flunitrazepam (Rohypnol®). Flunitrazepam, dubbed the "date rape drug" is marketed outside the United States as a sleeping pill. This is because it causes profound amnesia and lowered inhibitions as well as a decreased ability to resist a sexual assault. Unfortunately much of the publicity surrounding the drug educated some predatory males in the use of the drug. Flunitrazepam also produces muscle relaxation and has an elimination half-life of 16–35 hours allowing it to accumulate in the system. While not as toxic as barbiturates, when used with alcohol, it can be dangerous (NIDA Infofax, 1999; Smith, Wesson, & Calhoun, 1995). This benzodiazepine, although legal in approximately 60 countries, is illegal in the United States. Also known as "roofies," "rophies," "ropes," and "roches," it is many times more powerful than Valium® and sold on the street for $5 to $10 (Marnell, 1997). (*Also see Chapter 4.*)

GHB (gamma hydroxybutyrate). GHB is a sedative-hypnotic that was originally used as a sleep inducer but is now popular on the "rave" club scene. It has been touted as a drug that will lower inhibitions and make sex more pleasurable. It was widely available in health food stores in the 1980s and used by bodybuilders. The problem with GHB is that slight increases in amount used can mean large differences in the effects. Double the dose that induces a pleasant effect can induce, within 10–20 minutes (Morganthaler & Joy, 1994). Unfortunately the amnestic effects of the drug, which can be therapeutically valuable, can lead to high-risk sexual practices.

Alcohol

"One drink of wine and you act like a monkey, two drinks and you strut like a peacock, three drinks and you roar like a lion, and four drinks, you behave like a pig."
Henry Vollam Morton, 1936

More than any other psychoactive drug, alcohol has insinuated itself into the culture of romantic and sexual behavior—champagne to celebrate, the cocktail before sex, or beer swilled before a date. Alcohol's physical effects on sexual functioning are closely related to blood alcohol levels. Its mental effects, however, are less strictly dose related and have more to do with the psychological makeup of the user and the setting in which it is used. Often there are preexisting issues that are dealt with under the influence.

"It was making me feel better about myself. I was, like I was a grown woman. I could take any man I wanted. It was like, 'Honey, let's go have a drink,' and there was always

alcohol involved. And we would go to a bar and sit at a bar and then it was easy for them to invite me to a hotel for the night."
42-year-old recovering polydrug abuser

Effects of alcohol on sexuality vary from user to user, on the amount used, and the length of use.

Low-Dose Use

Males: Usually increases desire (lowered inhibitions, relaxation), slightly decreases erectile ability, delays ejaculation.
Females: Usually increases desire and intensity of orgasm (due to lowered inhibitions).

High-Dose Use

Males: Increases/decreases desire, greatly decreases erectile and ejaculatory ability, causes some impotence.
Females: Greatly lowers desire and intensity of orgasm (lowered inhibitions make a woman more susceptible to coercion and rape).

Prolonged Use

Males: Decreases desire, erectile ability, and ejaculatory ability; causes some impotence.
Females: Decreases desire, decreases intensity of orgasm, or blocks orgasm completely.

"Sure I could have sex without alcohol. I've just never had occasion to do it."
Problem drinker

Women & Alcohol

In most societies, more taboos and restrictions are placed on a woman's sexuality than on a man's. Many women who are heavy drinkers seem to associate their identity as a woman with their sexual activity. Inevitably, because alcohol diminishes sexual arousal, women suffer lowered self-esteem and feelings of inadequacy. Typically the alcoholic denies that what is happening to her sexuality is related to what is happening with her progressive alcohol use.

"I was quite drunk. It was a 'kegger' party and I remember sitting right next to the keg and just drinking constantly all night. I voluntarily went out to a car with a boy. I voluntarily had sex with that boy because I was quite drunk and I guess the thinking was that I wanted someone to hold me and love me and make me feel pretty."
24-year-old woman who is a heavy drinker

In one study of chronic female alcoholics, 36% said they had orgasms less than 5% of the time (Wilsnack, Klassen, Schur, et al., 1991). As drinking increases, menstrual disturbances, spontaneous abortions, and miscarriages increase, as do the adverse effects on fertility and sexual function (Mello, Mendelson, & Teoh, 1993).

In both men and women, as the drinking progresses, alcoholic behavior is reinforced and it is difficult for the alcoholic to do anything but drink. Sex is merely something to do while drinking.

Men & Alcohol

The familiar release of inhibitions both in words and deeds is the key to alcohol's dual effect on a man's sexual activity, i.e., more desire/less performance. In men a blood alcohol level of .05 (about three beers in one hour) has a very measurable physical effect on erectile ability and yet legal intoxication in most states is almost twice that amount. On the other hand, mentally even one drink can loosen the tongue. Physically alcohol diminishes spinal reflexes (thus decreasing sensitivity and erectile ability) and dilates blood vessels (interfering with the ability to have an erection or ejaculation). Even a few drinks lower testosterone levels, however, the long-term drinker shows a greater decrease in testosterone, an increase in female sex steroids, such as estradiol, and abnormalities in sex steroid metabolism (Wright, Gavaler, & Thiel, 1991; Zakhari, 1993).

Initially, however, alcohol gives men more confidence because it acts on the area of the brain that regulates fear and anxiety, thereby promoting, not decreasing, aggressiveness. As alcoholism progresses, many men feel less sexual (possibly due to decreased testosterone and preoccupation with alcohol) and tend to shy away from the bedroom and even become asexual. In one study, impotence was reported in 60% of heavy alcohol abusers (Crowe & George, 1989).

ALL AROUNDERS

Marijuana

Marijuana has been called the "**mirror that magnifies**" because many of its effects—sensory enhancement, seeming prolongation of time, increased affectionate bonding, disinhibition, diffusion of ego, and sexualized fantasy—suggest a preexisting desire for these sensations.

Most of the reported effects from marijuana are general comments, such as feelings of sexual pleasure, rather than specifics, like prolonged excitation or delayed orgasm. Marijuana, more than any psychoactive drug, illustrates the difficulty in separating the actual effects from the influence of the mind-set and setting where the drug is used. If the drug is shared in a social setting, at a party, or on a date, the expectation is that it will make people more relaxed, less inhibited, and more likely to do things they wouldn't normally do.

A problem with excessive marijuana smoking is that the user often forgets how to have sexual relations without being high, and so the cycle of excess use is perpetuated. (The loss of sexual interest in other cultures from hashish use is well-known.)

MDMA & MDA ("ecstasy," "rave")

A recent cover story on "ecstasy" in Time magazine said that although only 1% of the population used "ecstasy" in the past month and 8% of high school seniors have tried it, the numbers are growing. A recent bust in San Francisco netted 1/2 million pills (Time, 2000). Users say MDMA and MDA (at moderate doses), unlike methamphetamines, calm them, give them warm feelings toward others, and a heightened sensual awareness. The warm feelings supposedly make closer relations with those around them possible. The supposed neurological mechanism for some of the effects of MDMA are caused by its manipulation of serotonin—reportedly it controls the release of the neurotransmitter and then releases it in a big spurt. Supposedly excitement occurs more often when coming down from the drug (due to the serotonin release) than while under the influence (Meston & Gorzalka, 1992). However only 25% to 50% of the users report any of these reactions. Also most of the reports about the sexual effects of MDMA and MDA are anecdotal and since polydrug use is quite widespread (especially involving amphetamine, marijuana, and alcohol) and an exciting set and setting can enhance the effects, accurate data is lacking. Possible dangers from excess use include high blood pressure and rapid heart rate, seizures, overheating to the point of death, and the disruption of serotonergic activity in the central nervous system. For some the so-called emotional revelations brought on by the drug prove to be extremely upsetting. Use is followed by an emotional depression.

INHALANTS

"Poppers" (amyl & butyl nitrite)

Volatile nitrites are vasodilators and muscles relaxants. If inhaled just prior to orgasm, they seemingly prolong and enhance the sensation. Abused as orgasm intensifiers by both the gay and straight communities in the 1960s, they too gained the reputation of being yet another "love drug." They are also used because they relax anal sphincter muscles. The side effects, however, of dizziness, weakness, sedation, fainting, severe headaches, and loss of erection often end up counteracting the desired effects (Sharp & Rosenberg, 1997; O'Brien et al., 1992).

Nitrous Oxide (laughing gas)

Nitrous oxide has become popular at "rave" parties and "desert raves" for the giddiness it produces. However, it is not generally looked upon as a sexually enhancing substance. One study of 15 dental personnel who abused the substance over a period of time found impotence in 7 cases. The problem eventually was reversed when use of the gas was stopped (Jastak, 1991).

PSYCHIATRIC DRUGS

Most patients who use psychiatric medications have preexisting emotional problems that can impair sexual functioning. By treating the mental condition, the drugs can also affect the sexual problems of the user. For example, an antidepressant can make a patient more able to engage in intimate relations and sexual appreciation, capabilities that were impaired by the depression.

The neurotransmitter serotonin has been found to be involved with many aspects of sexual behavior. Depending on which serotonin receptor is involved, serotonin can either facilitate or inhibit sexual behavior.

Various studies involving tricyclic antidepressants, such as desipramine (Norpramine®) and amitriptyline (Elavil®), have linked them to decreased desire, problems with erection, and delayed orgasm. Initially, however, in many cases, the relief from depression makes the user more able to be sexually involved. Many of the newer antidepressants, known as "selective serotonin reuptake inhibitors" or "SSRIs," such as sertraline (Zoloft®), fluoxetine (Prozac®), and paroxetine (Paxil®), also cause delay or inhibition of orgasm and impaired erection ability (Kline, 1989; Goldberg, 1998). Delayed orgasm often goes away with time. Prozac® has also been associated with a significant incidence of sexual disinterest where sex is possible but interest diminishes (Meston & Gorzalka, 1992; PDR, 2000).

Antipsychotics, such as thioridazine (Mellaril®), inhibit erectile function and ejaculation. Chlorpromazine (Thorazine®) and haloperidol (Haldol®) can inhibit desire, erectile function, and ejaculation. Impaired ejaculation appears to be the most common side effect of the major tranquilizers (antipsychotics).

With lithium, there are some reports of decreased desire and difficulty maintaining an erection as the dosage increases.

APHRODISIACS

The search for true aphrodisiacs is complicated by the complexity of the sexual response. Are we talking about affection, love, or lust when we discuss drugs that enhance sexuality? Are we talking about drugs that change the mental or the physical aspects of sexuality? Is the drug expected to increase desire, prolong excitation, increase lubrication, delay orgasm, or improve its quality? Is a drug that lowers inhibitions an aphrodisiac?

Heroin sometimes delays orgasm, cocaine sometimes increases desire or prolongs an erection, and alcohol lowers inhibitions, thereby increasing desire.

As mentioned, Viagra® deals mostly with the ability to have an erection by increasing blood flow but hundreds of other substances have been tried over the centuries. Some purported aphrodisiacs, such as Spanish fly or ground rhinoceros horn, work by irritating the urethra and bladder, promoting a pseudosexual excitement. But Spanish fly (cantharidin derived from a beetle) is actually toxic. The scent or odor of **pheromones**, human hormones discovered in perspiration, has been shown to increase desire and sexual stimulation. Yohimbine is an alkaloid obtained from several plant sources including the yohimbe tree in West Africa. This psychedelic produces some hallucinations and a mild euphoria. It has been used in high doses as a treatment for impotence in men by increasing blood pressure and heart rate, thereby increasing penile blood flow. It can produce acute anxiety at low dosages (Morganthaler & Joy, 1994).

One problem with purported sexual enhancers is that the body adapts to any drug, so that its effectiveness decreases with time. Another problem with illegal substances is that controlled use is difficult and side effects start to over-

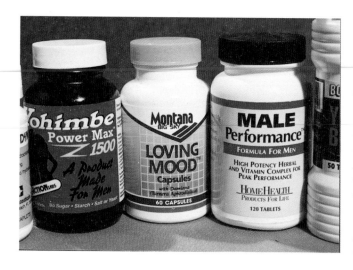

Besides Viagra®, the number of over-the-counter and prescription drugs that contain yohimbe, ginseng, and some other herbal stimulants (and promise sexual performance) has grown.

whelm any benefits. Third, and perhaps most important, the psychological roots of most feelings are quite complex and generally more important to sexual functioning than mere enhancement of sensations. Drugs can distort, magnify, or eliminate feelings involved with erotic activities.

SUBSTANCE ABUSE & SEXUAL ASSAULT

"These people were my friends that I've known for six or seven years, that I went to high school with and they did this to me. And they took advantage of me when I passed out at a party and I was sleeping on the couch. And I woke up and they were doing stuff to me that they shouldn't have been doing. And I went to school the next day and everybody's like, 'Oh Julie, I heard about you,' and I was so upset and so humiliated."

34-year-old female who was raped in high school

One in every three women in this country will be a victim of sexual violence in her lifetime. In one study of sexual assaults, victims reported using drugs or alcohol in 51% of the cases while substance use by the assailants was about 44% of the cases (Seifert, 1999). Another study found that approximately 60% of sexual offenders were drinking at the time of the offense (Roizen, 1997). Sexual assault has much

to do with the existing tendencies or character traits of the user and how the specific effects of the drugs exaggerate or alter those characteristics.

"He definitely had been drinking. I don't know him well enough to know whether he was drunk. However when I replay all the events of that night I feel like he knew exactly what was going to happen or how he was going to attempt each move that led to me being assaulted [raped]. That included offering me and giving me alcohol. And that's a really hard thing to say. That's the thing I blame myself for. I don't think I was scared until I realized what was happening to me, until I realized that he was raping me. And at that point I started screaming, although I did not hear myself screaming at all."

26-year-old woman

Some generalizations about the effects of psychoactive drugs on sexual behavior can be made.

◇ Alcohol lowers inhibitions and muddles rational thought, making the user more likely to act out irrational or inappropriate desires.

◇ Cocaine and amphetamines increase confidence and aggression, making the male user more likely to assault his date.

◇ Sedatives lower inhibitions, making users more prone to sexual advances or making the woman less able to resist.

◇ Marijuana makes users more suggestible to sexual activity and more sensitive to touch.

◇ PCP and heroin make users less sensitive or indifferent to pain, making them more liable to damage their partners or themselves.

◇ Steroids can increase aggression and irrational behavior.

"I've seen freshman girls drunk, so drunk that they couldn't even stand up and guys totally grabbing on to them on the dance floor. And it saddens me because we should be able to have that privilege to go out and have fun, drink a few beers or whatever and not have to worry about having someone taking advantage of us that night or waking up in a strange room and not knowing where you are."

22-year-old female who was raped

In most cases, the male user already has tendencies towards improper or aggressive behavior and the alcohol or other drug is the final trigger. The trigger can also be an emotion such as anger, hate, or in some cases, lust.

"In some men, alcohol can disinhibit their aggressive tendencies and they become violent when they drink alcohol but the violence was sitting in them and residing in their psyche way before they picked up that first drink."

Jackson Katz, Executive Director, MVP Strategies Inc. (Male Violence Prevention)

For example, with date rape, the man may just intend to have sex but when he is refused or doesn't get his way, he becomes angry and takes what he feels is his right. In the final analysis, rape is motivated by a need to overpower, humiliate, and dominate a victim not a desire to have sex.

"Sexual abuse is very much a prevalent thing in domestic violence situations. We estimate through statistics that probably 50% of all women who are battered are raped by their intimate partners."

Karen Darling, Director, Domestic Violence Education Center, Asante Health Services

What also occurs with sexual abuse and domestic violence is that the emotional pain and trauma intensify the need to block one's feelings leading to intensified use of the drug.

"I remember being beat up physically and being emotionally abused and drinking a gallon of wine and feeling like I just wanted to be out of it. And for me that was the way to deal with the pain. And I think women tend to do those things—take drugs to be able to continue to have some kind of relationship."

38-year-old counselor at the Haight-Ashbury Detox Clinic

SEXUALLY TRANSMITTED DISEASES (STDs), NEEDLE-TRANSMITTED DISEASES, HEPATITIS, & AIDS

The World Health Organization (WHO) estimates that worldwide, 333 million cases of sexually transmitted diseases occur each year. About one percent of those will eventually die from their STD. In contrast 33.6 million people are infected with the HIV virus that eventually becomes AIDS. And although survival time is increasing, almost all of them will die. There were 5.6 million new cases of HIV infection in 1999. By the end of 1999, 16.3 million people had died from AIDS (WHO, 2000). The three main routes for the transmission of HIV are heterosexual sex, homosexual sex, and drug use (IV use and unsafe sex).

Epidemiology

The dangers of sexually transmitted diseases, such as chlamydia, gonor-rhea, syphilis, and trichomoniasis (the four most common), along with genital herpes, genital warts, and hepatitis B, are well-known as are the mortal dangers of HIV disease. However, in spite of this knowledge and in spite of a growth in unwanted pregnancies, the practice of unsafe and unprotected sex by high school students, college students, and young adults continues. About 85% of all STDs occur in persons between the ages of 15 and 30. Very often, alcohol and other drugs are involved (CDC, 1999).

A study by the Center on Addiction and Substance Abuse at Columbia University that examined the habits of 34,000 teenagers from grades 7–12, found that students who drank and used drugs were five times more likely to be sexually active, starting sexual intercourse as early as middle school. They were three times more likely to have had sex with four or more partners in the previous two years (CASA, 2000).

The use of "crack" cocaine, methamphetamine, and marijuana increases high-risk sexual activity due to stimulation of sensations, lowering of inhibitions, and impaired judgment. In addition the very nature of sexual activity clouds judgment, as do most drugs. Drugs also affect memory, so even if users do something dangerous while under the influence, they might not remember it or if they do, they will see it in a more benign light and not appreciate the risks they took, thus laying the groundwork for repetition of that behavior.

With this mix, it is no wonder that almost half of all teenagers who are very active sexually have had chlamydia, the fastest-spreading sexually transmitted disease. In fact experts think that as many as 4 million Americans have caught the disease (often without knowing it). Perhaps 20% of all very sexually active men and women have genital herpes. Even syphilis, which had diminished dramatically in the last 50 years, has started to climb again. Most ominously there were 47,000 new cases of AIDS in the United States from July 1998 through June 1999 (CDC, 2000).

"This woman was pregnant, she was living on the street, she was prostituting, was HIV positive, and had a $250-a-day habit. I mean she's not a bad looking woman but she was definitely into her 'smack' and her cocaine. She told me she had to sleep with at least five guys a day, minimum, to support her habit. I wonder how many people she's given her diseases to."

AIDS patient

The increased risk of STDs, including HIV disease, among the drug-abusing population is also much higher because drug abuse requires money and people will often do anything to raise money to avoid a cocaine crash or heroin withdrawal symptoms. Trading sex for drugs is an all-too-common practice.

"I was selling dope and made $3 or $4 thousand a week. I had women coming to me. I never 'tossed' a woman in my life. Those women were coming after me. I mean, you've got to look at both sides of it."

22 year old recovering "crack" dealer/user

One thing to remember about sexually transmitted diseases is that there is a delayed incubation period before symptoms show up and the disease can be transmitted to others. There are also some diseases where symptoms aren't evident but the illness is still transmittable.

Needle-Transmitted Diseases

Many of the same illnesses that are transmitted sexually can be transmitted through contaminated hypodermic needles when drugs are taken intravenously. And since high-risk sex is often associated with drug use, the risk of transmitting diseases is even greater.

Needle kits are called "outfits," "fits," "rigs," "works," "points," and many other names. Intravenous drug use is also called "mainlining," "geezing," "slamming," or "hitting up." Problems with needle use come from several sources. Besides putting a large amount of the drug in the bloodstream in a short period of time, needles also inject other substances like powered milk, procaine, or even Ajax® that are often used to cut or dilute drugs. They can also inject dangerous bacteria and viruses.

Hepatitis A, B & C. Some of the most common diseases transmitted by needle are the various types of hepatitis, viral infections of the liver. These are the most common disease in needle users. Hepatitis A is often transmitted by fecal matter and is associated more with unsafe sex and poor hygiene than drug use. The two main types of hepatitis associ-

TABLE 8–6　SEXUALLY TRANSMITTED DISEASES

Disease	First Symptoms	Typical Symptoms
Chlamydia or NGU (nonspecific urethritis)	7–21 days	Discharge from genitals or rectum
Pelvic inflammatory disease (PID)	Highly variable	Infection of uterus, fallopian tubes, and ovaries, a potential cause of infertility
Gonorrhea ("clap," "dose")	2–30 days	Discharge from genitals or rectum, pain when urinating, sometimes no symptoms
Herpes simplex I or II (cold sore, fever blister)	2–20 days	Painful blisters/sores on genitals or mouth, fever, malaise, swollen lymph glands
Venereal warts (genital warts)	30–90 days (even years)	Itch, irritation, and bumpy skin growths on genitals, anus, mouth, throat
Syphilis ("syph," "bad blood," "lues")	10–90 days	Primary stage: chancre on genitals, mouth, anus; secondary stage: diffuse rash, hair loss, malaise
Hepatitis B and C (serum hepatitis)	60–90 days (hepatitis B) up to 20 years (hepatitis C)	Yellow skin and eyes, dark urine, severe malaise, weight loss, abdominal pain
Trichomonas vaginalis (vaginitis)	7–30 days	Women: vaginal discharge, itching, burning; men usually have no symptoms
Pubic lice ("crabs," "cooties")	21–30 days	Itching, tiny eggs (nits) on pubic hair
Scabies (7-year itch)	14–45 days	Itching at night, bumps and burrows on skin
Monila (candidiasis, yeast)	Highly variable	White, thick vaginal discharge and itching in women; men most often have no symptoms
Bacterial vaginosis (gardnerella, nonspecific vaginitis)	Highly variable	Vaginal discharge, peculiar odor in women; men most often have no symptoms
HIV infection (leads to AIDS)	Many months (up to 5 years)	Weight loss, fever, swollen glands, diarrhea, fatigue, severe malaise, recurrent infections, sore throat, skin blotches

(Venereal Disease Action Council of Portland, Oregon)

ated with drug use, specifically IV drug use, are hepatitis B and hepatitis C. Hepatitis B is marked by inflammation of the liver and general debilitation but it is treatable with a convalescence of 1–5 months. More than 75% of IV drug users test positive for hepatitis B. Of those, about 10% are chronic carriers, guaranteeing the continued spread of the disease (Novick, Haverkos, & Teller, 1997). As discussed in Chapter 4, the blood-borne hepatitis C virus (HCV) is more dangerous and can cause liver disease including cancer. Some people will carry the disease for 10–20 years without symptoms. Symptoms include lack of appetite, jaundice, abdominal pain, and a general malaise. The only way to be sure is to test for HCV antibodies. Chronic flareups can cause inflammation and scarring of the liver, along with liver cancer in 1% to 5% of the cases.

◇ The HCV positive rate in IV drug users is 50% to 90%.

◇ Of those that get infected with HCV, 20% to 40% will develop liver disease while 4% to 16% will develop liver cancer.

(Novick, Reagan, Croxson, et al., 1997; Cahoon-Young, 1997)

The HCV problem has become so severe that NIDA issued a special alert to increase counseling, treatment, and prevention.

◇ About 4 million Americans are infected with the virus with a majority of those young adults aged 20–29, although chronic infections are highest among 30–39 year olds. Since HCV has a 10-20 year incubation period, many more people are currently infected and do not know it.

◇ Between 8,000–10,000 die each year from the disease.

◇ Sharing needles is responsible for almost 2/3 of the infections.

◇ New IV drug users acquire HCV at an alarming rate with 50% to 80% becoming infected within 6–12 months. (The average incubation period is 6–7 weeks.)

◇ HCV has also been transmitted by the sharing of drug-snorting paraphernalia.

◇ The risk of sexual transmission of HCV is much lower than the risk of IV drug use, although 20% of the cases are supposedly due to sexual activity, particularly among multiple partners. In long-term monogamous relationships the rate is very low (0% to 4%).

◇ The risk of an infected mother passing the infection on to her fetus is about 5% to 6%.

(NIDA Bulletin, 2000)

Endocarditis. Another common problem is endocarditis, a sometimes fatal condition caused by certain bacteria that lodge and grow in the valves of the heart. IV cocaine users seem to have a higher rate of endocarditis, perhaps because the ups and downs of cocaine require many more injections than heroin or methamphetamines (Wartenberg, 1998).

Abscesses, Cotton Fever, and Flesh-Eating Bacteria. Needle use can also cause abscesses at a contaminated injection site or they can inject bits of foreign matter in the bloodstream that can lodge in the spine, brain, lungs, or eyes and cause an embolism or other problems. Needle users can also contract cotton fever, a very common disease. The symptoms are similar to those of a very bad case of the flu. Its cause is unknown, though some believe that it results from bits of cotton (used to filter the drug) that lodge in various tissues or from infections (viral or bacterial) carried into the body by cotton fibers injected into the blood. Starting in the mid- to late-1990s, more and more cases of necrotizing fasciitis (a flesh-eating bacteria and wound botulism or gangrene) have been reported.

"I started using drugs when I got together with my ex-boyfriend but then I quit using them because I would get these big abscesses on my arms and stuff and my veins—like when I go to the doctor to get blood drawn now, they can't use my veins in my arms."
22-year-old recovering heroin user

Typically veins of the arms, wrists, and hands are used first. As these veins become hardened due to constant sticking, the user will inject into the veins of the neck and the legs. As it becomes difficult to locate usable veins, addicts will also shoot under the skin ("skin popping") or into a muscle in the buttocks, shoulder, or legs ("muscling"). If they become desperate as they run out of places to shoot themselves, they will inject into the foot and males will even inject in the dorsal vein in the penis.

HIV Disease & AIDS

HIV means "human immunodeficiency virus," the virus that causes AIDS. AIDS stands for "acquired immune deficiency syndrome." AIDS is identified by the incidence of one or more of a group of serious illnesses, such as pneumocystis carinii pneumonia, Kaposi's sarcoma cancer, or tuberculosis, that develop when the HIV virus has taken control of the patient's body. However, since 1993, a new definition of AIDS has been added. AIDS is now also defined as "having a T-cell count below 200." T-cell counts measure the level of effectiveness of one's immune system (Alcamo & Wistreich, 1994).

AIDS is fatal because the HIV virus destroys the immune system, making it impossible for the body to fight off serious illnesses, such as pneumonia. Usually death occurs from a combination of many diseases and infections. Many needle users test positive for the HIV (AIDS) virus because they shared a needle used by someone already infected (JAMA, 1999).

"I know I'm really lucky that I didn't get AIDS 'cause a lot of people that I knew used my needles and then they would put them back in my clean needles and I didn't know that they were using them. And I just thank God that I didn't get any diseases or I'm not dead right now."
22-year-old heroin user

It is impossible to overemphasize the danger of using infected needles because IV use of a drug bypasses all the body's natural defenses such as body hairs, mucous membranes, body acids, and enzymes. And the HIV virus itself destroys the body's last line of defense, the immune system. In fact recent research shows that, in and of themselves, opioids and other drugs of abuse can weaken the immune system (Des Jarlais, Hagan, & Friedman, 1997). This, coupled with the malnutrition and unhealthy habits that compulsive drug use promotes, makes the body unable to fight off any illness.

"I told this guy that was sharing some 'speed' with me that I had AIDS and that he should clean the needle but he was so strung out and anxious to shoot up that he pulled a knife on me and made me give him the needle."

Intravenous cocaine user

Epidemiology of HIV & AIDS

Worldwide, 2/3 of those infected with AIDS are from Sub-Saharan Africa. About 16 million have already died from the epidemic, 2.6 million in 1999 alone. Most contract the infection by the age of 25 and die before their 35th birthday (WHO, 2000).

By comparison, approximately 700,000 in the United States are infected with the HIV virus or have AIDS while 420,000 have already died from the disease since it first appeared on the scene in 1981 (CDC, 2000). Another 27,000 got AIDS from having unprotected sex with an infected IV drug user.

Through July 1999, 179,228 intravenous (IV) drug users had either died from AIDS or were living with the infection as a result of injecting themselves with HIV-infected needles. This is about 26% of the total AIDS cases in the United States since the beginning of the epidemic. Some estimates of the HIV infection rate among IV drug users approach 80%. Infected needle drug users spread the disease to nondrug users through unsafe sexual practices. Even in Russia and the Ukraine, the use of infected needles has doubled the rate of HIV infection,

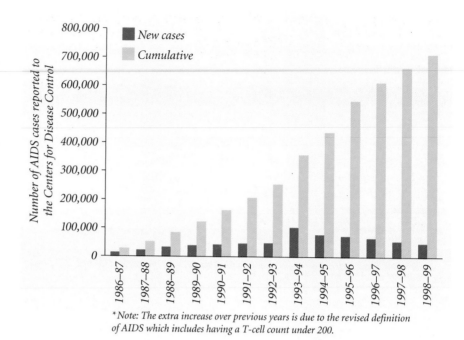

Note: The extra increase over previous years is due to the revised definition of AIDS which includes having a T-cell count under 200.

Figure 8-8•

The Centers for Disease Control and Prevention keep track of all infectious diseases in the United States.

reaching a total of 360,000 in 1999 (UNAIDS, 2000).

Men who have sex with other men are still the greatest cause of AIDS cases in the United States. In 1998, Washington, DC had the highest new AIDS cases rate while New York was second in rate but first in sheer numbers (Table 8-7).

Prevention of HIV & AIDS

It is important to remember the pattern of the spread of communicable diseases. They start slowly but then rage through the most susceptible groups. In the case of HIV and AIDS in the United States, the gay community that practiced unsafe sex was the most vulnerable compared to other countries where heterosexual high-risk sexual activity spread the disease.

Once the most vulnerable have been infected, there is usually a lull in the increase of the disease. During such lulls, a false sense of security, along with clouded judgment, build up a new upwelling of infection. The majority of new cases of HIV in the United States

(as in the rest of the world) will be in the heterosexual and drug-using communities. Continuing public education and public health prevention activities are crucial to stem the spread of AIDS and, for that matter, all sexually transmitted diseases.

"The only way the attitudes and practices towards AIDS would change is if everybody got these diseases, you hear what I'm saying? It doesn't really sink in unless it strikes close to you. Once the virus is in your own backyard, you become very serious. Kids wanna wear rubbers once they find out their father has it, you know what I mean? People are concerned once they find out their mother has it, or their brother has it, or they have it."

Recovering 43-year-old heroin addict who is HIV positive

Several strategies exist to stop the spread of AIDS, particularly in the drug-using community. Some of them are

TABLE 8–7   NEW AIDS CASES (STILL LIVING) & NUMBER OF CASES & RATES UNITED STATES JULY 1998–JUNE 1999 FROM ALL SOURCES

Selected States	Cases	Rate per 100,000
New York	7,655	42.1
California	5,737	17.6
Florida	5,683	38.1
Texas	3,715	18.8
New Jersey	2,061	25.4
Pennsylvania	1,806	15.0
Maryland	1,634	31.8
District of Columbia	750	143.4
U.S.: new AIDS cases 7/98–6/99	**47,083**	**17.1**
U.S.: total AIDS living	681,306	
U.S.:total AIDS deaths	420,201	
U.S.: total AIDS cases	**1,101,507**	
World: total AIDS/HIV living	33,600,000	
World: total AIDS deaths	16,300,000	
World: total AIDS/HIV cases (12/99)	**49,900,000**	

(CDC, 2000; WHO, 2000)

In studies by the Center for Disease Control and other agencies, drug abuse treatment, along with education and needle exchange programs that are tied to outreach components, seems to be the most effective HIV disease or AIDS prevention strategies.

Harm Reduction

In San Francisco several groups, including the HIV Prevention and Research Services of the Haight-Ashbury Free Clinics, have outreach programs meant to reach IV drug users who are not in treatment. Outreach workers from the Clinic, armed with AIDS educational materials, free bottles of bleach, and free condoms, go out to the "shooting galleries," "crack/rock houses," "dope pads," and other areas to distribute these materials and provide treatment referrals if requested. Other groups distribute free needles. It's an intervention into drug-related behavior without intervening into drug

◇ improved diagnosis and treatment of STDs;

◇ treatment on demand for drug addiction to encourage users to give up drugs;

◇ availability of AZT and other drugs for pregnant women who are HIV positive;

◇ needle exchange programs to control transmission of the disease;

◇ education and counseling programs that teach about the dangers of AIDS and that teach the use of bleach to clean needles;

◇ vocational training to counteract poverty, a predisposing factor to drug use and HIV infection;

◇ creation of outreach activities to get high-risk drug users into contact with the treatment community;

◇ education programs that teach about high-risk sexual activities;

◇ easy access to condoms at a reasonable price;

◇ interdiction and law enforcement activities to limit the flow of drugs into the community;

(UCSF, 1998)

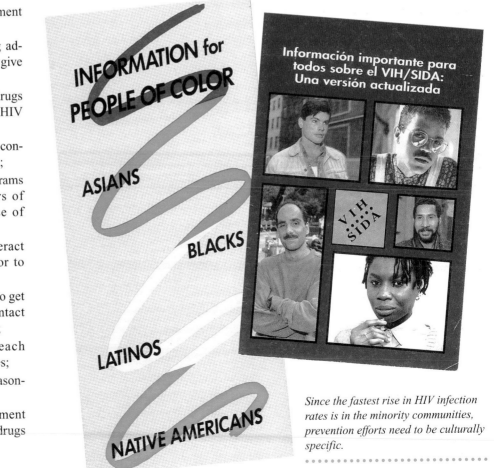

Since the fastest rise in HIV infection rates is in the minority communities, prevention efforts need to be culturally specific.

use. The drug use intervention part of the total policy is handled by the other sections of the Clinic.

The problem with tying education about the risks of sharing needles too close to treatment is that it may miss the larger segment of IV drug users who are not ready for treatment and therefore at highest risk for AIDS. Users alienated by the treatment community or in denial are hard to educate. Some clinics have a more tolerant policy toward relapses and toward users who can't clean up during their first few tries. The idea is at least the user is occasionally in contact with a treatment facility that can intervene, present important information, and eventually get the client into treatment, which is the best way to slow the spread of AIDS.

Education however does work. In San Francisco, in just a short period of time, drug users' awareness about the dangers of AIDS and the need to clean their needles jumped from a few percent to 85%. The HIV positive segment of the IV drug-using population in San Francisco is 15–17% compared to 60–80% in New York. Part of this difference in HIV infection rate between the two coasts seems to be due to the educational effort of the clinics, the San Francisco Health Department, and the gay community. Other differences seem to be the greater presence of "shooting galleries" in New York, the limited number of treatment facilities, the difficulty in obtaining clean needles, and language barriers (CDC, 1998).

Recently many new drugs besides AZT, one of the original AIDS drugs, have been developed and are showing promise in slowing or even halting the spread of the HIV virus in the body. Antiretroviral drugs and protease inhibitors seemed more effective but the complicated regime of dozens of pills that have to be taken daily and the severe side effects have faded some of the early promise.

In addition studies have shown that people who test positive for HIV, who stay clean and sober and maintain a healthy lifestyle with plenty of rest, good food, and exercise will avoid full-blown AIDS for years longer. And those who have an AIDS diagnosis will live months to years longer. The refinement of many techniques to treat the opportunistic infections that can be so lethal to immune systems weakened by AIDS can give years of life to infected clients (Haverkos, 1998).

"As I've started going into recovery and learning that I'm worth something and learning that I can have a life even though I'm HIV positive, yeah, it scares me to go back out there 'cause I know that when I use, I have unsafe sex, bottom line. And when I'm high, I'm not going to put on a condom. When I'm high, I will let people do things to me that I normally wouldn't let them do."

Recovering methamphetamine user who is HIV positive

DRUGS AT WORK

The concept of the drug-free workplace that includes preemployment drug testing, employee assistance programs, and a greater understanding of the effect drug abuse has on the bottom line, has led to a reduction in drug use and associated problems in the workplace.

Contrary to the popular picture of the unemployed drug or alcohol user

◇ 70% of illicit drug users age 18–49 work full-time, however, only about 15% of addicts are employed full-time;

◇ of the full-time workers in 1998, 6.2 million (7.9%) were heavy alcohol users;

◇ about 1.6 million of these workers were both heavy alcohol and illicit drug users;

◇ the percentage of all full-time workers who used illicit drugs in the past month fell from 17.5% in 1985 to 6.4% in 1998;

◇ 21.4% of full-time workers drank at least five drinks at one sitting in the last two weeks while 7.9% were classified as heavy drinkers.

(SAMHSA, 1999)

The highest rates of illicit drug use are in the construction industry and food preparation, and among waiters and waitresses, helpers, and laborers. The lowest rates are among police and detectives (SAMHSA/OAS, 1996).

COSTS

Studies on the impact of alcohol and other drug abuse in the American workplace have resulted in estimates that substance abuse cost our industries about $43 billion in 1979, $60 billion in 1983, and $140 billion in 1995 of which $60 billion was for drug-related costs and $80 billion for alcohol-related costs (ONDCP, 2000; NIDA/NIAAA, 1998). Detailed analysis of these substance abuse-related costs reveals not only an impact on industry but also an impact on the substance abusers themselves, their families, and their coworkers.

Loss of Productivity

Compared to a nondrug-abusing employee, a substance-abusing employee is

◇ late 3–14 times more often;

◇ absent 5–7 times more often and 3–4 times more likely to be absent for longer than eight consecutive days;

◇ involved in many more job mistakes;

◇ likely to have lower output, make a less-effective salesperson, experience work shrinkage, i.e., less productivity despite more hours put forth;

◇ likely to appear in a greater number of grievance hearings.

(Mercer, Meidinger, Hansen, 1988; SAMHSA/OAS, 1996; Mangione et al., 1998)

About 21% of workers report being injured, having to redo work or to cover for a coworker, needing to work harder, or being put in danger due to other's drinking. However 60% of alcohol-related work performance problems can be attributed to occasional binge drinkers rather than alcoholics or alcohol-dependent employees (USDL, 1990).

Medical Cost Increases

Substance abusers as compared to nondrug-abusing employees

◇ experience 3–4 times more on-the-job accidents;

◇ use 3 times more sick leave;

◇ overutilize health insurance for themselves and for their families;

◇ file 5 times more workman's compensation claims;

◇ increase premiums for the entire company for medical and psychological insurance;

◇ endanger the health and well-being of coworkers.

(Bernstein & Mahoney, 1989; USDL, 1990; Becker, 1989; Drug Strategies, 1995)

Legal Cost Increases

As tolerance and addiction develop, a drug-abusing employee often enters into some form of criminal activity. Crime at the workplace brought about by drug abuse results in

◇ direct and massive losses from embezzlement, pilferage, sales of corporate secrets, and property damaged during commission of a crime;

◇ increased cost of improved company security, more personnel, urine testing costs, product monitoring, quality assurance, intensified employee testing and screening;

◇ more lawsuits, both internal and external, expanded legal fees, court costs, and attorney expenses;

◇ loss of customer good will and negative publicity from drug use and trafficking at the workplace, employee arrests, the perception that there are more substance abusers than just those arrested, and manipulation of client contracts or goods.

(Drug Strategies, 1995)

PREVENTION & EMPLOYEE ASSISTANCE PROGRAMS (EAPs)

Businesses attempt to control drug abuse in two ways. One method is through preemployment and on-the-job drug testing. The other is through employee assistance programs (EAPs).

Workplace Drug Testing

The various drug-testing programs used by industry have shown a decrease in positive results.

◇ Since 1987 the percentage of positive drug tests among American workers dropped from 18% down to 5% in 1997. The National Household Survey has shown a very similar drop.

◇ The most common drug found in those testing positive, by far, is marijuana (59.1%), compared to cocaine (17.8%), and opiates (7.9%).

◇ In safety-sensitive industries such as transportation, the rate is about 1/2 that of the general workforce.

◇ Positive results from preemployment testing have gone from 3.4% in 1993 to 3.9% in 1997.

◇ About 10% of those tested for cause, tested positive for an illicit drug.

◇ The highest positive rates came from southern rural areas rather than from big cities like New York, Chicago, or Los Angeles.

(SmithKline, 1997)

Employee Assistance Programs (EAPs)

In response to the increased problem of drugs in the workplace and the resultant drain on profits and productivity, many employers have instituted an employee assistance program, or EAP. Successful EAP programs balance the needs of management to minimize the negative impact that drug abuse has on their business with a sincere concern for the better health of employees. Once the benefits of EAPs were recognized, many companies initiated programs. In 1980 there were 5,000 EAPs; in 1990 that number had grown to 20,000 and the number of covered employees grew from 12% to over 35%. Today 45% of full-time employees are covered. In large companies with over 500 employees, 70% are covered (Englehart, Robinson, & Kates, 1997).

Designed as an employee benefit, an EAP can assist with a wide range of life and health issues and not just substance abuse problems. These programs often encourage self-referral for the employee as well as a supervisor's referral as an alternative to more stringent discipline for poor work performance. The successful EAP brings to the workplace a broad-based strategy to address the full spectrum of substance abuse prevention needs. The most successful EAPs share two overall design features.

1. They frame the EAP drug abuse services as part of a full-spectrum prevention program that minimizes employee attraction to drugs and helps those with problems get into treatment.

2. They provide a diverse range of services for a wide spectrum of employee problems (emotional, relationship, financial, wage garnishment, and burnout).

These two design features lessen employees' apprehension about being labeled as a drug abuser. They prevent drug problems before they start and they identify drug problems for employees in denial who don't accept the fact that they have a problem and often first approach the EAP about another problem area. The EAP is comprised of six basic components:

1. prevention/education/training;

2. identification and confidential outreach;

3. diagnosis and referral;

4. treatment, counseling, and a good monitoring system (including drug testing);

5. follow-up and focus towards aftercare (relapse prevention);

6. confidential record system and effectiveness evaluation.

(SAMHSA/OAS, 1997; EAPA, 1990; Balzer & Pargament, 1988)

In a full-spectrum prevention program, the EAP provides primary, secondary, and tertiary prevention.

Primary Prevention.   In the most effective EAP programs, both corporate and individual denial are addressed with a systems-oriented approach to prevention. Education and training about the impact of substance abuse are provided at all levels in the corporation: to the administration, unions, and line staff. These segments agree on a single corporate policy on drug and alcohol abuse.

Secondary Prevention.   Both education and training focus on drug identification, major effects, and early intervention that are incorporated into the prevention curriculum. The corporation's legal, grievance, and escalating discipline policies are redesigned in light of EAP goals. Security measures (testing, staff review, monitoring, etc.) are established in a manner that is legal and humane. These measures operate both as deterrents to use as well as methods of identifying the abusers and getting them help.

Tertiary Prevention.   The EAP formalizes its intervention approach, allowing for confidential self-referral, peer referral, and supervisor-initiated referral to the EAP. A diagnostic process is established, along with a number of appropriate treatment referrals. Treatment is confidential but the EAP monitors treatment to insure for proper follow-up aftercare and continued recovery efforts. The employment status of workers is evaluated on work performance and not on their participatory effort in the EAP.

Effectiveness of EAPs

Well-conceived successful programs that strike a balance between the corporation's security needs and a genuine concern for the health and welfare of each individual employee have demonstrated great effectiveness and cost savings to businesses. For every $1 spent in an EAP, employers save anywhere from $5 to $16. The cost of providing EAP services ranges from $12 to $20 per employee per year (USDL, 1990). Several studies in major corporations have documented a 60–85% decrease in absenteeism, a 40–65% decrease in sick

time utilization and personal/family health insurance usage, and a 45–75% decrease in on-the-job accidents as well as other cost savings once the EAP system was put into operation.

◇ Northrup Corporation saw a 43% increase in productivity in its first 100 employees who entered an alcohol treatment program.

◇ Employees in the Philadelphia Police Department going through treatment reduced sick days by 38% and injury days by 62%.

◇ In Oldsmobile's Lansing, Michigan plant, lost man-hours declined by 49%, health care benefits by 29%, sick leaves by 56%, grievances by 78%, disciplinary problems by 63%, and accidents by 82%.

(Campbell & Graham, 1988)

DRUGS IN THE MILITARY

One example of reducing the use of psychoactive drugs in the workplace is the experience of the military. Since 1980, the use of illicit drugs has dropped nearly 90%. In the same period, cigarette smoking dropped by 1/3. Unfortunately the rate of heavy drinking showed a smaller drop. In a survey of American military personnel, psychologist Robert Bray of the Research Triangle Institute in North Carolina found that from 1980–1995, 30-day illicit drug use dropped from 27.6% to just 3% of military personnel (Bray, 1995).

The reasons for the drop are varied. Probably the strongest reason was an intensified program of urine testing, starting in the early 1980s, with a positive result as grounds for referral to rehabilitation or, if that fails, discharge. The military does about 3 million drug tests each year. The message was zero tolerance. In the past, drug users had been treated and kept in the military but with zero tolerance, they decided that there was no margin for having impaired people. A second reason for the drop in drug use was that drugs, in general, became less popular in society over that period of time. The drop in smoking from 51% to 32% over the same period of time was attributed to

military smoking bans, an end to free cigarettes for GIs, and stop-smoking programs as well as a general smoking decline in society as a whole. Heavy drinking still occurs at a higher rate than the general public: 17.1% in the military vs. just 12% in the general public. The highest rate is in the Marine Corps and the lowest in the Air Force. Part of the difficulty in reaching heavy drinkers who are mostly among young enlistees is because there is a high turnover rate in the ranks and, historically, drinking has been acceptable.

The military has the advantage of being able to discharge almost anyone they define as being dangerous to other military personnel. In addition, because it is the military, they can conduct testing whenever and almost wherever they choose.

During the Vietnam War, drug use, particularly heroin and marijuana, was high. It was readily available, stress was extremely high, and the environment was strange and permissive (Robins, 1994). During the war in the Persian Gulf, drugs and alcohol were difficult to obtain and as a result there were a lot fewer disciplinary problems among the troops (O'Brien et al., 1992).

DRUG TESTING

Increasingly, drug testing has appeared in all walks of life not just in business. Drug testing has long been used to determine the blood or breath alcohol level of drivers suspected of drunk driving. Testing has been expanded to include

◇ pre-employment testing,

◇ reasonable cause testing,

◇ random testing,

◇ post-accident testing,

◇ periodic testing,

◇ rehabilitation testing of ex-convicts or felons on probation, or others suspected of a crime,

◇ testing to determine social benefits (e.g., food stamps, general assistance) eligibility,

◇ testing for compliance in addicts who are in treatment,

◇ testing by medical examiners to determine the cause of death.

The federal government issued mandates in 1988 and 1998 for a drug-free workplace. Although there is more consensus on effective methods of testing there have been a number of regulations and laws promulgated over the past 10 years that limit random testing of special groups, testing of job applicants, testing of all federal employees, and even random testing of teachers and students.

At present the most widespread use of drug testing is in the military, in pre-employment drug testing, and in drug treatment facilities. Most medium and large businesses routinely use preemployment testing to keep drug users out because, once they are hired, the problems they engender can be very expensive. Because of the many challenges to random testing, many businesses are leery of using it. However, random testing is still used in jobs involving public safety—jobs such as bus drivers, policemen, and pilots.

THE TESTS

Many different laboratory procedures are used to test for drugs in the urine, blood, hair, saliva, sweat, and even different tissues of the body. Each test possesses inherent differences in sensitivity, specificity, and accuracy as well as other potential problems. The drugs that are most often tested for are amphetamines, cannabinoids, cocaine, opioids, and phencyclidine (PCP). Another group of drugs that are commonly tested for are barbiturates, benzodiazepines, methadone, propoxyphene (Darvon®), methaqualone, MDMA, and ethanol (alcohol). Those that can be tested for but are usually not include LSD, fentanyl, psilocybin, MDA, and designer drugs (DHHS/SAMHSA, 1997).

Currently, some two dozen methods are used to analyze body samples for the presence of drugs. None is totally foolproof. The following are the most common methods (Vereby & Buchan, 1997).

Chromatography, Especially Thin Layer Chromatography (TLC)

TLC searches for a wide variety of drugs at the same time and is fairly sensitive to the presence of even minute amounts of chemicals. The major drawback is its inability to accurately differentiate drugs that may have similar chemical properties. For example, ephedrine, a drug used legally in over-the-counter cold medicines, may be misidentified as an illegal amphetamine.

Enzyme-Multiplied Immunoassay Techniques (EMIT), Radio Immunoassay (RIA), Enzyme Immunoassay (EIA)

Immunoassays use antibodies to seek out specific drugs. EMIT tests are extremely sensitive, very rapidly performed, and fairly easy to operate. However they cannot usually distinguish the concentration of the drug present. Also, a separate test must usually be run for each specific suspected drug. Immunoassay techniques are used for many home-testing kits. Some can test for several drugs at once (e.g., Ascend Multimmunoassay [AMIA]).

EMIT tests can also mistake nonabused chemicals for abused drugs, mistaking, for example, opioid alkaloids in the poppy seeds of baked goods for heroin or another opioid. The chemical in Advil® or Motrin® may be mistaken for marijuana and the form of methamphetamine in Vick's Inhaler® is sometimes mistaken as "crank." This method can be so sensitive that breathing air at most rock concerts will show a positive trace of marijuana even though the testee didn't smoke. This oversensitivity is corrected by raising the sensitivity level of the test so only current users will test positive.

Gas Chromatography/Mass Spectrometry Combined (GC/MS) & Gas Liquid Chromotography (GLC)

The GC/MS test is currently the most accurate, sensitive, and reliable method of testing for drugs in the body. It uses gas chromatography separation and mass spectrometry fragmentation patterns to identify drugs. Being very sensitive, it can detect even trace amounts of drugs in the urine and therefore requires skilled interpreters to differentiate environmental exposure from actual use. However it is very expensive, requires highly trained operators, and is a very lengthy and tedious process in comparison to other methods.

The GLC test separates molecules by migration similar to TLC. This process is somewhat less accurate than GC/MS.

Hair Analysis

Hair analysis employs hair samples to detect drugs of abuse. Chemical traces of most psychoactive drugs are stored in human hair cells, so the drugs can be detected almost as long as the hair stays intact, even decades after the drug has been taken. This gives a picture of the degree of drug use (to differentiate occasional use from addictive use) and decreases the frequency of testing, although the ability to discover drug history has been questioned (Henderson, Harkey, & Jones, 1993). RIA techniques are used for screening of hair samples and GC/MS techniques are used for confirmation. More research needs to be done on the accuracy of hair testing, although a number of businesses, such as casinos in Nevada, are using it in preemployment drug testing.

Saliva, Sweat, & Breath

Less accurate tests look for traces of drugs in saliva, sweat, or exhaled air. The advantage of these tests is that they are less invasive, however, they are much more prone to contamination by environmental traces of drugs. Saliva and breath tests can be useful in on-the-spot testing of drivers involved in accidents or suspected of driving under the influence. Confirmation tests are almost mandatory because of the inaccuracy of the tests and because of probable court challenges.

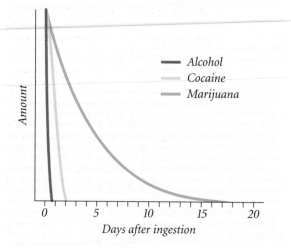

Blood Levels (approximations)

— Alcohol
— Cocaine
— Marijuana

Amount

0   5   10   15   20

Days after ingestion

Figure 8-9•

This graph compares the length of time cocaine, marijuana, and alcohol remain in the blood. For purposes of testing, there is a cutoff level when testing for certain drugs, so that even when there is still some of the drug in a person's blood or urine, it will not be detected by the standard test.

more common drugs of abuse are shown in Table 8-8. Again these are merely rough estimates with wide individual variations. Thus an individual delaying a urine test five days because of cocaine abuse will probably, but not definitely, test negative for cocaine.

Redistribution, Recirculation, Sequestration, & Other Variables

Long-acting drugs like PCP, ethchlovynol (Doriden®), and possibly marijuana can be distributed to certain body tissues or fluids, concentrated and stored there, then be recirculated and concentrated back into the urine. While not common, this can result in a positive test following negative tests after several months of abstinence.

DETECTION PERIOD

Many factors influence the length of time that a drug can be detected in someone's blood, urine, saliva, or other body tissues. These include an individual's drug absorption rate, metabolism rate, rate of distribution in the body, excretion rate, and the specific testing method employed. With a wide variation of these and other factors, a predictable drug detection period would be, at best, an educated guess. Despite this, the public interest requires that some specific estimates be adopted. For urine testing, these estimates can be divided into three broad periods: latency, detection period range, and redistribution.

Latency

Drugs must be absorbed, circulated by the blood, and finally concentrated in the urine in sufficient quantity before they can be detected. This process generally takes about 2–3 hours for most drugs except alcohol, which takes about 30 minutes. Thus someone tested just 30 minutes after using a drug would probably (but not always) test negative for that drug. A chronic user or addict, however, should have enough chemicals already present to test positive even if tested within 30 minutes (Johnson & Quander, 1998).

Detection Period Range

Once sufficient amounts of a drug enter the urine, the drug can be detected for a certain length of time by urinalysis. The rough estimates for the

ACCURACY OF DRUG TESTING

Despite many claims of confidence in the reliability of drug testing, independent blind testing of laboratory re-

TABLE 8–8   DETECTION PERIOD RANGE CHART

Alcohol	1/2–1 day
Amphetamine	2–4 days
Methamphetamine	2–4 days
Barbiturates	
amobarbital, pentobarbital	2–4 days
phenobarbital	up to 30 days
Benzodiazepines	
e.g., alprazolam (Xanax®),	up to 30 days
flunitrazepam (Royhypnol®)	
Cocaine ("coke," "crack")	12–72 hours
Marijuana	
single use	1–3 days
casual use to 4 joints per week	5–7 days
daily use	10–15 days
chronic, heavy use	1–2 months
Opioids	
codeine	2 days
hydromorphone (Dilaudid®)	2–4 days
propoxyphene (Darvon®)	6–48 hours
heroin (morphine is measured)	2–4 days
methadone	2–3 days
PCP	
casual use	2–7 days
chronic, heavy use	several months

(PharmChem, 1999; JAMA, 1987)

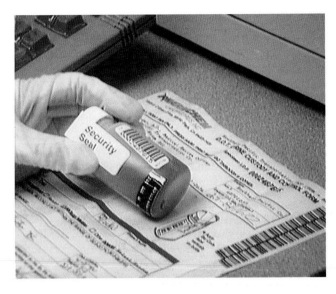

There is a rigid chain of custody for urine samples in good drug-testing laboratories. Detailed paperwork follows each sample.

rect observation of the body specimen collection and a rigid chain of custody over the sample. It would also include using the most accurate testing methods available (e.g., GC/MS) with a mandatory second confirmatory test via a different method and testing for a wide range of abused drugs. It would include the use of a medical review officer, along with a detailed medical and social history, in the interpretation of lab results. The American Association for Clinical Chemistry (AACC) lists 14 guidelines when choosing a lab and checking its accuracy.

1. Require that laboratory-testing methodologies should meet specific testing needs.
2. Correctly target drugs, threshold levels, and methods of screening.
3. Verify the laboratory's drug-testing experience.
4. Review the credentials of key laboratory personnel.
5. Require laboratory quality assurance measures.
6. Review the laboratory's chain of custody procedures.
7. Require advance written notification of changes in methods or thresholds.
8. Evaluate laboratory-reporting procedures.
9. Require timely reporting of test results.
10. Review the specimen storage procedures.
11. Review the policy on contested test results.
12. Check laboratory licensing and accreditation.
13. Continue to monitor the quality of the testing program.
14. Require a complete description of all laboratory fees and charges in advance.

(AACC, 1999)

Consequences of False Positives & Negatives

Concerns about false positive test results are well publicized, debated, and

sults continues to document high error rates for some testing programs. For this reason many companies and agencies use a **medical review officer (MRO)** to review positive results and rule out any errors in procedure, environmental contamination, or alternative medical explanations. The MRO usually interviews the testee, checks the chain of custody, or asks for retesting to search for explanations of a positive result since the consequences can greatly affect the person's future. In some cases the MRO will look at indeterminate results where manipulation of the specimens is suspected (e.g., when the urine sample is too dilute suggesting tampering) (Macdonald & Dupont, 1998).

False positive tests could result from the limitations of testing technology. For example, phenylpropanolamine and dextromethorphan, found in many cold products, have been misidentified as amphetamines and opioids respectively. Herbal teas have been implicated in producing a false cocaine-positive result.

Errors also can result from the mishandling of urine and other specimen samples taken. Tagging the specimen with the wrong label, mixing and preparing the testing solutions incorrectly, errors in calculations, coding the samples and solutions and logging and reporting of results as well as exposure of samples to destructive conditions or to drugs in the laboratory have all resulted in inaccurate tests.

False negative results, not false positives, constitute the bulk of urine-testing errors. These result from laboratories being overly cautious in reporting positive results and from specimen manipulation by the testee. Many manipulations, some effective and some just folklore, have been used by drug abusers to prevent the detection of drugs in their urine. Substitution methods include use of synthetic urine, urine from a clean donor, or even dog urine via a concealed container, injection into the bladder, or catheterization

Attempts to manipulate urine testing have grown to such proportions that "clean pee" (drug-free urine) has become a profitable black market item. Substances such as aspirin, goldenseal tea, niacin, zinc sulfate, bleach, Klear®, water, ammonia, Drano®, hydrogen peroxide, lemon juice, liquid soap, vinegar, and even Visine® have been tried. Most are ineffective. Further, recent designer drugs create a major problem in drug testing. Many have no standard to test against and some are so potent (the effective dose so small) that they will be impossible to identify in the body. Inaccurate tests also result from disease states, pregnancy, medical conditions, interference of prescribed drugs, and individual metabolic conditions.

With the technology available at this time, the best chance for a reliable drug-testing program would include di-

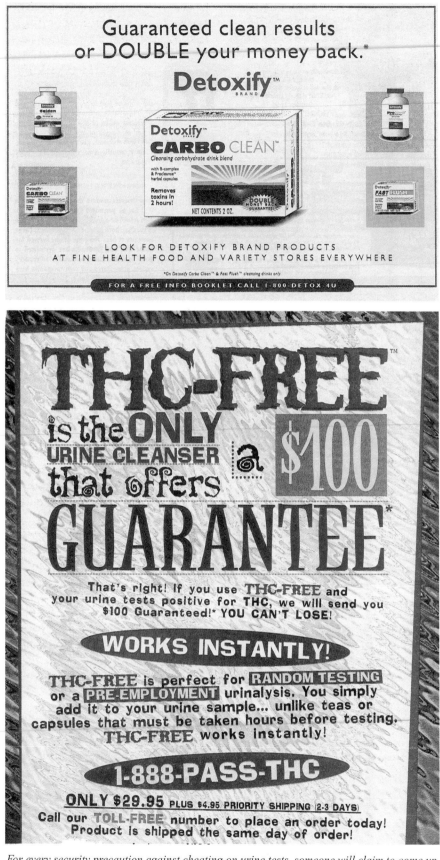

For every security precaution against cheating on urine tests, someone will claim to come up with a method to try to bypass it.

feared. People could lose their jobs, be denied employment, be disqualified from the Olympics, or even risk prison following an erroneous positive result. Less publicized or feared, but just as critical, are the false negative results. These prevent the discovery of drug abuse and feed the already strong denial process in the user. They permit the addict to become progressively more impaired and dysfunctional until a major life crisis occurs.

Nevertheless drug testing is still an effective intervention, treatment, and monitoring tool, especially when used to intervene with heavy users and to discourage casual use. Addicts often state that they wished they had been tested and identified before their lives had been destroyed. Drug abusers in treatment often request increased urine testing to help them focus on abstinence and resist peer pressure. They can say, "Hey, I can't use. I have to be tested." Treatment programs use testing to overcome denial and dishonesty in addicts during early treatment. Recovering addicts in jobs that expose the public to high risk would not be acceptable without a reliable drug-testing program.

DRUGS & THE ELDERLY

"As I started to get older in life and started to gain more experience in life, I started to realize that I was doing a lot of wrong things and it had affected a lot of other people's lives as well as destroying my own. I tried to hide from that pain."
65-year-old recovering heroin addict

SCOPE OF THE PROBLEM

Overall Drug Use

The number of elderly Americans has doubled since 1950. At present, 15% of the U.S. population is 65 years or older and that figure will increase to 21% by the year 2030. By 2050, 80

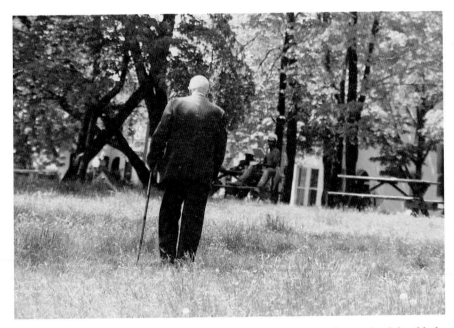

Isolation, ill health, and financial worries are some of the problems that can lead the elderly to drug abuse.

million Americans will be over the age of 65 (U.S. Bureau of the Census, 1996). As the population grows, the problems with drug overuse, abuse, and addiction will grow as well.

This is mostly due to the increased use of prescription drugs, over-the-counter drugs, and alcohol. The use of street drugs decreases with age. For example, in 1998, 30-day use of drugs by Americans over 35 years of age was significantly lower than those aged 26–34. Further

◇ marijuana use was 2.5%, vs. 5.5% for 26 to 34 year olds;

◇ cocaine use was 0.5% vs. 1.2%;

◇ cigarette use was 23.4% vs. 32.5%;

◇ alcohol use was 53.1% vs. 60.9%.

(SAMHSA, 1999)

From 363 million filled prescriptions in 1950 to over 3 billion in 1998, the increase in the use of prescribed medications has been fueled by a larger medical care system, greater life span, and the discovery of hundreds of new compounds (PhRMA, 1999). This surfeit of available remedies for the illnesses and problems of the aging process have also increased the chances of adverse reactions from medications, along with the chances of abuse of drugs with psychoactive properties. In addition peak use of over-the-counter medications occurs after the age of 65 and these too can have adverse reactions and interactions with other drugs. Since more than four out of five elderly suffer from some chronic disease by age 65, 83% of them take at least one prescription drug, however, an astonishing 30% take eight or more (Sheahan, Hendricks, & Coons, 1989).

Chemical Dependency

Up to 17% of adults age 60 and older abuse alcohol and legal drugs (ASAM, 1998). Often the elderly abuse psychoactive drugs to deal with physical or psychological problems, their feelings of loneliness, being unwanted, not respected, and rejected by their families and the workplace. Events such as the death of a spouse, retirement, illness, loss of physical appearance, financial worries, and ageism can also increase drug use and abuse. Although most older adults (87%) see physicians regularly, it is estimated that 40% of those who are at risk do not self-identify or seek services for substance abuse problems on their own

(Raschko, 1990). Unfortunately physicians have a tough time identifying alcoholism or drug abuse. In one study only 37% of alcoholics were identified compared to a 60% identification rate in younger patients (Geller, Levine, Mamon, Moore, Bone, & Stokes, 1989). This is partly because most older adults live in the community and fewer than 5% live in nursing or personal care homes where supervision and physician contact is greater (Altpeter, Schmall, Rakowski, Swift, & Campbell, 1994). In addition many manifestations of drug abuse can be attributed to other chronic illnesses often present in those over 55 and since so many drugs are being used legally, adverse reactions due to the misuse of psychoactive drugs can be masked. Even family members can misattribute the symptoms of drug abuse to the normal effects of aging or the effects of legal prescription drugs.

To compound these problems, the attitude of society is often one of, "They've lived a full life and made their contribution to society, so why disturb their lives now? If they want to abuse drugs at this age, whom will it harm?" This attitude assumes that the unhindered abuse of psychoactive drugs is desirable. But since addiction is a progressive illness for the elderly as well as the young, continued use leads to progressive physiological, emotional, social, relationship, family, and spiritual consequences that users find intolerable. Addiction means unhappiness and lack of choice, no matter what the age of the addicted person.

Costs mount up for untreated elderly chemical abusers. Failure to prevent and then treat chemical abuse among this population leads to huge costs in treating high blood pressure, cardiac and liver disease, gastrointestinal problems, and all the other diseases resulting from the abuse of drugs.

PHYSIOLOGICAL CHANGES

"When I was young, nobody told me what really happens to your body when you grow old and now that I'm here, it's a shock. The physical part I can

accept, although the constant arthritis makes me an aspirin addict. It's the mental part that's difficult, being closer to the end than the beginning. Wine and beer used to be my favorite psychiatric drug, better than Prozac®, but at my age, my liver and body can only handle a couple of drinks and I nod off."

68-year-old male

The human body's physiological functioning and chemistry are not as efficient in the elderly as they are in young people and midlife adults. This results in an abnormal response to drugs compared to younger adults. Generally elderly people's enzymes and other bodily functions become less active, conditions that impair their ability to inactivate or excrete drugs (Smith, 1998). This makes drugs more potent in older people. For example, Valium® is deactivated by liver enzymes but after the age of 30, the liver slowly loses its ability to make the necessary enzymes. Thus a 10-milligram dose of Valium® taken by someone age 70 will result in an effect equal to a dose of about 30 milligrams taken by a 21 year old.

Older people are also more likely to have concurrent illnesses that may greatly alter the effects of drugs in their bodies or make them more sensitive to the toxic and adverse side effects. Conditions like diabetes and liver, heart, and kidney disease all affect or are affected by drug abuse. Further, drugs used to treat these concurrent illnesses, along with a greater use of over-the-counter drugs, give rise to a greater potential for drug interactions.

The most commonly abused drugs in the elderly besides alcohol are prescription sedatives (e.g., Valium®), codeine, Darvon® and other opioid analgesics, narcotic cough syrups, and over-the-counter sedatives or sleep aids. One change that has reduced the abuse of psychoactive drugs has been the increased use of psychiatric medications, e.g., fluoxetine (Prozac®), sertraline (Zoloft®), and buspirone (BuSpar®). Because older adults are less likely to use psychoactive medications nontherapeutically, many problems with drugs fall into the misuse category. A major problem is not understanding directions, especially when several medications are involved, often from multiple physicians unaware of a colleague's treatments.

Age does not endow a person with immunity to the negative effects of drugs or chemical dependence. Six percent to 11% of elderly patients who are admitted to hospitals display symptoms of alcoholism. This figure goes up to 14% for emergency room admissions, 20% for elderly patients in psychiatric wards, and as high as 49% in some nursing homes, though this high figure may result from the use of nursing homes as short-term alcoholism treatment facilities (JAMA, 1996). Thus prevention education and treatment services targeted for the aged are as important as those for adolescents.

In addition age-related changes significantly affect the way an older person responds to alcohol, the main drug of abuse:

◇ a decrease in body water,

◇ an increased sensitivity and decreased tolerance to alcohol,

◇ a decrease in the metabolism of alcohol in the gastrointestinal tract.

The decrease in body water means that, for a given dose of alcohol, the concentration of alcohol in the blood system is higher in an older person than in a younger person. For this reason the same amount of alcohol that previously had little effect can now cause intoxication (Smith, 1995).

PREVENTION ISSUES

Primary Prevention

Because social drinkers and even abstainers develop late onset alcoholism, often in response to problems of aging, older people need to be reeducated about the dangers of excessive use of alcohol or other psychoactive drugs. Elderly people need to receive information and counseling about ways to manage the problems associated with growing older without using psychoactive drugs at all or at least, in the case of alcohol, in moderation. Community volunteerism, an active social life, continuing education are also ways that primary prevention can work for this group. Information about primary prevention, customized for the elderly, needs to be given to those who provide services to this population, such as nurses, physicians, and social workers.

Secondary Prevention

Secondary prevention for this age group focuses on recognition of early stages of alcoholism or drug abuse and appropriate intervention tactics. Frequently, there is strong denial by this age group, particularly because many of this generation see alcohol and other drug abuse as a sin or moral failure. Drug abuse tends to be secretive or hidden, particularly because of the seclusion and solitude many live in, so a mobile professional staff and vigorous outreach program are necessary. Home visits are particularly effective. It is especially important to recognize alcoholism and addiction as primary diseases that must be treated.

In addition to healthcare workers recognizing signs of addiction, friends and family of older adults, along with drivers and volunteers from senior centers who see older adults on a regular basis and are intimately acquainted with their habits and daily routines, should also be aware of signs. Other venues and activities where problems can be identified are clubs, health fairs, congregate meal sites, and senior day care programs.

Tertiary Prevention

Treatment frequently involves different procedures from those used with younger clients. This age group is not responsive to abrupt, coercive, confrontational therapies. The pace of therapy has to be slow, patient, and reassuring. Bringing in the entire family to create an understanding sympathetic support group helps. Detoxification needs more time as does the period for recovery, often two years or more.

Thereafter outpatient counseling, peer group work, and a protective environment (safe from alcohol and other drugs) provide continuing care and reinforce recovery (CSAT, 1998). The least-intensive treatment options are recommended. Although these less-intensive options will not resolve the elderly patients' alcohol or drug problems, they can move them into specialized treatment by helping them overcome their denial or resistance to change (Johnson, & London, 1997).

CONCLUSIONS

NO SIMPLE SOLUTION

The major difficulty with prevention efforts at this time is to provide a measurement of long-term effectiveness for the strategies involved. Studies cannot conclusively show the effectiveness of a campaign since so many factors are involved and it can be hard to differentiate inevitable trends in society with specific efforts. However to do nothing is worse. A second, seemingly successful, recent direction is the use of massive advertising campaigns that are more effective, more honest, and more pervasive than earlier efforts. The reasoning is that if multiple ads and marketing campaigns can get people to eat unhealthy food, drink beer, and smoke cigarettes, why can't they do the opposite.

There is profound disagreement about drugs and drug policy in our society. Some see all drugs as inherently evil substances that must be regulated by laws. Some see drug use as a matter of choice (of free choice in the case of legal drugs) or eventual decriminalization and even legalization in the case of illicit drugs. Some see drug abuse as a pathological disease requiring treatment.

CURRENT PROMISING DIRECTIONS

As we begin the twenty-first century, prevention is seen as a shared responsibility. The most promising approaches are the ones in which various segments of a community work in unison—youth, merchants, police, professionals, schools, parents, the government, and the media. An entire community arrives at a consensus about what it must do to prevent drug abuse, then agrees on the specific models that would best serve individuals and the whole community.

People are at risk throughout their lives. If they are going to be exposed from cradle to grave, then prevention efforts also must extend over a lifetime.

◇ Early primary prevention can treat a pregnant mother that uses drugs, so the child is not born addicted. Prenatal care programs can provide parenting skills, teaching her to give unconditional love, showing the importance of holding her baby, and making her aware of other resources available to her. Toddlers can be given activities that increase bonding with their parents or caregiver. If the child has been exposed to drugs in the womb, intensive care can minimize long-term effects.

◇ Parents may decide not to drink or use during their child-rearing years especially and model life-enhancing behavior. The family is a crucial prevention delivery system in childhood.

◇ Grammar schools can integrate prevention into the curriculum. Developmental skills can be taught, including resistance and decision-making skills. Students can be taught how to process moral dilemmas and how to talk about feelings. Activities that build and promote self-esteem need to be included.

◇ By middle school, many children stop listening to adults and start listening to other children. Peer educator programs can identify natural leaders who will serve as models, leaders, teachers, and guides for in-school peer-prevention efforts.

◇ In high school and college, since there is greater exposure to drugs, prevention must assume a higher level of sophistication to counter

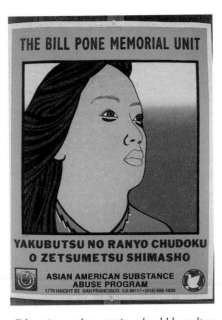

Education and prevention should be culturally specific.

experimentation, social use, and habituation. Prevention at this level must make a continual effort involving curriculum infusion, support services, environmental change, policy formulation, and enforcement as well as alternatives to alcohol and other drug use in social occasions.

◇ For the work force, prevention needs to be continued through EAPs. They must be proactive and provide ongoing prevention, referral, and treatment opportunities. Prevention education should be provided in the normal course of job training.

◇ Programs should be developed that address and publicize many of the health effects of drugs, such as sexually transmitted diseases including HIV and hepatitis C from needle use as well as lung disease from cigarettes.

◇ For older people preretirement training sessions and grief counseling can help prevent alcohol and other drug use. Outreach programs need to take the prevention message to the people who are housebound or are not part of the school-workplace-community avenues of access.

◇ Finally prevention must be adapted to the needs of specific audiences. A program for a rural midwestern town may not be consistent for a school in inner-city Los Angeles.

Secondary prevention designed for experimenters who need to know effects of drugs might actually stimulate experimentation in a primary audience. Since no single pre-

vention program can demonstrate universal, reproducible results, modifications of existing programs must be made to fit a particular situation.

CHAPTER SUMMARY

INTRODUCTION

1. Psychoactive drugs affect people at all ages from the "crack"—affected baby to the elderly woman who borrows a friend's prescription painkiller. Thus prevention needs to address all ages.

PREVENTION

Concepts of Prevention

2. The goals of prevention are to prevent abuse before it begins, stop it where it has begun, and treat people where abuse and addiction have taken hold.

3. The three methods of prevention are supply reduction, demand reduction, and harm reduction.

4. About 1/3 of the National Drug Control Budget is aimed at demand reduction.

5. Historically prevention has wavered between temperance and prohibition. In the 1920s and 1930s, Prohibition did reduce problems associated with alcohol, although it was repealed 14 years after being put into law.

6. Scare tactics, drug information programs, skill-building and resiliency programs, environmental change programs, and the public health model programs are some of the prevention tactics that have been tried.

7. The public health model uses the concepts of the host (the actual user), the environment (the social climate), and the agent (the psychoactive drug) to explain all the combinations of prevention programs.

8. The most effective prevention programs involve the family.

Prevention Methods

9. Supply reduction by law enforcement and other government agencies, augmented by the passage of antidrug laws, are aimed at reducing the supply of drugs on the streets. The effectiveness of supply reduction is open to debate.

10. Demand reduction tries to reduce people's desire for drugs either through primary, secondary, or tertiary prevention (which includes treatment).

11. Primary prevention for drug-naive young people aims at preventing experimentation and social use.

12. Secondary prevention seeks to halt drug use once it has begun through education, intervention, and skill building.

13. Tertiary prevention, usually some form of treatment, seeks to stop further damage from drug abuse and addiction. Through intervention, individual and group therapy, medical intervention, cue extinction, and promotion of a healthy lifestyle, recovery is encouraged.

14. The primary goal of harm reduction is not abstinence but rather reduction of the harm that addicts do to themselves and to society.

15. Drug substitution programs, designated driver programs, and outreach needle exchange programs are some examples of harm reduction. These programs conflict with zero tolerance government programs.

Challenges to Prevention

16. The legality of alcohol and tobacco, along with heavy advertising, limits the effectiveness and believability of many prevention programs.

17. Prevention that works takes time, must be carried on throughout people's lifetimes, and must be adequately funded.

FROM CRADLE TO GRAVE

Patterns of Use

18. The age of first use of drugs has gotten lower and lower, particularly since 1992. Caffeine, cigarettes, inhalants, and alcohol are generally the first drugs used.

19. Neither level of intelligence, income, nor social class protects one from abuse and addiction.

Pregnancy & Birth

20. Up to 37% of fetuses are exposed to some psychoactive drug, particularly alcohol, tobacco, and marijuana, during pregnancy.

21. Drugs are particularly dangerous to the fetus because its defense mechanisms, e.g., drug-neutralizing metabolic system, immune system, and mature organs, are not yet developed. For example, each surge of effects from a drug the mother takes gives multiple surges to the defenseless fetus.

22. Major problems from drug use during pregnancy include a higher rate of miscarriage, blood vessel damage, severe withdrawal symptoms, and a much higher risk of

Bry, B. H., McKeon, P., & Pandina, R. J. (1982). Extent of drug use as a function of number of risk factors. *Journal of Abnormal Psychology, 91*(4), 273–279.

Bufum, J. (1982). Pharmacosexology: The effects of drugs on sexual function, a review. *Journal of Psychoactive Drugs, 14*(1–2), 5–43.

Cahoon-Young, B. (1997). Prevalence of hepatitis C virus in women: Who's getting it, why and co-infection with HIV. Perspective on the epidemiology. *Treatment and Interventions for the Hepatitis C Virus.* San Francisco: Haight-Ashbury Free Clinics.

Campbell & Graham. (1988). *Drugs and Alcohol in the Workplace: A Guide for Managers.* New York: Facts on File Publications.

Carlson, B. (1998). Addiction and treatment in the criminal justice system. In A. W. Graham & T. K. Schultz (Eds.), *Principles of Addiction Medicine* (2nd ed., pp. 405–419). Chevy Chase, MD: American Society of Addiction Medicine, Inc.

CASA. (2000). *Dangerous Liaisons: Substance Abuse and Sex.* Centers on Addiction and Substance Abuse: New York: Columbia University.

CDC. (1998). *Trends in the HIV & AIDS Epidemic.* Centers for Disease Control and Prevention. Rockville, MD: Department of Health and Human Services.

CDC. (2000). *HIV/AIDS Surveillance Report 11*(1). Atlanta: Centers For Disease Control and Prevention. Rockville, MD: Department of Health and Human Services.

CDC. (1999). Sexually Transmitted Disease Surveillance, 1989. Centers for Disease Control and Prevention. http://www. wonder.cdc.gov.

Centrella, M. (1994). Physician addiction and impairmentæ Current thinking: A review. *Journal of Addictive Disease, 13*, 91–105.

Cherukuri, R., Minkoff, H., Feldman, J., Parekh, A., & Glass, L. (1989). A cohort study of alkaloidal cocaine ("crack") in pregnancy. *Obstetrics and Gynecology, 72,* 145–151.

Clarren, S. K. (1999). Interview with publisher. November, 1999. Authors files.

Comerci, G. D. (1998) Office assessment and brief intervention with the adolescent suspected of substance abuse. In A. W. Graham & T. K. Schultz (Eds.), *Principles of Addiction Medicine* (2nd ed., pp. 1145–1146). Chevy Chase, MD: American Society of Addiction Medicine, Inc.

Cook, P. C., Petersen, R. C., & Moore, D. T. (1994). *Alcohol, tobacco, and other drugs may harm the unborn.* Rockville, MD: U.S. Department of Health and Human Services, Public Health Service.

Crowe, L., & George, W. (1989). Alcohol and sexuality. *Psychological Bulletin, 105,* 374–386.

CSAT. (1998). *Substance Abuse Among Older Adults* (CSAT Treatment Improvement Protocol No. 26). Rockville, MD: Center for Substance Abuse Treatment.

CSAT. (1994). Final Report of the National Structured Evaluation of Alcohol and Other Drug Abuse Prevention. Unpublished report. Rockville, MD: Center for Substance Abuse Prevention.

Day, N. L., Richardson, G. A., Goldschmidt, L., et al. (1994). Effect of prenatal marijuana exposure on the cognitive development of offspring at age three. *Neurotoxicology and Teratology, 16,* 169–175.

DEA (Drug Enforcement Administration). (1998). NNICC Report on the Supply of Illicit Drugs to the United States, 1997. *http://www.usdoj.gov/dea/pubs/intel/nnicc 97.htm.*

Des Jarlais, D. C., Hagan, H., & Friedman, S. R. (1997). Epidemiology and Emerging Public Health Perspectives. In J. H. Lowinson, P. Ruiz, R. B. Millman, & J. G. Langrod, (Eds.), *Substance Abuse: A Comprehensive Textbook* (3rd ed., pp. 591–596). Baltimore: Williams & Wilkins.

DHHS/SAMHSA. (1997). Department of Health and Human Services Substance Abuse and Mental Health Services Administration *National Laboratory Certification Program.* Rockville, MD: SAMHSA.

Dielman, T. E. (1995). School-based research on the prevention of adolescent alcohol use and misuse: Methodological issues and advances. In G. M. Boyd, J. Howard, & R. A. Zucker (Eds.), *Alcohol Problems Among Adolescents: Current Directions in Prevention Research.* Hillsdale, NJ: Lawrence Erlbaum Associates.

DOJ (Department of Justice). (2000). *Drugs, Crime, and the Justice System.* Bureau of Justice Statistics. *http://www.doj.gov.*

Drug Strategies. (1995). Keeping score. Washington, DC: Drug Strategies.

EAPA. (1990). Standards for employee assistance programs. Employee Assistance Professionals Association, Inc. *Exchange, 20*(10).

Englehart, P. F., Robinson, H., Kates, H. (1997). The workplace. In J. H. Lowinson, P. Ruiz, R. B. Millman, & J. G. Langrod, (Eds.), *Substance Abuse: A Comprehensive Textbook* (3rd ed., pp. 875–884). Baltimore: Williams & Wilkins.

Ennett, S. T., Tobler, N. S., Ringwalt, C. L., & Flewelling, R. L. (1994). How effective is drug abuse resistance education? A meta-analysis of project DARE outcome evaluations. *American Journal of Public Health, 84,* 1394–1401.

Eriksson, M., Larsson, G., Zetterstrom, R. (1981). Amphetamine addiction and pregnancy. *Acta Obstetrics and Gynecology Scandinavia, 60,* 253–259.

Eyler, F. D., Behnke, M., Conlon, M., Woos, N. S., & Wobie, K. (1998). Birth outcome from a prospective, matched study of prenatal crack/cocaine use; II. Interactive and dose effects on neurobehavioral assessment. *Pediatrics, 101,* 237–241.

Feacham, R. G. A. (1995). Valuing the Past . . . Investing in the Future. Evaluation of the National HIV/AIDS Strategy 1993–94 to 1995–96. Canberra, Australia: Australian Government Publishing Service.

Finnegan, L. P., & Ehrlich, S. M. (1990). Maternal drug abuse during pregnancy: Evaluation and pharmacotherapy for neonatal abstinence. *Modern Methods of Pharmacological Testing in the Evaluation of Drugs of Abuse, 6,* 255–263.

Finnegan, L. P., & Kandall, S. R. (1997). Maternal and neonatal effects of alcohol and drugs. In J. H. Lowinson, P. Ruiz, R. B. Millman, & J. G. Langrod, (Eds.), *Substance Abuse: A Comprehensive Textbook* (3rd ed., pp. 513–533). Baltimore: Williams & Wilkins.

Fleming, M. F., Barry, K. L., Manwell, L. B., Johnson, K., and London, R. (1997). Brief physician advice for problem alcohol drinkers: A randomized controlled trial in community-based primary care practices. *Journal of the American Medical Association, 277,* 1039–1045.

Fried, P. A. (1995). The Ottawa Prenatal Prospective Study (OPPS): Methodological issues and findings: it's easy to throw the baby out with the bath water. *Life Sciences, 56,* 2159–2168.

Fried, P. A., O'Connel, C. M., & Watkinson, B. (1992). 60- and 72-month follow-up of children prenatally exposed to marijuana, cigarettes, and alcohol: Cognitive and language assessment. *Developmental and Behavioral Pediatrics, 13,* 383–391.

Fried, P. A., & Watkinson, B. (1997). Reading and language in 9- to 12-year-olds prenatally exposed to cigarettes and marijuana. *Neurotoxicology and Teratology, 19,* 171–183.

Fried, P. A., Watkinson, B., & Gray, R. (1998). Differential effects on cognitive functioning in 9 to 12 year olds prenatally exposed to cigarettes and marijuana. *Neurotoxicology and Teratology, 120,* 293–306.

Fulroth, R., Phillips, & Durand, D. J. (1989). Perinatal outcome of infants exposed to cocaine and/or heroin in utero. *American Journal of Disabled Children, 143,* 905–910.

Gambert, S. R. (1997). The elderly. In J. H. Lowinson, P. Ruiz, R. B. Millman, & J. G. Langrod, (Eds.), *Substance Abuse: A Comprehensive Textbook* (3rd ed., pp. 692–698). Baltimore: Williams & Wilkins.

Geller, G., Levine, D. M., Mamon, J. A., Moore, R. D., Bone, L. R., and Stokes, E. J. (1989). Knowledge, attitudes, and reported practices of medical students and house staff regarding the diagnosis and treatment of alcoholism. *Journal of the American Medical Association 261,* 3115–3120.

Gerstein, D. R., Johnson, R. A., Harwood, H., Fountain, D., Suter, N., & Malloy, K. (1994). *Evaluating Recovery Services: The California Drug and Alcohol Treatment Assessment (CALDATA)*. Sacramento, CA: California Department of Alcohol and Drug Programs

Gold, M. S., & Miller, N. S. (1997). Cocaine (and "crack"): Clinical Aspects. In J. H. Lowinson, P. Ruiz, R. B. Millman, & J. G. Langrod, (Eds.), *Substance Abuse: A Comprehensive Textbook* (3rd ed., p. 188). Baltimore: Williams & Wilkins.

Goldberg, R. J. (1998). Selective serotonin reuptake inhibitors: Infrequent medical adverse effects. *Archives of Family Medicine, 7*, 78–84.

Gomby, D. S., & Shiono, P. H. (1991). Estimating the number of substance-exposed infants. In *The Future of Children*. Los Altos, CA: Center for the Future of Children.

Greenfeld, L. A. (1998). *Alcohol and Crime: An Analysis of National Data on the Prevalence of Alcohol Involvement in Crime*. Washington, DC: U.S. Department of Justice.

Hans, S. L. (1998). Developmental outcomes of prenatal exposure to alcohol and other drugs. In A. W. Graham & T. K. Schultz (Eds.), *Principles of Addiction Medicine* (2nd ed., pp. 1223–1236). Chevy Chase, MD: American Society of Addiction Medicine, Inc.

Hansen, W. B., & Graham. J. (1993). Preventing alcohol, marijuana, and cigarette use among adolescents: Peer pressure resistance training versus establishing conservative norms. *Prevention Medicine, 20*, 414–430.

Harvard. (1998). Cocaine Before Birth. *The Harvard Mental Health Letter, 15* (6), 1–4.

Haverkos, H. (1998). HIV/AIDS, tuberculosis, and other infectious diseases. In A. W. Graham & T. K. Schultz (Eds.), *Principles of Addiction Medicine* (2nd ed., pp. 825–832). Chevy Chase, MD: American Society of Addiction Medicine, Inc.

Hazelden. (1993). *Refusal Skills*. Center City, MN: Hazelden Foundation.

Hechtman, L. (1989). Teenage mothers and their children: risks and problems. *Canadian Journal of Psychiatry, 34*, 569–575.

Henderson, G. L., Harkey, M. R., & Jones, R. (1993). Hair analysis for drugs of abuse. Final report, grant No. NIJ 90-NU-CX-0012. Rockville, MD: NIDA.

Himelein, M. J. (1995). Risk factors for sexual victimization in dating. *Psychology of Women Quarterly, 19*, 31–48.

Hird, S., Khuri, E. T., Dusenbury, L., & Millman, R. B. (1997). Adolescents. In J. H. Lowinson, P. Ruiz, R. B. Millman, & J. G. Langrod, (Eds.), *Substance Abuse: A Comprehensive Textbook* (3rd ed., pp. 683–691). Baltimore: Williams & Wilkins.

Hoffman, K. (1998). Fitting prevention into the continuum of care. In A. W. Graham & T. K. Schultz (Eds.), *Principles of Addiction Medicine* (2nd ed., pp. 233–245). Chevy Chase, MD: American Society of Addiction Medicine, Inc.

Hubbard, R. L., Craddock, S. G., Flynn, P. M., Anderson, J., & Etheridge, R. M. (1997). Overview of one-year follow-up outcomes in DATOS. *Psychology of Addictive Behavior.*

Jaffe, J. H. (1995). Prohibition of alcohol. In J. H. Jaffee (Ed.), *Encyclopedia of Drugs and Alcohol* (Vol. 2, pp. 885–888). New York: Simon & Schuster Macmillan.

Jaffe, J. H., & Shopland, D. R. (1995). Tobacco: Medical Complications. In J. H. Jaffee (Ed.), *Encyclopedia of Drugs and Alcohol* (Vol. 2, pp. 1045–1046). New York: Simon & Schuster Macmillan.

JAMA (Journal of the American Medical Association). (1987). Scientific issues in drug testing. *JAMA, 257*(22), 3112.

JAMA. (1996). Council on Scientific Affairs. Alcoholism in the elderly. *JAMA, 275*(10), 797–801.

JAMA. (1999). HIV infection and AIDS. *JAMA Education & Support Center.*

Jastak, J. T. (1991). Nitrous oxide and its abuse. *Journal of the American Dental Association, 122*, 48–52.

Johnson, B. L., & Quander, J. D. Esq. (1998). Overview of drug-free workplace programs. In A. W. Graham & T. K. Schultz (Eds.), *Principles of Addiction Medicine* (2nd ed., pp. 1241–1254). Chevy Chase, MD: American Society of Addiction Medicine, Inc.

Jones, K. L., & Smith, D. W. (1973). Recognition of the Fetal Alcohol Syndrome in early infancy. *Lancet, 2*, 999–1001.

Joseph, H., & Paone, D. (1997). The homeless. In J. H. Lowinson, P. Ruiz, R. B. Millman, & J. G. Langrod, (Eds.), *Substance Abuse: A Comprehensive Textbook* (3rd ed., pp. 733–743). Baltimore: Williams & Wilkins.

Juliana, P, & Goodman, C. (1997). Children of substance-abusing parents. In J. H. Lowinson, P. Ruiz, R. B. Millman, & J. G. Langrod, (Eds.), *Substance Abuse: A Comprehensive Textbook* (3rd ed., pp. 665–671). Baltimore: Williams & Wilkins.

Kaltenbach, K., & Finnegan, L. P. (1989). Children exposed to methadone in utero: assessment of developmental and cognitive ability. *Annual; New York Academy of Science, 562*, 360–362.

Kaminer, Y. (1994). Adolescent substance abuse. In M. Galanter, & H. D. Kleber (Eds.), *Textbook of Substance Abuse Treatment*. Washington, DC: The American Psychiatric Press.

Kandall, S. R. (1998). Treatment options for drug-exposed neonates. In A. W. Graham & T. K. Schultz (Eds.), *Principles of Addiction Medicine* (2nd ed., pp. 1211–1222).

Chevy Chase, MD: American Society of Addiction Medicine, Inc.

Kandall, S. R. (1993). *Improving Treatment for Drug-Exposed Infants* (Treatment Improvement Protocol Series). Rockville, MD: Center for Substance Abuse Treatment, 14–15.

Kandall, S. R., Gaines, J., Habel, L., Davidson, G., & Jessop, D. (1993). Relationship of maternal substance abuse to sudden infant death syndrome in offspring. *Journal of Pediatrics, 123*, 120–126.

Klein, L., & Goldenberg, R. L. (1990). Prenatal Care and its Effect on Pre-Term Birth and Low Birth Weight In I. R. Markets, & J. E. Thompson. (Eds.), *New Perspectives on Prenatal Care* (pp. 511–513). New York: Elsevier.

Kline, M. D. (1989). Fluoxetine and anorgasmia. *American Journal of Psychiatry, 146*, 804–805.

Kumpfer, K. L. (1994). *Promoting Resiliency to AOD Use in High Risk Youth*. Rockville, MD: Center for Substance Abuse Prevention.

Kumpfer, K. L., Goplerud, E., & Alvarado, R. (1998). Assessing individual risks and resiliencies. In A. W. Graham & T. K. Schultz (Eds.), *Principles of Addiction Medicine* (2nd ed., pp. 207–214). Chevy Chase, MD: American Society of Addiction Medicine, Inc.

Lender, E. M., & Martin, J. K. (1987). *Drinking in America*. New York: Free Press.

Macdonald, D. I., & DuPont, R. L. (1998). The role of the medical review officer. In A. W. Graham & T. K. Schultz (Eds.), *Principles of Addiction Medicine* (2nd ed., pp. 1255–1262). Chevy Chase, MD: American Society of Addiction Medicine, Inc.

Marnell, T. (Ed.). (1997). *Drug Identification Bible* (3rd ed.). Denver, CO: Drug Identification Bible Publishing.

Mangione, T. W. et al. (1998). *New Perspectives for Worksite Alcohol Strategies: Results from a Corporate Drinking Study*. Boston: JSI Research & Training Institute.

Marques, P. R., & McKnight, A. J. (1991). Drug abuse risk among pregnant adolescents attending public health clinics. *American Journal of Drug and Alcohol Abuse, 17*, 399–414.

Martin, J. C. (1992). *The effects of maternal use of tobacco products or amphetamines on offspring*. Baltimore: The Johns Hopkins University Press.

May, P. A. (1996). Research issues in the prevention of fetal alcohol syndrome and alcohol-related birth defects. *Research Monograph 32, Women and Alcohol: Issues for Prevention Research*. Bethesda, MD: National Institute on Alcohol Abuse and Alcoholism.

Mayes, L., Grillon, C., Granger, R., & Schottenfeld, R. (1998). Regulation of arousal and attention in preschool children exposed to cocaine prenatally. *Annals of the New York Academy of Sciences, 846,* 144–152.

Mello, N. K., Mendelson, J. H., & Teoh, S. K. (1993). An overview of the effects of alcohol on neuroendocrine function in women. In S. Zakhari (Ed.), *Alcohol and the Endocrine System.* NIAAA Research Monograph No. 23, NIH Pub. 93-3533. Bethesda, MD: NIAAA.

Meston, C. M., & Gorzalka, B. B. (1992). Psychoactive drugs and human sexual behavior: The role of serotonergic activity. *Journal of Psychoactive Drugs, 24*(1), 1–40.

Metzger, D. S., Woody, G. E., McLellan, A., et al. (1993). Human immunodeficiency virus seroconversion among intravenous drug users in and out of treatment: An 18th month prospective follow-up. *Journal of Acquired Immune Deficiency Syndrome, 6,* 1049–1056.

Milberger, S., Biederman, J., Faraone, S. V., & Jones, J. (1998). Further evidence of an association between maternal smoking during pregnancy and attention deficit hyperactivity disorder: Findings from a high-risk sample of siblings. *Journal of Clinical Child Psychology, 27,* 352–358.

Miller, L. J. (1998). Treatment of the addicted woman in pregnancy. In A. W. Graham & T. K. Schultz (Eds.), *Principles of Addiction Medicine* (2nd ed., pp. 1199–1210). Chevy Chase, MD: American Society of Addiction Medicine, Inc.

Morganthaler, J., & Joy, D. (1994). *Better Sex Through Chemistry: A Guide to the New Prosexual Drugs.* Petaluma, CA: Smart Publications.

Moskowitz, J. (1989). The primary prevention of alcohol problems. A critical review of the research literature. *Journal of Studies on Alcohol, 50*(1), 54–88.

Mumola, C. (1998). *Substance Abuse and Treatment, State and Federal Prisoners, 1997.* Washington, DC: Bureau of Justice Statistics.

NIAID. (1995). *AZT and Pregnant Women (ACTG 076).* Washington DC: National Institute of Allergy and Infectious Diseases.

NIDA/NIAAA. (1998). The Economic Costs of Alcohol and Drug Abuse in the United States. *http://www.nida.nih.gov/Economic-Costs/Chapter1.html#1.10*

NIDA. (1994). *Annualized Estimates from the National Pregnancy Health Survey.* Washington, DC: National Institute on Drug Abuse.

NIDA Bulletin. (2000). Hepatitis C: NIDA Community Drug Alert Bulletin. http://www.drugabuse.gov.

NIDA Media Advisory. (1998). Prevention Could Save $352 Million Annually. *http://www.nida.hih.gov/MedAdv/98/MA-1022.htm.*

NIDA Infofax. (1999). Rohypnol and GHB. NIDA Infofax. *http://www.nida.nih.gov/Infofax/RohypnolGHB.html.*

Noble, A., Vega, W. A., Kolody, B., Porter, P., Hwang, J., Merk, G. A., & Bole, A. (1997). Prenatal substance abuse in California: Findings from the perinatal substance exposure study. *Journal of Psychoactive Drugs, 29*(1), 43–53.

Novick, D. M., Haverkos, H. W., & Teller, D. W. (1997). The medically ill substance abuser. In J. H. Lowinson, P. Ruiz, R. B. Millman, & J. G. Langrod, (Eds.), *Substance Abuse: A Comprehensive Textbook* (3rd ed., pp. 534–550). Baltimore: Williams & Wilkins.

Novick, D. M., Reagan, K. J., Croxson, T. S., Gelb, A. M., Stenger, R. J., & Kreck, M. J. (1997). Hepatitis C virus serology in parenteral drug users with chronic liver disease. *Addiction, 92*(2), 167–171.

NRC (National Research Council), & NIM (National Institute of Medicine). (1995). *Preventing HIV Transmission. The Role of Sterile Needles and Bleach.* Washington, DC: National Academy Press.

Nurco, D. N., Hanlon, T. E., Bateman, R. W., & Kinlock, T. W. (1995). Drug abuse treatment in the context of correctional surveillance. *Journal of Substance Abuse Treatment, 12*(1), 19–27.

O'Brien, R., Cohen, S., Evans, G., & Fine, J. (1992). *The Encyclopedia of Drug Abuse* (2nd ed.). New York: Facts On File.

ONDCP. (2000). *National Drug Control Strategy: 2000 Annual Report.* Office of National Drug Control Policy. Bethesda, MD: National Drug Clearinghouse.

ONDCP. (1999). National Drug Control Strategy: 1999 Annual Report. Office of National Drug Control Policy. Bethesda, MD: National Drug Clearinghouse.

ONDCP. (1999). *Remarks by Barry R. McCaffrey,* Director, Office of National Drug Control Policy to the Dante B. Fascell North-South Center. University of Miami, Florida, 2-11-99. Bethesda, MD: National Drug Clearinghouse.

ONDCP/Prevention. (2000). *Evidence-based principles for substance abuse prevention.* Office of National Drug Control Policy. *http://www.whitehousedrugpolicy.gov.*

Paria, B. C. et al. (1999). Fatty-acid amide hydrolase is expressed in the mouse uterus and embryo during the periimplantation period. *Biology of Reproduction, 60,* 1151–1157.

Paria, B. C., Das, S. K., & Dey, S. K. (1995). The preimplantation mouse embryo is a target for cannabinoid ligand-receptor signaling. *Proceedings of the National Academy of Sciences, 92,* 9460–9464.

Partnership. (1998). Partnership for a Drug Free America. *http://www.drugfreeamerica.org.*

PDR. (2000). *Physicians' Desk Reference* (54th ed.). Montvale, NJ: Medical Economics Co.

Perkins H. W., Meilman P. W., Leichliter J. S., Cashin J. R., & Presley, C. A. (1999). Misperceptions of the norms for the frequency of alcohol and other drug use on college campuses. *Journal of American College Health, 47*(6), 253–258.

PhRMA. (1999). Industry Profile, 1998. PhRMA (Pharmaceutical Research and Manufacturers of America) Publications. *http://www.phrma.org/publications/industry/profile98.*

Plessinger, M. A., & Woods, J. R. Jr. (1998). Cocaine in pregnancy: Recent data on maternal and fetal risks. *Obstetrics and Gynecology Clinics of North America, 25*(1), 99–112.

Quinn, T. (1996). Global burden of the AIDS epidemic. *Lancet, 348,* 99–106.

Raschko, R. (1990). "Gatekeepers" do the case finding in Spokane. *Aging, 361,* 38–40.

Richardson, G. A. (1998). Prenatal cocaine exposure: A longitudinal study of development. *Annals of the New York Academy of Sciences, 846,* 144–152.

Richardson, G. A., Day, N. L., & Goldschmidt, L. (1995). Prenatal alcohol, marijuana, and tobacco use: Infant mental and motor development. *Neurotoxicology and Teratology, 17,* 479–487.

Robins, L. N. (1994). Lessons from the Vietnam Heroin Experience. The Harvard Mental Health Letter. *http://www.mentalhealth.com/mag1/p5h-sbo3.htm.*

Roizen, J. (1997). Epidemiological issues in alcohol-related violence. In M. Galanter (Ed.), *Recent Developments in Alcoholism* (Vol. 13). New York: Plenum Press.

Rusche, S. (1995). Prevention movement. In J. H. Jaffee (Ed.), *Encyclopedia of Drugs and Alcohol* (Vol. 2, pp. 856–861).

Rush, D., & Callahan, K. R. (1989). Exposure to passive cigarette smoking and child development: A critical review. *Annals of New York Academy of Sciences, 562,* 74–100.

SAMHSA. (2000). *Patterns of alcohol use among adolescents and associations with emotional and behavioral problems.* Substance Abuse and Mental Health Services Administration. *http//www.samhsa.gov.*

SAMHSA. (1999). *Summary of findings from the 1998 National Household Survey on Drug Abuse, H-9 & H-10.* Rockville, MD: National Clearinghouse for Alcohol and Drug Information.

SAMHSA. (1999). *National Household Survey on Drug Abuse, Main Findings, H-11.* Rockville, MD: National Clearinghouse for Alcohol and Drug Information.

SAMHSA. (1998, 1999). *Substance Abuse and Mental Health Statistics Source Book, 1998.* Rockville, MD: National Clearinghouse for Alcohol and Drug Information.

SAMHSA/CSAT. (1999). *Worker Drug Use and Workplace Policies and Programs:*

Results from the National Household Survey on Drug Abuse. Rockville, MD: National Clearinghouse for Alcohol and Drug Information.

SAMHSA/OAS. (1996). *Drug use Among U.S. Workers: Prevalence and Trends by Occupation and Industry Categories.* Rockville, MD: National Clearinghouse for Alcohol and Drug Information.

Schmid, P. C. et al. (1997). Changes in anandamide levels in mouse uterus are associated with uterine receptivity for embryo implantation. *Proceedings of the National Academy of Sciences, 94,* 4188–4192.

Seifert, S. A. (1999). Substance use and sexual assault. *Substance Use & Misuse, 34*(6), 935–945.

Sharp, C. W. & Rosenberg, N. L. (1997). Inhalants. In J. H. Lowinson, P. Ruiz, R. B. Millman, & J. G. Langrod, (Eds.), *Substance Abuse: A Comprehensive Textbook* (3rd ed., pp. 246–264). Baltimore: Williams & Wilkins.

Sheahan, S. L., Hendricks, J., & Coons, S. J. (1989). Drug misuse among the elderly: A covert problem. *Health Values 13*(3), 22–29.

Shen, W. W., & Sata, L. S. (1983). Neuropharmacology of male sexual dysfunction. *Journal of Clinical Pharmacology Research Communication, 3.*

Sher, K. J. (1997). Psychological characteristics of children of alcoholics. *Alcohol Health & Research World, Children of Alcoholics, 21*(3), 247–254.

Sher, K. J. (1999). Drug paraphernalia laws and injection-related infectious disease risk among drug injectors. *Research Briefs.* 5-21-99.

Smith, D. E., Wesson, D. R., & Apter-Marsh, M. (1984). Cocaine- and alcohol-induced sexual dysfunction in patients with addictive diseases. *Journal of Psychoactive Drugs, 16,* 359–361.

Smith, D. E., Wesson, D. R., & Calhoun, S. R. (1995). Rohypnol: Quaalude of the nineties? *CSAM News. Newsletter of the California Society of Addiction Medicine, 22*(2).

Smith, J. W. (1995). Medical manifestations of alcoholism in the elderly. *International Journal of the Addictions 30*(13 & 14), 1749–1798.

Smith, J. W. (1998). Special problems of the elderly. In A. W. Graham & T. K. Schultz (Eds.), *Principles of Addiction Medicine* (2nd ed., pp. 833–854). Chevy Chase, MD:

American Society of Addiction Medicine, Inc.

SmithKline. (1997). *SmithKline Beecham Drug Testing Index, 1997.* Collegeville, PA: SmithKline Beecham Clinical Laboratories.

Sokol, R. J., & Clarren, S. K. (1989). Guidelines for use of terminology describing the impact of prenatal alcohol on the offspring. *Alcoholism: Clinical & Experimental Research, 13,* 597–598.

Time. (2000). The lure of ecstasy. *Time Magazine* (6-5-00). *http://www.time.com.*

UCSF. (1998). *Does HIV prevention work?* Center for AIDS Prevention Research, University of California in San Francisco. *http://www.caps.ucsf.edu.*

U.S. Department of Agriculture. (1999). *Tobacco facts.* U.S. Department of Agriculture's Economic and Statistics System. Washington, DC: U.S. Printing Office.

USDHHS. (1988). *The Health Consequences of Smoking: 25 Years of Progress. A Report of the Surgeon General.* Rockville, MD: Office on Smoking and Health.

UNAIDS. (2000). *Report of the Global HIV/AIDS Epidemic.* New York: United Nations Publications.

University of Michigan. (1999). *Monitoring the Future Study.* Rockville, MD: SAMHSA. *http://www.MonitoringThe Future.org.*

U.S. Bureau of the Census. (1996). *65+ in the United States.* Current Population Reports, Special Studies, Number P23-190. Washington, DC: U.S. Government Printing Office.

USA Today. (8-12-98). Hands Off Pregnant Drug Users. *USA Today* Study.

USDL. (1990). *What Works: Workplaces Without Drugs.* Rockville, MD: U.S. Department of Labor.

Vereby, K. G., & Buchan, B. J. (1997). Diagnostic laboratory: Screening for drug abuse. In J. H. Lowinson, P. Ruiz, R. B. Millman, & J. G. Langrod, (Eds.), *Substance Abuse: A Comprehensive Textbook* (3rd ed., pp. 369–376). Baltimore: Williams & Wilkins.

Wartenberg, A. A. (1998). Management of common medical problems. In A. W. Graham & T. K. Schultz (Eds.), *Principles of Addiction Medicine* (2nd ed., pp. 731–740). Chevy Chase, MD: American Society of Addiction Medicine, Inc.

Wechsler, H., Kelley, K., Weitzman, E. R., Giovanni, J. P. S., & Seibring, M. (2000).

What colleges are doing about student binge drinking: A survey of college administrators. *Journal of American College Health, 48,* 219–226.

Wechsler, H., Lee, J. E., Kuo, M., & Lee, H. (2000). College binge drinking in the 1990s: A continuing problem. *Journal of American College Health, 48,* 199–210.

White, W. L. (1998). *Slaying the Dragon: The History of Addiction Treatment and Recovery in America.* Bloomington, IL: Chestnut Health Systems/Lighthouse Institute.

WHO (World Health Organization). (1999). Burden of disease by sex, cause, and WHO region, estimates for 1998. *The World Health Report, 1999. http://www.who. int/emc.hiv/.*

WHO. (2000). AIDS epidemic update: December, 1999. *http://www.who.int/ asd/figures/Global_report.htm.*

Wilsnack, S. C., Klassen, A. D., Schur, B. E., et al. (1991). Predicting onset and chronicity of women's problem drinking. *American Journal of Public Health, 61*(3), 305–318.

Wodak, A., & Lurie, P. (1997). A tale of two countries: Attempts to control HIV among injecting drug users in Australia and the United States. *Journal of Drug Issues, 27*(1), 117–134.

Worth, D. (1991). American women and poly-drug abuse. In P. Roth (Ed.), *Alcohol and Drugs are Women's Issues* (Vol. 1). Metuchen, NJ: Women's Action Alliance and the Scarecrow Press.

Wright, H. I., Gavaler, J. S., & Thiel, D. H. (1991). Effects of alcohol on the male reproductive system. *Alcohol Health and Research World, 15*(2), 110–114.

Young, N. K. (1997). Effects of alcohol and other drugs on children. *Journal of Psychoactive Drugs, 29*(1), 23–42.

Zakhari, S., (Ed.). (1993). *Alcohol and the Endocrine System.* NIAAA Research Monograph No. 23. NIH Pub. No. 93-3533. Bethesda, MD: National Institute on Alcohol Abuse and Alcoholism.

Zuckerman, B., Frank, D. A., Hingson, G., et al. (1989). Effects of maternal marijuana and cocaine use on fetal growth. *New England Journal of Medicine, 320,* 762–768.

Treatment

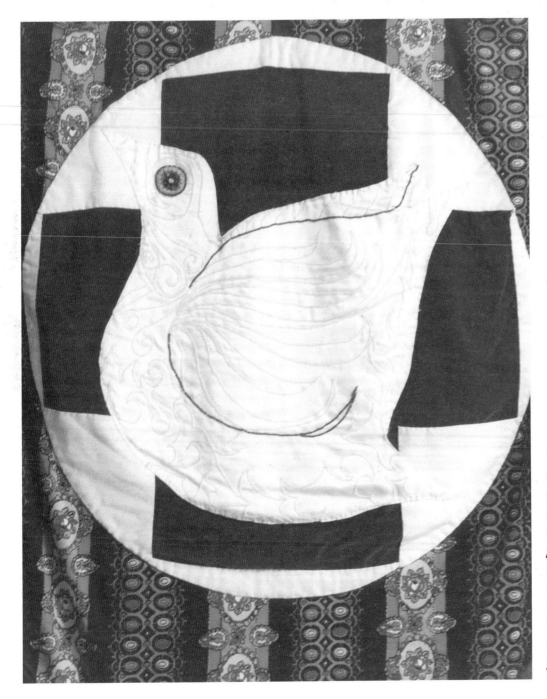

T *his is the symbol of the Haight-Ashbury Free Clinics that opened their doors in 1967 to help take care of the influx of young people during the "Summer of Love." Since that time, they have treated more than 100,000 clients with one of the highest success rates in the country. There are 130 people on staff.*

- **Introduction:**
  - ◊ **A Disease of the Brain:** The most prevalent mind disorder is substance abuse. It causes more illness, death, and social disruption than any other mental illness.
  - ◊ **Current Issues in Treatment:**
    1. The rapidly expanding use of medications to treat detoxification, withdrawal symptoms, craving, and to promote short- and long-term abstinence;
    2. The use of imaging techniques and other new diagnostic techniques to visualize the physiological effects of addiction on the human brain;
    3. The lack of resources to provide the treatment that has been proven to be effective;
    4. The conflict between abstinence-oriented recovery and harm reduction as philosophies of treatment. Historically, America has vacillated between temperance, individual abstinence, and societal prohibition. Much of the conflict is due to varying definitions of harm reduction—is it a complete philosophy of treatment or merely some techniques such as methadone maintenance and needle exchange that can reduce risks and encourage recovery?

- **Treatment Effectiveness:** Treatment has a 50% success rate and saves $7 to $20 for every $1 of treatment costs especially in prison costs. About 20% to 25% of inmates have been convicted of drug crimes.

- **Principles & Goals of Treatment:** Certain principles for effective treatment include having a wide variety of treatment programs that are readily available, using medications in conjunction with individual and group therapy, and treating any coexisting conditions, not just the addiction itself. Goals include motivating clients towards abstinence and reconstructing their lives in ways that exclude drug abuse.

- **Selection of a Program:** Correct diagnosis, a delicate process with drug abuse, helps treatment professionals match the client to the best program.

- **Broad Range of Techniques:** Providing a wide range of treatment approaches, plus customizing treatment for culture, sex, ethnic, and other target populations, dramatically improves outcomes. Programs include medical model detoxification, social model detoxification, social model recovery, therapeutic communities, and harm reduction programs. About $1^1/_2$ million people are treated for substance abuse each year.

- **Beginning Treatment:** Breaking through denial is the crucial first step in treatment. Hitting bottom, especially when health, family, work, financial, or legal problems are involved, often gets the user into treatment. Direct intervention, often using an intervention specialist, is also used to get the person into treatment.

- **Treatment Continuum:** Once addiction has occurred, treatment becomes a lifetime process.
  - ◊ **Detoxification** uses medical care, emotional support, and medications to control withdrawal symptoms, reduce craving, and help the client to begin abstinence.
  - ◊ **Initial Abstinence** uses counseling, anticraving medications, drug substitution, and desensitization techniques to rebalance body chemistry, continue abstinence, and prevent relapse due to environmental triggers.
  - ◊ **Long-Term Abstinence** involves participation in group, family, and 12-step programs to prevent relapse and to recognize that relapse is a lifelong danger.
  - ◊ **Recovery** is a lifelong process that involves rebuilding one's lifestyle to live sober and drug free.
  - ◊ **Outcome & Follow-Up** studies are used to judge the effectiveness of treatment programs.

- **Individual vs. Group Therapy:** Individual counseling, peer groups, 12-step groups, facilitated group therapy, and educational groups are all used in treatment.

- **Treatment & the Family:** Treatment should involve the whole family. The problems of codependency, enabling, and being a child of an alcoholic/addict must be addressed.

- **Drug-Specific Treatment:** Certain psychoactive drugs call for specialized medical and counseling treatment techniques, e.g., methadone maintenance, stimulant abuse groups, or dual diagnosis groups. A behavioral addiction like gambling is treated with many of the same techniques that are used for substance addiction.

- **Target Populations:** Treatment should be culturally specific (i.e., address ethnicity, sex, language); treatment techniques vary between men and women, old and young, and among Black, White, Hispanic, Asian, and Native American people.

- **Treatment Obstacles:** Developmental arrest, lack of cognition, conflicting goals, poor follow-through, and lack of facilities are the main problems in treatment.

- **Medical Intervention Developments:** More than 60 medications are being developed. They focus on such aspects of treatment as detoxification, replacement or agonist therapies, antagonist or vaccine effects, anticraving effects, metabolism modulation, and restoration of homeostasis.

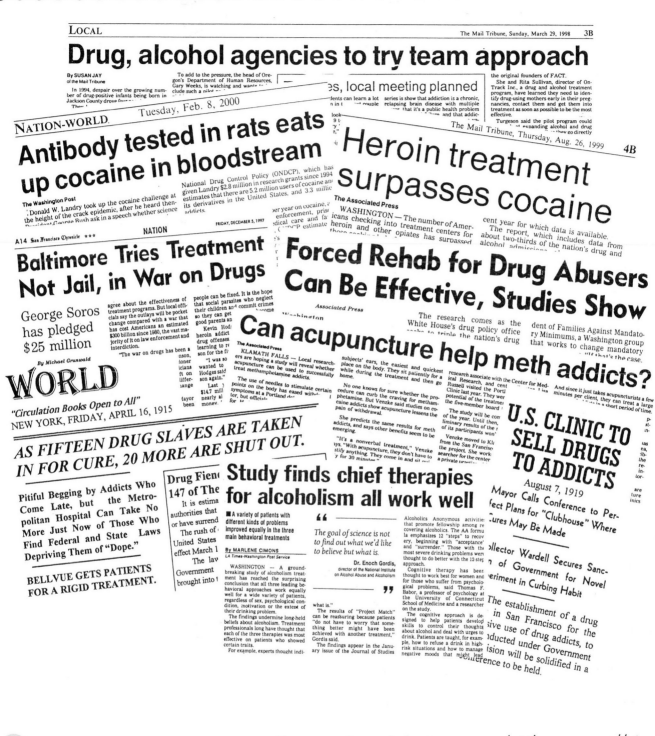

INTRODUCTION

"I've been in the Haight-Ashbury program for a year now. And I was in the Glide Memorial Church program for six months before that. And what changed me was I learned about myself.

I learned how to stay clean and sober. I was given tools I can use to stay clean."

38-year-old recovering female polydrug abuser

"Treatment is effective. Scientifically based drug addiction treatments typically reduce drug abuse by 40% to 60%. These rates are not ideal, of

course, but they are comparable to compliance rates seen with treatments for other chronic diseases, such as asthma, hypertension, and diabetes. Moreover treatment markedly reduces undesirable consequences of drug abuse and addiction, such as unemployment, criminal activity, and

HIV/AIDS or other infectious diseases, whether or not patients achieve complete abstinence."

Alan I. Leshner, Ph.D., Director, National Institute on Drug Abuse (NIH, 1999)

A DISEASE OF THE BRAIN

Mental illnesses, nervous system diseases, brain tumors, and physical head trauma come to mind when one thinks of pathological conditions of the human mind but in reality chemical dependency and addiction are more prevalent and have a much greater impact on the social fabric of society. For example, from the ages of 18–54, the one-year prevalence rate of

◇ anxiety disorders is 16.4%;

◇ schizophrenia is about 1.3%;

◇ mood disorders (major depression, bipolar disease, affective disorders) is about 7.1%;

◇ any mental disorder is about 21%.

(Public Health Service, 1999; Regier, Narrow, & Rae, 1999)

This compares to

◇ alcoholism, alcohol dependence, or problem drinking that affects 6% to 10% of the U.S. population over the age of 15;

◇ addiction to heroin or cocaine, devoid of alcohol problems, that affects another 2% to 3%;

◇ any substance abuse/dependence disorder besides nicotine that is found in about 11% of the population;

◇ and nicotine addiction that occurs in about 25% of the population over the age of 12.

(SAMHSA, 1999; Kessler, McGonagle, Zhao, et al., 1994; NIAAA, 1997)

Chemical dependency may also be America's number one continuing public physical health problem.

◇ More than 418,000 Americans die prematurely every year due to nicotine addiction;

◇ another 130,000 die prematurely from alcohol dependence, abuse, and overdose, or from associated diseases;

◇ 6,000 to 10,000 die of cocaine, heroin, and recently methamphetamine dependence;

◇ inhalant abuse kills 1,200 "huffers" every year;

◇ 35% to 40% of all hospital admissions are related to nicotine-induced health problems;

◇ 25%, of all hospital admissions are related to alcohol-induced health problems.

(CDC, 1996; SAMHSA, 1998, 1999)

These figures are startling when compared to other major health problems like AIDS, prostate or breast cancer, and even stroke, all of which are often the result of drug abuse and addiction. America ended the 1990s with a major crisis in health care. Perhaps this is due in part to our neglect of treating the root cause of many health problems—substance abuse.

Finally, psychoactive drug abuse has profound effects on social systems, family relationships, crime, violence, mental health, and a dozen other areas of daily life. Certainly if we could reduce the impact of addiction, we would have a major impact on the quality of life in the United States and around the world.

CURRENT ISSUES IN TREATMENT

At the start of the twenty first century, four aspects of treatment for substance and behavioral addictions dominate research and discussion.

1. The rapidly expanding use of medications to treat detoxification, withdrawal symptoms, craving and promote short- and long-term abstinence

Because addictive use of substances causes changes in brain chemistry, there is an increasing effort to find medications that can correct or lessen the impact of those chemical and structural changes, such as

CROQUIS D'ÉTÉ

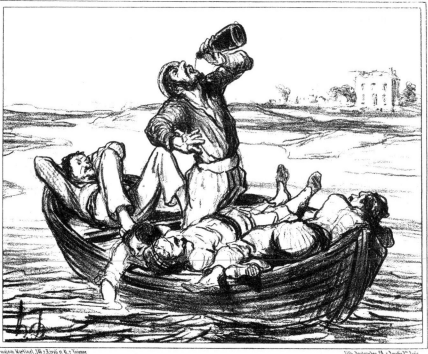

Descendant joyeusement le fleuve de la vie .

This etching by Honoré Daumier, circa 1840, titled "Joyously going down the river of life," is a reminder that alcohol has been around for millennia but it's mostly the attitude towards drunkenness, temperance, and sobriety that has changed.

◊ nutritional supplements to stimulate neurotransmitter production;

◊ antidepressants to increase serotonin activity and relieve depression;

◊ substitute medications that are less damaging than the primary substance of abuse including methadone and LAAM;

◊ drugs to lessen withdrawal symptoms, such as phenobarbital for alcohol withdrawal and antipsychotics to control stimulant-induced psychosis;

◊ and drugs to lessen craving (bromocryptine for stimulants and naltrexone, buprenorphine, or clonidine for heroin).

2. The use of imaging techniques and other new diagnostic techniques to visualize the physiological effects of addiction on the human brain

Until the advent of sophisticated imaging techniques, gene identification technologies, and sensitive neurochemical measurement methodologies, addiction was easy to deny because compulsion was considered a mental disease with few physical indicators that could be examined. There are four common imaging techniques used at research centers such as NIDA's Regional Imaging Center at Brookhaven National Laboratory; the Amen Clinic for Behavioral Medicine in Fairfield, California; Johns Hopkins Medical Institution in Baltimore; McLean Hospital's Brain Imaging Center near Boston; Massachusetts General Hospital Department of Psychiatry and Radiology; Harbor-UCLA Medical Center; and the Addiction Research Center at the University of Pennsylvania in Philadelphia (Meuller, 1999).

◊ CAT (computerized axial tomography) scans use x-rays to show structural changes in brain tissues due to drugs.

◊ MRI (magnet resonance imaging) uses the positioning of magnetic nuclei to give two- and three-dimensional images of brain structures in great detail; it can record subtle alterations of brain tissues due to psychoactive drug use or brain anomalies that indicate a susceptibility to drug abuse. For example, an MRI study at the University of Southern California showed a smaller prefrontal cortex (11% smaller on average) in those prone to rage and violence with antisocial personality disorder, a diagnostic technique that proved as accurate as psychological testing techniques (Raine, Phil, Lencz, et al., 2000). Since antisocial personality disorder is a significant risk factor for drug abuse, this becomes a valuable diagnostic technique. There are variations of MRI techniques such as magnetic resonance spectroscopy (31P MRS) that measures abnormal brain activity due to chronic drug use and fMRI (functional MRI) that records blood flow changes to visualize the effects of drugs.

◊ PET (positron emission tomography) scans use the metabolism of radioactively labeled chemicals that have been injected into the bloodstream to measure glucose metabolism, blood flow, and oxygenation. This shows where drugs and naturally occurring neurotransmitters act and any changes that occur when drugs are involved.

◊ SPECT (single photon emission computed tomography) scans also use radioactive tracers to measure cerebral blood flow and brain metabolism to show how a brain functions or doesn't function when using drugs; they are similar to PET scans but less expensive and easier to use.

(Mathias, 1999)

"There's so much these scans and looking at the brain can offer the field of addiction. Number one, it helps us to understand what the drugs actually do to the brain function and physiology. The second thing is education. We can show children, teenagers, and adults that drugs have an impact on their brain. It's much more powerful than showing them a picture of fried eggs and bacon. It's very helpful in denial to actually sit in front of a computer screen with somebody that has been using drugs and they go, 'Oh, there are really no problems.' And you can go, 'Let's look at yours.' And what I've seen—it's really turned many people around."
Daniel Amen, M.D., Founder, Amen Clinic for Behavioral Medicine (Amen, 1998)

3. The lack of resources to provide the treatment that has been proven to be effective

Many states are doing outcome studies to assess the effectiveness of treatment. Those that have been completed show that for every $1 spent on treatment, $7 to $20 are saved, mostly in prison costs, lost time on the job, health problems, and extra social services (Gerstein, Johnson, Harwood, et al., 1994; Hubbard, Craddock, Flynn, et al., 1997). Other research has shown the greatly increased effectiveness of matching treatment modalities to each client's needs (McLellan, Grissom, Zanis, et al., 1997; Nielsen, Nielsen, & Wrae, 1998). Finally, studies have shown that the more services, such as health care, psychological care, and social support, that are available, the better the outcome (Fiorentine, 1999). The problem is that because of limited community, state, and federal resources, more reliance on managed care and a general reluctance to spend money on treatment for so-called drug addicts, cities, counties, and states cannot provide sufficient treatment even for those who desperately want it. In San Francisco and Baltimore, two cities where the concept of treatment on demand was seriously studied, waiting lists for treatment slots still remain excessively high.

4. The conflict between abstinence-oriented recovery and harm reduction as philosophies of treatment

Most treatment personnel believe that users who have crossed the line into uncontrolled use of drugs or compulsive behaviors can refuse the first drink, injection, or bet but they are unable to refuse the second. For these treatment personnel, abstinence is absolutely necessary for recovery because the very definition of addiction is based on the concept of loss of control. In various studies, the Haight-Ashbury Clinic found that when a client **slipped,** e.g., had a drink, smoked one "joint," or smoked one cigarette, it turned into a full **relapse** in 95% of the cases (O'Malley, Jaffe, Chang, et al., 1992). The full relapse might take an hour, a day, a month or occasionally more, but in 19 out of 20 users who have crossed the line into addiction, it will occur. Even in 1879 a recovering alcoholic and temperance lecturer and author, Luther Bensen, was aware of his susceptibility to uncontrolled use.

"Moderation? A drink of liquor is to my appetite what a red-hot poker is to a keg of dry powder.... When I take one drink, even if it is but a taste, I must have more, even if I knew hell would burst out of the earth and engulf me the next instant."

Luther Bensen, 1879 (Bensen, 1879)

Conversely there is a growing group of chemical dependency personnel who believe that harm reduction is a viable treatment alternative. The problem with evaluation of the effectiveness of harm reduction is that it means different things to different groups. One definition of harm reduction is "a willingness to work for incremental changes rather than to require complete behavior change" (Morris, 1995). Another is "any steps taken by drug users to reduce the harm of their behavior including changing the route of administration, substituting less harmful drugs for more harmful ones, and promoting moderate or nondependent use of all drugs" (Marlatt, 1995; Marlatt & Tapert, 1993). Harm reduction can also include drug replacement therapy, such as methadone maintenance instead of heroin use or methylphenidate maintenance instead of co-

caine use. Harm reduction also includes needle exchange, the use of less harmful drugs for more harmful ones drug decriminalization/legalization through legislation, and the most controversial techniques, controlled drinking/drug use through behavior modification. Numerous studies have been done on controlled drinking and again the problem is definitions that obscure reported data. What constitutes controlled drinking? Was the patient an alcoholic or an abuser before starting treatment? Is the patient's self-reporting of the amount being drunk and the consequences accurate (Peele, 1995)? Long-term follow-up strongly suggests that true controlled drinking does not work (Vaillant, 1995). For some, harm reduction consists of individual techniques that will help advance the addict to full (abstinent) recovery while to others, harm reduction is an all-encompassing philosophy of treatment and drug use.

It is difficult to measure treatment outcome. Is it measured in days of abstinence, amount of drug used, reduction in hospital visits, improvement in marital and other relationships, or amount of money saved by society? This lack of consensus can further aggravate the argument (Geller, 1997).

More on Abstinence vs. Harm Reduction (temperance, to abstinence, to prohibition)

In his excellent book, *Slaying the Dragon,* on the history of addiction treatment in America, William White shows that this controversy has been around for 230 years. The temperance movement started at the end of the eighteenth century as America emerged from its revolution against England and coincidentally changed its drinking habits. From 1792 to 1830, the per capita consumption went from 2.5 gallons of pure alcohol per year to an unbelievable 7.1 gallons or two standard drinks for every man, woman, and child every day of the year (Cherrington, 1920). (In the year 2000, per capita consumption is back down to 2.2 gallons.) The

initial goal of the **temperance movement** was just to limit the amount drunk but as consumption and public drunkenness increased, that goal shifted from temperance to **abstinence,** that is, complete avoidance by the alcoholic of any and all alcoholic beverages (White, 1998). Even then many people thought of alcoholism as a disease.

"The remedy we would suggest, particularly to those whose appetite for drink is strong and increasing, is a total abstinence from the use of all intoxicating liquors. This may be deemed a harsh remedy, but the nature of the disease absolutely requires it."

From an 1811 temperance pamphlet (Dascus, 1877)

A large segment of the abstinence movement then expanded the goal to make society as a whole abstinent (**prohibition**), not just those who couldn't limit their consumption. This way alcohol would just not be available, at least legally.

"Our main object is not to reform inebriates, but to induce all temperate people to continue temperance, by practicing total abstinence. The drunkards, if not reformed, will die, and the land be free."

Dr. Justin Edwards, 1824 (Dorchester, 1884)

This shift from simply treating the addict to reforming society confused the perception of the problem of how to treat alcoholism and addiction. The question became "Should a substance that triggers uncontrolled harmful use in 5% to 10% of the population (25% to 50% for tobacco) be banned, allowed, or controlled?" In wanting to allow controlled use of a psychoactive substance, some advocates of harm reduction ignore the nature of addiction. Conversely some advocates of abstinence and/or prohibition overreact to any use of a psychoactive substance, even in that 90% of the population with a lower susceptibility to uncontrolled

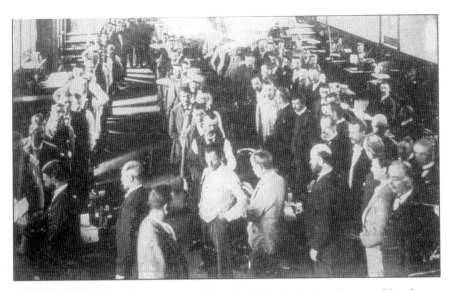

Patients at a Keeley Institute who were addicted to alcohol and other drugs would go for a four-week cure. Part of the treatment was daily injections of a secret formula to help subdue the pains of withdrawal and keep the patient in treatment. Though the formula was kept secret, various laboratories suggested that the medicine contained a number of ingredients, some of which were psychoactive. These included alcohol, strychnine, willow bark, ginger, ammonia, belladonna, atropine, hyoscine, scopolamine, coca, opium, and morphine.
Courtesy of Keeley Collection. © Illinois State Historical Library

use. In many of the arguments on the subject, both sides confuse ideas about the effectiveness of abstinence-based treatment and effective harm reduction techniques with arguments about freedom, politics, and morality.

The recent advocacy of harm reduction started in the late 1980s and early '90s in response to the inaccessibility of treatment to many segments of society infected with the HIV virus, hepatitis C, and other diseases who continued to spread the diseases or infect themselves through dirty needles, contaminated drugs, and unsafe sex. Needle exchange programs, free condoms, food incentives, and social service referral information enabled outreach workers to come in contact with homeless street kids, illicit drug users, prostitutes, and others living on the fringes of society to engage them in prevention efforts that would slow the spread of these diseases. The contact also gave the outreach workers an opportunity to engage them in drug treatment or, at the very least, increase their knowledge of drug abuse and addiction.

The harm reduction people were willing to accept small changes in drug use status in order to protect the addict and society from further infection. What happened was that, as in the past, the harm reduction concept became an end in itself for certain treatment personnel rather than a transitory step for clients on the way to abstinence and full recovery. Interest in harm reduction also came from health care insurers and managed care systems who saw harm reduction as a more economical way to cover their obligations to provide treatment for chemical dependency problems (Morris, 1995).

One item that has added to the controversy surrounding harm reduction is confusion about the difference between abuse and addiction. The key is that there is a qualitative difference between those two levels of drug use, not just a quantitative difference. Many of the successes of harm reduction have been in users who had not crossed that line into loss of control that is the hallmark of addiction, and so harm reduction in some of those cases was sustainable.

But even there, since addiction is a progressive disease and intensifies with use, continued abuse will often become addiction. Some advocates of harm reduction will point to treatment of obesity as proof that harm reduction works but most studies on weight-loss programs show that the failure rate is 97%, just a little more than the percentage of addicts in treatment who let a slip become a relapse.

To a certain extent all treatment is harm reduction since rebounding from relapses is part of the recovery process. Most people try a number of times to become abstinent before it is sustainable while others will continue to have periods of abstinence between relapses where their physical and mental health improves, along with their socioeconomic status. Those periods of harm reduction marked by abstinence are generally longer and of higher quality than those marked by controlled use.

The Haight-Ashbury Clinic has an abstinence-based philosophy of treatment that also incorporates many harm reduction techniques. The rest of this chapter reflects that philosophy.

TREATMENT EFFECTIVENESS

Even though chemical dependency is America's and possibly the world's number one health and social problem, it is also the most treatable. Several studies have confirmed that treatment outcomes for drug and alcohol abuse result in long-term abstinence, along with tremendous health, social, and spiritual benefits to the patient.

"Everything that I am and everything that I have in me is invested in what I'm doing today in recovery— everything."
56-year-old recovering heroin addict

What is often overlooked when local, state, and federal governments vote on how much money should be al-

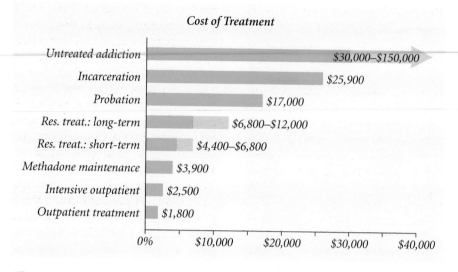

Figure 9-1 •

The cost of treatment for an addict utilizing outpatient treatment if less than 1/10 the cost of incarceration.

(Estimates by authors, 1999)

listed heroin as their primary drug of choice. Cocaine users' outcomes fell between these two drugs.

◇ Better treatment outcomes were linked to program modifications directed at being culturally consistent with a specific target population. For example, programs that targeted women and added child care services to their treatment programs had much better outcomes than generic treatment programs for women. Those programs that added transportation services had better outcomes than those that just had child care. Every additional innovation that was target-group specific improved the outcome of treatment.

(Gerstein, Johnson, Harwood, et al., 1994; Mecca, 1997)

lotted for treatment is the undeniable fact that treatment saves money—large sums of money (Fig. 9-1).

TREATMENT STUDIES

The CALDATA (California Drug and Alcohol Treatment Assessment) Study

Studies conducted by the Rand Corporation and the Research Triangle Institute support the current findings of the CALDATA Study, the most comprehensive and rigorous study on treatment outcome conducted by the State of California and duplicated by several other states. All of these studies monitored the effect of treatment on several hundred thousand addicts and alcoholics treated in a variety of programs.

The CALDATA Study monitored patients for a period of three to five years following treatment. Continual abstinence in these patients approached 50% of all those treated. It further demonstrated that crime was abated in 74% of those treated and that the state enjoyed actual savings of $7 for every $1 spent on treatment. For more expensive programs, there was a savings of $4 and for the inexpensive programs, the savings were $12. California spent $209 million on treatment between

October, 1991 and September, 1992 and saved an estimated $1.5 billion, much due to crime reduction and reduced use of health care facilities. The study found that "crack" use declined almost 1/2, heroin use declined by 1/5, and alcohol use fell by 1/3. The only negative side of the equation was that those in recovery lost income while undergoing treatment and their financial condition did not improve immediately after treatment. The study also looked at a number of variables that, when examined, supported many concepts and practices in the treatment field.

◇ Treatment was most effective when patients were treated continuously for a period of six to eight months.

◇ Shorter periods of time resulted in poorer outcomes and longer treatment duration resulted in continuously better outcomes but not at the same rate. There is a point of diminishing returns.

◇ Group therapy was shown to be much more effective than individual therapy.

◇ Drug of choice also seemed to affect outcomes. For example, those who listed alcohol as their primary drug of choice had treatment outcomes twice as good as those who

DATOS (Drug Abuse Treatment Outcome Study)

An earlier study of the effectiveness of treatment, the Drug Abuse Treatment Outcome Study (DATOS) tracked 10,010 drug abusers in 100 treatment facilities in 11 cities who began treatment from 1991–1993. The study compared pre- and post-treatment drug use, criminal activity, employment, and thoughts of suicide (Hubbard et al., 1997). The four common types of drug abuse treatment studied were outpatient methadone programs, long-term (several months) residential programs, short-term inpatient (up to 30 days) programs, and outpatient drug-free programs. Researchers found that the use of all drugs after treatment was reduced by 50% to 70%. The final level of drug use after treatment was about the same level for all four programs. Short- and long-term residential programs seemed to have the greatest effect. As expected low retention rates were most prevalent in clients with greater problems (Mueller & Wyman, 1997). Unfortunately, most patients said they did not receive the services they thought they needed. The study found a decrease in the number of services offered over the past decade (Ethridge, Craddock, Dunteman, & Hubbard, 1995).

TREATMENT & PRISONS

On January 1, 2000, 1,983,084 Americans were in federal, state, and local prisons while another 4.3 million were on parole or probation. Of those on probation, 24% were for a drug law violation and 17% for driving while intoxicated. Average time served increased from 22 months to 27 months. About 20% to 25% of all inmates are drug offenders—convicted of drug crimes—while another 40% to 65% committed their crime under the influence of alcohol or drugs (ONDCP, 1999).

The percentage of arrestees testing positive for drugs (not including alcohol) is many times the percentage of drug use in the general population. Arrests for actual drug offenses more than tripled from 1980 to 1998. Juvenile arrests for drug crimes doubled from 1990 to 1998. Despite the high percentage of drug problems among the inmate population, treatment is available for only about 10% of inmates who have serious drug habits (DOJ, 1999). Various studies of inmate populations with drug problems have found a comparatively low percentage have had contact with the treatment community (Mahon, 1997). About 8% of all admissions for substance abuse treatment are prison inmates (SAMHSA/ TEDS, 1999). One of the positive changes in the criminal justice system has been the increased use of drug courts where first-time drug offenders can be diverted to treatment rather than incarceration. Defendants who complete the program can have their charges dismissed or probation sentences reduced. In 1999 about 500 drug courts were operating in the United States. Of the more than 100,000 people who had entered drug courts, 70% graduated or remain active participants. These courts keep felony offenders in treatment at about double the retention rate of community drug programs. Two of the reasons are that there is much closer supervision and there is the threat of incarceration (Belenko, 1998). The most effective drug courts are those that work in close cooperation with community facilities.

Recent studies of prisoners and those involved with the criminal justice system have shown that drug abuse treatment reduces recidivism dramatically when the treatment is linked to community services rather than strictly in-jail services. Normally about 62% of criminals are rearrested within three years after being released from prison. Community-linked drug abuse addiction treatment lowers that number to only 20% (DOJ, 1999). Since the cost of keeping a felon in jail runs between $25,000 to $40,000 a year, not including any assistance for the felon's family, compensation for human and property damage, and a dozen other liabilities, the savings for keeping people out of prisons is quite large (Fig. 9-2). In contrast, outpatient treatment costs between $1,800 to $4,000 a year depending on the treatment approach (Osborne et al., 1998).

"In California during the early '90s, we built nine new prisons but we built no new universities and actually suffered a decrease in drug treatment slots due to reduced funding. Yet 80% to 85% of our prisoners listed a drug problem as a major reason for their offense. I think we have our priorities backwards."
Ⅽalifornia education consultant

PRINCIPLES & GOALS OF TREATMENT

PRINCIPLES OF EFFECTIVE TREATMENT

In a recent 1999 publication by NIH (National Institutes of Health), *Principles of Drug Addiction Treatment,* 13 principles of effective treatment were listed. These principles are applicable to any treatment facility, program, or therapy.

1. **No single treatment is appropriate for all individuals.** Matching treatment settings, interventions, and services to each individual's particular problems and needs is critical to his or her ultimate success in returning to productive functioning in the family, workplace, and society.

2. **Treatment needs to be readily available.** Because individuals who are addicted to drugs may be

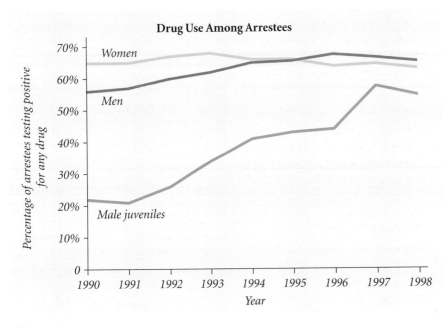

Drug Use Among Arrestees

Percentage of arrestees testing positive for any drug

Women

Men

Male juveniles

70%
60%
50%
40%
30%
20%
10%
0

1990 1991 1992 1993 1994 1995 1996 1997 1998
Year

Figure 9-2 •

Testing at jails and prisons is for illicit drugs and excludes alcohol. Besides alcohol the most common drugs found in arrestees are marijuana and cocaine (ADAM, 1999).

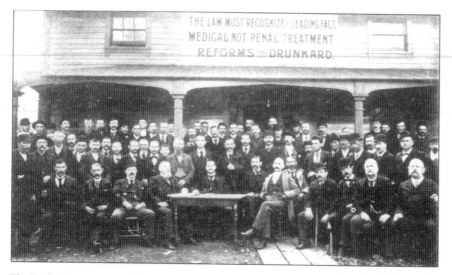

The Keeley League, started in 1891, preceded the modern self-help and 12-step groups that were started by Alcoholics Anonymous in 1934. The Keeley Leagues put greater emphasis on community involvement but their main purpose of supporting the recovering addict was the same as all modern self-help groups. The sign above attendants at an open-air session in Dwight, Illinois emphasized treatment rather than incarceration.

Courtesy of Keeley Collection. © Illinois State Historical Library

uncertain about entering treatment, taking advantage of opportunities when they are ready for treatment is crucial. Potential treatment applicants can be lost if treatment is not immediately available or is not readily accessible.

3. **Effective treatment attends to multiple needs of the individual not just his or her drug use.** To be effective, treatment must address the individual's drug use and any associated medical, psychological, social, vocational, and legal problems.

4. **An individual's treatment and services plan must be assessed continually and modified as necessary to ensure that the plan meets the person's changing needs.** In addition to counseling or psychotherapy, a patient at times may require medication, other medical services, family therapy, parenting instruction, vocational rehabilitation, and social and legal services.

5. **Remaining in treatment for an adequate period of time is critical for treatment effectiveness.** Research indicates that for most patients, the threshold of significant improvement is reached at about three months in treatment.

6. **Counseling (individual and/or group) and other behavioral therapies are critical components of effective treatment for addiction.** In therapy, patients address issues of motivation, build skills to resist drug use, replace drug-using activities with constructive and rewarding nondrug-using activities, and improve problem-solving abilities and social skills.

7. **Medications are an important element of treatment for many patients, especially when combined with counseling and other behavioral therapies.** Methadone, LAAM, naltrexone, bupropion, and a number of other medications can help with detoxification as well as short- and long-term abstinence. For patients with mental disorders, both behavioral treatments and medications can be critically important.

8. **Addicted or drug-abusing individuals with coexisting mental disorders should have both dis-**

orders treated in an integrated way. Because addictive disorders and mental disorders often occur in the same individual, patients presenting for either condition should be assessed and treated for the co-occurrence of the other type of disorder.

9. **Detoxification is only the first stage of addiction treatment and by itself does little to change long-term drug use.** While detoxification alone is rarely sufficient to help addicts achieve long-term abstinence, for some individuals it is a strongly indicated precursor to effective drug addiction treatment.

10. **Treatment does not need to be voluntary to be effective.** Sanctions or enticements in the family, employment setting, or criminal justice system can significantly increase both treatment entry and retention rates and the success of drug treatment interventions.

11. **Possible drug use during treatment must be monitored continuously.** The objective monitoring of a patient's drug and alcohol use during treatment, such as through urinalysis or other tests, can help the patient withstand urges to use drugs. Such monitoring can also provide early evidence of drug use so that the individual's treatment plan can be adjusted.

12. **Treatment programs should provide assessment for HIV/AIDS, hepatitis B and C, tuberculosis and other infectious diseases, and counseling to help patients modify or change behaviors that place themselves or others at risk of infection.** Counseling can help patients avoid high-risk behaviors. Counseling also can help people who are already infected manage their illness.

13. **Recovery from drug addiction can be a long-term process and frequently requires multiple episodes of treatment.** Addicted individuals may require prolonged treatment and multiple episodes of treatment to achieve long-term ab-

stinence and fully restored functioning. Participation in self-help support programs during and following treatment is often helpful in maintaining abstinence.

(Adapted from NIH, 1999)

The problem with this list is that to fully implement most of the concepts is costly. Many local, state, and federal governments and health care systems are unable or reluctant to commit the necessary funds to provide a full range of services.

GOALS OF EFFECTIVE TREATMENT

Most treatment experts agree that the two most important goals for treatment outcome are first, to motivate clients towards abstinence from their drugs of abuse and second, to reconstruct their lives once their focus is redirected away from substance abuse.

To accomplish these and other goals, several elements need to be addressed through an understanding that addiction treatment is a lifelong process for the addict. Treatment merely motivates, initiates, and provides some tools that help them to have uninterrupted abstinence from their addiction throughout their lives.

"Well, basically, I'd like to stay off drugs. I'd like to get my family life together again and have a relationship with my children—a good one—and if nothing else, I'd just like to know that when I do die, I did have a life, you know, aside from being just another dope fiend in the gutter."
24-year-old recovering heroin addict

Primary Goals

A comprehensive treatment model will include the capacity to accomplish the following:

Motivation Towards Abstinence. Components of these efforts consist of education, counseling, and involvement with 12-step or self-help groups. This might include harm reduction approaches like methadone maintenance whereby an addict is provided with an alternate medically controlled drug to promote abstinence from the street drug of choice.

Creating a Drug-Free Lifestyle. This covers all aspects of an addict's life, including the ability to address social/environmental issues, like homelessness, relationships, family, and friends, in order to develop drug-free life interactions. They are connected to drug-free activities, like clean and sober dances, and most important, they learn relapse prevention skills, such as stress reduction, cue resistance, coping, decision making, and conflict resolution.

Supporting Goals

Enriching Job or Career Functioning. Often neglected in treatment, jobs and career comprise a major portion of someone's life. This goal is accomplished through vocational services, management of personal finances, and maintenance of a drug-free workplace.

Optimizing Medical Functioning. Besides treatment of withdrawal and other acute medical problems associated with addiction, many addicts have undiagnosed or existing medical problems that have been neglected through their use of drugs. The comprehensive treatment program includes the ability to assess and treat such conditions.

Optimizing Psychiatric & Emotional Functioning. Many studies suggest that greater than 50% of all substance abusers also have a coexisting psychiatric condition. Identification and appropriate treatment of psychiatric problems are an essential element of the modern treatment program (*see Chapter 10*).

Addressing Relevant Spiritual Issues. Although the inclusion of either spirituality or religious beliefs in addiction treatment is controversial, the most effective long-term treatments of addiction are the spiritually based 12-step Alcoholics Anonymous and Ad-dictions Anonymous programs. Further many of the other treatment programs in operation base their interventions on the 12-step traditions. Thus it has become essential for programs to at least help clarify this issue with their clients and provide appropriate referrals.

(Schuckit, 1994)

"I don't have hopes of living forever. I never have. I mean, to be my age is a complete shock to me, so it's not about that but the issue is about the quality of life."
40-year-old recovering heroin addict

SELECTION OF A PROGRAM

Most program selections occur on the spur of the moment based upon cost, familiarity, location, and convenience of access. The current era of managed health care has made pretreatment assessments essential because they can better match addicts to programs that address their specific needs and thus promote better outcomes.

In making a program selection, one should be knowledgeable about the addicted person's specific needs, his or her resources to afford treatment, the specific components and deficiencies of available programs, and the ultimate client goal of these potential programs.

It is important to note that program selection should be completed before a formal intervention is performed on an addicted person. Successfully getting someone to accept and address a drug problem can be completely undermined by having no immediate resource for the addict to address his or her problems.

DIAGNOSIS

Once addiction is suspected, various diagnostic tools can be used to help verify, support, or clarify the potential diagnosis of chemical addiction. Several diagnostic criteria have been developed to assist clinicians in making a diagnosis of chemical dependence (Mersy, 1991; Lewis, Dana, & Blevins, 1994). The following are some of the more common ones used.

◊ *The American Psychiatric Association Diagnostic and Statistical Manual of Mental Disorders (DSM-IV)* relies on the pattern and duration of drug use, the negative impact of drugs on the social or occupational functioning of the user, and the pathological effects (e.g., tolerance or withdrawal symptoms) to confirm a diagnosis of addiction.

◊ *The Selective Severity Assessment (SSA)* evaluates 11 physiologic signs (e.g., pulse, temperature, and tremors) to confirm the severity of the addiction in an addict.

◊ *The National Council on Alcoholism Criteria for Diagnosis of Alcoholism (NCA CRIT)* and its *Modified Criteria (MODCRIT)* outline two bases on which to make the diagnosis of alcoholism:
  1. physical and clinical parameters,
  2. behavioral, psychological, and attitudinal impact.

◊ *The Addiction Severity Index (ASI)* represents the most comprehensive and lengthy criteria for the diagnosis of chemical dependency. One hundred and eighty items cover six areas that are affected by substance use and abuse.

◊ A simple diagnostic aid, the *Michigan Alcoholism Screening Test (MAST)*, uses just 25 questions that are primarily directed at the negative life effects of alcohol on the user (*see Chapter 5*). There is also the *Short Michigan Alcohol Screening Test* with just 13 questions.

◊ The simplest self-assessment tool for problem drinking is the *CAGE* questionnaire that consists of just 4 questions.
  1. Have you felt the need to <u>C</u>ut down on your drinking?
  2. Do you feel <u>A</u>nnoyed by people complaining about your drinking?
  3. Do you ever feel <u>G</u>uilty about your drinking?

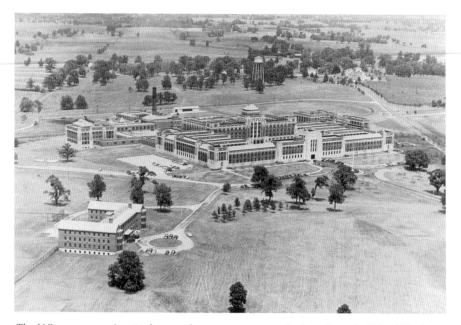

The U.S. government's attitude towards most treatment methods at the end of World War I limited the facilities available for addicts. In 1929 the government allocated funds for two "narcotic farms" to house and rehabilitate addicts who had been convicted of violating federal drug laws or those who wished to commit themselves voluntarily. The Lexington Kentucky Narcotics Farm opened in 1935 and the second facility in Fort Worth, Texas in November, 1938. The Lexington facility shown in this picture had about 1,000 inmates. Treatment protocol included tapered withdrawal, convalescence, and rehabilitation. Treatment could last up to a year or more. A study of effectiveness showed that 90% to 96% of addicts returned to active addiction, most within six months of discharge (White, 1998).
Courtesy DHHS (Department of Health and Human Services), Program Support Center

4. Do you ever drink an <u>E</u>ye-opener in the morning to relieve the shakes?

Two or more affirmative responses suggest that the client is a problem drinker.
(Allen, Eckardt, & Wallen, 1988)

BROAD RANGE OF TECHNIQUES

"Let the experiment be fairly tried; let an institution be founded; let the means of cure be provided; let the principles on which it is to be founded be extensively promulgated and, I doubt not, all intelligent people will be satisfied of its feasibility . . . let the principle of total abstinence be rigorously adopted and enforced . . . let

appropriate medication be afforded . . . let the mind be soothed . . . let good nutrition be regularly administered— this course, rigorously adopted and pursued, will restore nine out of ten in all cases."

Dr. Samuel Woodward, 1833 (Grinrod, 1886)

The nineteenth-century expert on mental health Dr. Samuel Woodward thought that society should support recovery and proposed one kind of facility. Addiction is a complex interaction between biologic, social, and toxic factors—heredity, environment, and psychoactive drugs. Given these multiple influences, treatment has evolved along various paths, all of which enjoy some success. However, since each person is unique and the level of addiction different, no treatment has proven to be universally effective for everyone who has an addiction. Often, effective treatment requires a variety of techniques in a variety of settings.

"I'm considering going into inpatient treatment. I've talked it over with my counselor and he said 'Anybody can stay clean in the closet.' I'm good as far as bullshitting and manipulating. I could pass a 30-day and probably a 60-day situation. But you know, when I come outside, there's things that I'm going to have to deal with, so an outpatient program still makes sense."

24-year-old "crack" addict in group therapy meeting

Besides matching the treatment protocol to the level of addiction and the user's personality, it is very important to factor in the physical withdrawal syndrome produced by a drug or a combination of drugs because withdrawal from drugs, especially alcohol and sedative-hypnotic drugs (e.g., Valium® or Klonopin®), may produce life-threatening seizures that require medical and hospital management. Cocaine or amphetamine withdrawal usually requires less medical intervention but clients need intense psychosocial intervention to prevent relapse.

"My mother swore off the gin and the Valium® for my wedding. She was too good to her word. She started withdrawing and having convulsions at my reception and almost died in the ambulance. It put somewhat of a damper on the honeymoon."

23-year-old bride

TREATMENT OPTIONS

"Someone asked me, 'Where would you go to get off drugs? Where would you feel comfortable?' If I had everything I needed, lifetime supplies, and I was shipwrecked on an island, that would be fine."

Recovering 22-year-old methamphetamine abuser

A wide range of options exists for the treatment of alcohol or other chemical addiction. The range is

◇ from "cold turkey" or "white knuckle" dry outs to medically assisted detoxification;

◇ from expensive medical or residential approaches to free peer groups, 12-step groups, or social model group therapy;

◇ from outpatient treatment, to halfway houses, to residential programs;

◇ from long-term residential treatment (two years or more) to seven-day hospital detoxification with aftercare;

◇ and from methadone maintenance or other harm reduction techniques to acupuncture, aversion therapies, or a dozen other treatment modalities.

"I believed there were only AA and NA for my 'crank' use and I knew—I just knew these wouldn't work. Then after a particularly nasty run, which I thought I kept from my probation officer, he gave me a choice of getting into treatment or going back to prison. I was startled when he handed me a full-page list of different places I could go. There was a medical program. There was a NA program made up of 'speed freaks' like myself. There was a mental health program near my apartment. There were places I could go to live while kicking."

35-year-old recovering "crank" addict

Treatment programs that focus their development on a specific target population and provide culturally relevant services have demonstrated the ability to attract, bond, and shepherd addicts into a recovery process much better than a general program with no specific focus. Models for such an approach have been developed based on ethnicity, age, sex, profession, sexual orientation, mental status, drug of choice, and even specifically for those with HIV infection or AIDS.

In many of the studies on the effectiveness of different types of programs, what is sometimes forgotten is the

process of **treatment self-selection.** This means that addicts will often end up in a program that works and drop out of those that feel uncomfortable, are not relevant to their problem, or that they are not ready for based on the stage of their addiction. So a statistic might read that "this program is only effective for 10% of all addicts," and that's true as far as it goes. However, it could be read, "this type of program works for 10% of the addicted population and luckily there are a dozen other programs and if each one is only effective with 10% of the population, then we can offer recovery to most addicts." It also means that we can't put all treatment hopes in just one type of therapy be it drug replacement therapy, a therapeutic community, or 12-step groups. A simile would be that treatment for a heart condition could be diet change, coronary artery bypass, angioplasty, or in the extreme, a heart-replacement operation.

There are dozens of different types of treatments and treatment facilities available. Many of the facilities will provide a variety of programs and therapies or shift the patient among programs. The following describes the most widely used programs.

Medical model detoxification programs can be hospital inpatient, residential, or outpatient. The treatment in medical model programs is supervised and managed by medical professionals. Medications useful to the treatment of the patient can be administered in conjunction with traditional recovery-oriented counseling and educational approaches. These are usually the most expensive types of programs but have the advantage of being able to do a more comprehensive assessment and treatment of the addict's overall physical and mental health. Inpatient medical model programs can cost $3,000 to $25,000 depending on the length of stay (3–28 days) while outpatient medical model programs range from $1,500 to $5,000, again depending on the length of stay (1–6 months). Methadone maintenance is considered a medical model treatment program.

Social model detoxification programs are nonmedical programs that can be either inpatient or outpatient. These programs are also short term (7–28 days) and aimed at providing a safe and sober environment for addicts to rebalance their body and brain chemistry that was disrupted by abuse of drugs. This then enables them to enter into a full recovery program.

Social model recovery programs (also called "outpatient drug-free programs") are outpatient programs that use a wide variety of approaches to move a client toward recovery. Since social model programs are totally nonmedical, the client usually must be abstinent from drugs for 72 hours before they will be admitted. Approaches include cognitive behavioral therapy, insight-oriented psychotherapy, problem-solving groups, and 12-step programs. Clients may stay in these programs for months or longer (Dodd, 1997).

Therapeutic communities are generally long-term (1–3 years), self-contained residential programs that provide full rehabilitative and social services under the direction of the facility. These include daily counseling, drug education, vocational and educational rehabilitation, and case management, including referrals to social and health services. Many peer counselors, administrators, and role models in therapeutic communities are ex-addicts. The goals of this type of program are

◇ habilitation or rehabilitation of the total individual;

◇ changing negative patterns of behavior, thinking, and feeling that predispose drug use; and

◇ development of a drug-free lifestyle.

(Institute of Medicine, 1990)

Because of funding limitations and availability, variations of the long-term therapeutic community concept have developed, e.g., short-term communities (3–6 months), modified therapeutic communities (6–9 months), adolescent therapeutic communities for juveniles that focus on the specific problems of youth, and jail-based therapeutic communities (Crowe & Reeves, 1994).

Many addicts are often put off by making such a long commitment to

being cut off from society. Many programs divide the treatment into 3–6 month phases that permit making commitments to each phase of treatment rather than the full 1–3 years all at one time.

Halfway houses permit addicts to keep their jobs and outside contacts while being involved in a residential treatment program. Addicts receive educational and therapeutic interactions after work hours and live within the facility. Weekends or nonworking days are reserved for more intensive program work that continues for a long duration (1–3 years). Several new religious movements (NRMs) also use the halfway house concept to treat addiction. They are controversial because some critics say that joining a religious movement is exchanging one compulsion for another while the other side says that a spiritual awakening is necessary for true recovery and a NRM halfway house can provide that structure (Muffler, Langrod, Richardson, & Ruiz, 1997).

Sober-living or transitional-living programs are generally for clients who have completed a long-term residential program. They consist of apartments or cooperatives for groups of recovering addicts with strong house rules to maintain a clean and sober living environment that is supportive of each person's recovery effort. Minimal to moderate treatment structure is provided for those living arrangements and programs merely monitor compliance to protocols that allow the addicts to reenter the broader society with a drug-free lifestyle.

Partial hospitalization and day hospitals are medical outpatient programs that involve the client in therapeutic activities for four to six hours per day while the client still lives at home. These programs provide medical services for detoxification and for medically assisted recovery with medications that either treat withdrawal symptoms, modify craving, or help prevent relapse. Counseling and education are part of these programs. Intensive outpatient programs are a less intense (six to eight hours per week) modification of this model.

Harm reduction programs, as discussed earlier in this chapter, consist mainly of pharmacotherapy maintenance approaches (also called "agonist maintenance treatment"), particularly methadone maintenance clinics that substitute a long-acting synthetic opioid that is taken orally to prevent opioid withdrawal, block the effects of illicit opioids, and reduce opioid craving. LAAM is an even longer-acting opioid antagonist that is used in this kind of treatment. Another harm reduction program that is less successful is controlled drinking or drug use taught through behavioral training programs. There are also education programs that teach how to minimize problems from drug use; partial detox clinics to minimize damage to the user; and even designated driver programs that seem to sanction heavy drinking by some (Morris, 1995).

In 1997 a total of 1,477,881 people were treated in various programs and facilities. It is estimated that another 2,000,000 hard-core users also needed treatment and possibly another 3,500,000 problematical users needed some kind of treatment. The totals mean that in 1997 about 7 million Americans had serious enough drug and alcohol problems to need treatment.

BEGINNING TREATMENT

It is vital to remember that addiction is a dysfunction of the mind caused by actual biochemical changes in the central nervous system that can originate at birth, be changed by environmental influences, and be further manipulated by psychoactive drugs and/or compulsive behaviors. Brain cells, unlike all other cells, are generally nonrenewable, although recent research has shown that there is a reservoir of immature brain cells, called "stem cells," that can regenerate into new brain cells when needed (Snyder et al., 1999). We are born with most of the brain cells we will ever have (including the reservoir

TABLE 9–1 PAST-YEAR ADMISSIONS BY TREATMENT FACILITY IN THE UNITED STATES—1997

Type of Facility	All Admissions	Alcohol Only	Alcohol & Other Drug	Opiates (Heroin)	"Crack" Cocaine	Other Cocaine	Marijuana	Methamphetamine or Amphetamine
TOTAL (numbers)	1,477,881	401,961	311,778	232,452	163,211	58,790	191,724	66,461
Percent of each drug category that uses a particular type of facility								
Ambulatory (%)	**63.8%**	**63.2%**	**60.6%**	**63.4%**	**53.2%**	**59.3%**	**79.7%**	**58.3%**
Outpatient	50.5	53.8	50.1	37.7	39.3	47.5	66.3	48.2
Intensive outpatient	9.3	8.7	9.7	3.8	12.9	11.3	12.6	9.4
Detoxification	4.0	0.6	0.8	21.6	0.9	0.5	0.9	0.8
Residential/Rehab (%)	**18.4%**	**12.2%**	**22.9%**	**12.4%**	**29.6%**	**26.6%**	**16.4%**	**28.2%**
Short-term (<31 days)	9.0	7.2	13.4	4.8	12.1	10.9	7.6	11.0
Long-term (31 + days)	8.3	3.8	8.4	6.8	16.8	13.5	7.8	16.3
Hospital (nondetox)	1.1	1.2	1.2	0.7	0.7	2.3	1.0	1.0
Detoxification (%)	**17.9%**	**24.6%**	**16.5%**	**24.6%**	**17.2%**	**14.1%**	**3.8%**	**13.5%**
Free-standing residential	15.8	22.1	14.9	19.7	16.3	12.1	3.5	13.2
Hospital inpatient	2.1	2.5	1.6	4.9	0.9	2.0	0.3	0.4

Source: Treatment Episode Data Set: 1992-1997 (SAMHSA/TEDS, 1999)

TABLE 9–2 ONE DAY CENSUS OF CLIENTS IN TREATMENT BY INSTITUTION

Type of Institution	1980	1987	1993	1997
Free-standing/outpatient	250,378	368,775	565,293	507,683
Mental health services	106,157	99,184	150,519	225,777
Physical health services	57,365	79,889	94,368	125,981
Other community services & settings	62,860	56,841	95,682	10,968
Correctional services & settings	12,143	9,434	37,368	56,677
Totals	**488,903**	**614,123**	**943,230**	**927,086**

◇ 72% of all clients were male.

◇ 4.9% of female clients were pregnant.

◇ Close to half of all clients resided in urban areas.

◇ 1/4 of all clients were IV drug users at the time of admission.

◇ 12% were under 20 years old.

◇ 76% were between 21–44 years old.

◇ 11% were between the ages of 45 and 64.

◇ 1% were over 65 years old.

Source: Uniform Facility Data Set Survey, 1995–1997 (UFDS, 1998); National Drug and Alcoholism Treatment Unit Survey 1980–1993 (NDATUS, 1994)

of immature stem cells) unlike tissues such as skin cells that are totally replaced every eight days or so. Thus the brain cell disease of addiction is a chronic progressive process that can be treated and arrested but not one that can be reversed to any great extent or cured. The Haight-Ashbury Clinic rec-ognizes that recovery is a lifelong process since the brain cells have been permanently changed. Addicts (those who have lost control of their drug use) must refrain from ever abusing and, in most cases, even using small amounts of any psychoactive drug if they want to avoid relapsing into addiction.

"Friday I was feeling good. I even went to a meeting. I'd been in this program for two years. I thought I could have one drink to relax with some friends I ran into. I had about five scotches and ended up using all night long in a hotel with two prostitutes. I went through

about $700 and was broke and then I stole $150 from my roommate. I was ripped off a couple of times buying stuff and at the end of it, I was tweaked and I still wanted more."
Recovering 24-year-old "crack" user

RECOGNITION & ACCEPTANCE

Treatment starts with a recognition and acceptance of addiction by the addict. This self-diagnosis often requires the addict to hit bottom or be the subject of an intervention with an assessment to support and validate the need for treatment. Only then can an addict be entered into a continuum of lifelong processes to assist her or him in a quest for recovery.

Hitting Bottom

Addiction is a progressive illness that leads to severe life impairment and dysfunction when left to proceed without disruption.

"It really took my soul. I really feel it took my soul. As a human being, it's important to have a soul and I think I was just a hollow shell, man. It took my family, it took my kids, it took my self-esteem, which is probably the most important facet of all because without that, everything else was just temporary anyway.
Recovering heroin abuser

The earlier it is recognized, accepted, and treated, the more likely the addict will have a rewarding life and good health. All too often, users come in for treatment after they have hit rock bottom, leaving their hopes for a quality life handicapped. Hitting bottom doesn't have to be life threatening, it can simply be hopelessness.

"I got up and I looked at my pipe. And then I said, 'No,' and I put it down and I put it in the trash—I didn't break it—and I rocked myself and I said, 'No dope, no dope, no dope,' and I rocked myself until I could not rock myself any more."
Recovering "crack" addict

Denial

Overcoming denial, the essential first step in all treatment, is also the most difficult to accomplish. Denial is the universal defense mechanism experienced not only by addicts but also by their families, friends, and associates. Denial prevents or delays the proper recognition and acceptance of a chemical dependency or compulsive behavioral problem. **Denial** is a refusal to acknowledge the negative impact that the drug use is having on one's life. It is also assigning the reason for negative consequences to other causes rather than the drug use or compulsive behavior.

One problem is that many people are unwilling to make the diagnosis or they just don't recognize the signs and symptoms. In particular the medical profession has a tendency to deny or overlook addiction. How often does a physician inquire about a patient's alcohol or other drug use history? How often is a caffeine-intake assessment done by a physician who is treating anxiety and insomnia in a patient? A study of physician awareness in Boston found that about 45% of 1,440 patients with a substance abuse problem said that their physician was unaware of their illness. Uninsured clients, those with a history of medical illness, or those who had been previously treated for substance abuse or mental illness

Protocol for Client Intake

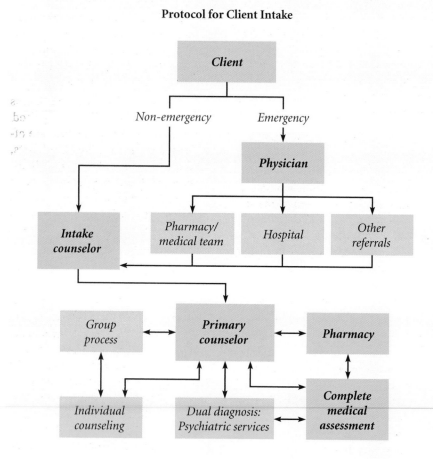

Figure 9-3 •

This is the protocol for the Haight-Ashbury Detox Clinic (medical model outpatient program). It emphasizes the complexity of treating a compulsive drug user who comes in for treatment, particularly if other problems such as medical complications, mental problems (dual diagnosis), or HIV disease are involved. The limiting factor for many clinics is their budget.

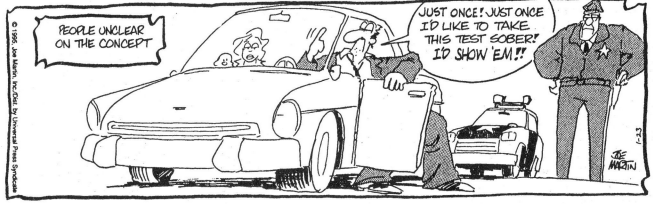

MISTER BOFFO *Joe Martin*

PEOPLE UNCLEAR ON THE CONCEPT

JUST ONCE! JUST ONCE I'D LIKE TO TAKE THIS TEST SOBER! I'D SHOW 'EM!!

MR. BOFFO ©1995, Joe Martin. Reprinted, by permission. Distributed by Universal Press Syndicate.

were even more unlikely to be diagnosed correctly by their physician (Saitz, Mulvey, Plough, & Samet, 1998).

"I woke up after passing out in a friend's home, and they had taken my money away from me, and they had posted somebody at the door, and my mother came and said, 'I will not watch your children for you while you go out and party. If you do something about your problem, I'll take care of your kids for a week.' That was the first time anybody had said to me I had a problem and that was the first time anybody said, 'Stop. You can't do this anymore.'"
37-year-old recovering "speed" user

Breaking Through Denial

Denial plus the toxic effects that psychoactive drugs have on judgment and memory make the addict likely to be the last person to recognize and accept her or his addiction. Usually those closest to the addict, the family or spouse, have the best chance to make the earliest recognition of addiction (not just use) and to help the person break through denial. Besides close relations, others able to recognize addiction include friends, coworkers, employers, ministers, medical professionals, the IRS, and the law. On the other hand, addiction is the only illness that requires a self-diagnosis for treatment

to be effective. Normally when physicians tell patients that they have high blood pressure, they usually accept that diagnosis without question and make changes in their lives to improve their health. But when addicts are first confronted with their addiction, they almost always deny any drug problem and continue to abuse drugs.

There are several ways to break through denial.

◇ Legal Intervention: The threat of loss of property, professional licensure, or freedom forces users to accept that they are having a problem with drugs. Legal requirements may mandate treatment while incarceration limits drug use and promotes abstinence in prisons where drug trafficking is kept to a minimum. Unfortunately some prison personnel estimate that, if tested, from 10% to 30% of inmates would test positive for an illicit psychoactive drug.

◇ Workplace Intervention: Poor performance and the threat of the loss of one's livelihood may break through denial. Strong employee assistance programs can work with the at-risk employee.

◇ Physical Health Problems: Deteriorating health and doctors' warnings can make the user consider drug problems as a possible cause or complicating factor. The existence of lung cancer, high blood pressure,

or heart, liver, kidney, and other diseases caused by drug toxicity can be a powerful tool to confront a patient's denial to addiction.

◇ Mental Health Problems: Emotional and mental traumas, like depression, anger, and mental confusion, that affect day-to-day functioning can also act as a warning signal.

◇ Financial Difficulties: Problems such as paying bills, buying food, or covering the rent, which are affected by escalating drug costs force the user either to deal drugs, turn to other crimes, or cut back on use, thus compelling the user to recognize the financial damage of addiction.

(Miller & Hester, 1989; Heather, 1989)

Table 9-3 shows the sources of referral for people who have entered substance abuse treatment. Some interesting observations: first is that overall, about 1/3 are self-referred and another 1/3 are referred by the justice system, usually court-ordered treatment; the percentage of self-referrals for marijuana is almost 1/2 of the number of referrals for other drugs (except heroin); while criminal justice or DUI referrals for marijuana are almost double the number of referrals for other drugs (SAMHSA, 1999).

"My dad's an alcoholic. I've tried so many things just to get him into treatment but no matter how much I try, he

TABLE 9–3   ADMISSIONS BY SOURCE OF REFERRAL IN THE UNITED STATES

Source of Referral	All Admissions	Alcohol Only	Alcohol w/ Other Drug	Heroin	"Crack"	Other Cocaine	Marijuana	Metham-phetamine
Total # of Admissions	1,436,635	390,511	303,082	214,919	158,821	56,316	185,928	65,006
Individual (self)	33.4%	26.2%	27.8%	65.6%	35.9%	33.3%	18.3%	31.8%
Criminal justice/DUI	34.9%	45.1	35.1	10.9	25.2	30.5	52.3	38.0
Substance abuse provider	12.9%	10.8	17.1	13.2	18.6	14.0	7.2	7.5
Other health care provider	7.2%	8.4	7.8	5.0	7.5	7.8	5.6	6.8
School (educational)	1.5%	0.8	1.2	0.1	0.1	0.4	5.2	0.7
Employer/EAP	1.3%	1.5	1.3	0.4	0.1	2.3	1.9	1.0
Other community referral	8.8%	7.2	9.6	4.9	11.7	11.8	9.4	14.2

Source: Treatment Episode Data Set: 1992–1997 (SAMHSA/TEDS, 1999)

just doesn't listen. So I'm not gonna let him take me down from my recovery. I just told him, you know, 'Forget it. And if you want to be with me, you're going to have to be clean.' And he only loves two things and that's me and my brother. And if we take one of those away, he might want to quit."

Recovering 15-year-old recovering polydrug abuser

Intervention

Special strategies have been developed to attack the denial in drug abusers and addicted people and help them recognize their dependence on drugs. Generally referred to as "intervention," these strategies have been documented since the late 1800s to effectively bring those who are addicted into treatment and hold them there. Further there are now specialists who help to organize and implement intervention (Mersy, 1991). The current style of formal intervention was developed by Dr. Vernon Johnson in the 1960s and refined by a number of treatment professionals.

"Intervention is a process by which the harmful, progressive, and destructive effects of chemical dependency are interrupted and the chemically dependent person is helped to stop using mood-altering chemicals and to develop new healthier ways of coping

with his or her needs and problems. It implies that the person need not be an emotional or physical wreck (or hit bottom) before such help can be given."

Vernon E. Johnson, Founder, Johnson Institute (Johnson, 1986)

Generally a formal intervention should be tried after informal interventions have failed or if a professional feels that the wall of denial is too great.

Most intervention strategies consist of the following elements:

Love. An intervention should always start and end with an expression of love and genuine concern for the well-being of the addicted person. Multiple participants should be recruited from various aspects of the addicted person's life—all of whom share a sense of true affection for the user but recognize the progressive impairment of the addiction and are bold enough to commit themselves to participation in the intervention. Generally this intervention team consists of two or more of the following: family members, close friends and coworkers, other recovering addicts, a representative of the user's spiritual community (clergy or community leader), and a lead facilitator.

Facilitator. A professional intervention specialist or a knowledgeable chemical dependency treatment professional is selected to organize the inter-

vention, educate the participants about addiction and treatment options, train and assist team members in the preparation of their statements, and support or confirm the diagnosis of addiction. The team meets and prepares its intervention without revealing their activities to the user.

Intervention Statements. Each team member prepares a statement that he or she will make to the addicted person at the time of the intervention. Each statement consists of four parts:

1. a declaration of how much they love, care for, and respect the user;

2. specific incidents they have personally witnessed or experienced related to the addiction and the pain they have personally experienced from the incidents;

3. personal knowledge that the incidents occurred not because of the user's intent but because of the effects that the drug has caused on the user's behavior;

4. reassurance of their love, concern, and respect for the user with a strong request that he or she recognize and accept the illness and enter treatment immediately.

Anticipated Defenses & Outcomes. The facilitator prepares the team to deal with expected defense mechanisms like denial, rationalization, minimization, anger, and accusations. The team also prepares for all logistics (reserving a program or hospital admission, packing clothing and toiletries, covering work and home duties) so that the user will have no excuse or delay in entering treatment immediately should a successful intervention ensue. The team also prepares for contingencies and alternative treatments other than the ones they selected should the addict refuse to accept their first recommendation. It is important that the user accepts one of the treatment programs selected by the team and not delay entry by selecting a different program.

The Intervention. Timing, location, and surprise are crucial components of the actual intervention. A neutral, nonthreatening, and private location must be secured for the intervention. It should occur at a time (usually early Sunday morning) when the user is most likely to be sober or not under the influence of a drug. The evidence presented in statements should include current incidents. A reliable plan should be developed to get the addicted person to the location that does not cause her or him to suspect what is about to occur. Finally the facilitator should prepare the order of the statements that have been rehearsed by the team prior to the intervention.

Contingency. Successful or not, it is important for the intervention team members to continue to meet after the intervention to process their experiences. This also provides the opportunity for team members (especially family members) to explore their own support or treatment needs for issues such as codependency, enabling, or adult children of addicts syndrome.

Despite the inherent risks of anger or rejection that may result from an unsuccessful intervention, the potential benefits from these strategies far outweigh the risks. At a very minimum, the pathological effects of secrecy that pervade an addiction have been brought out to all those who are most affected by it, allowing a chance for successful treatment.

TREATMENT CONTINUUM

"I know it sounds strange but the best thing that ever happened to me was that I became an addict. That's because my addiction forced me into treatment and the recovery process and through recovery I found what was missing in my life."
Nurse with 20 years of recovery time

The chronic, progressive, and relapsing nature of addiction is a depressing and degrading process. Results of a Beck's Depression Inventory (BDI) evaluation of patients entering into treatment at the Haight-Ashbury Clinic demonstrated that 34% to 38% tested for maximum depression. Admission interviews also demonstrated that 30% to 34% had made at least one suicide gesture prior to seeking help for their addiction (Haight-Ashbury Clinic, 1996). Fortunately recovery is a spiritually uplifting and motivating process through which individuals gain a sense of purpose, community, and meaning for their lives. Recovery is also a gradual process and a client passes through several changes, no matter which therapy is used. The treatment should address four major phases that lead one to health: **detoxification, initial abstinence, sobriety,** and **continuous recovery.** It is necessary for the addict to become and remain abstinent through all phases of treatment to be successful, however, slips and relapses are part of the addiction process and often occur during treatment. For this reason they need to be accepted and processed by the client and counselor or therapist.

The four steps to recovery are the ones used at the Haight-Ashbury Detox Clinic and have been valuable during the 33 years to tens of thousands of clients who have been treated.

DETOXIFICATION

The first step is to get the drug out of the body's system if the client is still using. The user's body chemistry has become so unbalanced that only abstinence will give it time to metabolize the drug and begin to normalize neurochemical balance. Detoxification will also help clients' thinking processes to normalize so they can participate fully in their own recovery. It takes about a week to completely excrete a drug such as cocaine and perhaps another 4 weeks to 10 months until the body chemistry settles down. Certain drugs, including marijuana and PCP, take longer to be excreted from the body. Some treatment programs will assist in the detoxification process but most require several days of abstinence prior to admission.

The initial detoxification process is usually through a process called "white knuckling" where addicts or abusers stop taking the drug on their own and suffer through physical and mental withdrawal symptoms. It can also be done on an outpatient basis, an intense outpatient basis, a residential facility that is medically supervised, or a medically managed inpatient facility that can include treatment in the emergency room of a hospital if the client is in crisis (Chang & Kosten, 1997).

For those facilities (including the Haight-Ashbury Clinic) that assist in detoxification, assessment of the severity of addiction is important to determine if medical detoxification is necessary and, if so, which facility should be used. The level of intoxication, the potential for severe withdrawal symptoms, the presence of other medical or psychological problems, the patient's response to treatment recommendations, the potential for relapse, and the environment for recovery need to be determined.

Severe physical dependence on alcohol or sedatives, major medical or psychiatric complications, and pregnancy are all indications for initiating detoxification in a hospital-based program.

"Something told me I had to stop, so I did. And I stopped by myself for seven days straight. I didn't know what I was going through. I was having flashes, I heard people talking to me,

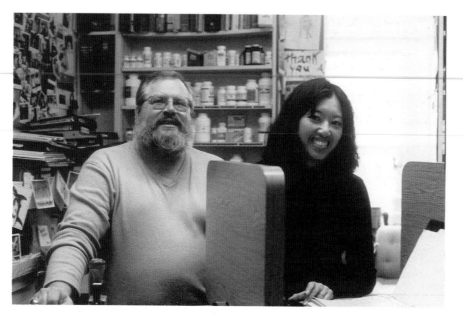

Chief pharmacist Greg Hayner, Pharm.D., and Karen Dang, Pharm.D. of the Haight-Ashbury Clinic dispense a wide variety of medications used for detoxification, abstinence, anticraving, and relapse prevention in conjunction with individual and group counseling. Medication therapy is becoming a larger part of treatment therapies.

and I was sweating. I had the shakes real bad, so I called General Hospital. They gave me poison control and they transferred me to the Haight-Ashbury Clinic."

23-year-old recovering cocaine addict

Medication Therapy for Detoxification

A variety of specific medications are used during the detoxification phase to ease the symptoms of withdrawal and minimize the initial drug cravings that occur. (*There is more thorough coverage of potential treatment medications at the end of this chapter.*)

◇ Clonidine (Catapres®) dampens the withdrawal symptoms of opioids, alcohol, and even nicotine addiction.

◇ Phenobarbital is used to prevent withdrawal seizures and other symptoms associated with alcohol and sedative-hypnotic dependence.

◇ Methadone is the federally approved medication for opioid addiction treatment (for detoxification and maintenance) while

l-alpha acetyl methadol (LAAM) and buprenorphine are being developed as alternatives for methadone in the detoxification (or maintenance) of opioid addictions.

◇ Antipsychotic medications, like halperidol (Haldol®), and antidepressants, including desipramine and imipramine (Tofranil®), have been used in the initial detoxification of cocaine, amphetamine, or other stimulant drug addictions.

◇ Bromocriptine (Parlodel®), amantadine (Symmetrel®), and L-Dopa® have been used to treat the craving associated with cocaine and stimulant drug dependence; naltrexone (Revia®) and acomprosate have been used to decrease alcohol cravings.

◇ Nicotine patches (Nicoderm® or Prostep®) are approved to treat the withdrawal symptoms of tobacco whereas nicotine-laced gum (Nicorette®) helps to lessen craving.

◇ Antabuse® (disulfiram) helps to prevent alcoholism relapse by creating unpleasant side effects if alcohol is used while it is being taken.

◇ Naltrexone (Revia®) blocks the effects of opioids. The addict will have no response to heroin if she or he happens to slip while in treatment. It is also being used to prevent craving in recovering alcoholics.

◇ Finally, a number of amino acids are used individually or in combination with each other to alleviate withdrawal and craving symptoms from addiction to various drugs. The theory is that the brain uses these amino acids to make neurotransmitters that were depleted by the drug addiction. It is believed that the imbalance or depletion of neurotransmitters is the cause of the withdrawal and craving. Common amino acids used for this purpose are tyrosine, taurine, tryptophane, d,l-phenylalanine, lecithin, and glutamine.

Psychosocial Therapy

Medical intervention alone is rarely effective during the detoxification phase. Indeed most programs forego medical treatment when the addict is not in any physiological or psychological danger from drug withdrawal. Intensive counseling, group work, and 12-step group participation have proven to be the most effective measures of engaging addicts into a recovery process and should be the main focus of all phases of treatment despite the many medical innovations being developed.

Psychosocial client interactions during detoxification are usually intense (daily encounters in an outpatient program) and highly structured for a two to six week duration. The aim of this treatment phase is to break down residual denial and engage the client into the full recovery process. This is accomplished through mandated participation in educational sessions, task-oriented group work, therapy groups, peer recovery groups, 12-step groups, and individual counseling.

Treatment focuses on helping the addict to learn about the disease concept of addiction, the harmful effects of the disease, and the intensity of detoxification symptoms being experienced by the addict. The clients also receive information about their treatment and any medications used in detoxification. Clients develop their recovery or treatment plan with their primary counselor and initiate activities to accomplish their goals. Some programs have also begun to use structured treatment manuals that have a developed curriculum for each phase of treatment with individual daily lesson plans, exercises, and homework assignments.

"I knew I could do it myself. I tried those programs in AA. I stopped using drugs a million times and I never needed one of those programs. I figure if you're going to do it, you're going to do it anyway."
Heroin addict dying from AIDS

INITIAL ABSTINENCE

Once the addicts have been detoxified, their body chemistry must be given the opportunity to regain balance. Continued abstinence during this phase is best promoted by addressing both the continuous craving for drugs and the problems in their lives that may put them at risk for relapse.

Anticraving medications, such as those used during the detoxification phase, can be continued during the initial abstinence phase when more traditional approaches, like voluntary isolation (staying away from slippery places like bars, slippery people like co-users, and slippery things like drug paraphernalia), counseling, group and 12-step meetings, are ineffective in controlling the episodic drug hunger.

Medication Therapies for Initial Abstinence

Medical approaches like Antabuse® or alcoholism, naltrexone for opioids and alcohol, and various amino acids like tyrosine or d,l-phenylalanine for many of the drug addictions have been used to support the work of the self-help groups. They suppress or reverse the pleasurable effects of drugs or decrease the drug craving, all of which

helps encourage the addict to stay clean (O'Brien, 1997; Gatch & Lal, 1998).

Recently an injection of a benzodiazepine antagonist, flumazenil (Mazicon®), has been used for the treatment of benzodiazepine overdose (Valenzuela & Harris, 1997). Research into a cocaine vaccine and a true alcohol antagonist may lead to treatments for these addictions in the same manner that naltrexone is effective in preventing readdiction to opioids.

Environmental Triggers, Relapse Prevention, & Cue Extinction

"When I'm smelling the marijuana here in the building where I live, I smell the 'primos,' which is 'crack' cocaine laced with marijuana, the cravings do come back. And what I do is I call my sponsor. I go to a meeting. I go to a NA and AA meeting and I mostly talk to my sponsor and I tell her what I'm feeling and I pray to God to give me the strength not to go out to buy me any kind of drugs to use."
38-year-old recovering polydrug abuser

Environmental triggers or cues often precipitate drug cravings. These triggers have been classified into two broad categories: intrapersonal and interpersonal factors (internal states and external influences). Internal (intrapersonal) states that have the greatest impact are negative emotional and physical states or attempts to regain control and use. External influences include relationship conflict, social pressure, lack of support systems, negative life events, and so-called slippery people, places, and things (Marlatt, 1995; Carter & Tiffany, 1999). Some other factors that help lead to relapse are exhaustion, dishonesty, impatience, argumentativeness, depression, frustration, self-pity, cockiness, complacency, expecting too much from others, letting up on disciplines, use of any mood-altering drugs, overconfidence (PRO, 1999). Addicts have discovered this by themselves and long ago developed handy acronyms like HALT (hungry, angry, lonely, tired) and RID (restless, irritable, & discontent) to remind themselves of the triggers which lead them into relapse.

Relapse prevention has become the focus of almost every treatment pro-

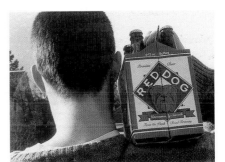

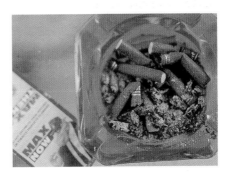

Environmental cues that trigger drug craving can include paraphernalia, drug-using partners, old neighborhoods, and especially money.

gram. There are a number of strategies and themes that are used in this process.

◇ Addicts must understand the process of relapse and then learn to recognize their personal triggers that can be anything from drug odors, seeing friends who use, having money in one's pocket, and even hearing a song about drugs.

◇ They must then develop mechanisms to avoid external cues. These include avoiding old neighborhoods and dealers, changing one's circle of friends, limiting the amount of money that's carried, and not going into bars or gatherings where drugs are readily available.

◇ They must learn to cope with or be prepared with a strategy to prevent themselves from using when their craving is activated by internal or external cues that they can't avoid. These include developing a support system, developing coping skills for negative emotional states and cognitive distortions, developing a balanced lifestyle, and possibly using anticraving medications (Daley & Marlatt, 1997).

It is important to note that drug craving is a true psychological response that is manifested by actual physiological changes of increased heart rate and blood pressure, sweating, dilation of the pupils, specific electrical changes in the skin, and even an immediate drop of two degrees or more in body temperature.

Deconditioning techniques, stress reduction exercises, expressing one's feelings, and long walks or cold showers are all strategies used by addicts to dissipate the craving response when it arises.

A technique such as Dr. Anna Rose Childress's Desensitization Program retrains brain cells to not react when confronted by an environmental cue. The procedure involves exposing an addict to progressively stronger environmental cues over 40–50 sessions in a controlled setting. This technique gradually decreases response to the cues until there are no physiologic

signs of a craving response even when the addict is exposed to heavy triggers. Every time an addict refrains from using while craving a drug, it lessens the response to the next trigger experience. Desensitization has also been called "cue extinction" (Childress, McClellan, Ehrman, & O'Brien, 1988).

"I did it myself. Every day I would take out my Librium® pills and look at them, touch them, and even smell them. Then I would put them back in the bottle because I knew I couldn't ever use them again. After a while I lost interest in them altogether."
Recovering Librium® addict

Psychosocial Support

Initial abstinence is also the phase during which addicts start to put their lives back in order, working on all the things they neglected to take care of while practicing their addiction. A comprehensive analysis of an addict's medical health, psychiatric status, social problems, and environmental needs must be conducted and a plan developed to address all issues presented.

Most importantly addicts need to build a support system that will give continuing advice, help, and information when the user returns to job and home and is subject to all the pressures and temptations that made drug abuse begin. The support groups and 12-step programs like AA (Alcoholics Anonymous), NA (Narcotics Anonymous), CA (Cocaine Anonymous), and others are essential to maintaining a clean, sober, drug-free lifestyle. Involvement in group therapy and continued recovery counseling have been demonstrated to have the most positive treatment outcomes during the initial abstinence phase.

Acupuncture

The use of acupuncture to relieve withdrawal symptoms and reduce craving has been on the increase in the last 27 years since it was first observed to reduce opium withdrawal symptoms (Wen & Cheung, 1973). The hypothesis as to

why acupuncture works is that by stimulating the peripheral nerves, messages are sent to the brain to release natural (endogenous) endorphins that promote a feeling of well-being (Pomeranz, 1987). Acupuncture has also been shown to alter levels of other neurotransmitters, specifically serotonin and norepinephrine, as well as the hormones prolactin, oxytocin, thyroxin, corticosteroid, and insulin (Boucher, Kiresuk, & Trachtenberg, 1998; Steiner, May, & Davis, 1982). Besides opiate detoxification, it has been used to reduce craving for alcohol and stimulants with varying results. As with all initial abstinence and detoxification techniques, acupuncture is not effective when used as the sole treatment or modality. It is imperative that it be combined with counseling, group therapy, education, and peer interaction. It can also be used with detox medication. The problem with acupuncture is that since it is not a replacement therapy for other modalities, it can be expensive and adds an additional therapeutic cost to the treatment process.

LONG-TERM ABSTINENCE

The pivotal component of this phase occurs when an addict finally admits and accepts her or his addiction as lifelong and surrenders to the long-term, one-day-at-a-time treatment process. Continued participation in group, family, and 12-step programs is the key to maintaining long-term abstinence from drugs. The addict must accept that addiction is chronic, progressive, incurable, and potentially fatal and that relapse is always possible.

"We always say, 'I know that I have another relapse in me. I don't know if I have another recovery in me.'"
7-year member of Alcoholics Anonymous

It is also vital for recovering addicts to accept that their condition is chemical dependency or drug compulsivity and not just that of alcoholism, or cocainism, or opioidism. Individuals who manifest addiction to a particular drug, such as cocaine, are well advised to abstain from the use of all psychoactive substances, especially alcohol. Even a seemingly benign flirtation with marijuana will probably lead to other drug hunger and relapse. It is a common clinical observation that compulsive drug abusers often switch intoxicants only to find the symptoms of addiction resurfacing through another addictive agent. Drug switching does not work with recovery-oriented treatment. A study of men and women in treatment found that 80% had taken two or more substances during their lifetimes, either concurrently or sequentially (Carrol, 1980).

RECOVERY

Treatment and a continued focus on abstinence are not enough to assure recovery and a quality lifestyle. Recovering addicts also need to restructure their lives and find things they enjoy doing that give them satisfaction and that give them the natural highs instead of the artificial highs they came to seek through drugs. Without this they may have sobriety but they will not have recovery. This integral phase of treatment has been validated experimentally by Dr. George Vaillant, Professor of Psychiatry, in studies in 1983. He indicates four components necessary to change an ingrained habit of alcohol dependence. In the following model, the generic term "drug" is substituted for Dr. Vaillant's specific reference to alcohol:

1. offering the client or patient a non-chemical substitute dependency for the drug, such as exercise;

2. reminding her or him ritually that even one episode of drug use can lead to pain and relapse;

3. repairing the social, emotional, and medical damage done;

4. restoring self-esteem.

Continued and lifelong participation in the fellowship of 12-step programs, along with the concerted effort to seek out natural, healthy, nondrug, rewarding experiences, is the formula that most recovering addicts have found to be successful in achieving their treatment goals (Vaillant, 1995).

"I found in sobriety that I love people. I found in sobriety that I have real feelings. I found in sobriety that I have real emotions. I found in sobriety that there's a world of people out there in society that's willing, that's been there all along for me, to assist me. I just never knew it."
56-year-old recovering heroin addict

Natural Highs

"Getting high on life is a skill and just like any other skill—athletic, artistic, musical, or professional—the more you practice it, the more you can improve."
George Obermeier, drug educator

Since psychoactive drugs create sensations or feelings that have a natural counterpart in the body, so human beings can create virtually all of the sensations and feelings they try to get through drugs by concentrating on the feelings they experience from natural life situations. Athletic competition releases the same neurotransmitters as cocaine and amphetamine. Experiencing a second wind or the runner's high from jogging comes from opiate receptor activation. Traveling or experiencing new environments activates the same area of the brain that marijuana affects. Being in touch with the natural or drug-free highs available to the brain is what being alive is all about. In recovery it's about getting to a quality lifestyle.

OUTCOME & FOLLOW-UP

Primarily promoted by government and other funding sources to justify spending for addiction treatment, client outcomes and follow-up evaluations have become a major element in treatment program activities. What seems to be neglected by this process is an opportunity for treatment programs to utilize the data obtained to modify their treatment protocols and interventions to promote better outcomes for clients. Since addiction by nature is a chronic,

multivaried, and relapsing condition, there is a need to develop outcome measures that evaluate different phases of the recovery process including long-term follow up.

Indications most often evaluated for successful addiction treatment include:

◊ prevalence of drug slips and relapses (duration of continuous sobriety);

◊ retention in treatment;

◊ completion of treatment plan and its phases;

◊ family functioning;

◊ social and environmental adjustments;

◊ vocational or educational functioning, including personal finance management;

◊ criminal activity or legal involvement.

What is important to note is that, in general, all types of addiction treatment have demonstrated positive client outcomes when evaluated by rigorous scientific methods.

"These abscesses came through my addiction to heroin. Never cleaned my

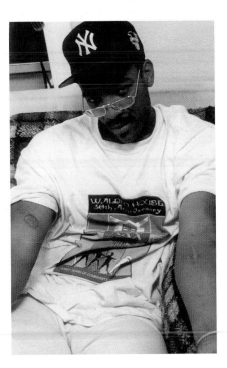

arm, let alone my body. My wake up-call was just getting tired, man, you know. So where I stand today is that I realize that I'm a better person than that. I don't need that garbage. I got a beautiful lady that's very supportive of me. It gives me a reason not to want to use. You know, not just saying it in my head but inside my heart. I didn't love myself. I didn't care about nobody because I didn't care about me. Now I care about myself and it allows me to care about other people too."

35-year-old recovering addict

INDIVIDUAL VS. GROUP THERAPY

There are two main integrated components of addiction treatment: psychosocial therapy and medical (especially medication) therapy. Recent developments in understanding the neurobiological process of addiction have resulted in an explosive growth of medication treatments and the new medical specialty of addiction medicine. However, it is important to remember those treatments are not effective unless they are integrated with psychosocial therapies. There are two general types of counseling therapies: individual and group. Most treatment facilities will use a combination of these counseling therapies.

INDIVIDUAL THERAPY

Individual therapy is a process usually conducted by trained chemical dependency counselors often credentialed to work with substance abusers. They deal with clients on a one-to-one basis to explore the reasons for their continued use of psychoactive substances and identify all areas of intervention needs. This may lead to a referral for specialized treatment, such as psychiatry, medical care, family counseling, and others. The therapist is able to work with addicts to help them gain a perspective on their usage and to identify tools and mechanisms that will keep them abstinent from drugs. The most common individual therapies are cognitive-behavioral therapy, reality therapy, aversion therapy, psychodynamic therapy, art therapy, assertiveness training, and social skills training to name a few (Stevens-Smith & Smith, 1998).

A treatment plan is developed with the client to guide in this process and individual treatment may continue from one month to several years. Although the majority of treatment is based on group and peer interaction, individual treatment may be more effective for certain types of drugs such as heroin and sedatives.

A drug counselor and a heroin addict in a counseling session at the Haight-Ashbury Detox Clinic in San Francisco

Addict: "When I'm going through withdrawal, it's a physical thing, and then after I'm clean, I have the mental problem having to say no every time I get money in my hands: 'Should I or shouldn't I? No, I shouldn't. Go ahead, one more time won't hurt.' After I've passed withdrawal, and I pass by areas where I used to hang out, and I see other people nodding, in my mind, I start feeling like I'm sick again. I want to stay clean."

Counselor: "You can stay clean for a while. Is that what you want? You want to stay clean for a while or for the rest of your life?"

Addict: "I want to stay clean permanently."

Counselor: "Permanently drug free?"

Addict: "But I can do it without attending those [Narcotics Anonymous] meetings."

Counselor: "All by yourself?"

Addict: "I mean with the medication that I take."

Counselor: "But the medications are only going to last you 21 days. They'll help you for a little while with the withdrawal of getting off heroin but what are you going to do when the urges come up?"

Addict: "I guess I'll deal with that when the time comes."

Counselor: "So you're just going to wait for it? You're going to wait for the urges to come on and start using then?"

Addict: "Nah, I can deal with it."

Counselor: "You're being highly uncooperative. As a matter of fact, we're going to stop the medications today because we know you're still using heroin and we can't have you using on the program."

Addict: "I need those medications."

Counselor: "What for? It's just another drug. What you're doing is using it like another drug. I'd like for you to come back to get into that group meeting we have at three o'clock. Also I want you to go to a NA (Narcotics Anonymous) meeting every day. I want you to go to these meetings and participate. Talk every opportunity you can. And also what I want you to do is bring back the signed participation card that you attended. I want you to do that. That's just part of the requirement of being in the program. See, I'm going to assume that you want to stop using drugs."

Addict: "Why can't I just get the detoxification drugs?"

Counselor: "Because we're not just a medication program. It's a counseling and full recovery program too."

It is also observed that individual treatment is less threatening for many individuals and therefore can be used as a short-term initial treatment in addiction.

GROUP THERAPY

There are several types of group therapies. They are facilitated, peer, 12-step, educational, topic specific, and targeted. Generally a major focus of group therapy is having clients help each other to break the isolation that chemical dependency induces so they know they are not alone. Addicts are able to gain experience and understanding from each other about their addiction and learn different ways to combat craving that help prevent their abuse or relapse. As peers they are also better equipped to confront one another on issues that may lead to relapse or continued use.

"The group keeps me honest with myself. I get to look at a lot of things and behaviors that are going on with me and I try and keep in the now. I keep thinking about staying clean today, and the group keeps me focused on my goal of each day trying to stay clean."

Recovering "crack" cocaine user

Facilitated Groups

Group therapy usually consists of six or more clients who meet with one or more therapists on a daily, weekly, or monthly basis. Therapists may facilitate the group by actively leading it, bringing up topics to be discussed, and processing all issues with their clinical insight. The facilitator (counselor) helps to establish a group culture where sharing, trust, and openness become natural to the participants.

Stimulant abuse peer group which uses confrontational techniques and a facilitator

William: "I have two sets of friends. People I use with and people who don't use at all. We've got together and had dinner and so forth."
Facilitator: "That's real safe for you, William. Listen to me, William. They don't know what to look for.

They don't know what to expect and you can manipulate them real easy."
Maria: "The same thing happened to me. You still think you can sit around with alcoholics, with people who drink, like you think you can hang around with dope dealers?"
William: "So the only people I can associate with are people in recovery?"
Maria: "I had to give up my sister."
William: "Okay, admit it. Everybody out there doesn't have a problem."
Maria: "But you do."
William: "That's true."
Facilitator: "Let me ask you a question. Can you see your ears?"
William: "No."
Facilitator: "So that means we can see something you can't see, right? Okay. So far, this group, with your issues, we're batting a thousand. Yes or no?"
William: "Yes."

Peer Groups

Peer group therapy consists of therapists playing a less active role in the dynamics. They observe interaction and are available to process any conflicts or areas of need but they do not direct or lead the process.

Drug abuse recovery peer group

John: "I didn't want to come here this morning and then to come here and be faced with, 'Well, you gotta think whether you really want to be here.' It's like I'm ready. And I'm scared."
Counselor: "What's scaring you?"
John: "I feel like I'm failing myself."
Bob: "When did you fail before?"
John: "When have I failed before? Oh, I would say the last time was when I got busted buying 'crack'. Just going out there is failing. Knowing I shouldn't be doing that."

Bob: "You gotta put that out there. You gotta deal with that."
John: "The thing is I'm scared of when I'm going to snap again."

Self-Help Groups & Alcoholics Anonymous (12-step group)

The concept of abstinence-based self-help groups goes back hundreds of years in America to fraternal temperance societies and reform clubs where recovering alcoholics could go to maintain their abstinence by discussion, prayer, and social activities. One of the earliest groups was the Washingtonian Revival, started in 1840 by six members of a drinking club in Baltimore, Maryland. They started a temperance meeting that met on a weekly basis and instead of debates, drinking games, and speeches, their main activity was sharing their experiences, starting with confessions of a debasing lifestyle caused by their excessive drinking and of their personal recovery. New members, still in the throws of their addiction, were encouraged to tell their own story and sign a pledge of abstinence. This working-class movement spread its message rapidly and chapters formed throughout the country. At the peak of the Washingtonian movement, more than 600,000 pledges were signed. Some meetings had thousands of participants, almost like a revival. The women's auxiliary was called the "Martha Washington Society." The Washingtonian program of recovery closely mirrored that of Alcoholics Anonymous that was created 90 years later.

The program of recovery included

◇ public confession,
◇ public commitment,
◇ visits from older members,
◇ economic assistance,
◇ continued participation in experience sharing,
◇ acts of service toward other alcoholics,
◇ sober entertainment.

The demise of the movement seven years after its inception was somewhat of a mystery although everybody had an explanation—that they mostly ignored religion in the movement, that they had a weak organizational structure, that they were too sensationalistic, that they didn't have a sustainable recovery program, and that prosperity made them less essential. However, the example of the Washingtonians encouraged other fraternal temperance societies and reform clubs, groups that included the Order of the Good Samaritans, the Order of Good Templars, the Black Templars, the Independent Order of Rechabites, and Osgood's Reformed Drinkers Club. There was continuing debate over whether Prohibition was the real answer to alcoholism. Over the next 50 years, many types of organizations were tried, such as those with a religious basis like rescue missions and the Salvation Army (White, 1998).

It was the evolution and refinement of these groups coupled with the end of Prohibition, the closing down of many drying out institutions and treatment hospitals, along with the beginning of the Great Depression, that eventually led to Alcoholics Anonymous in the 1930s, the most widespread recovery movement in history. It is a peer group concept based on 12 steps of recovery. These groups have no professional therapist present to interact with their members. Each group is independent and relies on each other's knowledge and successes to help curb alcohol and other drug use. The parent group provides literature, suggestions for meeting format, and general structure. The core book is called "*Alcoholics Anonymous*" (usually referred to as "*The Big Book*") that was written by Bill Wilson and Dr. Bob Smith, the founders of AA, along with 100 recovering alcoholics who tell their stories (Trice, 1995).

"When I went to my first meeting, a 30-year-old beautician was running [telling] her story about how her drinking started, the pain she suffered because of it, and what happened to change her. I was a 49-year-old male with my own business and yet her story was my story. Her reaction to al-

cohol was the same as mine. Her helplessness after the first drink was mine. Her denial was mine. Her divorce was mine. Her reaction to life's problems were mine. The familiarity and the sheer power of her running her story have kept me in the group for five and one-half years. In AA they say, 'We only have our stories and all we can do is tell what worked for us to stay sober."

Recovering 54-year-old alcoholic

Some of the other 12-step groups that have formed besides AA, CA, and NA are Marijuana Anonymous (MA), Gamblers Anonymous (GA), Overeaters Anonymous (OA), Sexaholics Anonymous, Emotions Anonymous, Relationships Anonymous, and Shoppers Anonymous. In addition Al-Anon (for familes of alcoholics), Adult Children of Alcoholics (ACoA), and Alateen (for teenage drinkers), use the 12-step process.

All 12-step programs are free. They pay their minimal costs through voluntary donations. The only requirement for membership is a desire to stop the addiction.

The 12-step process engages addicts at their level of addiction, breaks the isolation, guilt, and pain, and shows them they are not alone. The process also fully supports the idea that addiction is a lifelong disease and must be dealt with for the remainder of a person's life. It promotes a program of honesty, open-mindedness, and willingness to change. Those are the key elements in sustaining lifelong abstinence from drugs, alcohol, and other addictive behaviors. It breaks down denial and supplies a structure through which people can continue to work on their addiction. The 12-step programs are based on the concept of solution of problems through personal spiritual change, a concept articulated by the Oxford Group, a popular spiritual movement of the 1920s and 1930s (AA, 1935; Nace, 1997; Miller, 1998).

"People misunderstand spirituality. They mistake it for religion.

Spirituality is people's personal relationship with their higher power as they define him, her, or it. Religion is the way they practice their spirituality. My higher power is God as I learned of him in my youth. For others their higher power could be an ideal, a philosophy, the goodness within them, a great person they met in their lives, the stars, or the members of the 12-step group itself. It's something outside of themselves that they can turn to, to get help for their smothering addiction, and to reconstruct their lives. It's only when they give up the need to try to control everything in their lives and give up control to their higher power that they gain the power to overcome their addiction and say no to the first drink."

51-year-old ex-priest who gives talks on spirituality and his recovery from alcoholism

Although most 12-step groups understand and accept spirituality, some users cannot accept the idea of a higher power. For those people *The Big Book* of Alcoholics Anonymous says to take what you want and leave the rest.

The 12 Steps of Alcoholics Anonymous

Step 1: We admitted we were powerless over alcohol [cocaine, cigarettes, food, gambling, etc.] and that our lives had become unmanageable.

Step 2: Came to believe that a power greater than ourselves could restore us to sanity.

Step 3: Made a decision to turn our will and our lives over to the care of God as we understood Him.

Step 4: Made a searching and fearless moral inventory of ourselves.

Step 5: Admitted to God, to ourselves, and to another human being the exact nature of our wrongs.

Step 6: Were entirely ready to have God remove all these defects of character.

Step 7: Humbly asked Him to remove our shortcomings.

Step 8: Made a list of all persons we had harmed and became willing to make amends to them all.

Step 9: Made direct amends to such people wherever possible, except when to do so would injure them or others.

Step 10: Continued to take personal inventory and when we were wrong promptly admitted it.

Step 11: Sought through prayer and meditation to improve our conscious contact with God as we understood Him, praying only for knowledge of His will for us and the power to carry that out.

Step 12: Having had a spiritual awakening as the result of these steps, we tried to carry this message to alcoholics and to practice these principles in all our affairs.

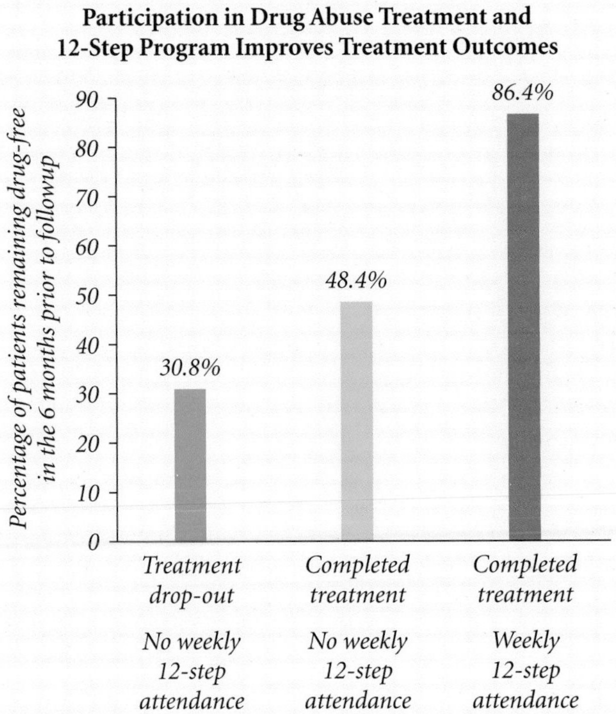

In a study of 12-step programs at UCLA by Dr. Robert Fiorentine and his colleagues, it was found that participation in meetings after completing treatment increased the abstinence rate twofold and presumably the recovery rate (Fig. 9-4) (Fiorentine, 1999). The same study found that increasing counseling sessions (four group sessions and one individual session more per month) reduced drug use by 40%.

"I'm not the same person that I was when I entered this fellowship.
Through my recovery and the 12 steps,
I have found meaning and purpose in my life. It feels especially good with my kids because they know that I'm here for them. There's no catch-up anymore. I keep my promises. The challenge of a sober parent is keeping promises."
Recovering heroin addict

What came to be understood is that the 12 steps work for any addictive behavior. This is because the roots of addiction lie first in the character and lifestyle of the user and second in the use of psychoactive substances.

There are also secular versions of the peer group process used in 12-step groups. These groups do not believe that a higher power is necessary for recovery.

Participation in Drug Abuse Treatment and 12-Step Program Improves Treatment Outcomes

Figure 9-4 •
Weekly attendance at 12-step meetings after treatment almost doubles the abstinence rate of patients (48% vs. 86.4%).

A group like **Rational Recovery (RR)** believes that if you learn to like yourself for who you are, then you will not need to drink or use other drugs. They believe that all addictions come from the same roots. Their approach is based on rational emotive therapy developed by Albert Ellis.

Another group, **Secular Organization for Sobriety (SOS),** also makes no distinction among the various chemical addictions. Their goal is sobriety, one-day-at-a-time, like AA's and NA's goal.

Women for Sobriety (WFS) does have a spiritual basis but feels that AA principles work better for men. WFS emphasizes the power of positive emotions. **Men for Sobriety (MFS)** has also been formed.
(Horvath, 1997)

Educational Groups

These groups focus primarily on providing information about the addictive process in recovery. Trained counselors provide the education and often bring in other experts to promote individual lesson plans to help addicts gain knowledge about their conditions.

Homework assignments are often included to help addicts understand the information. A variety of workbooks and manuals have been written to assist this process. They also teach relapse prevention, coping skills, and even support therapy.

Targeted Groups

These groups can either be part of a formal program or a nonfacilitated peer group and are directed at specific populations of users. Such targeted groups include men's groups, women's groups, gay and lesbian groups, physician groups, dual diagnosis groups, bad girls groups (targeted at prostitutes), and priest/minister/rabbi groups (targeted at the clergy). The key element to the success of any group is its ability to develop a group culture that provides relevant, meaningful, acceptable, and insightful knowledge for that selective gathering of participants.

Topic-Specific Groups

Whereas target groups are aimed at certain cultures, topic groups are aimed at certain issues, e.g., AIDS recovery, early recovery, relapse prevention, recovery maintenance, relationships, and codependency. The advantage of these groups is that they allow the participants to focus on key specific issues that are a threat to their continued recovery.

"I think confrontation is crucial in counseling but it's how it's done. I think that if it's done where the client knows that you're giving them information to help them, not just to put them down or to shame them or to make them feel bad—that it's something we need to talk about—then it's different."
Haight-Ashbury Detox Clinic counselor

From most studies, group therapies seem to promote better outcomes and sustain abstinence more than individual therapies. Specifically, alcohol and cocaine addictions are more responsive to the group process than to individual counseling. From an administrative standpoint, group processes are also much more cost-effective since a large number of clients can be served by a minimal amount of staffing.

Ten Common Errors Made in Group Treatment by Beginning Counselors or Substance Abuse Workers

(Adapted from Geoffrey L. Greif, D.S.W., Associate Dean and Professor, University of Maryland)

1. Failure to have a realistic view of group treatment

Preconceived expectations about the effectiveness of group therapy may cause a new therapist to become impatient with the group's progress when the reality is that each group moves at a different rate of progress from extremely slowly to explosive movement.

Possible solutions: Supervision teaches the therapist to adopt a longer-term perspective. In addition a thorough understanding of the behaviors caused by the specific drug, the way the other groups in the agency function, the cultural backgrounds, and gender-related behaviors of the members make for realistic expectations.

"I think that no matter who you're treating, no matter who you're working with, I think language and culture need to be respected. I think they need to know they're not bad people trying to be good. They're sick people and they can get better. Unconditional love, empathy, warmth, and confrontation, lots of confrontation, lots of humor."
Haight-Ashbury drug counselor

2. Self-disclosure issues and the failure to drop the "mask" of professionalism

New leaders are often challenged by the group members to test the therapist's understanding and/or personal experience with substance abuse.

Possible solutions: A response to any challenge by group members needs to be prepared in advance since too much disclosure by the therapist of personal experience can be as bad as too little disclosure. The leader needs to accept the humanity of their clients as well as disclosing their own.

3. Agency culture issues and personal style

Different methods of running the groups can confuse clients and make them feel trapped between styles. Group culture vs. facility culture can cause dissonance.

Possible solutions: The therapist needs to make his or her approach consistent with the agency style. Personal styles of treatment that are not contradictory to other counselors' styles should be developed with the help of the supervisor and more experienced therapists.

4. Failure to understand the stages of therapy

Groups pass through specific stages during the recovery process and failure to see the progression can hamper the group process.

Possible solutions: There must be a thorough understanding of the various stages of recovery and how to respond with appropriate and timely exercises and thoughts.

5. Failure to recognize counter-transference issues

Often an inexperienced group leader or therapist will let personal feelings about group members show through or affect their performance, particularly if the age, gender, ethnic background, or lifestyle is different.

Possible solutions: The novice therapist must be aware of and accept such feelings as a normal part of the therapist-client relationship—they should just avoid acting on those feelings in a nontherapeutic manner.

6. Failure to clarify group rules

The largest mistake is failure to clarify group rules (e.g., confidentiality, coming to the group high, arriving late, meeting outside of groups, making personal attacks on other members).

Possible solutions: A written handout that contains clear explanations of the procedures followed by a discussion of the rules will give the group a solid base of understanding.

7. Failure to do group therapy by focusing on individual problem solving

In trying to please individual members of the group by giving insightful and helpful suggestions, the therapist can weaken the group.

Possible solutions: Let the group solve individual problems rather than giving individual help and advice. This gives meaning, purpose, and power to the group.

8. Failure to plan in advance

When the leader decides to wing it and doesn't quite know what the group will be doing, less is accomplished.

Possible solutions: The therapist should have a plan for each session and possibly a backup plan so the group doesn't feel directionless.

9. Failure to integrate new members into the group

If a new member enters the group, integrating them into the established

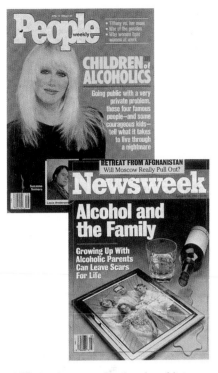

Addiction is not confined to the addicts.

· ·

TREATMENT & THE FAMILY

"I got put into treatment and got out of treatment, you know. I just bullshitted my whole way through treatment. I told them what they wanted to hear and got out and just relapsed again because my dad was like, 'Here, you want to smoke some 'weed'? You want to drink a beer?' It's kinda hard to say no when your dad's sitting there asking you. It makes you feel like it's okay."

15-year-old recovering polydrug abuser

Addiction is a family disease. Abuse of drugs and alcohol greatly impacts every member of addicts' families regardless of whether or not they also abuse psychoactive substances. Analysis of employed addicts and alcoholics demonstrates that their families use the employer's health insurance much more than the families of nonaddicts. This is indicative of the great emotional, physical, and social strain that addicts place on their families.

"Addicts don't have families, they take hostages."

John DeDomenico, family therapist, Haight-Ashbury Detox Clinic

Despite this well-established relationship, the family is often ignored and neglected in the treatment of addictive disease. This has resulted in family members seeking treatment on their own through traditional family and mental health services or through self-help family treatment systems, like Tough Love, Al-Anon, or Nar-Anon.

More importantly, continued stress from family problems or troubled family members makes it difficult for the recovering addict to remain abstinent.

"A family is ruled by its sickest member."

Moss Hart, dramatist

flow can slow the group down. Conversely, if new members are instantly integrated, they don't have time to develop naturally and feel part of the group.

Possible solutions: The therapist can use the opportunity to have the group reevaluate its progress and recommit to the group.

10. Failure to understand interactions in the group as a metaphor for drug-related issues occurring in the group member's family of origin

A new therapist may believe that reactions among group members that are based on a client's familial relationships are true reactions. They might not realize the source of the reactions and so lose an opportunity to use that information to help the client.

Possible solutions: The therapist needs to take the time to establish strong bonds with members of the group, so issues and insights raised by group interactions can be used to help the clients.

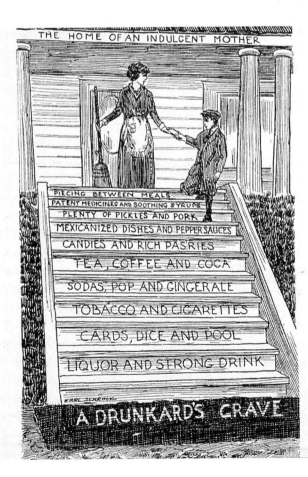

In the past, many problems such as alcoholism were blamed on indulgent parents and especially mom. Many such temperance charts were popular 100 years ago.

Courtesy of Illinois Addiction Studies Archives

· · · · · · · · · · · · · ·

GOALS OF FAMILY TREATMENT

Treatment of addicts and their families has four major goals:

1. acceptance by all family members, including the addicts themselves, that addiction is a treatable disease not a sign of moral weakness;

2. establishing and maintaining a drug-free family system that often includes treatment of the spouse's drug problems or those of the addict's children;

3. developing a system for family communication and interaction that continues to reinforce the recovery process of the addict. This is accomplished by integrating family therapy into addiction treatment;

4. processing the family's readjustment after cessation of drug and alcohol abuse.

"I burnt every bridge that I've got with pretty much everybody in my whole life. The family sessions here are helping a little bit, you know. My mom comes in—my stepdad doesn't want anything to do with me but my mom comes in; we're working, we're listening, you know. We're not just fighting anymore. She's not yelling at the top of her lungs. I'm not telling her to f***- off anymore. We're actually working together. It feels good. I might, you know, I might be able to get a life."
18-year-old recovering male polydrug abuser

DIFFERENT FAMILY APPROACHES

Family therapists employ a wide variety of techniques and tools to accomplish these goals once all family members have been motivated to participate. The following are some of the more commonly used models.

Family Systems Approach

This model explores and recognizes how a family regulates its internal and external environment making note of how these interactional patterns change over time. Three major areas of focus of this approach are daily routines, family rituals (e.g., holidays), and short-term problem-solving strategies. The drug or drinking problem is seen as an integral part of the functioning of all members of the family not just the person with the problem. Some family system therapists use 12-step groups as part of their therapy while many feel that correcting family relationships corrects much of the substance abuse problem (Berenson & Schrier, 1998).

Family Behavioral Approach

This approach operates under the concept that interactional behaviors are learned and perpetuated by reinforcements for continuing the behavior. Thus the therapist works with the family to recognize those family behaviors associated with drug use; to categorize the interactions as either negative or positive in reinforcing drug usage; and then to provide specific interventions to support and reinforce those behaviors that promote a drug-free family system. Some of the specific strategies used are couples sessions, homework, self-monitoring exercises, communications training, and the development of negotiating and problem-solving skills. A couple might even enter into a behavior change agreement (O'Farrell & Cowles, 1989). Some who use the behavioral approach will focus more on working with the nonabusing spouse.

Family Functioning Approach

This approach first helps the addict or treatment programs classify the family system into one of four different types, then uses the classification as a guide for a therapeutic intervention best suited to the functioning of that system.

1. **Functional family systems** are those in which the family of the addict has maintained healthy interactions. Interventions in this system are therefore targeted directly at the addict. Other family members receive limited education and advice to support the recovery of the addict.

2. **Neurotic or enmeshed family systems** usually require intensive family treatment aimed at restructuring the way the family interacts.

3. **Disintegrated family systems** call for a separate yet integrated treatment of addicts and their families. The family may attend Al-Anon while an alcoholic is engaged in an intensive medical detoxification program. Though separated in treatment, this approach needs to be integrated at some point into the common goal of maintaining a drug-free lifestyle by the addict.

4. **Absent family systems** are those in which family members are not available for treatment.

Social Network Approach

This approach focuses mainly on the treatment of the addict but also establishes a concurrent and integrated support network for the family to assist them with the issues caused by the addiction. Through participation in multiple family support or therapy groups, the family breaks their isolation and develops skills that help them support the recovery effort of its addicted member.

Tough Love Approach

Though controversial, this movement has grown on the West Coast. The Tough Love approach addresses the major obstacle of denial in both the addict and his or her family. When the addicted family member refuses to accept or deal with dysfunctional drug-using behavior, the family members seek treatment and support from other families experiencing similar problems. The family learns to establish limits for their interaction with the addict. This has even included kicking that family member out of the home and severing all contact until the addict agrees to treatment.

OTHER BEHAVIORS

"Even though it was my dad that drank till he got sick, doing the intervention was harder for me than for

him. I knew he denied his drinking. I didn't realize that I did too even though I didn't drink myself and that I had almost as many problems as he did."
31-year-old adult child of an alcoholic (ACoA)

The stress of living with an alcoholic or drug abuser causes dysfunctional behaviors in the nonusing family members. The most prevalent conditions are

◇ codependency,

◇ enabling,

◇ and manifesting symptoms caused by being children of addicts or adult children of addicts.

Codependency

Just as addicts are dependent upon a substance, codependents are dependent on the addicts to fulfill some need of their own. For example, a wife may be dependent on her husband maintaining his addiction in order for her to hold power over the relationship. As long as he's addicted, she has an excuse for her own shortcomings and problems. In this way it creates dysfunction in the addict because it promotes the addiction. Codependency can also be extremely subtle. For example, a person who has been abstinent from alcohol for a week or so has a spouse who offers a drink as a reward for the abstinence. In this kind of household, the chances of recovery are greatly reduced unless the codependents are willing to accept their role in the addictive process and submit to treatment themselves (Gorski, 1993; Liepman, 1998).

"I was clean for 16 months. My husband had only been clean for 6 weeks. And I tried to show him that being clean and sober does work. Because my husband—he's not an alcoholic—he basically just smokes 'crack.' And I think he saw what the program was doing for me and that I wasn't going back out or relapsing and buying

drugs for him. [In the past] he would sit here and think I would get up and feel sorry for him and go, 'Okay, honey, you're craving, let's get high together.'"
38-year-old recovering polydrug abuser

Enabling

When a family becomes dependent upon the addiction of a family member, there is a strong tendency to avoid confrontation about the addictive behavior and a subconscious effort to perpetuate the addiction, often led by a person who benefits greatly from that addiction, the "chief enabler." Although enablers may be disgusted with the addict and the addictive behavior, they continue paying off drug debts, paying rent, providing money, or even continuing emotional support for a practicing addict. As with codependents, the enablers need to accept the role they are playing in this cycle and seek therapy so they can be more effective in the addict's recovery.

Children of Addicts & Adult Children of Addicts

Many studies have found coping problems in a large percentage of the children of addicts and alcoholics. About 11 million children of alcoholics are under the age of 18 years and about 3 million of those will develop alcoholism, other drug problems, and other serious coping problems (Windle, 1999). (These statistics also mean that about 3/4 of children of alcoholics do not develop addiction or serious coping problems.)

Many children of addicts take on predictable behavioral roles within the family that "co" the addiction and often continue on into their adult personalities. In addict families, the roles taken on by the children are usually one or more of the following:

◇ Model child: These children are high achievers and are overly responsible. They become chief enablers of addicted parents by taking over their roles and responsibilities.

◇ Problem child: These children experience continual, multiple per-

sonal problems and often manifest early drug or alcohol addiction. They demand and get most of what attention is left from parents and siblings.

◇ Lost child: These children are withdrawn, "spaced-out," disconnected from the life and emotions around them. Often avoiding any emotionally confronting issues, they are unable to form close friendships or intimate bonds with others.

◇ Mascot child or family clown: These children use another avoidance strategy, which is to make everything trivial by minimizing all serious issues. They are well liked and easy to befriend but are usually superficial in all relationships, even those with their own family members.

What is important to remember about children of alcoholics/addicts is that although they may not abuse drugs, their behavior and emotional reactions can be as dysfunctional as those of an addict. Often they learn very early on that they cannot control the addiction of a loved one, so they often resort to trying to control all other aspects of their life, leading to strained and inappropriate relationships later in life.

Adult children of alcoholics (ACoA) or addicts also

◇ are isolated and afraid of people and authority figures;

◇ are approval seekers who lose identity in the process;

◇ are frightened by angry people and personal criticism;

◇ become or marry alcoholics or find another compulsive person to fulfill abandonment needs;

◇ feel guilty when standing up for themselves instead of giving in to others;

◇ become addicted to excitement and stimulation;

◇ confuse love and pity; tend to "love" people that can be pitied and rescued;

◇ repress feelings from traumatic childhoods and lose the ability to feel or express feelings;

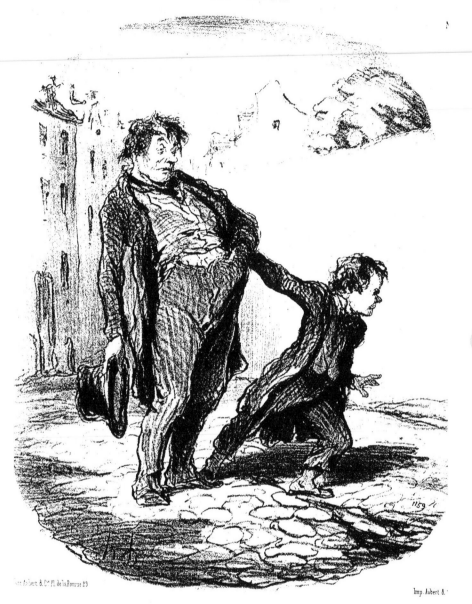

LES PAPAS.

Un fils modèle.

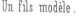

The etching by Henri Daumier is titled "The Fathers" *while the caption reads,* "A model son."

◇ judge themselves harshly and have low self-esteem;

◇ are reacters rather than actors.
(Sher, 1997; Adger, 1998)

ACoA is a 12-step group to help adult children of alcoholics work through the emotional baggage that followed them into adulthood. ACoA and other similar groups try to help members

◇ understand the disease of addiction and alcoholism because understanding is the beginning of the gift of forgiveness;

◇ put themselves on top of their priority list;

◇ detach with love;

◇ feel, accept, and express feelings and build self-esteem;

◇ learn to love themselves, thus enabling them to love others in healthy ways.

Al-Anon and **Nar-Anon** are 12-step-oriented groups targeted for the families of addicts or alcoholics. They involve peer interaction and often the addict is not present. The group meets to support and provide resources to families of addicts to deal with their addicted relatives or lovers. It is common for families to participate in these groups prior to their addicted family member participating in any treatment. **Alateen** is a division of the Al-Anon Family Group. Alateen focuses mostly on 14 to 17 year olds who have an alcoholic in their family and feel more comfortable with just their peers.

DRUG-SPECIFIC TREATMENT

POLYDRUG ABUSE

Experience at the Haight-Ashbury Detox Clinic and treatment centers across the United States shows that although addicts may identify a drug of choice, they are more often than not polysubstance abusers who are using a wide range of substances either concurrently or intermittently. The profile of alcoholics, for example, often includes sedatives, cocaine, and even opioids in addition to their abuse of alcohol. Treatment programs need to be aggressive about identifying the total drug profile of their clients. Heroin addicts will often minimize or lie about their use of alcohol even though their use of that drug may be at a problematic level. Many substance abusers will also be practicing a behavioral addiction such as gambling, compulsive eating, or even Internet addiction.

"I have cleaned up off of dope though I've been a drug addict for 23 years. And I have no desire whatsoever to do drugs but alcohol is still there and I do it out of boredom."
42-year-old recovering heroin addict

By addressing addiction as chemical dependency rather than a drug-specific problem, treatment is effective in promoting recovery, preventing relapse, and preventing a switch to alternate drug addictions. When treatment doesn't address all addictions, a heroin addict might come back as an alcoholic a few months later.

"The cravings were just continuous. It was just like—if I was coming off of 'speed,' I wanted heroin. If I was coming off heroin, I wanted to snort cocaine and if I was coming off that, I wanted to stay numb. I wanted to just go from one drug to another."
38-year old recovering polydrug abuser

Given the similarity of the roots of addiction, each drug still has unique effects and problems that should be specifically addressed.

STIMULANTS (cocaine & amphetamines)

A wide range of psychiatric symptoms often accompanies stimulant abuse. Acute paranoia, schizophrenia, major depression, and bipolar disorder are often the initial presentations by a stimulant addict, particularly at the end of a long run. These symptoms require psychiatric intervention to prevent harm and to assess whether they have been caused by the drug itself or whether the mental illnesses are preexisting and will continue to be a problem after detoxification and initial abstinence.

Besides psychoactive symptoms or dual diagnosis, other key symptoms to watch out for in cocaine or amphetamine abusers who are detoxifying are **prolonged craving, anergia** (exhaustion), **anhedonia** (lack of an ability to feel pleasure), and **euthymia** (a feeling of elation that occurs three to five days after stopping use). Euthymia makes users feel that they never were addicted and that they don't need to be in treatment. The anergia and anhedonia start to overtake the euthymia at about two weeks after starting detoxification and these feelings, particularly the total lack of ability to feel pleasure, often lead to relapse (Gawin, Khalsa, & Ellinwood, 1994).

"I think when you're using the drug, it's real easy to deny everything that's going on and put everything on the shelf and not cope with it. Your whole world becomes the acquiring of whatever drug you happen to be using. But when you stop, it's all there waiting for you. And eventually you have to deal with it."
Methamphetamine user

Detoxification & Initial Abstinence

After detoxification and treatment for any psychotic symptoms and any life-threatening symptoms, such as extremely high blood pressure and heart rate, the vast majority of stimulant abusers respond positively to traditional drug counseling approaches.

However, a number of stimulant addicts have not been able to respond to these traditional approaches and initially require a more intensive medical approach to bridge the detoxification/ withdrawal period prior to their engagement into recovery.

Medical treatments include the use of antidepressant agents, such as imipramine, desipramine, amitriptyline, doxepin, trazodone, or fluoxetine (Prozac®). These affect serotonin, the neurotransmitter in the brain that deals with both depression and mood.

Antipsychotic medications, such as haloperidol (Haldol®), chlorpromazine (Thorazine®), and others, are also used to buffer the effects of unbalanced dopamine. Sedatives, including phenobarbital, chloral hydrate, flurazepam (Dalmane®), chlordiazepoxide (Librium®), or even diazepam (Valium®), are prescribed very carefully, on a short-term basis, to treat anxiety or sleep disturbance problems.

Nutritional approaches aimed at enhancing the production of those neurotransmitters that have been depleted by heavy stimulant use have been used to decrease craving and counteract many of the withdrawal symptoms seen in stimulant addiction. Tyrosine, phenylalanine, and tryptophane are proteins

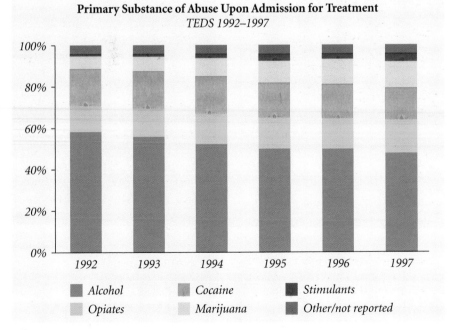

Primary Substance of Abuse Upon Admission for Treatment
TEDS 1992–1997

Legend:
- Alcohol
- Cocaine
- Stimulants
- Opiates
- Marijuana
- Other/not reported

Figure 9-5 •

While the number admitted for primary alcoholism treatment and primary cocaine treatment has declined since 1992, marijuana treatment admissions have more than doubled as have methamphetamine admissions. Opiate admissions went up 50%.

(TEDS, 1999)

used by brain cells to manufacture dopamine, adrenaline, and serotonin that are depleted by stimulant abuse.

Long-Term Abstinence

A lot of work is currently being put into the treatment of craving and particularly stimulant craving. Two major types of craving have been addressed: endogenous craving and environmentally triggered craving.

Endogenous craving is believed to be caused by the depletion of dopamine in the nucleus acumbens of the limbic system. To treat this situation, many medications, like amantadine, bromocryptine, and L-Dopa®, have been used to simulate dopamine in the nucleus acumbens, thereby diminishing craving for stimulants. Acupuncture is also used to stimulate dopamine release. Animal research suggests that the dopamine imbalance may last for up to 10 months after cessation of cocaine or amphetamine use (Ricaurte, Seiden, & Schuster, 1984).

Environmentally triggered craving is particularly intense in stimulant addiction. It is more likely to lead to relapse than endogenous craving and has to be treated by intense counseling, group sessions, or desensitization techniques. This type of craving may last throughout one's life but evidence indicates that continued abstinence weakens the craving response. This weakening can lead to the extinction of craving caused by environmental triggers.

In a NIDA-funded investigation of 1,600 cocaine-dependent patients with moderate to severe problems, researchers found that an absolute minimum of three months of treatment was needed to achieve lasting results (eight months maximized effectiveness). About 2 1/2 times more patients relapsed after leaving short-term treatment (38% relapsed) than those leaving long-term residential treatment (15% relapsed) (Simpson, Joe, Fletcher, et al., 1999).

TOBACCO

The only guaranteed successful therapy when it comes to tobacco is to never smoke, chew, or use it in any form. Abstinence is necessary because many of the neurologic and neurochemical alterations that cause nicotine addiction are permanent. This means that even 10 years after cessation of smoking, a single cigarette can trigger the nicotine craving.

The failure rate for most therapies to stop smoking is 70% to 80%, this in spite of the fact that 80% of all smokers want to quit. In the past the focus on treatment was the psychological components of addiction, particularly the "habit" of smoking. Unfortunately these approaches didn't fully take into account the lifetime nature of nicotine addiction and, therefore, recovery. They tried to apply short-term fixes (e.g., 21-day smoking cessation programs) to a long-term problem.

Recently, in recognition of the very real alterations in brain chemistry that trigger nicotine craving during withdrawal, the treatment community has focused on pharmacological treatments.

Nicotine Replacement

Since the main mechanism that causes craving is the drop in blood levels of nicotine that then triggers withdrawal symptoms such as irritability, anxiety, drowsiness, and light-headedness, research has been aimed at nicotine replacement systems. The purpose of these systems is to slowly reduce the blood plasma nicotine levels to the point where cessation will not trigger withdrawal symptoms that will cause the smoker to relapse (Thompson & Hunter, 1998).

The four types of nicotine replacement systems are transdermal nicotine patches, nicotine gum, nicotine sprays, and nicotine nasal inhalers. One of the main advantages of all of these systems is that users are no longer damaging their lungs with some of the 4,000 chemicals found in cigarette smoke. This alone could save almost 200,000 lives per year in the United States. The main problem is that if relapse prevention, counseling, and self-help groups are not used in conjunction with nico-

tine replacement therapy, then the chances of smokers returning to their old habits are high (Rustin, 1998).

Nicotine Patches. Nicotine patches, such as Nicoderm® and Habitrol®, are nicotine-infused adhesive patches that are applied to the skin. Patches can be worn intermittently (daytime only) or continuously. Most of them contain enough nicotine to last for 24–72 hours. The advantages of patches are the steady rate of release of nicotine, the ease of compliance, and the lack of toxic effects to tissues in the mouth or digestive track. The disadvantages are the cost, the inability to alter the amount being absorbed, and the 4–6 hours it takes for a patch to raise the nicotine level enough to dull nicotine craving. Also, if the user starts smoking while wearing the patch, extremely

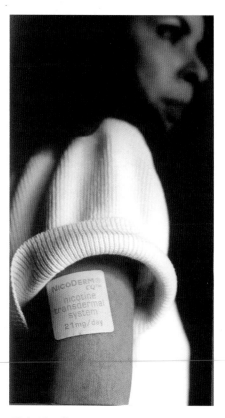

With 47 million Americans addicted to cigarettes, the potential market for devices and drugs, such as a nicotine patch, to help kick the habit is huge, much larger than the $59 million in tobacco subsidies voted by Congress in 1996.

high and dangerous plasma levels of nicotine can occur.

Nicotine Gum. Nicotine gums, such as Nicorette®, have the advantage of slowing the rise in nicotine levels that smoking brings. The 10-second rush of an inhaled cigarette gives way to the 15- to 30-minute slow rise that nicotine gum provides when absorbed through the gums and other mucosal tissues. A slower rise means that craving, which is triggered by the sudden drop in nicotine levels after smoking, doesn't occur. The 15- to 30-minute rise, however, is considerably faster than the 4–6 hours it takes for a transdermal patch to work, so the user has more control over the dose. The disadvantages are that the user can cram a lot of gum into the mouth or not use it at all; the gum can irritate mucosal tissues; and an oral habit is maintained (users are still putting something in their mouths when the craving hits or when they are agitated).

Nasal Spray. Nasal sprays (still undergoing clinical trials) are self-administered and reach the brain in 3–5 minutes, thereby giving more instant relief to the nicotine craving and giving more control to the user. Disadvantages include irritation to the nasal passages and reinforcement of nicotine addiction.

Nicotine Inhalers. Nicotine inhalers (still undergoing clinical trials) give the fastest relief of nicotine craving without involving the inhalation of all the other toxic chemicals present in smoke. The problem seems to be that misuse can produce plasma levels similar to those produced by smoking, thereby perpetuating the addictive process.

Treating the Symptoms

The purpose of symptomatic treatment is to reduce the anxiety, depression, and craving that accompany nicotine withdrawal and therefore trigger relapse. Benzodiazepines, clonidine, bupropion (Zyban®), buspirone, fluoxetine (Prozac®) and other antidepressants, mecamylamine, propranolol, naltrexone, and naloxone have been used to try to alleviate the symptoms of nicotine withdrawal. Even clonidine, often used to control symptoms of heroin withdrawal, has been used effectively to control nicotine withdrawal (Rustin, 1998).

Most behavioral therapies, which include one-on-one counseling, group therapy, educational approaches, aversion therapy, hypnotism, and acupuncture, have a one-year success rate of 15% to 30% Many of the techniques used in stimulant abuse recovery are directly applicable to quitting smoking. These include

◇ desensitizing the smoker to environmental cues that trigger craving;

◇ practicing alternate methods of calming oneself when under stress or going through withdrawal;

◇ avoiding environments and situations, such as bars, where smoking is rampant;

◇ finding other ways of getting the small rush or mild euphoria that nicotine provides;

◇ teaching the smoker the physiology of nicotine use and addiction, along with the medical consequences of smoking or chewing tobacco;

◇ and teaching the smoker the extraordinary benefits of quitting.

OPIOIDS

Along with treatment for nicotine addiction, treatment for opioid addiction has the highest rate of relapse. This is partially because physical withdrawal from opioids is more severe than withdrawal from stimulants. For this reason most opioid abusers who want to recover need to be involved in a detoxification and treatment program.

Detoxification

Programs may use mild opioids like Darvon® to detoxify and taper the habit. This allows addicts to have less fear of the pain of withdrawal, less pain during withdrawal, and it encourages them to stay in treatment. An alternative is clonidine, a drug that quiets the part of the brain that gets hyperactive when one goes through withdrawal. Methadone and LAAM are used for detoxification (or for long-term substitution treatment known as **"maintenance pharmacotherapy"**).

"The physical part of the treatment for opioid addiction is only a tiny portion of the process. It's what happens after you get off—after you detox—that's important. Everyone around you is using and in a lot of cases you may have financial problems. You may not even have a place to stay. There are other kinds of things that build up and cause you to use again."
Drug counselor

Initial Abstinence & Long-Term Abstinence

Long-lasting opioid antagonists, such as naltrexone (Revia®), that decrease craving for the drug and block opioids from activating brain cells are used after detoxification to insure abstinence.

As with all other treatments, initial abstinence and long-term abstinence are supported by participating in individual counseling sessions, group sessions, or self-help groups such as Narcotics Anonymous. During the first four to eight weeks of abstinence, daily attendance in these programs is crucial in maintaining a drug-free state when the craving is strongest. As successful treatment continues, fewer sessions are necessary.

Recovery

Since opioid addiction is so time consuming and involving, the key to recovery from heroin or other opioid addiction is learning a new lifestyle. Instead of waking up every morning with the need to raise $100 to $200 to support a heavy habit, instead of nodding off or feeling drugged, and instead of trying to get clean needles to avoid HIV infection, addicts have to learn how to enjoy nondrug activities. They have to learn how to have a relationship and even how to get a driver's license.

"I'm not used to having a room. For the last two years, I was on the streets. I spent $200 a day on heroin and couldn't even manage to find enough money to get a room at the end of the night. That's pretty sick. I've never actually had a checking account and such because I started using and dealing heroin when I was 12 and I always had to hide my finances."

Recovering 42-year-old heroin addict

Other Opioid Treatment Modalities (methadone maintenance)

Recently there has been an effort to expand the use of methadone to treat heroin and opiate addiction. A consensus statement by the National Institutes of Health recommended less regulation for dispensing methadone, wider dispensing authority for trained physicians rather than just at methadone clinic settings, and improved training in medical schools and for physicians on how to diagnose and treat opiate addiction (NIH-CDC, 1997).

Much controversy has always swirled around the concept of opiate or opioid substitution ever since morphine addiction became a problem in the nineteenth century. Because of the large number of morphine addicts following the Civil War, opiate maintenance clinics multiplied. At this time morphine was used in China to treat opium addiction. In the early 1900s, heroin was used to treat morphine addiction in Europe. This practice of using opiates to treat opiate addiction was ended in the United States (though it continued in England and other countries) in the 1920s and not revived until **methadone maintenance** was developed in the late 1960s in New York City by Vincent Dole and Marie Nyswander (Dole & Nyswander, 1965; Payte, 1997). This treatment modality eventually spread to hundreds of methadone maintenance

clinics nationwide in the '70s and '80s. Today there are more than 115,000 heroin addicts in methadone maintenance programs (NIH-CDC, 1997).

The theory is that methadone, a synthetic opiate, while not as intense as heroin, is longer lasting, and thus will keep the user from having heroin-like withdrawal symptoms for 36–48 hours. Heroin, on the other hand, causes withdrawal symptoms in a few hours, so the user goes through the roller coaster of highs and lows and the pain of withdrawal on a daily basis (Lowinson, Payte, Salsitz, et al., 1997).

With methadone maintenance, the highs and lows that promote addiction are avoided. The user doesn't have to hustle for money to pay for a habit, get drugs and needles on the street, or be exposed to a high-risk lifestyle. With HIV and hepatitis C infection rates in

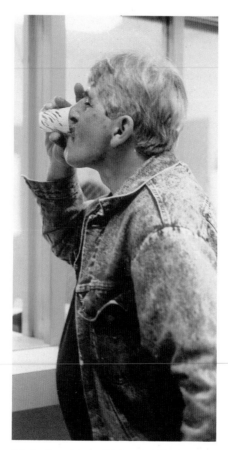

Methadone is usually dispensed in juice and drunk on the spot to make sure it is being taken properly and is not being diverted to street sales.

intravenous heroin users as high as 80%, this method of harm reduction has certain benefits. These include forcing the addict to come to a certain location every day where counseling, medical care, and other services are available, thus reducing the harm addicts do to themselves and others (Payte & Zweben, 1998). Balancing the dose used is a continuing problem with the use of methadone. Constant monitoring for symptoms of withdrawal is necessary.

Methadone client being examined by a registered nurse at the health facility that works with the methadone clinic

Client: "I don't feel good. I feel like I have the flu or something."
Nurse: "Can you describe it?"
Client: "Aches, pains, sweats, real bad, like I'm real anxious—shaking, quivers, hair standing on end."
Nurse: "And you've been on methadone . . . ?"
Client: "For about five years."
Nurse: "About 80 milligrams for well over a year now?"
Client: "Yeah. He drew blood for a methadone level."
Nurse: "You look a little calmer since you've dosed, since you first came in."
Client: "Yeah, the shakes are gone."
Nurse: "Your methadone dose may need to change and need to go up. Everything else is OK. Your lungs sound fine. Your pulse is fine. You might just need to go up a couple of milligrams to meet your needs."

The controversy over the use of methadone maintenance arises because many chemical dependency treatment personnel don't believe drug abuse should be treated with another addicting drug on a long-term basis. Since many users seek treatment after only a short period of addiction while their dose is still relatively low, the immediate use of methadone will further in-grain their opioid addiction. In fact a recent study has shown that a higher dose of methadone is more effective in reducing illegal opioid and heroin use than a moderate dose (Strain, Bigelow, Liebson, & Stitzer, 1999).

The pro-methadone advocates believe that keeping addicts from their harmful lifestyle is more important than focusing on total recovery from opioid addiction that, in any case, is extremely difficult. It also reduces crime and other social problems by providing access to stabilized doses of a legal drug. Methadone maintenance has often been referred to as a "political solution for a medical problem."

LAAM. Recently the use of LAAM (levo acetyl alpha methadol), a long-acting methadone-like drug, has been used in much the same manner. LAAM will stay in the body for up to three days, so users further avoid withdrawal and the ups and downs of opioid addiction. Also they do not have to go to a clinic every day. The negative side of LAAM is that it is still an addictive drug and though fewer clinic visits mean lower treatment costs, they also means fewer opportunities to encourage recovery.

Buprenorphine. Another drug that is being tried for treating opioid addiction is buprenorphine. It is an opioid agonist-antagonist. What this means is that at low doses it is a powerful opioid, almost 50 times as powerful as heroin, but strangely it blocks the opioid receptors at high doses. It enables an addict to be started on methadone, then switched to buprenorphine as a transition to a true antagonist, like naltrexone.

SEDATIVE-HYPNOTICS (barbiturates, benzodiazepines)

The majority of tranquilizer and sedative abusers tend to be older, white (85% to 89%), and female (59% to 60%). Most enter treatment through individual referral. In addition about 41% of primary tranquilizer admissions and 33% of sedative admissions reported concurrent use of alcohol while 18% reported concurrent use of marijuana (SAMHSA/TEDS, 1999).

Withdrawal from sedative-hypnotic addiction results in life-threatening seizures if not medically managed. Thus intensive medical assessment and specific medical treatment is a necessity when treating people who have become addicted to sedative-hypnotics such as "reds" (secobarbital), Xanax® (alprazolam), other benzodiazepines, or even muscle relaxants like Soma® (carisoprodal) (Hayner, Galloway, & Wiehl, 1993).

Detoxification

Substitution therapy (using a drug that is cross-tolerant with another drug) is needed to detoxify a sedative-hypnotic addict. Although many drugs in this class of substances can be used, outpatient programs often utilize phenobarbital because of its long duration of action and its more specific anti-seizure activity. A dose of phenobarbital sufficient to prevent any withdrawal symptoms without causing major drowsiness or sedation is established as a baseline to begin detoxification. Butabarbital is also used as an alternate to phenobarbital in the detoxification process. Phenytoin (Dilantin®) may be added to either medication therapy to further prevent any seizures from developing.

The initial detoxification from sedative-hypnotics requires intensive and daily medical management that also provides the opportunity to get the addict into intensive counseling and social services that are vital to recovery once detoxification is completed.

Initial Abstinence

Continued abstinence from sedatives requires intensive participation in group, individual, and educational counseling as well as specific self-help groups or Narcotics Anonymous. Many sedative addicts, and especially those addicted to benzodiazepines, complain of bizarre and prolonged symptoms such as taste or visual distortions for several months after detoxification.

Also many experience inappropriate rage or anger during the early months of abstinence that requires skilled mental health intervention.

After detoxification some sedative addicts experience the reemergence of withdrawal-like symptoms even though they have remained totally abstinent. This reaction can occur anywhere from one to several months after detoxification and may occasionally require medical intervention in treatment.

Two controversial explanations have been offered to explain this phenomena. One asserts that long-acting benzodiazepines, like diazepam (Valium®) or alprazolam (Xanax®), produce active metabolites that persist in the body, resulting in additional withdrawal symptoms once their levels decrease, even after several months of abstinence from the parent drug. Another explanation asserts that these are not true withdrawal symptoms but merely the reemergence of an original anxiety disorder that was controlled by the use of sedatives. Under this second explanation, psychiatrists need to initiate maintenance pharmacotherapy treatment to address the underlying psychiatric problems. Since many antianxiety medications are abusable sedative-hypnotics, this requires skillful medical management to prevent excessive inappropriate use or relapse to sedative-hypnotic addiction (Eickelberg & Mayo-Smith, 1998).

Although flumazenil (Mazicon®) has been developed as an effective benzodiazepine antagonist, it is currently available only in injectable form to treat overdoses of these drugs. Future developments may lead to effective oral and long-acting benzodiazepine or barbiturate antagonists to help those addicted to sedative-hypnotics to accomplish initial abstinence.

Recovery

Continued participation in self-help or Narcotics Anonymous groups has been the most effective means of promoting continuous abstinence and recovery in sedative-hypnotic addiction.

As with cocaine and other addic-

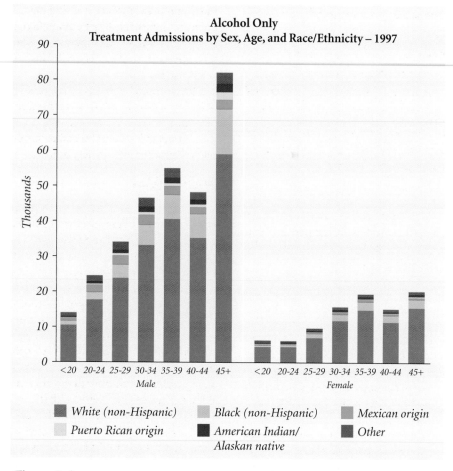

Alcohol Only
Treatment Admissions by Sex, Age, and Race/Ethnicity – 1997

White (non-Hispanic)   Black (non-Hispanic)   Mexican origin
Puerto Rican origin   American Indian/   Other
Alaskan native

Figure 9-6 •
Since alcohol dependence takes a longer time to develop than dependence with other drugs, admissions for treatment grow later in the life of an alcoholic, peaking after the age of 45 (SAMHSA/TEDS, 1999).

tions, the sedative-hypnotic addicts are vulnerable to environmental cues that trigger drug hunger and relapse throughout their lifetimes. Treatment that includes cue or trigger recognition, avoidance tools, and coping mechanisms is vital to addressing sedative-hypnotic addiction.

ALCOHOL

Denial

Denial on the part of the alcoholic or compulsive drinker is the biggest hindrance to beginning treatment. One reason that denial is so common with the use of alcohol is the long time it can take for social or habitual drinking to advance to abuse and addiction (10 years on the average). Denial also oc-

curs because alcoholics have no memory of the negative effects they experienced while in an alcoholic "blackout." Thus they don't believe that alcohol has harmed them. Further, alcohol impairs judgment and reason in all users, making them less likely to associate any problem with their drinking.

Detoxification

For a heavy drinker physical withdrawal is very uncomfortable but usually not dangerous. Symptoms can often be handled by aspirin, rest, liquids, and any one of hundreds of hangover cures that have been handed down from generation to generation.

For the alcoholic the potentially life-threatening symptoms of with-

drawal can be medically managed with a variety of sedating drugs, e.g., barbiturates, benzodiazepines such as chlordiazepoxide (Librium®), paraldehyde, chloral hydrate, and the phenothiazines. Since several of these drugs are addictive, they should be used sparingly and on a very short-term basis. Normally tapering is done on a 5–7 day basis but can be extended to 11–14 days.

Along with emergency medical care, withdrawal and detoxification can be handled through emotional support and basic physical care, such as rest and nutrition (thiamin, folic acid, multi-vitamins, amino acids, electrolytes, and fructose). Many of the problems will start to abate with detoxification but for the long-term drinker, some damage is irreversible: liver disease, enlarged heart, cancer, and nerve damage among others (Wiehl, Galloway, & Hayner, 1994).

Initial Abstinence

A common treatment for initial abstinence is the use of Antabuse®, a drug that will make people ill if they drink alcohol. This is used for about 6 months or longer to help get alcoholics through initial abstinence when they're most likely to relapse. A more important part of this process is encouraging them to go to Alcoholics Anonymous meetings or other support group meetings in addition to individual therapy. One procedure is to have the user go to 90 Alcoholics Anonymous meetings in 90 days (called a "90/90 contract").

In 1996 naltrexone (Revia®) was approved by the FDA for the treatment of alcohol addiction. When used during the first 3 months of the recovery process, it decreased alcohol relapse by 50% to 70% when combined with a comprehensive treatment program. Unfortunately naltrexone can be hard on the liver and needs to be used under strict supervision.

Long-Term Abstinence & Recovery

In treatment one often encounters someone known as a "dry drunk." This means that the person is not actually drinking alcohol but still has the behavior and mind-set of an alcoholic. Thus the purpose of this stage of treatment, besides avoiding relapse, is to begin healing the emotional scars, confusion, and immaturity that had kept the person drinking for so many years.

Many treatment centers advertise 30-day drying out programs, implying that detoxification is the key to recovery rather than being a small initial step in a long process As with all addictions, working on recovery throughout one's lifetime is necessary to prevent relapse. Brain cells have been permanently changed by years of drinking, so the recovering alcoholic is always susceptible to relapse.

PSYCHEDELICS

For hallucinogens such as LSD, MDMA, "'shrooms," and ketamine, the overwhelming majority of users in treatment are male, White, and below the age of 24. For marijuana smokers, the majority who are in treatment are male and below the age of 24 but more evenly divided ethnically (SAMHSA/TEDS, 1999).

Many psychedelics will mimic mental conditions, such as schizophrenia, and so the clinician or intake counselor has to make a tentative diagnosis when first seeing the patient and give the drug time to clear before making a more definite diagnosis. Antipsychotic medications, sedatives, and other medications are used to stabilize the client.

Bad Trips (acute anxiety reactions)

The amount of "acid" or other psychedelic taken, the surroundings, the user's mental state and physical condition all determine the reaction to all arounders. Because of their effect on the emotional center in the brain, a user is open to the extremes of euphoria and panic. Inexperienced or even experienced users who take too high a dose of LSD or other psychedelic can feel acute anxiety, paranoia, fear over loss of control, delusions of persecution, or feelings of grandeur leading to dangerous behaviors like bungee jumping without a cord.

"In the 8th grade I started doing 'acid' and drinking a lot and when I was about 15, I took too much 'acid' one night and I tripped out and I cut my arm. Got a big old scar on my arm and took off my clothes and ran down the street naked. Just tripped out. So then I went to rehab after that. I spent four days in the hospital."
Ex-"acid" user

Over the years the Haight-Ashbury Detox Clinic has developed a set of steps to help detoxify a psychedelic user having a bad trip.

There are two things to remember when using the ARRRT talk-down technique.

◇ First if the user seems to be experiencing severe medical, physical, or even emotional reactions that are not responding to the talk-down, medical intervention is needed. Get the person to a hospital or bring in emergency medical personnel experienced in treating that kind of reaction.

◇ Second, although most psychedelic bad trip reactions are responsive to ARRRT, PCP and ketamine may cause unexpected and sudden violent or belligerent behavior. Caution must be exercised in approaching a "bum tripper" suspected of being under the influence of these drugs.

The best treatment for someone on a bad trip is to talk him or her down in a calm manner without raising one's voice or appearing threatening. Avoid quick movements and let the person move around, so there is no feeling of being trapped.

Some of the "rave" club drugs, like MDMA, "ecstasy," GHB, and ketamine, have created addictive behaviors in users that are treated with traditional counseling, education, and self-help groups.

MARIJUANA

Since the 1980s there has been a steady increase in the number of people entering treatment for marijuana dependence. While much of the increase nationally has been because of court-mandated treatment referrals (Fig. 9-7), those entering the Haight-Ashbury Clinic on an increasing basis are predominantly self-referred. Thus through the eyes of marijuana smokers as well as the eyes of the law, there is a growing problem with marijuana dependence. These facts seem to challenge the continued perception that marijuana is a benign drug. Experience at the Haight-Ashbury Clinic has shown that marijuana has a true addiction syndrome encompassing both physical and emotional dependence.

"I ain't gonna say I can quit any time. But if I had to stop, I could stop. I ain't gonna say I could quit. I can't go just cold turkey just like that. I could go maybe three days without and then I smoke a joint. And then maybe I go like three or four days without, and then

---

TABLE 9–4   TREATMENT FOR BAD TRIPS

The Haight-Ashbury Detox Clinic uses the following ARRRT guidelines in dealing with a person experiencing a bad trip:

A acceptance: first gain users' trust and confidence;

R reduction of stimuli: get users to quiet nonthreatening environments;

R reassurance: educate users that they are experiencing a bad trip and assure them that they are in a safe place, among safe people, and that they will be all right;

R rest: assist users to relax using stress-reduction techniques that promote a calm state of mind;

T talk-down: discuss peaceful, nonthreatening subjects with users, avoiding any topic that seems to create more anxiety or a strong reaction.

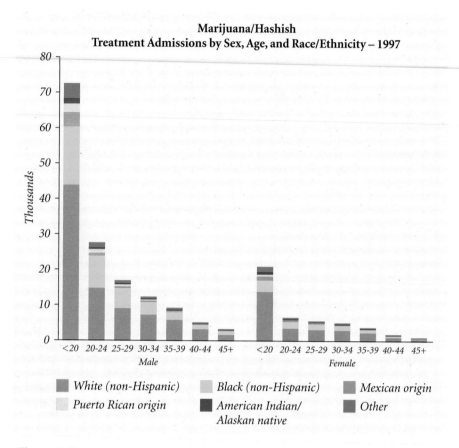

**Marijuana/Hashish
Treatment Admissions by Sex, Age, and Race/Ethnicity – 1997**

Legend:
- White (non-Hispanic)
- Black (non-Hispanic)
- Mexican origin
- Puerto Rican origin
- American Indian/ Alaskan native
- Other

Figure 9-7 •

The vast majority of those entering treatment for marijuana dependence are under the age of 20. The reason is that over 1/2 of the referrals for treatment are court mandated while only 18% are self-referred. (SAMHSA/TEDS, 1999)

maybe I'll smoke a joint but that'd take some work."

33-year-old chronic marijuana abuser

The physical withdrawal symptoms, though uncomfortable, rarely need medical treatment. They consist of major sleep and appetite disturbances, irritability, anxiety, emotional depression, and even mild muscular discomfort. Craving persists for several months to years upon abstinence. One of the main reasons for the lack of acceptance of these withdrawal symptoms is that their onset is delayed from three weeks to several months after cessation of use. Marijuana has a wide distribution in body tissues and especially in fat, thus enabling it to persist in the system over a prolonged period of time. Even urine tests of chronic marijuana users remain positive sometimes for three weeks to several months. The persistence accounts for the delayed onset of withdrawal.

"After I stopped smoking, it took me about three or four months before I really came out of the fog and really started getting a grasp of what was going on around me . . . and another month or so after that is when I really started to understand that I could do this. And then I started really enjoying it.

28-year-old recovering compulsive marijuana smoker

Treatment for marijuana dependence or addiction is evolving along the same lines as those developed for alcohol dependence and addiction. Psychosocial interventions, education, and peer support have been the most effective in helping people abstain and pre-

vent relapse. Currently treatment for marijuana addiction is made difficult because much of society still views marijuana as nonproblematic and therefore views those in treatment as overreacting to their use of the drug. This often undermines the treatment process. Further the 12-step process and other peer-support systems, invaluable in the treatment of other drug dependencies, have not evolved fully when marijuana dependence or addiction is involved.

INHALANTS

The treatment of those who use inhalants excessively involves immediate removal from exposure to the drug to prevent them from aggravating the dangerous effects of the drug, such as lack of oxygen to the brain, damage to the respiratory system, and injuries from accidents. Patients must then be monitored for potential adverse psychiatric conditions that may require the use of major antipsychotic medications targeted to treat psychoses and suicidal depression. Many inhalants can also produce physical dependence that is similar to the dependence that occurs with sedative-hypnotic drugs. Thus they should be monitored for withdrawal seizures and treated with appropriate anticonvulsant medication when warranted. Each inhalant has its own physical toxic effects. Some may lead to heart, liver, lung, kidney, and even blood diseases. These must be evaluated and treated. These substances are reinforcing and can cause psychic dependence and often require long-term psychosocial interventions targeted to prevent relapse into addiction.

Since the majority of these inhalants are commercially available and relatively cheap, they are easily accessible to adolescents and therefore the majority of abusers are under the age of 20. Almost 1/3 of inhalant admissions had used inhalants by the age of 12 and another 1/3 by the age of 14 (SAMHSA/ TEDS, 1999). What this means in treatment is that there are major developmental problems as well that must be addressed. Treatment specialists talk about the need to habilitate rather than rehabilitate the "huffer."

About 2/3 of inhalant abusers admitted for treatment reported use of other drugs as well, primarily alcohol (44%) and marijuana (41%) (SAMHSA/TEDS, 1999). These figures emphasize the need to evaluate addiction to other drugs.

TREATMENT FOR BEHAVIORAL ADDICTIONS

It has become increasingly recognized that behavioral addictions that result from a predisposition to addiction, an environment that further predisposes one to compulsive behaviors, and pleasurable reinforcement from the activity itself follow similar brain pathways as drug addiction. These behavioral addictions, such as compulsive gambling, sexual addiction, compulsive Internet use, compulsive shopping, and eating disorders (anorexia, bulimia, compulsive overeating), require the same intensity of intervention and treatment as substance abuse disorders.

Since many behavioral addictions have not been studied and treated to the same extent as drug abuse and addiction, there is a scarcity of research data, treatment facilities, and qualified treatment personnel. Besides treatment at mental health facilities, the front line of treatment has been the evolution of self-help and 12-step support groups.

Compulsive Gambling

The number of compulsive gamblers has have grown dramatically with the increase in games of chance in every state but Utah. The sheer availability of gambling facilities has contributed to the growth of the industry and to multiple relapses during treatment. In one of the few before and after studies, the percentage of Iowans reporting a gambling problem at some time in their lives went from 1.7% in 1989 to 5.4% in 1995 and probably even more today—a three- to four-fold increase (Harden & Wardson, 1996). Even the gaming industry estimates that 25% to 40% of their revenue comes from that 6% to 8% who are compulsive or problem gamblers. The figures are probably much higher for certain types

of gambling, e.g., poker machines in Oregon where it is estimated that 7% of the people spend 60% to 80% of the money generated by this industry.

"I was at a Gamblers Anonymous meeting in Reno and about 50 people were there. The longest abstinence in that meeting was just four months. In meetings I've been to in other states, many people have years of abstinence. The only difference I see is that in Reno, gambling is everywhere and the triggers are everywhere, and the temptation is everywhere."

44-year-old recovering compulsive gambler (three years clean)

With so many compulsive gamblers, there is a startling lack of facilities to treat this addiction. Until a few years ago, many states didn't even have a single gambling addiction specialist. Society has been slow to recognize compulsive gambling as a compulsion as powerful as any drug addiction.

Compulsive gambling has been described as one of the purest addictions since the only substance involved is money. Denial is therefore very powerful in compulsive gamblers and until a devastating bottom has been reached, most gamblers are reluctant to seek treatment, let alone admit that they have a problem. Outside interventions, especially those triggered by legal problems (e.g., arrest for embezzlement or declaring bankruptcy), are usually necessary. To most gamblers their trouble is a cash flow problem (Brubaker, 1997).

"I figured I was losing $500 here and there, you know, a week. I never thought it was that big a deal because I always thought of myself as going to be successful, going to get a better job down the road where I'll make all this money back . . . so why quit now?"

21-year-old recovering sports gambler

The Charter Hospital of Las Vegas that treats compulsive gamblers reports withdrawal symptoms similar to alco-

holism, including restlessness, irritability, apprehension about well-being, anger, abdominal pain, headaches, diarrhea, cold sweats, insomnia, tremors, and above all an intense desire to return to gambling.

"I don't want to sit here and tell anybody anything that's unrealistic. I miss gambling. I miss it still. It brought a sense of—like a power or a satisfaction. I'm learning how to treat it and how to deal with it but that doesn't mean it's over."

42-year-old relapsing compulsive gambler

The standard assessment test for compulsive gambling is the South Oaks Gambling Screen (SOGS), usually accompanied with an in-depth assessment and formal diagnosis. Treatment options developed over the last 30 years include self-help groups such as Gamblers Anonymous (Blume, 1997).

"Going to GA groups helps me—seeing people who have gone through the same struggles and seeing how every one of them wishes they had quit when they were my age so they didn't have to go through the struggles."

21-year-old recovering sports gambler

The Gamblers Anonymous program parallels the 12-step process used by Alcoholics Anonymous. It also employs sponsors, mandatory group meetings, commitment to complete abstinence, and contact numbers and support to help the gambler through the initial 90-day phase. Additional support groups include Gam-Anon for the families of compulsive gamblers and also a group for children of pathological gamblers called Gam-A-Teen.

"It's not just an addiction to a substance . . . it's a whole way of thinking. It's a whole lifestyle and you have to change everything you do and everything about it."

Wife of compulsive gambler

Outpatient along with inpatient or residential treatment programs are available (and very rare), though insurance companies seldom pay for a primary diagnosis of compulsive gambling. It usually takes a diagnosis of a mood disorder or other coexisting condition to get insurance coverage for treatment. Frequently, compulsive gamblers have already lost their jobs and insurance coverage before they seek help for their addiction. In the last few years, a few states that have government-controlled lotteries, gambling machines, and various scratch-off games are recognizing their responsibility in providing treatment for the compulsive gamblers. The state of Connecticut spends the most money in treatment. Next is Oregon that passed a bill allotting 1.0% of its gross revenues or $2 million a year towards treatment. California, with 12 times the population, only allots about $500,000 towards treatment.

Even with gambling, several addictions are always involved. Gambling often coexists with drinking, compulsive spending, and a few other disorders. The gambling can replace another addiction. Many alcoholics switched to gambling when they quit drinking. The gambling quickly became compulsive (McElroy, Soutullo, & Goldsmith, 1998).

Eating Disorders

One of the main elements for effective treatment of all three eating disorders is early intervention. The longer the disorder continues, the more deeply ingrained the behavior and the more physiological and psychological damage. A number of steps are recommended for treating eating disorders:

◊ diagnose and treat any medical complications—hospitalization if necessary;

◊ encourage attendance at Overeaters Anonymous 12-step groups or other groups to give support to the client;

◊ encourage the client to eat a balanced diet as well as educate them as to the components of proper nutrition and exercise;

◊ use behavioral and group therapies to encourage weight gain in anorexics and weight loss in bulimics and overeaters;

◊ use cognitive and other therapies to change false attitudes and perceptions of body image and eating;

◊ enhance self-esteem, independence, and development of a stronger identity;

◊ treat and educate the whole family.

In addition to the general guidelines, each of the three eating disorders has unique problems.

Anorexia. Most severely ill anorexic patients have to be admitted to a hospital because of the extreme weight loss, disturbed heart rhythms, extreme depression, and often suicidal ideation. It usually takes 10–12 weeks for full nutritional recovery. Unfortunately most health insurance only covers 15 days. During the hospital or home care stay, besides taking care of medical problems and nutritional deficiencies, weight gain of one to two pounds a week are necessary even if the patient or family wants to lower those goals. Exercise is also recommended. The complexities of anorexia require a team approach since so many problems are involved: physicians for medical complications, dietitians, therapists, counselors, and trained nurses.

Bulimia. Clients with bulimia usually have more long-term health problems than those with anorexia, such as atherosclerosis and diabetes, and rarely need hospitalization but often need continuing medical care. Because of the strong link between depression and bulimia and the similarity in serotonin disruption, antidepressants are often used, including tricyclic antidepressants, MAO inhibitors, and selective serotonin reuptake inhibitors (e.g., Prozac® and sertraline) (Goldbloom, 1999).

Compulsive Overeating (including binge-eating disorder). As with bulimia, serotonin reuptake inhibitors, and other medications used to treat depression are prescribed. Support groups including Overeaters Anonymous (OA), TOPS (Take Off Pounds Sensibly), Weightwatchers, and others are crucial in maintaining weight loss and encouraging recovery. A number of professionals and overeaters believe that abstaining from certain foods, particularly refined carbohydrates (e.g., sugar, refined flour, alcohol, and pasta) or fatty substances, act on the same reward systems that reinforce compulsive drug-use behavior.

"If I am eating those reward foods and sugars, I can't engage in my treatment. It's almost as if I'm drunk. When I abstain, I can refuse the first bite."
58-year-old compulsive overeater

Sexual Addiction

One theory of sexual addiction suggests that predisposed individuals experience an intense form of sexual stimulation when young, identify it with a parent (usually the mother), and come to anticipate that sexual behavior can provide pleasure or relieve pain or tension. The experience is often in conjunction with covert or overt seduction. Because of the relationship between early childhood sexual experiences, the treatment inevitably has to deal more with childhood development rather than the mechanics of the addiction. The treatment often includes behavior modification (e.g., aversion therapy), cognitive-behavioral therapy, groups, family or couple therapy, psychodynamic psychotherapy, and medications (Goodman, 1997). Again the concurrent use of addictive substances is more prevalent than in the general population because predisposing factors in all addictions are so similar and because psychoactive drugs are often used to affect sexuality, e.g., lower inhibitions or enhance arousal. In addition the client will be in recovery for a lifetime because the predisposing factors are so ingrained just like other substance addictions.

Sexaholics Anonymous. As with compulsive gambling, sexual addiction is difficult to treat. The sense of being alone in their addiction or what they consider unique behavior is alleviated when they realize there are millions of others with the same problems. The introduction to the Sexaholics Anonymous handbook says,

"When we came to SA, we found that in spite of our differences, we shared a common problem—the obsession of lust, usually combined with a compulsive demand for sex in some form. We identified with one another on the inside. Whatever the details of our problem, we were dying spiritually—dying of guilt, fear, and loneliness. As we came to see that we shared a common problem, we also came to see that for us, there is a common solution—the Twelve Steps of Recovery practiced in a fellowship and on a foundation of what we call sexual sobriety."

Sexaholics Anonymous, 1989

Internet Addiction

Internet addiction crosses the line into other addictions: cybersexual addiction, cyberrelationship addiction, online gambling and day trading, information overload (compulsive web surfing), computer addiction (game-playing), or any combination of the above (Netaddiction, 2000). Along with compulsive gambling, Internet addiction is the fastest growing addiction exploding from virtually nonexistant five years ago. Because it is so new, treatment personnel and treatment facilities are rare. Unfortunately the Internet has become so much a part of life and work situations, it is hard to give up use altogether. The problems with Internet addiction treatment are similar to the problems with all addictions.

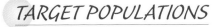

TARGET POPULATIONS

MEN VS. WOMEN

Research at the Haight-Ashbury Detox Clinic has discovered that the

process of addiction and especially recovery varies dramatically for men and women. Men are often external attributers, blaming negative life events like addiction on things outside their control whereas women are more often internal attributers blaming problems on themselves. For example, if a man slips on a banana peel, he might say, *"Who's the idiot who left that peel on the ground?"* A woman who slips on a banana peel might say, *"I should have looked where*

I was going. Boy, am I clumsy." When this is extended to their views of addiction, men often blame a wide variety of external forces for their dependence on drugs whereas women often blame themselves for being bad or crazy.

The counseling and intervention used in treatment have focused on early confrontation to break down addicts' denial and make them accept their condition. While appropriate for men, this treatment approach merely reinforces

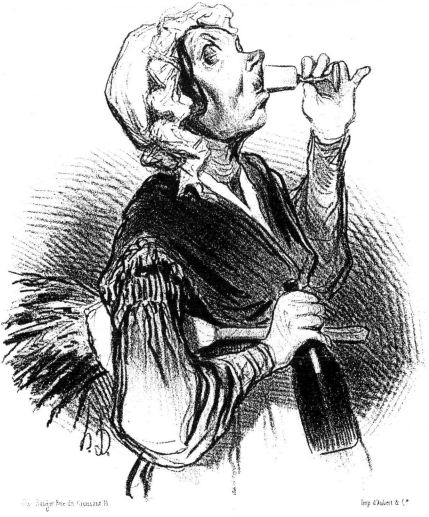

SILHOUETTES.

LA FEMME DE MÉNAGE.

Ainsi nommée par anti-phrase, parceqn élle ne ménage ni les meubles, ni la vaisselle, ni le vin de ses pratiques.

This etching by Honore Daumier says roughly, "Thus called [Housekeeper], she is the opposite because she takes care of neither the furniture nor the dishes, nor the wine of her employers."

women's guilt and shame and often prevents them from engaging in treatment or has them leave treatment early. Treatment approaches that are more supportive and less confrontative result in better outcomes for women.

Women have been also found to be the primary childcare provider in a family, so for a woman to be able to participate in treatment, childcare must be provided. Further it has been found that women lack transportation more often than their male counterparts. Therefore bus tokens, vans, car pooling, or other means of transportation provided to women clients also result in higher success rates.

YOUTH

Young people often have the perception of invulnerability to drugs and therefore are often in much greater denial about their addiction than adults. Further, studies confirm that young people are much less willing to accept guidance or intervention from adults but are more willing to listen to their peers (Hird, Khuri, Dusenbury, & Millman, 1997). Both of these factors call for programs to develop around peer interaction and guidance to other youth. Normal adult programs do not work with young people. Specific youth-directed programs have to be provided.

One of the biggest problems with treating teenagers is that they are present-oriented, that is they have problems recognizing consequences that are not immediate. The idea that a three-month flirtation with cocaine will necessitate a lifetime of recovery is beyond their scope. They also seek instant gratification, much more than even adult addicts, and expect rewards from treatment immediately. Youth programs that include reward incentives for accomplishing different phases of treatment result in better long-term outcomes. Part of the reward structure is that they get included in a group that they can feel a part of.

OLDER AMERICANS

Because many older Americans view addiction as a character flaw rather than a disease, they are less likely to seek help for any problematic use of alcohol or other drugs. In addition signs of addiction are often misinterpreted as part of the aging process or reaction to prescription medications that are common among the elderly. Also, because of less physical resiliency in those over 55, problematic use of alcohol or other drugs occurs at lower dosages than with younger people. The House Select Committee on Aging has reported that about 70% of hospitalized elderly persons show evidence of alcohol-related problems (although they might be in the hospital for some other condition). About 2.5 million older adults are addicted to alcohol, drugs, or both.

At present there are few treatment programs aimed specifically at older Americans but as the percentage of older Americans grows and as the baby boomers begin to retire, the need will grow. As with other special groups, older Americans with a substance abuse problem seem to do better in groups with others their own age although mixed groups will work.

Of nine centers set up by NIDA to study addiction, one has been designated specifically to investigate this problem in older Americans. It is located at the University of Florida in Gainesville.

ETHNIC GROUPS

Recognition of cultural variances between groups provides better treatment outcomes. Studies continue to verify that treatment specifically targeted to different ethnic groups promotes continued abstinence better than general treatment programs (Perez-Arce, Carr, & Sorensen, 1993). Cultural competency and culturally consistent treatment are now key components of successful programming. It is imperative to note that culture includes a diverse constellation of vital elements: customs, values, rituals,

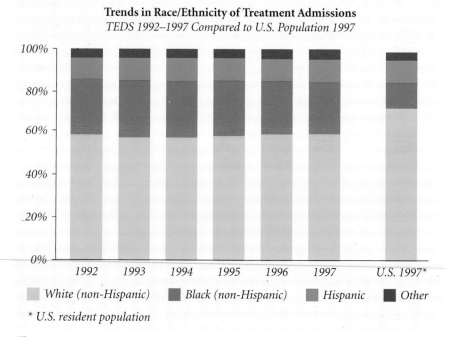

Trends in Race/Ethnicity of Treatment Admissions
TEDS 1992–1997 Compared to U.S. Population 1997

White (non-Hispanic)   Black (non-Hispanic)   Hispanic   Other

* U.S. resident population

Figure 9-8 •

The racial composition of admissions to drug treatment programs has remained fairly consistent since 1992 and proportionally it is somewhat different than the actual composition of the U.S. population. Whites are 73% of the U.S. population but only 61% of admissions while Blacks are 12% of the population but 25% of admissions to drug programs (SAMHSA/TEDS, 1999).

norms, religious beliefs, and ideals. You can't just base a culture upon the color of the skin or general area of the world. Thus the more specific the program is, the more effective it will be.

African American

The following ideas as to the differences in the treatment/intervention needs of inner-city, African American substance abusers are the result of years of experience working with the African American community in San Francisco by members of the Haight-Ashbury Detox Clinic and the Black Extended Family Program at Glide Memorial Church (Smith, Buxton, Bilal, & Seymour, 1993).

Higher Pain Threshold. Historically African Americans have developed a high pain threshold to help them survive in a harsh and painful environment. Unfortunately this greater tolerance for suffering delays a cry for help, leading to more severe addiction and other life problems before entering treatment. One solution to lowering the pain threshold and getting addicts to treatment sooner is educating the African American community to the true impact of drugs.

◇ In some urban areas, an alarmingly high number of African American babies are born drug affected.

◇ African American teenagers have a greater chance of dying from "crack"-related crime than they do from being hit by a car.

◇ There are more African American men in their 20s who are in jail from drug-related offenses than are in college.

◇ Since African American women are using "crack" at a greater rate than any other drug except alcohol, the family structure is dissolving at an alarming rate.

◇ Many neighborhoods with a high African American population have an alarmingly high infant mortality rate due to drug use by pregnant women who abuse or are addicted to substances like "crack" and heroin.

Drugs as an Economic Resource. Few economic windfalls are available to inner-city African American communities. Reducing drug dealing here means a loss of income to many families. This is in contrast to the European American community where drug/alcohol abuse usually drains the finances of families.

The true economics of the process need to be taught. For example, once the dealer becomes a user, the economic drain starts. Other members of the community are devastated and become dysfunctional; crime is brought to their own backyard.

"Most African Americans come into recovery by way of the criminal justice system, very late in the whole process of addiction, and are compelled to come to programs like Glide or Haight-Ashbury by the courts. So you have a whole different attitude from a person who has hit rock bottom and has decided they've got to seek help. The kids are more concerned about just finishing their term and finishing whatever sentence they have and getting out. They don't want to deal with counselors. They don't want to deal with advice. So what you've got is a chance, at that point, to try to hook them into some kind of system that allows them to get back into the society with a greater chance of success."
Youth drug counselor

Crime Leads to Chemical Dependency. Most often crime is the first entry into the chemical dependency subculture rather than drug use itself as with the European American community. Often in the African American community, the pattern is to make sales first and then sample the wares.

Strong Sense of Boundaries. Intervention is viewed as an inappropriate imposition or violation of one's space. There is resistance from within the community to approaching some-one with a chemical dependency problem because that would violate the person's boundaries or turf but not approaching someone also perpetuates denial.

These problems are the most difficult to address. They need a major attitudinal change, i.e., is it better to respect one's turf or to attempt interventions and try to do something about the problem?

Chemical Dependency: Primary or Secondary Problem? Chemical dependency is most often viewed in the African American community as a secondary problem and not a primary one. Minority communities often cite underemployment, poor housing, and lack of social/recreational resources as the primary problems instead of chemical dependency. This perpetuates denial and prevents many addicts from getting into treatment early. Drug users must understand that no other issues can be tackled successfully without tackling recovery first. The community needs to accept chemical dependency as a primary problem.

"Recovery is a lifetime process. That's a very difficult thing for African Americans to focus on. We're sprinters. We're real good at the 50-yard dash and the 100-yard dash and we have a feeling that, 'Okay, it's a drug problem. Once I stop using and I put it behind me, I can forget it and go about my business.' But no, recovery is a lifetime process and you have to think more in terms of being a marathoner."
Rafiq Bilal, former Director, Black Extended Family Program

Conspiracy Theory. The belief that "the rapid spread of 'crack' (and AIDS) into the African American community is deliberate genocide" is very widely held in the African American community. Given the history of slavery, segregation, and defacto segregation, it is understandable. Whether or not the conspiracy theory is true, addiction is a disease that must be treated in the individual as well as in society as a whole.

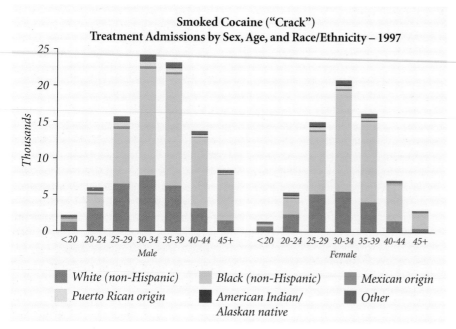

Smoked Cocaine ("Crack")
Treatment Admissions by Sex, Age, and Race/Ethnicity – 1997

Legend:
- White (non-Hispanic)
- Black (non-Hispanic)
- Mexican origin
- Puerto Rican origin
- American Indian/Alaskan native
- Other

Figure 9-9 •

The impact of "crack" on the African American community has, in fact, been much stronger than other drugs, particularly among women (SAMHSA/TEDS, 1999).

Revelations. In the African American community, organized spirituality has been found to be a key to promoting recovery. Treatment programs based in church settings have been shown to be more effective than more traditional treatment settings.

"The African American community is very spiritually oriented whether from involvement with the church or from historical associations. Most interesting is a recovery pattern of consecutive periods of clean time/relapse, clean time/relapse, until a revelation or 'snapping' occurs that results in a continuous sustained recovery effort. This is different from the more classic, 'expanding periods of sobriety, leading towards more sustained, long-term recovery.'"

Rafiq Bilal, former Director, Black Extended Family Program

The Black Extended Family Program under the guidance of Reverend Cecil Williams uses the concept and emotional force of the extended family to help keep people in treatment and give them an alternative to the lonely life of the addict. This concept reestablishes the family, spirituality, and self-worth, qualities that have been weakened by drug use. The Terms of Resistance, a 10-step equivalent of the 12 steps, was developed by Reverend Williams in 1992.

1. I will gain control over my life.
2. I will stop lying.
3. I will be honest with myself.
4. I will accept who I am.
5. I will feel my real feelings.
6. I will feel my pain.
7. I will forgive myself and forgive others.
8. I will rebirth a new life.
9. I will live my spirituality.
10. I will support and love my brothers and sisters.

(Smith et al., 1993)

Hispanic

With Hispanics it is important to understand the cultural diversity and the differences between groups as well as the similarities.

The most common similarities are

◊ Spanish language,
◊ Catholic background,
◊ Indian or African traits,
◊ Iberian heritage,
◊ strong family structure.

The differences are

◊ number of years or generations they have lived in the United States;
◊ country of origin; the three most prevalent being Mexico, Puerto Rico, and Cuba;
◊ level of education;
◊ economic status, e.g., are they Mexican migrant workers who immigrate to survive poverty and help their family back home; are they upper-class Mexicans or Costa Ricans looking to protect their wealth; are they middle- and upper-class Cubans who fled Fidel Castro a generation ago and have become a driving force in the Florida economy; or are they lower-, middle-, and upper-class Puerto Ricans (American citizens) who have moved to the East Coast to find a better life for their families?

After addressing any emergency physical or mental health needs, the first thing a treatment facility has to determine is the level of acculturation of any Hispanic clients coming in for treatment. For example, how well do they speak English; are they newly arrived immigrants; how integrated are they in the predominantly Anglo society; are they first, second, or third generation Hispanics who have stayed aware of their cultural heritage and kept contact with relatives and friends at home; or are they caught between two cultures without a solid home base?

In New York the rapid influx of Puerto Ricans in the 1950s, '60s, and '70s often caused a fragmentation of the extended family system, a polarization between generations, a loss of many aspects of the Puerto Rican culture, and an identity crisis. These stressors, along with language differences, were found responsible (in a New York State survey) for increases in substance abuse. With Cuban Americans, however, the rapid integration into American society has resulted in a level of drug use about half that of the Mexican American and Puerto Rican communities (Ruiz & Langrod, 1997).

What this means in terms of treatment is that programs have to be flexible, have a diverse staff that has a preponderance of Spanish-speaking and/or bilingual and bicultural counselors and administrators, and be willing to treat the whole family since the family is so important in Hispanic cultures. Because Hispanic American families have excellent networking systems, these systems can be used extensively in the treatment process. In addition the treatment facility should be aware of the roles that each member in the family plays. This is in contrast to many Anglo families where the roles of each member can be quite variable.

The core aspect of Hispanic cultures are *dignidad, respeto, y carino*—dignity, respect, and love. Even the concept of urine testing can be a touchy subject because the request for a urine test implies a lack of trust. Another aspect is the strong role spirituality plays in Hispanic culture. In addition to a Catholic heritage, many Hispanic cultures have nonorthodox religious beliefs, such as Spiritualism, Santeria, Brujeria, and Curanderism. Pentecostal and Jehovah's Witness churches are also strong in Hispanic communities.

"Some of the recent Mexican immigrants I've worked with who have an alcohol problem didn't start drinking heavily until they came to this country at the age of 25 or 30. At home they had to care for their families and had little money. Here, they are separated from their families and have more money, and so the use of alcohol and other drugs escalates. The other thing I've found is that even if an Hispanic client speaks perfect English, the fact that I'm bilingual and bicultural increases participation in treatment."

Hispanic specialist drug counselor from Washington state

Asian American

With Asian Americans, as with Hispanics, there are a wide variety of cultures.

The differences include

◇ a variety of distinct and separate ethnic groups, like Japanese, Filipino, Cambodian, Indian, and Samoan;

◇ a variety of languages, such as Korean, Chinese, Tagalog, and hundreds more;

◇ a variety of religions from Buddhism and Hinduism to Animism, Islam, and Christianity;

◇ a variety of strong cultural characteristics based on thousands of years of history;

◇ a great variety of cultures even within immigrants from the same country, e.g., Cantonese, Shanghaiese, and Taiwanese;

◇ different levels of acculturation depending on the number of generations they have been in the United States. For example, many Chinese Americans and Japanese Americans stretch back four or five generations while the newer immigrants, such as Laotians, Vietnamese, Koreans, and Thai, go back only one or two generations.

(Westermeyer, 1997)

The similarities are

◇ they are along the Pacific Rim;

◇ they have a strong regard for family;

◇ they generally have a high respect for education;

◇ they are less demonstrative or open in their communication about personal issues;

◇ they are more reserved about expressing accomplishments because they feel this would be a form of arrogant boasting;

◇ they are reluctant to discuss health issues or death because they superstitiously believe that it would make those problems occur.

These and other similarities affect treatment.

Asian Americans respond more to credentialed professionals than to peer counselors and prefer individual counseling to group counseling. They rely more on their own responsibility to handle their addiction rather than a higher power or external control. They also feel that if they were to complain about their issues, they would be imposing on others. They feel that saving face and individual honor are important issues and so they are, therefore, less responsive and will avoid confrontation. They prefer alternative ways of being able to express their feelings, like creative or expressive arts therapy. They require a strong incorporation of family therapy. Finally, they have strongly developed gender roles, so separate male and female groups are more effective than mixed groups.

For Asian Americans, entry into treatment usually occurs late since an admission of addiction is an admission of loss of control. Another problem is that addicts live for the addiction and for themselves rather than for the family and the community as they have been taught. Finally, the sense of family shame often keeps the family enabling and rescuing the addict again and again. On the other hand, the strong sense of family makes for greater compliance with protocols once treatment, which incorporates family therapy, has been started.

Available Programs. Because of the wide variety of Asian American cultures, the historical importance and availability of certain drugs, and the wide geographic distribution in cities and states of various groups, treatment personnel must do surveys of their neighborhoods to make treatment relevant. For example, the utilization of treatment services by Asian Americans in San Francisco was extremely low in the 1980s. This was misinterpreted to mean that Asian Americans had fewer drug problems than other ethnic groups.

Community reports however found as high an incidence of drug abuse in the Asian community as in other ethnic groups, the difference being that the

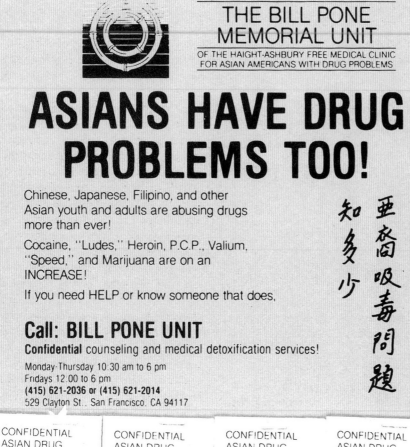

THE BILL PONE MEMORIAL UNIT
OF THE HAIGHT-ASHBURY FREE MEDICAL CLINIC
FOR ASIAN AMERICANS WITH DRUG PROBLEMS

ASIANS HAVE DRUG PROBLEMS TOO!

Chinese, Japanese, Filipino, and other Asian youth and adults are abusing drugs more than ever!

Cocaine, "Ludes," Heroin, P.C.P., Valium, "Speed," and Marijuana are on an INCREASE!

If you need HELP or know someone that does,

Call: BILL PONE UNIT
Confidential counseling and medical detoxification services!

Monday-Thursday 10:30 am to 6 pm
Fridays 12:00 to 6 pm
(415) 621-2036 or (415) 621-2014
529 Clayton St., San Francisco, CA 94117

知多少　亞裔吸毒問題

CONFIDENTIAL ASIAN DRUG DETOX SERVICES
Mon-Thurs 10:30 am-6 pm
Friday 12 pm-6 pm
CALL (415) 621-2036 or (415) 621-2014

CONFIDENTIAL ASIAN DRUG DETOX SERVICES
Mon-Thurs 10:30 am-6 pm
Friday 12 pm-6 pm
CALL (415) 621-2036 or (415) 621-2014

CONFIDENTIAL ASIAN DRUG DETOX SERVICES
Mon-Thurs 10:30 am-6 pm
Friday 12 pm-6 pm
CALL (415) 621-2036 or (415) 621-2014

CONFIDENTIAL ASIAN DRUG DETOX SERVICES
Mon-Thurs 10:30 am-6 pm
Friday 12 pm-6 pm
CALL (415) 621-2036 or (415) 621-2014

Educational material and promotion of a clinic's programs have to be directed at specific communities.

Asian American's drugs of choice were sedatives, particularly street Quaaludes® and Soma® (sedating muscle relaxant) that weren't focused on in most treatment programs. When the Haight-Ashbury Detox Clinic developed a specific Asian American program incorporating family therapy, treatment of sedative abuse, and personnel who were bicultural and bilingual, it resulted in a dramatic increase of Asian Americans coming into treatment at a level consistent with their overall population in the city.

Programs for Asian Americans must involve the family in any treatment or the chances of success are greatly lowered. In addition cultural connections must be recognized and utilized to make the treatment relevant.

Native American

Native American groups have a wide variety of cultural traditions. For example, the five eastern nations (tribes) of Oklahoma, who are literate, complex, and successful, have low rates of alcoholism. This is in comparison to some western mountain tribes who, in one study, were found to have a rate of alcoholism seven times the national average. In addition drugs with an historical context, such as tobacco and peyote, are used more often in ceremonies than as recreational drugs, so the introduction of different drugs, particularly alcohol and inhalants, with no cultural tradition of restricted use, has caused numerous problems.

Bicultural and bilingual treatment personnel greatly increase the chances of successful treatment. Many nations incorporate cultural traditions in healing, including talking circles, purification ceremonies, sweat lodges, meditative practices, shamanistic ceremonies, and even community "sings."

Detoxification centers, halfway houses, outpatient programs, and hospital units have been funded by the Indian Health Service and certain state and county governments. However over 60% of Native Americans live away from traditional communities in multiethnic urban areas, so treatment centers in those locales should have the same diversity of bilingual and bicultural personnel for Native Americans as they do for other ethnic and cultural groups.

Talking circles have been used for hundreds of years in various Native American tribes as a way to solve problems and heal members of the tribe. The process is similar to peer groups, though instead of round robin talking with no interruptions, there is crosstalk and questions. The sessions usually last for two or three hours, though they can be much longer.

"On reservations, you get locked into a community where you don't grow and there is a minimum of interaction with other groups. There is virtually no middle class. You have a group who are highly religious who do not drink at all, you have a few who work for the Bureau of Indian Affairs or in limited industry and drink sparingly, and you have another group that lives to drink and drinks to live. There's not enough

work, nothing to do, and often nothing to look forward to for many in this group. You're just another Indian and you're not to be trusted. You have to want to be more than just another drunken Indian.

We have to be proud of who we are before we can reach recovery. In the Native American community, the family is very tight. Everyone is your cousin or aunt or uncle. A sense of pride in your people is part of the core of spirituality that helps us survive. As part of this, we've always looked to elders for guidance. The elders would talk to you about your drinking (a form of intervention) to get you to make changes in your life. The elders have a variety of approaches. They might even do a tough love approach and tell alcoholics to leave the reservation, finish their drinking, and come back when they are sober; or they might tell them to get honest with themselves and make a sobriety pledge to the medicine man or in a pipe ceremony.

We have a variety of tribes that I deal with here in Montana, such as Sioux, Northern Cheyenne, Blackfoot, and Crow. Each one has their own traditions. Unfortunately a number of clinic directors on reservations who are brought in from the outside have trouble understanding the traditions, so they rely more on standard psychosocial therapy, which is not as effective and breeds distrust. Adding to this is the fact that, for many Native Americans, hitting bottom is not as big a trigger for self-referral into treatment as it is in the Anglo community. Often they are not aware of what bottom is. It takes intervention or court mandate to make changes. On the other hand, once they get recovery, they are much less likely to let go. I tell them

that alcoholism is like the raven that has stolen your shadow. If your shadow is gone, your spirituality is gone. Be proud of who you are."

Bob Clarkson, Native American drug and alcohol counselor

Great Spirit, grant me the serenity of a dove to accept the things I cannot change, the courage of an eagle to change the things I can, and the wisdom of an owl to know the difference.

Native American version of the Serenity Prayer used in Alcoholics Anonymous

OTHERS

There are numerous groupings of Americans who require targeted treatment. Whether they are substance abusers who have physical disabilities, gays or lesbians, homeless, mentally challenged, elderly, or a dozen other groups, the key seems to be involvement with peer groups who have experienced the lifestyle, the problems, the prejudice, the homophobia, the shunning, the joys, the problems with self-esteem or relationships, and can speak and help based on personal experience.

The common point that needs to be recognized is that addiction is addiction. To imagine that problems with addictive behavior would disappear if only some other conditions or problems were taken care of is a sure path to continued addictive behavior. On the other hand, the other problems, such as racism and mental instability, have to be addressed and treated at the same time because many of the roots of compulsive use lie in a subconscious effort to avoid or cope with the pain experienced in these conditions or lifestyles.

Physically Disabled

For example, Americans with disabilities represent a much-neglected group of chemically dependent people. Some of the more common disabilities are blindness, deafness, head or brain injury (50,000 a year), and spinal cord injury (10,000–15,000 new cases a year). Despite passage of the Amer-

icans with Disabilities Act in 1990, most programs remain inaccessible to many with mobility impairment, visual impairment, and hearing impairment. In addition there is very little interdisciplinary training for working with physically disabled substance abusers (Heinemann, 1997). One problem that occurs is that the counselor can focus too much on the physical disability and miss signs and symptoms of relapse and additional problems or focus too strongly on the addiction and not take into account the extra stress that can be caused by the disability. Conversely the rehabilitation professional might feel unqualified or leery of handling substance abuse problems or might not even recognize the signs and symptoms. In addition society's attitude towards people with disabilities can promote the concept of learned helplessness and dependency on others and subsequently on drugs. One irony of substance abuse in people with physical disabilities is that substance use is a factor in up to 68% of traumatic disabling injuries (Heinemann, 1993). A thorough medical and drug history is helpful in judging whether the substance abuse predated the disability, was triggered by the disability, or occurred independently of the disability for other reasons.

Because physical disabilities often involve pain, there is an increased use of prescription medications that can be abused. Again it is a preexisting susceptibility to addiction or preexisting substance abuse that usually indicates that the person with a physical disability will have a dependence problem with pain medications, such as opioids or benzodiazepines (Schnoll, 1993).

In a study of 96 persons with long-term spinal cord injuries, 43% used prescription medications with abuse potential and 1/4 of those, or about 10% of the total, reported misusing the medications. The group that regularly misused the prescription medications was less accepting of their disability and more depressed. Another study found that the existence of a preexisting substance abuse problem made it more likely that the client would not participate fully in rehabilitation, thereby slowing recovery and increasing stress (Heinemann, 1993).

Gay & Lesbian

There has been a lack of research on substance abuse in the gay and lesbian communities, so the studies that have been done are not exhaustive, merely suggestive. The studies that have been done put the incidence of drug and alcohol in the gay community as significantly higher than in the general population (Bickelhaupt, 1995). A directory of gay and lesbian AA groups listed more than 800 meetings in the United States in the mid-'90s. One study showed that 42% of gay and bisexual men used alcohol and drugs at a level that implied use at risky or problematic levels. Alcohol was the preferred drug of choice but polydrug use was common. Marijuana was also used at a significantly higher level, almost 1/3 more than in the general population (Kelly, 1991).

The high incidence of HIV and AIDS in the gay male community is aggravated by drug or alcohol use for two reasons; the use of drugs lowers inhibitions and leads to unsafe sex and the use of contaminated needles also spreads the HIV virus quickly.

"I'd been using drugs for years and years but when I found out I was positive I said, 'Oh, I'm going to die,' and I just started 'slamming' dope faster and harder and I did that for two years and when I wasn't dead I said, 'Wait a minute, I'm not dying and I gotta keep going with my life and I started realizing that I could get clean, and I could stay as healthy as I could, and I could make something out of my life."

Gay recovering substance abuser with AIDS

Though many groups have to deal with society's hostility, indifference, fear, or misunderstanding and be subject to extra stress, it is still the roots of addiction that are the greater influence—genetics tempered by childhood stresses and inflamed by drug use.

"When I first came here, I was so nervous about being gay, one of the minority in the group 'cause there's a lot more straight men, but I really like it now because I can work on my issues about being heterophobic—I get fears around heterosexuals. I stereotype straight guys, 'Oh, they all hate me and they all think I'm less of a man.' And I get to find out that's not true and I get to find out that if someone does have that, then that's theirs. It ain't mine."

Gay recovering polydrug abuser in stimulant abuse group

Because of societal homophobia, internalized homophobia (the fear and hatred of one's homosexuality) is often one of the greatest barriers to long-term sobriety and recovery (Kominars, 1995). As with low self-esteem, it can be successfully treated. Fortunately, in recent years, there has been a decrease in these feelings, mostly due to a decrease in societal homophobia (Cabaj, 1997).

TREATMENT OBSTACLES

Denial and lack of financial or treatment resources have always comprised the biggest obstacles to addiction treatment. But as the treatment of addictive disease continues to evolve, other significant obstacles are being identified that require intervention for successful treatment outcomes.

DEVELOPMENT ARREST

The use of psychoactive drugs can delay user's emotional development and keep them from learning how to deal with life's problems. In terms of treatment, the counselors or other professionals have to be aware of the level of development in the individual. They have to be aware of how much of what they or others are teaching is being understood by the client. If a client is not fully detoxified or is not given time to start functioning normally, even the most sophisticated treatment can fall on deaf ears. More extensive assessment is one way to overcome these problems.

FOLLOW-THROUGH (monitoring)

Nothing is more indicative of poor treatment outcome than early program dropout or lack of compliance to the treatment protocol. Ironically client confidentiality that is so vital to the addiction treatment process has contributed to the problem of poor treatment compliance. Clients who have not or will not release information about their treatment progress can be noncompliant to protocols without the awareness of families, employers, or others until more destruction has resulted from their resumed addiction.

Professional licensing boards (medical, nursing, legal) now mandate release of confidentiality as a condition of retaining a license when addicts who are professionals are delivered to treatment after their addiction has been discovered. This practice, though assuring better program compliance, created another obstacle for the treatment professional. How could a therapist engage an addict into deep and sensitive issues about their addiction without being viewed as an extension of the licensing board, the family, or law enforcement? To address this obstacle, some licensing boards and employee assistance programs now employ a program monitor who oversees the progress of an addict in treatment to assure compliance to program protocols.

CONFLICTING GOALS

An individual addict's treatment goal may conflict with a program's goal. Some addicts may enter treatment merely to be able to better manage their abuse of drugs or to qualify for certain social benefits. Most treatment programs insist on an immediate commitment from their clients to a drug-free lifestyle. This difference between goals leads to a poor treatment outcome.

Program goals may conflict with society's goals for treating addicts. Programs naturally focus on the care of their clients using interventions which they hope will lead their clients to the best possible life outcome. Society is more interested in supporting programs that decrease the social costs of addiction (e.g. crime, health costs, accidents, and violence).

The problems of conflicting goals are best managed by development of clear program objectives and goals and better assessment and matching of clients to programs. Although these concepts seem straightforward and easy to practice, only now is investment in these two areas beginning to occur.

TREATMENT RESOURCES

The biggest obstacle continues to be lack of treatment resources. On a national basis, individuals who apply for treatment are put on a waiting list of 2 weeks to 3 months or longer before they can get into treatment. Studies have shown that for every 100 people put on a waiting list, 66% will never make it into treatment. Over the past 30 years, the Haight-Ashbury Detox Clinic has found that of those put on their waiting list, 80% never access treatment. What happens to those potential clients is a matter of deep concern. Many die from drugs or from suicide while waiting for treatment (O'Boyle & Brandon, 1998). Most become more heavily involved in drugs and a high proportion end up in the criminal justice system. Since treatment has been shown to be very effective, it is a national tragedy that we continue to have long protracted waiting periods for clients wanting to access treatment.

MEDICAL INTERVENTION DEVELOPMENTS

INTRODUCTION

Drug replacement therapies, medical pharmacotherapy, pharmacologic therapies, chemically assisted detoxification, drug-assisted recovery, antipriming medications, drug restoration of homeostasis, medication therapies in addiction, and other medical interventions currently in development to treat drug addiction would have been considered to be oxymorons in the field of recovery a few short years ago. Further these terms would have terrified chemical dependency treatment clinicians and recovering addicts as both recognized that the use of psychoactive drugs often resulted in relapse.

Advances in the understanding of the neuropharmacology of addiction during the 1990's Decade of the Mind has led to a virtual flood of medication developments targeted to treat chemical dependencies. By the year 2000, the number of new drugs being developed to treat addictions was second only to those in development to treat other mental health disorders and far outnumbered the drugs being developed to treat infections, heart disease, cancer, AIDS, and other illnesses (American Pharmacist, 1999). Chemical dependency treatment specialists now need to broaden their understanding and acceptance of medical therapies as they are certain to be incorporated into addiction treatment in the near future.

TYPES OF MEDICATIONS

The different types of medications being developed to treat addictions can be classified based on the targeted stage of recovery or by their effects on the nervous system and rest of the body:

◊ detoxification,

◊ rapid opioid detoxification,

◊ replacement or agonist effects,

◊ antagonist (blocking) or vaccines,

◊ mixed agonist-antagonist,

◊ anticraving and anticued craving,

◊ metabolism modulation,

◊ restoration of homeostasis,

◊ modulation of drug effects and antipriming.

(O'Brien, 1997; Vocci, 1999)

Detoxification

Medications that moderate or eliminate the withdrawal syndrome in addicts have been shown to be effective in engaging them into long-term treatment. Some examples of this detoxification development include buprenorphine and lofexidine to treat opioid withdrawal; selegiline and SSRI antidepressants (paroxetine) for cocaine and stimulant addiction; and phenobarbital or lorazepam for alcohol or sedative-hypnotic dependence (O'Brien, 1997; Vocci, 1999).

Rapid Opioid Detoxification

This technique uses various medications in combination with naloxone or naltrexone and has also been clinically developed to treat opioid addiction. Opioid antagonists like naloxone and naltrexone are used to precipitate immediate withdrawal and the other medications are used to mitigate the withdrawal symptoms. Clonidine is combined with naltrexone to accomplish physical detoxification from opioid tissue dependence within 2–3 days. The benzodiazepine sedative midazolam is used with naloxone and naltrexone to accomplish opioid detoxification in 24 hours. A benzodiazepine sedative is combined with clonidine, along with naloxone and naltrexone, to detoxify an opioid addict within 6–8 hours while they are anesthetized with propofol. These methods of rapid detoxification are medically dangerous and require intensive medical supervision. Further it is very important to remember that the techniques only accomplish physical detoxification and do not address the long-term behavioral and emotional components of addiction that are necessary to maintain abstinence and recovery (Lorenzi et al., 1999; Cucchia et al., 1998; Byrne, 1998; Dyer, 1998; Barter et al., 1996; Senft, 1991).

Replacement or Agonist Effects

Controversy over whether this type of therapy is more harm reduction than recovery remains very heated in the addiction treatment community. However, few can deny the effectiveness of methadone replacement therapy in producing positive benefits for both the addict (reduced morbidity and mortality while increasing overall life functioning) and for society (cost effectiveness and reduction in crime) (Ball & Ross, 1991). Positive results from methadone maintenance have stimulated the search for other replacement or agonist therapies. LAAM (levo-alpha acetyl methadol) and buprenorphine for opioid addiction, methylphenidate and pemoline for cocaine and stimulant dependence, and SSRI antidepressants and GHB (gamma hydroxybutyrate) for alcohol and sedative-hypnotic addiction are examples of replacement therapies in development to treat addictive disorders (O'Brien, 1997; Vocci, 1999).

Antagonist (blocking) Medications or Vaccines

Medications or vaccines that block the effects of addictive drugs without inducing their own major psychoactive effects are widely accepted as recovery-oriented treatment approaches. While on these types of agents, addicts will be unable to experience the effects of an abused drug should they have a "slip." This destroys the addict's motivation for using and promotes continued abstinence. Significant examples of this treatment approach are the development of depo-naltrexone for opioid addiction and UH-232 for cocaine addiction. A cocaine vaccine that produces antibodies for cocaine, preventing its action for up to 30 days, is also in development (O'Brien, 1997; Vocci, 1999; Carrera et al., 1996; Fox et al., 1996)

Mixed Agonist-Antagonist

A single medication can have an agonist effect at one receptor site and an antagonist effect at another site. Or a combination of drugs are used together that work independently at different receptor sites to accomplish the same overall agonist-antagonist goal. The agonist component of this approach is targeted to prevent withdrawal while the antagonist effects prevent craving by blocking any further drug use. Ex-

amples of this approach are the developments of butorphanol and buprenorphine in opioid addiction; cyclazocine in cocaine dependence; and the combination of low-dose nicotine with mecamylamine to treat nicotine addiction. Rapid opioid detoxification described previously also employs this technique of combining agonist with antagonist medication to treat heroin and other opioid addictions (O'Brien, 1997; Rose, Behm, Westman, et al., 1994).

Anticraving & Anticued Craving

Craving or drug hunger is now an established component of addiction. Negative emotional states (e.g., **h**ungry, **a**ngry, **l**onely, **t**ired—HALT; and **r**estless, **i**rritable, **d**iscontent—RID) as well as imbalances in brain chemistry due to drug use cause endogenous craving. Environmental cues or triggers (e.g., drug odors, white powders, paraphernalia, "crack" houses, drug-using acquaintances) also induce a great potential for relapse. Medications that can mitigate and reduce the craving and the cued-craving responses have witnessed dramatic development in treating addictions (O'Brien, 1977). Naltrexone has been fully approved as an anticraving treatment for alcoholism and is in development to block cocaine and opioid craving (O'Brien, 1997; Volpicelli, O'Brien, Atterman, & Hayashida, 1992; O'Malley et al., 1992). A concern regarding potential liver toxicity with naltrexone use has limited its use in treating alcohol dependence. Nalmefene, another opioid antagonist, has been shown to reduce alcohol craving without any liver toxicity and is now being developed to treat alcohol addiction (Mason, Ritvo, Morgan, et al., 1994; O'Brien, 1997).

Acamprosate, a nonopioid drug, also exhibits alcohol anticraving effects through modulation of GABA (gamma-aminobutyric acid) and dopamine neurotransmitters (O'Brien, 1997).

Mecamylamine appears to block cocaine-cued craving and is currently in development for this indication, along with its development as a nicotine anticraving medication (Reid, Mickalian, Delucchi, et al., 1999).

The FDA has approved bupropion, an antidepressant medication, for the treatment of nicotine-cued craving and it is also in development as a cocaine anticraving medication. Bupropion research demonstrated that it prevented nicotine craving in patients who did not have symptoms of depression which indicates that it mitigates craving by another unknown mechanism. Similarly SSRI antidepressants like paroxetine decrease alcohol use in even nondepressed alcoholics (O'Brien, 1997; Ferry, 1992).

The craving response is physiologically similar to a body stress reaction. This has led researchers to study drugs that can antagonize corticotropin releasing factor (CRF) that triggers the stress reaction in the brain. The hypothesis is that craving can be prevented by blocking the body's stress reaction. Ketoconazole and CP154,526 inhibit the release of CRF in the brain and are being developed to treat cocaine craving. Metynapone inhibits the synthesis of body corticoids, which are also involved in the stress reaction. It is also being developed as a drug to treat cocaine craving (Vocci, 1999).

Metabolism Modulation

Medications that can alter the metabolism of an abused drug to render it ineffective or noxious when used are also being developed. Historically disulfiram, used to treat alcoholism, has been the only drug developed in this class. Disulfiram blocks the metabolic processes of alcohol leading to a build-up of acetaldehyde. Acetaldehyde causes nausea, flushing, and negative body reactions. Thus alcoholics suffer immediate adverse consequences from drinking. The effectiveness of disulfiram relies upon the compliance of the alcoholic to take it in support of their stated desire for abstinence. It has therefore had limited success in treating alcoholism in the past. However, the increase of coercive treatments during the past decade (e.g., drug courts, contingency contracting, probation/parole requirements, and job or career threats) has improved disulfiram treatment compliance and increased positive outcomes (O'Brien, 1997; Keane et al., 1984; Keane & Fuller, 1986). This has increased interest in the metabolism modulation approach and some work has begun on the search for medications that can increase the metabolism of cocaine to render it ineffective when abused (Vocci, 1999).

Restoration of Homeostasis

Abuse of addictive drugs imbalances brain chemistry, which then reinforces the need to continue using the drug. Medications and nutrients that restore brain chemical imbalances are theorized to restore homeostasis and mitigate the need for continued drug use. Selegiline, drugs that have dopamine-activating effects in the brain (e.g., amantadine and pergolide), and antidepressants (e.g., desipramine, nefazodone, paroxetine, sertraline, and venlafaxine) that increase serotonin in the brain are all being developed to treat cocaine and alcohol addiction by restoring brain chemical homeostasis (Vocci, 1999).

Amino Acid Precursor Loading

This technique consists of administering protein supplements (e.g., tyrosine, taurine, d,l phenylalanine, glutamate, and tryptophan) to addicts in an effort to increase the brain's production of its neurochemicals and restore homeostasis. Though not yet established by rigorous research, many treatment programs report good patient treatment compliance and positive outcomes when amino acid precursor loading is added to the treatment process for cocaine, amphetamine, alcohol, and opioid dependence (Blum et al., 1989).

Modulation of Drug Effects & Antipriming

A fairly recent development is the use of medications that can modulate or blunt the pleasurable reinforcing effects of addictive drug use. Calcium channel-blocking medications prevent calcium ions from entering brain cells and increase the release of dopamine resulting in a mitigation of the reinforcing effects of cocaine, opioids, and alcohol. Nimodipine, acamprosate, amlodipine, nephedipine, and isadipine are all calcium channel blockers being developed to treat addiction to cocaine, opioids, and alcohol (Vocci, 1999; Shulman, Jagoda, Laycock, & Kelly, 1998).

Sodium Ion Channel Blockers

Medications like riluzole, phenytoin, and lamotrigine interfere with neuron transmission via this process and result in muting cocaine's reinforcing effects. Cyclazocine, a mixed opioid agonist-antagonist, also reduces cocaine reinforcement by interfering with cocaine's action on presynaptic neurons' sodium ion channels (Vocci, 1999).

Low Doses of Nicotine

This technique has been shown to decrease craving without reinforcing the need to increase its dosage or to continue its use. This effect is known as an "antipriming action" and it is the basis for the development of low-dose nicotine delivery systems, like the nicotine patch, to treat nicotine addiction.

Other Drugs

Some medications have clinically been shown to be useful in addiction treatment but by what mechanism they accomplish their positive benefit effect is unknown. Psychedelic drugs like ibogaine and ketamine are said to be effective in treating cocaine and opioid addiction even though the use of ibogaine to treat opioid addiction had resulted in some fatalities. Dextromethorphan (DM), a nonprescription anticough medication is being studied to treat opioid addiction. DM has been shown to be a weak glutamate agonist but its mechanism to decrease opiate withdrawal symptoms, craving, and relapse is unclear. Cycloserine, an antibiotic for the treatment of tuberculosis, is being studied for its ability to decrease opioid use by some unknown mechanism. Anticonvulsant medications like valproate and carbamazepine appear to diminish cocaine's craving and "kindling" effects. Smart drugs, also known as "nootropic agents," are believed to increase brain activity by unknown mechanisms and are also being tested to treat cocaine and stimulant addiction. Camitine/coenzyme Q10, ginkgo biloba, pentoxifylline, Hyydergine®, and piracetam are current nootropics being studied for use in cocaine addiction treatment. Tiagabine and gabapentin are anticonvulsant medications used in the treatment of epilepsy. They are believed to increase brain GABA activity but their ability to decrease cocaine addiction occurs by some yet-to-be-discovered mechanism. These and other clinical observations of drugs that lessen addiction or relapse liability indicate that there is a lot more still to be learned about the addicted brain (Vocci, 1999; O'Brien, 1997).

Some companies, such as Drug Abuse Sciences, Inc., are developing time-release delivery systems for naltrexone (Naltrel®), methadone (Methaliz®), and buprenorphine (Buprel®).

THE NEW DRUG DEVELOPMENT PROCESS

The federal Food and Drug Administration (FDA) has established a structured process for the approval of new drugs to treat specific therapeutic indications or the approval of existing drugs to be used for new therapeutic applications. This consists of three steps and four phases.

Step 1: Preclinical Research & Development

This step consists of the initial chemical development of a drug, along with animal studies to determine the general effects, toxicity, and projected abuse liability of the substance. If these results indicate that the drug is useful and marketable, the drug's sponsor will apply for an Investigational New Drug (IND) number that will permit them to conduct human research with the substance.

Step 2: Clinical Trials

Step 2 is comprised of three Phases that study the efficacy and safety of the drug in humans.

◇ Phase I: Initial Clinical Stage—a small number of human subjects are used to establish drug safety, dosage range for effective treatment, and the occurrence of side effects or adverse reactions.

◇ Phase II: Clinical Pharmacological Evaluation Stage—double-blinded studies (neither the researcher nor the test subject knows if they have received the actual test drug or a placebo) are used to evaluate the effects of the drug, determine side effects, and gauge the effectiveness of its use in treating a specific medical condition.

◇ Phase III: Extended Clinical Evaluation—the new drug is made available to a large number of researchers and patients with the indicated medical condition to further evaluate its safety, effectiveness, recommended dosage, and side effects.

Step 3: Permission to Market

If the drug successfully completes Steps 1 and 2 to demonstrate acceptable efficacy and safety, the FDA can allow the drug to be marketed under its patented name. The process from Step 1 to Step 3 takes up to 12 years to complete. After the drug is marketed, the FDA continues to monitor the drug for adverse or toxic reactions because it can take years for some negative effects to manifest and be discovered. This postmarketing scrutiny is often referred to as "Phase IV" because of the ability of the FDA to remove the drug from the market at any time if negative effects outweigh the positive benefits of using the drug (Hanson & Venturelli, 1998).

OVERVIEW OF MEDICATIONS

A partial list of medications in development for the treatment of addictive disorders was prepared by the authors using information gathered from a large number of references with consultation from the Pharmaceutical Research Center of the Haight-Ashbury Free Clinics. It should be noted that the many drugs being developed for cocaine addiction are also being studied to treat amphetamine and other stimulant dependence as well.

TABLE 9–5   MEDICATIONS IN DEVELOPMENT FOR ADDICTIVE DISORDERS

Drug	Brand Name	Current Medical Use	Proposed Use	Theoretical Action	Status
acamprosate			alcohol craving	calcium channel blocker, dopamine, GABA & glutamate modulation	Step 1, studied in Europe
amantadine	Symmetrel®	antiviral & Parkinsonism	cocaine addiction	dopamine agonist	Phase II
amlodipine	Lotrel® & Norvasc®	antihypertension	cocaine addiction	calcium channel blocker	clinical observation
baclofen		muscle relaxant	cocaine addiction	GABA & dopamine agonist	Phase II
BP 897			cocaine addiction	dopamine d2 & d3 antagonist inhibits cued craving	Step 1
bromocriptine	Parlodel®	antiprolactin	cocaine addiction	dopamine agonist	clinical observation
buprenorphine	Buprenex® & Subutex®	analgesia	opioid withdrawal & replacement	opioid agonist-antagonist	IND submitted
buprenorphine with naloxone	Suboxone®	analgesia	opioid withdrawal & replacement	opioid agonist-antagonist	Phase III
bupropion	Wellbutrin® & Zyban®	antidepressant	cocaine & nicotine addiction	anticued craving	Phase II, approved for nicotine
butorphanol	Stadol®	analgesia	opioid addiction	opioid agonist-antagonist	Phase II
cabergoline	Dostinex®	antiprolactin	cocaine addiction	dopamine agonist	Phase II
camitine/Co Q (coenzyme Q10)	Ubigold-10®	nootropic (smart drug)	cocaine addiction	mechanism unknown	Phase II
carbamazepine	Tegretol®	anticonvulsant	cocaine addiction	unknown mechanism	clinical observation
carbidopa with levodopa	Atimet® & Sinemet®	Parkinsonism	cocaine addiction	dopamine agonist	clinical observation
	CigRx®		nicotine replacement	low nicotine & carcinogen cigarette	Phase II
clonidine	Catapres®	antihypertension	opioid withdrawal	alpha 2 agonist	Phase II
cocaine vaccine	ITAC®		cocaine addiction	antibodies that prevent cocaine action for 30 days	Phase I
CP-154,526			cocaine addiction	CRF antagonist	Step 1
cyclazocine			cocaine addiction	opioid agonist-antagonist, cocaine mechanism unknown	Phase I

continued

TABLE 9–5 *CONTINUED*

Drug	Brand Name	Current Medical Use	Proposed Use	Theoretical Action	Status
cycloserine	Seromycin®	antibiotic	opioid addiction	mechanism unknown	Phase I
depo-naltrexone			opioid addiction	opioid antagonist in depo form blocks opioids for 14–30 days	Step 1
desipramine	Norpramine®	antidepressant	cocaine withdrawal	serotonin, dopamine, NE & E modulation	Phase II
dextroamphetamine	Dexedrine®	narcolepsy & ADD	cocaine replacement	CNS stimulant	Phase II
dextromethorphan	in various cough meds	anticough	opioid withdrawal & addiction	weak glutamate antagonist but opioid mechanism unknown	Phase II
disulfiram	Antabuse®	alcohol addiction	cocaine addiction	cocaine mechanism unknown	Phase II
dynorphan 1-13			opioid addiction	a naturally occurring opioid agonist	Phase II
enadoline			opioid & cocaine addiction	selective kappa opioid agonist, mechanism in cocaine unknown	Phase I & Phase II
ergot extract	Hydergine®	nootropic	cocaine addiction	dopamine agonist	Phase II
flupenthixol		antipsychotic	cocaine addiction	dopamine antagonist	Phase II
gabapentin	Neurontin®	anticonvulsant	cocaine addiction	mechanism unknown	Phase II
gamma hydroxy butyrate (GHB)			alcohol & opioid addiction	naturally occurring inhibitory neurotransmitter like GABA	clinical observation
GBR 12909			cocaine addiction	glutamate agonist	Phase I
ginkgo biloba	Bio Ginkgo®	nootropic	cocaine addiction	mechanism unknown	Phase II
	Gumsmoke®		smokeless tobacco addiction	tobacco-flavored chewing gum alternative to chewing tobacco	Phase II
ibogaine	Endabuse®		opioid & cocaine addiction	mechanism unknown, a toxic psychedelic	Phase I
isradipine	Dynacirc®	antihypertension	alcohol addiction	calcium channel blocker	clinical observation
ketamine	Ketalar®	anesthetic	alcohol addition	mechanism unknown	studied in Russia
ketoconazole	Nizoral®	antifungal	cocaine addiction	CRF antagonist	clinical observation
lamotrigine	Lamictal®	anticonvulsant	cocaine & opioid addiction	sodium channel blocker	Phase II & Phase I
lazabemide	Tempium®	Alzhemier's disease	nicotine addiction	MAO-B inhibitor	Phase III
levo-alpha acetyl methadol (LAAM)		opioid addiction	opioid replacement	opioid agonist	Approved for use
lobeline			nicotine addiction	autonomic ganglia agonist	Phase I
lofexedine			opioid addiction	calcium channel blocker	Phase II
mazindol			cocaine replacement	phenethylamine CNS stimulant	Phase II
mecamylamine	Inversine®	antihypertension	cocaine addiction	blocks nicotine-cued cocaine craving	Step 1
methylphenidate	Ritalin®	ADD & AD/HD	cocaine replacement	CNS stimulant	Phase II
metynapone			cocaine addiction	inhibits corticoid synthesis to inhibit cocaine craving	Step 1
nalmefene			alcohol & opioid addiction	opioid antagonist with no liver toxicity	Phase II
naltrexone	Revia®	alcohol addiction	opioid & cocaine addiction	opioid antagonist inhibits opioid & cocaine craving	Phase II
nefazodone	Serzone®	antidepressant	cocaine addiction	serotonin, dopamine, NE & E modulation	Phase II
nicotine with mecamylamine patch			nicotine addiction	antipriming & anticraving	Phase III
nicotine oral lozenge			nicotine addiction	antipriming & anticraving	Phase I

continued

TABLE 9–5 *CONTINUED*

Drug	Brand Name	Current Medical Use	Proposed Use	Theoretical Action	Status
nifedipine	Adalat® & Procardia®	vasospastic angina	alcohol, opioid, amphetamine, benzodiazepine & marijuana addiction	calcium channel blocker, increased dopamine to mitigate withdrawal and craving	clinical observation
nimodipine	Nimotop®	neurologic problems from ischemia	opioid addiction	calcium channel blocker	Phase II
NS 2359			cocaine addiction	dopamine agonist	Phase I
olanzapine	Zyprexa®	antipsychotic	cocaine addiction	benzodiazepine with antipsychotic effects	Phase II
OT-nicotine			nicotine addiction	antipriming, anticraving, replacement therapy	Phase II & III
paroxetine	Paxil®	SSRI antidepressant	cocaine & alcohol addiction	serotonin modulation, mechanism in alcoholism unknown	Phase II & clinical observation
pemoline	Cylert®	AD/HD	cocaine replacement	CNS stimulant	Phase II
pentoxifylline	Trental®	improve blood flow	cocaine addiction	mechanism unknown	Phase II
pergolide	Permax®	Parkinsonism	cocaine addiction	dopamine d1 & d2 agonist	Phase II
phenytoin	Dilantin®	anticonvulsant	cocaine addiction	sodium channel blocker	Phase II
piracetam	Nootropil®	nootropic	cocaine addiction	mechanism unknown	Phase II
pramipexole	Mirapex®	Parkinsonism	cocaine addiction	dopamine agonist	Phase II
propranolol	Inderal®	antihypertension	cocaine addiction	beta adrenergic blocker but cocaine mechanism unknown	Phase II
reserpine		antihypertension	cocaine addiction	dopamine, NE & E modulation	Phase II
riluzole	Rilutek®	ALS disease	cocaine addiction	sodium channel blocker	Phase II
risperidone	Risperdal®	antipsychotic	cocaine addiction	dopamine d2 & serotonin antagonist	Phase II
selegiline (IR & TS)	Eldepryl®	Parkinsonism	cocaine addiction	MAO-B inhibitor increased dopamine, NE & E	Phase I & III
sertraline	Zoloft®	SSRI antidepressant	cocaine & alcohol addiction	serotonin modulation, mechanism in alcohol unknown	Phase II & clinical observation
tiagabine	Gabitril®	anticonvulsant	cocaine addiction	GABA modulation	Phase II
tramadol	Ultram®	analgesia	opioid replacement	mu opioid receptor agonist	Phase I
tyrosine	nutritional supplement	amphetamine & cocaine addiction	increased dopamine	synthesis in the brain	Phase I
UH-232			cocaine addiction	nondysphoric cocaine antagonist	Step 1
valproate	Depacon®	anticonvulsant	cocaine addiction	GABA modulation, antikindling	Phase II
venlafaxine	Effexor®	antidepressant	cocaine addiction	serotonin & NE modulation	Phase II
verapamil	Calan®	angina	alcohol, opiates, amphetamine, benzodiazepine & marijuana addiction	calcium channel blocker	clinical observation

CHAPTER SUMMARY

Introduction

1. The most prevalent disease of the brain is addiction. Annually it causes over 1/2 million deaths and intense social disruption. The vast majority of deaths are from available legal drugs, like tobacco and alcohol.

2. Current issues in treatment include:

   ◇ the rapidly expanding use of medications to treat detoxification, control craving, and assist relapse prevention; medications include drugs to lessen withdrawal symptoms, nutritional supplements, antidepressants, substitute medications (e.g., methadone, and anticraving drugs);

   ◇ the use of imaging techniques and other new diagnostic techniques to visualize the physiological effects of drugs; CAT (computerized axial tomography), MRI (magnetic resonance imaging), PET (positron emission tomography), and SPECT (single photon emission computed tomography) are the four methods used. They help understand what drugs do, they help educate the general public, and they help break through denial;

◊ the lack of resources to provide the treatment that has been proven effective; studies have shown that treatment is effective but governments do not allot enough money to provide sufficient treatment;

◊ the conflict between abstinence-oriented recovery and harm reduction as philosophies of treatment; most treatment modalities say abstinence is absolutely necessary to recovery while harm reduction advocates say incremental changes are acceptable.

Treatment Effectiveness

3. Treatment is effective. It has a 50% success rate according to the DATOS and CALDATA studies.

4. Each $1 spent on treatment saves at least $7 to $20 in costs related to unchecked addiction.

5. Prison costs $25,000 to $40,000 per inmate a year compared to $2,000 to $3,900 for outpatient treatment or methadone maintenance.

6. Almost 2/3 of arrestees test positive for psychoactive drugs, particularly cocaine and marijuana.

Principles & Goals of Treatment

7. NIH listed 13 principles of effective treatment, e.g., no single treatment is appropriate for all individuals, treatment needs to be readily available, and effective treatment attends to multiple needs of the individual.

8. The two key treatment goals are motivation towards abstinence and creating a drug-free lifestyle. The secondary goals have to do with creating a better lifestyle by improving job, medical, psychiatric, emotional, and spiritual functioning.

Selection of a Program

9. Programs are chosen because of cost, familiarity, location, and convenience of access.

10. Diagnosis of the type and level of addiction is ascertained through interviews and diagnostic tests, particularly the Addiction Severity Index (ASI).

Broad Range of Techniques

11. Treatment options include medical model detoxification, social model detoxification, social model recovery, therapeutic communities, halfway houses, sober-living or transitional-living programs, partial hospitalization, and harm reduction programs.

12. About $1\frac{1}{2}$ million clients are treated each year for drug abuse. About 930,000 are in treatment on any given day.

13. Two million more hard-core abusers need treatment.

Beginning Treatment

14. Recognition and acceptance of addiction by the client is crucial to recovery. Breaking through denial is the crucial first step to begin treatment.

15. Denial can be overcome when the addict hits bottom or through a direct intervention (e.g., legal system, family, workplace supervisor, physician).

16. The elements of a formal intervention are love, a facilitator, intervention statements, anticipated defenses and outcomes, the intervention itself, and contingency plans.

17. The two major sources of referral are self-referral and legal referrals by the criminal justice system.

Treatment Continuum

18. Treatment starts with detoxification and escalates through initial abstinence, long-term abstinence, and recovery.

Detoxification

19. Drugs can be cleared from the system through abstinence, medication therapy, and psychosocial therapy.

20. Detoxification medications include clonidine, phenobarbital, methadone, antipsychotics, and others.

Initial Abstinence

21. This phase is supported through anticraving medications (e.g., naltrexone, bromocryptine, and nicotine replacements), individual counseling, and group therapy.

22. Environmental triggers cause relapse. Cue extinction or desensitization is one way to avoid relapse.

23. Psychosocial support to help the clients put their lives back in order is crucial: job support, physical and mental health problems support, and housing searches.

24. Acupuncture can help calm withdrawal symptoms and reduce craving to some extent.

Long-Term Abstinence

25. Addicts must accept that treatment for addiction is a lifelong process and that chemical dependency extends to a variety of substances not just the drug of choice.

26. Long-term abstinence uses individual and group therapy and 12-step groups to prolong abstinence.

Recovery

27. Recovery entails restructuring one's life, not just staying abstinent.

Outcome & Follow-Up

28. Follow-up is important not just to satisfy government funding agencies but to know which programs work.

29. Follow-up helps tailor programs to match the client and identify clients who need to be treated again for a relapse.

Individual vs. Group Therapy

30. Individual therapy, conducted by a trained counselor, helps the recovering client address specific issues.

31. Some individual therapies include cognitive-behavioral therapy, reality therapy, psychodynamic therapy, and aversion therapy.

32. Group therapy can be facilitated, peer, 12-step, educational, topic-specific, or targeted.

33. Various 12-step groups, such as Alcoholics Anonymous, Narcotics Anonymous, and Overeaters Anonymous, use sponsors, spirituality, and the power of people telling their own stories to teach a clean and sober lifestyle.

34. There are a number of errors that novice counselors make in groups, e.g., unrealistic view of group treatment, self-disclosure confusion, and failure to plan in advance.

Treatment & the Family

35. Addiction affects the whole family, so good treatment should involve the whole family.

36. There are a number of family treatment approaches including the family systems approach and the family behavioral approach.

37. Codependency and enabling, whereby family members support the addict in his or her addiction, must be addressed in treatment.

38. Adults who were raised in addictive households carry many of their problems into adulthood and must face those problems in treatment.

39. Groups such as Al-Anon, Nar-Anon, and ACoA help support and educate the family and friends of alcoholics and addicts.

Drug-Specific Treatment

40. Most people coming in for treatment are polydrug abusers even though they have a drug of choice.

41. Stimulant detoxification often initially presents treatment professionals with symptoms of psychosis and paranoia.

42. Anticraving medications and therapy help overcome anergia, euthymia, and craving in stimulant treatment.

43. Because smoking addiction involves nicotine craving, nicotine replacement therapies help taper tobacco craving.

44. Heroin and other opioid treatments usually need medications to soften withdrawal during detoxification.

45. Methadone maintenance is a harm reduction therapy that substitutes a controlled opioid for an illicit, problem-causing street opioid.

46. Alcohol or sedative-hypnotic withdrawal can be life-threatening unless assisted with medical therapy that includes an antiseizure medication like phenobarbital.

47. Peer groups and 12-step groups are vital to both long-term abstinence and recovery from alcoholism or any other addiction.

48. Talk-downs with emotional support and time for the drug to leave the body are the usual treatments for bad trips due to LSD or other psychedelics. Antipsychotic or antianxiety medications are also used when needed.

49. There has been a steady increase in people going into treatment for marijuana. The majority of referrals are court ordered.

50. The majority of inhalant abusers are under 20 years old compared to older abusers of other drugs.

51. The treatment for behavioral addictions is similar to the treatment for drug addiction.

52. Sufficient facilities and personnel for treating compulsive gamblers are sorely lacking. With 7.5 million problem gamblers, there are only a handful of inpatient facilities and a lack of truly qualified treatment personnel.

53. Early intervention for eating disorders is very important in treating anorexia, bulimia, and compulsive overeating.

54. Sexual addiction is most often treated by getting at the psychodynamic roots of their compulsion.

55. Internet addiction includes cybersexual addiction, cyberrelationship addiction, information overload, and computer addiction (playing games).

Target Populations

56. Treatment must be tailored to specific groups based on gender, sexual orientation, age, ethnic group, job, and even economic status.

57. Treatment for men should be different than for women. Men often blame external forces and women often blame themselves for their addiction.

58. Older Americans are a fast-growing segment of those with a substance abuse problem and are often reluctant to seek treatment because they view addiction as a character flaw not a disease.

59. Treatment for different ethnic groups requires bilingual and/or bicultural counselors, culture-specific treatment protocols, and acceptance of addiction as a disease.

60. African American, Hispanic American, Asian American, and Native American treatment often requires strong family involvement and accessing the spiritual roots of each community.

61. Little research has been done on treatment for those with physical disabilities. Too much focus is on the handicap and not on the addiction.

62. There is also a lack of research for the gay and lesbian communities. The use of alcohol and drugs lowers inhibitions and abets the spread of disease including HIV. Homophobia and heterophobia complicate substance abuse treatment.

Treatment Obstacles

63. Being aware of the emotional maturity of clients, doing follow-ups

to make sure the client is following the program, resolving goal conflicts, and making sure there are enough treatment slots to meet demand are vital to the effectiveness of treatment programs.

Medical Intervention Developments

64. The fastest-growing field in treatment is the development of new medications. Drugs are being developed for: detoxification, replacement therapy (agonist effects), antagonist effects, vaccines, mixed agonist-antagonist effects, anticraving, metabolism modulation, restoration of homeostasis, and modulation of drug effects and antipriming.

65. There are three steps in the new drug development process including preclinical research and development, clinical trials, and permission to market.

REFERENCES

AA. (1935, 1976). *Alcoholics Anonymous: The Story of How Many Thousands of Men and Women Have Recovered From Alcoholism.* New York: Alcoholics Anonymous World Services, Inc.

ADAM (Arrestee Drug Abuse Monitoring). (1999). *Annual Reports on Adult and Juvenile Arrestees, 1992, 1993, 1994, 1995, 1996, 1997, 1998.* National Institute of Justice. *http://www.adam-nij.net.*

Adger, H. (1998). Children in alcoholic families. Family dynamics and treatment issues. In A. W. Graham & T. K. Schultz, T. K. (Eds.), *Principles of Addiction Medicine* (2nd ed., pp. 1111–1114). Chevy Chase, MD: American Society of Addiction Medicine, Inc.

Allen, J. P., Eckardt, M. J., & Wallen, J. (1988). Screening for alcoholism: techniques and issues. *Public Health Reports, 103,* 586–592.

Amen, D. (1998). *Interview on May 18, 1998 with author.*

American Pharmacist. (1999). Top-selling drugs in the United States. *American Pharmacist Magazine, January, 1999.*

American Psychiatric Association (APA). (1994). *Diagnostic and Statistical Manual of Mental Disorders* (4th ed.). Washington, DC: American Psychiatric Association Press.

Ball, J. C., & Ross, A. (Eds.). (1991). *The Effectiveness of Methadone Maintenance Treatment.* New York: Springer-Verlag.

Barter, T. et al. (1996). Rapid opiate detoxification, *American Journal of Drug and Alcohol Abuse, 22*(4), 489–495.

Belenko, S. (1998). Research on drug courts: a critical review. *National Drug Court Institute Review, 1*(1). *http://www.drugcourt.org/.*

Bensen, L. (1879). *Fifteen Years in Hell: An Autobiography* (pp. 128–129). Indianapolis: Douglas & Carlon.

Berenson, D, Schrier, E. W. (1998). Current Family Treatment Approaches. In A. W. Graham & Schultz, T. K. (Eds.), *Principles of Addiction Medicine* (2nd ed., pp. 1115–1125). Chevy Chase, MD: American Society of Addiction Medicine, Inc.

Bickelhaupt, E. E. (1995). Alcoholism and drug abuse in gay and lesbian persons: A review of incidence studies. In R. J. Kus, *Addiction and Recovery in Gay and Lesbian Persons* (pp. 5–14). New York: Harrington Park Press.

Blum, K. et al. (1989). Cocaine therapy: The reward-cascade link. *Professional Counselor, Jan/Feb 1989,* 27.

Blume, S. B. (1997). Pathological Gambling. In J. H. Lowinson, P. Ruiz, R. B. Millman, & J. G. Langrod (Eds.), *Substance Abuse: A Comprehensive Textbook* (3rd ed., pp. 330–337). Baltimore: Williams & Wilkins.

Boucher, T. A., Kiresuk, T. J., & Trachtenberg, A. I. (1998). Alternative Therapies. In A. W. Graham & Schultz, T. K. (Eds.), *Principles of Addiction Medicine* (2nd ed., pp. 371–394). Chevy Chase, MD: American Society of Addiction Medicine, Inc.

Brubaker, M. (1997). *Compulsive Gambling & Recovery.* Casa Grande, AZ: Brubaker & Associates (800/636-9788).

Byrne, A. (1998). Rapid opiate detoxification. *British Journal of Psychiatry, 172, 451, 316*(7126), 170.

Cabaj, R. P. (1997). Gays, lesbians, and bisexuals. In J. H. Lowinson, P. Ruiz, R. B. Millman, & J. G. Langrod (Eds.), *Substance Abuse: A Comprehensive Textbook* (3rd ed., pp. 725–732). Baltimore: Williams & Wilkins.

CALDATA Study. (1994). State of California.

Carrera, M. R. et al. (1996). *Nature, 378,* 727.

Carrol, J. E. (1980). Uncovering drug abuse by alcoholics and alcohol abuse by addicts. International. *Journal of Addiction, 15,* 591–595.

Carter, B. L., & Tiffany, S. T. (1999). Meta-analysis of cue-reactivity in addiction research. *Addiction, 94*(3), 327–340.

CDC. (1996). *Cigarette smoking related mortality.* TIPS, Office on Smoking and Health, Centers for Disease Control and Prevention, unpublished data.

Chang, G., Kosten, T. R. (1997). Detoxification. In J. H. Lowinson, P. Ruiz, R. B. Millman, & J. G. Langrod (Eds.), *Substance Abuse: A Comprehensive Textbook* (3rd ed., pp. 377–381). Baltimore: Williams & Wilkins.

Cherrington, E. (1920). *The Evolution of Prohibition in the United States.* Westerville, Ohio: The American Issue Press.

Childress, A. R., McClellan, A. T., Ehrman, R., & O'Brien, C. P. (1988). Classically conditioned responses in opioid and cocaine dependence: A role in relapse? In B. A. Ray (Ed.), *Learning Factors in Substance Abuse, NIDA Research Monograph 84.* Rockville, MD: National Institute on Drug Abuse.

Crowe, A. H., & Reeves, R. (1994). *Treatment for Alcohol and Other Drug Abuse: Opportunities for Coordination.* Technical Assistance Publication Series #11. Rockville: SAMHSA.

Cucchia, A. T. et al. (1998). Ultra-rapid opiate detoxification using deep sedation with oral midazolam: Short and long-term results. *Drug & Alcohol Dependency, 52*(3), 243–250.

Daley, D. C., & Marlatt, G. A. (1997). Relapse Prevention. In J. H. Lowinson, P. Ruiz, R. B. Millman, & J. G. Langrod (Eds.), *Substance Abuse: A Comprehensive Textbook* (3rd ed., pp. 458–467). Baltimore: Williams & Wilkins.

Dascus, J. (1877). *Battling with the Demon: The Progress of Temperance.* Saint Louis: Scammell & Company.

Dodd, M. H. (1997). Social model of recovery: Origin, early features, changes, and future. *Journal of Psychoactive Drugs, 29*(2), 133–140.

DOJ (Department of Justice). (1999). *Bureau of Justice Statistics Special Report: Substance Abuse and Treatment, State and Federal Prisoners, 1998, http://www.ojp.usdoj.gov/bjs/crimoff.ht m#recidivism.*

Dole, V. P., & Nyswander, M. E. (1965). A medical treatment for diacetylmorphine (heroin) addiction: A clinical trial with methadone hydrochloride. *Journal of the American Medical Association, 193*(8), 646–650.

Dorchester, D. (1884). *The Liquor Problem in All Ages.* NY: Phillips & Hunt.

Dyer, C. (1998). Addict died after rapid opiate detoxification. *British Medical Journal, 316*(7126), 170.

Eickelberg, S. J., & Mayo-Smith, M. F. (1998). Management of sedative-hypnotic intoxication and withdrawal. In A. W. Graham & T. K. Schultz, T. K. (Eds.), *Principles of Addiction Medicine* (2nd ed., pp. 441–454). Chevy Chase, MD: American Society of Addiction Medicine, Inc.

Ethridge, R. M., Craddock, S. G., Dunteman, G. H., & Hubbard, R. L. (1995). Treatment services in two national studies of community-based drug abuse treatment programs. *Journal of Substance Abuse, 7*, 9–26.

Ferry, L. H. (1992). *Circulation, 86*, 1671.

Fiorentine, R. (1999). After drug treatment: Are 12-step programs effective in maintaining abstinence? *American Journal of Drug and Alcohol Abuse, 25*(1), 93–116.

Fox, B. S. et al. (1996). *Nature Medicine, 2*, 1129.

Gatch, M. B., & Lal, H. (1998). Pharmacological treatment of alcoholism. *Progress in Neuro-Psychopharmacology and Biological Psychiatry, 22*(6), 917–944.

Gawin, F. H., Khalsa, M. E., & Ellinwood, Jr., E. (1994). Stimulants. In M. Galanter & H.D. Kleber (Eds.), *Textbook of Substance Abuse Treatment* (pp. 111–139). Washington, DC: American Psychiatric Press.

Geller, A. (1997). Comprehensive treatment programs. In J. H. Lowinson, P. Ruiz, R. B. Millman, & J. G. Langrod (Eds.), *Substance Abuse: A Comprehensive Textbook* (3rd ed., pp. 425–429). Baltimore: Williams & Wilkins.

Gerstein, D. R., Johnson, R. A., Harwood, H., Fountain, D., Suter, N., & Malloy, K. (1994). *Evaluating Recovery Services: The California Drug and Alcohol Treatment Assessment (CALDATA).* Sacramento, CA: California Department of Alcohol and Drug Programs (Executive Summary: Publication No. ADP94–628). (Copies of study available by calling 916/327–3728).

Gerstein, et al. (1997). *National Treatment Improvement Evaluation Study (NTIES) Final Report.* Rockville, MD: Center for Substance Abuse Treatment.

Goldbloom, D. S. (1999). *Pharmacotherapy of bulimia nervosa.* Medscape: Clarke Institute of Psychiatry.

Goodman, A. (1997). Sexual addiction. In J. H. Lowinson, P. Ruiz, R. B. Millman, & J. G. Langrod, (Eds.), *Substance Abuse: A Comprehensive Textbook* (3rd ed., pp. 340–354). Baltimore: Williams & Wilkins.

Gorski, T. T. (1993). *Addictive Relationships: Why Love Goes Wrong in Recovery.* Independence, MO: Herald House/Independence Press.

Grinrod, R. (1886). *Bacchus: An Essay on the Nature, Causes, Effects and Cure of Intemperance.* Columbus, OH: J&H Miller (Reprint of the 1840 edition).

Haight-Ashbury Clinic. (1996). Examination of clinic records.

Hanson, G., & Venturelli, P. (1998). Regulating the development of new drugs, Appendix B, in *Drugs and Society* (5th ed., p. 494), Sudbury, MA: Jones and Bartlett.

Harden & Wardson. (1996). Addiction: Are states preying on the vulnerable? *Washington Post, 3/4/96.*

Hayner, G., Galloway, G., & Wiehl, W. O. (1993). Haight-Ashbury Free Clinics' drug detoxification protocols - Part 3: benzodiazepines and other sedative-hypnotics. *Journal of Psychoactive Drugs, 25*(4), 331–335.

Heather, N. (1989). Brief intervention strategies. In R. K. Hester, & W. R. Miller (Eds.), *Handbook of Alcoholism Treatment Approaches* (pp. 93–116). Boston: Allyn and Bacon.

Heinemann, A. W. (1993). An introduction to substance abuse and physical disability. In A. W. Heineman (Ed.), *Substance Abuse & Physical Disability* (pp. 3–9), Binghamton, NY: The Haworth Press, Inc.

Heinemann, A. W. (1997). Persons with disabilities. In J. H. Lowinson, P. Ruiz, R. B. Millman, & J. G. Langrod (Eds.), *Substance Abuse: A Comprehensive Textbook* (3rd ed., pp. 716–724). Baltimore: Williams & Wilkins.

Hird, S., Khuri, E. T., Dusenbury, L., & Millman, R. B. (1997). Adolescents. In J. H. Lowinson, P. Ruiz, R. B. Millman, & J. G. Langrod (Eds.), *Substance Abuse: A Comprehensive Textbook* (3rd ed., pp. 683–692). Baltimore: Williams & Wilkins.

Horvath, A. T. (1997). Alternative support groups. In J. H. Lowinson, P. Ruiz, R. B. Millman, & J. G. Langrod (Eds.), *Substance Abuse: A Comprehensive Textbook* (3rd ed., pp. 390–395). Baltimore: Williams & Wilkins.

Hubbard, R. L., Craddock, S. G., Flynn, P. M., Anderson, J., & Etheridge, R. M. (1997). Overview of one-year follow-up outcomes in DATOS. *Psychology of Addictive Behavior,* in press.

Institute of Medicine. (1990). *Treating Drug Problems* (Vol. 1). Washington, DC: National Academy Press.

Johnson, V. E. (1986). *Intervention.* Minneapolis: Johnson Institute Books.

Keane, T. M. et al. (1984). *Journal of Clinical Psychology, 40*, 340.

Keane, T. M., & Fuller, R. K. (1986). *Journal of the American Medical Association, 256*, 1449.

Kelly, J. (Ed.) (1991). *San Francisco lesbian, gay and bisexual alcohol and other drugs needs assessment study: Vol. I.* Sacramento, CA: EMT Associates, Inc.

Kessler, R. C., McGonagle, K. A., Zhao, S. et al. (1994). Lifetime and 12-month prevalence of DSM-II-R psychiatric disorders in the United States. Results from the National Comorbidity Survey. *Archives of General Psychiatry, 51,* 8–19.

Kominars, S. B. (1995). Homophobia: The heart of the darkness. In R. J. Kus (Ed.), *Addiction and Recovery in Gay and Lesbian Persons.* New York: Harrington Park Press.

Lewis, J. A., Dana, R. Q., & Blevins, G. A. (1994). *Substance Abuse Counseling.*

(2nd ed.). Pacific Grove, CA: Brooks/ Cole Publishing Company.

Liepman, M. R. (1998). The Family in Addiction. In A. W. Graham & T. K. Schultz, T. K. (Eds.), *Principles of Addiction Medicine* (2nd ed., pp. 1093–1110). Chevy Chase, MD: American Society of Addiction Medicine, Inc.

Lorenzi, P. et al. (1999). Searching for a general anaesthesia protocol for rapid detoxification from opioids. *European Journal of Anaestheriology*, 10, 719–727.

Lowinson, J. H., Payte, J. T., Salsitz, E. A., Joseph, H., Marlon, I. J., & Dole, V. P. (1997). Methadone Maintenance. In J. H. Lowinson, P. Ruiz, R. B. Millman, & J. G. Langrod (Eds.), *Substance Abuse: A Comprehensive Textbook* (3rd ed., pp. 405–414). Baltimore: Williams & Wilkins.

Mahon, N. (1997). Treatment in prisons and jails. In J. H. Lowinson, P. Ruiz, R. B. Millman, & J. G. Langrod (Eds.), *Substance Abuse: A Comprehensive Textbook* (3rd ed., pp. 455–457). Baltimore: Williams & Wilkins.

Marlatt, G. A. (1995). Relapse prevention: theoretical rational and overview of the model. In G. A. Marlatt & Gorden, J. (Eds.), *Relapse Prevention: A Self-Control Strategy in the Maintenance of Behavior Change*. New York: Guiford.

Marlatt, G. A., & Tapert, S. F. (1993). Harm reduction: Reducing the risks of addictive behaviors. In J. S. Baer, G. A. Marlatt, & R. J. McMahon (Eds.), *Addictive Behaviors Across the Lifespan* (pp. 243–271). Newbury Park, CA: Sage Publications.

Mason, B. J., Ritvo, E. C., Morgan, R. O., et al. (1994). A double-blind, placebo-controlled pilot study to evaluate the efficacy and safety of oral nalmefene HCL for alcohol dependence. *Alcoholism, 18*, 1162–1167.

Mathias, R. (1999). The basics of brain imaging. *NIDA Notes, 11*(5).

McClellan, A. T., Grissom, G. R., Zanis, D., Randall, M., Brill, P., & O'Brien, C. P. (1997). Problem-service "matching" in addiction treatment: A prospective study in four programs. *Archives of General Psychiatry, 54*, 730–735.

McElroy, S. L., Soutullo, C. A., & Goldsmith, R. J. (1998). Other impulse control disorders. In A. W. Graham & T. K. Schultz (Eds.), *Principles of Addiction Medicine* (2nd ed.). Chevy Chase, MD: American Society of Addiction Medicine, Inc.

Mecca, A. M. (1997). Blending policy and research: The California Outcomes Study. *Journal of Psychoactive Drugs, 29*(2), 161–164.

Mersy, D. J. (1991). Interventions for recovery in drug and alcohol addiction. In N. S. Miller (Ed.), *Comprehensive Handbook of Drug and Alcohol Addiction* (pp. 1063–1077). New York: Marcel Dekker, Inc.

Meuller, M. D. (1999). NIDA-supported researchers use brain imaging to deepen understanding of addiction. *NIDA Notes, 11*(5).

Meuller, M. D., & Wyman, J. R. (1997). Study sheds new light on the state of drug abuse treatment nationwide (DATOS). *NIDA Notes, 12*(5).

Miller, W. R. (1998). Researching the spiritual dimensions of alcohol and other drug problems. *Addiction, 93*(7), 979–990.

Miller, W. R., & Hester, R. K. (1989). Treating alcohol problems: Toward an informed eclecticism. In R. K. Hester, & W. R. Miller (Eds.), *Handbook of Alcoholism Treatment Approaches* (pp. 3–13). Boston: Allyn and Bacon.

Morris, S. (1995). Harm Reduction vs. disease model: Challenge for Educators. Presented at Boston Conference: *International Coalition of Addiction Studies Educators (*INCASE).

Muffler, J., Langrod, J. G., Richardson, J. T., & Ruiz, P. (1997). Religion. In J. H. Lowinson, P. Ruiz, R. B. Millman, & J. G. Langrod (Eds.), *Substance Abuse: A Comprehensive Textbook* (3rd ed., pp. 492–295). Baltimore: Williams & Wilkins.

Nace, E. P. (1997). Alcoholics anonymous. In J. H. Lowinson, P. Ruiz, R. B. Millman, & J. G. Langrod (Eds.), *Substance Abuse: A Comprehensive Textbook* (3rd ed. pp. 383–389). Baltimore: Williams & Wilkins.

NDATUS. (1994). *National Drug and Alcoholism Treatment Unit Survey*. Bethesda, MD: SAMHSA.

Netaddiction. (2000). What is Internet addiction? Center for On-Line Addiction. *http://netaddiction.com*.

NIAAA. (1997). *Ninth Special Report to the U.S. Congress on Alcohol and Health*. U.S. Department of Health and Human Services, National Institute on Alcohol Abuse and Alcoholism.

Nielsen, B., Nielsen, A. S., Wrae, O. (1998). Patient-treatment matching improves compliance of alcoholics in outpatient treatment. *Journal of Nervous and Mental Disease, 186*(12), 752–760.

NIH (National Institutes of Health). (1999). *Principles of Drug Addiction Treatment*. National Institute on Drug Abuse. NIH Publication No. 99-4180. *http://www.nida.nih.gov/PODAT/PODATindex.html*.

NIH-CDC. (1997). *Effective medical treatment of heroin addiction. NIH Consensus Statement*. Bethesda, MD: National Institutes of Health.

O'Boyle, M., & Brandon, E. A. (1998). Suicide attempts, substance abuse, and personality. *Journal of Substance Abuse Treatment, 15*(4), 353–356.

O'Brien, C. P. (1997). A range of research-based pharmacotherapies for addiction. *Science, 278*(5335), 66–70.

O'Farrell, T. J., & Cowles, K. S. (1989). Marital and family therapy. In R. K. Hester, & W. R. Miller (Eds.), *Handbook of Alcoholism Treatment Approaches* (pp. 183–205). Boston: Allyn and Bacon.

O'Malley, S. S., Jaffe, A. J., Chang, G., Schottenfeld, R. S., Meyer, R. E., & Rounsaville, B. (1992). Naltrexone and coping skills therapy for alcohol dependence. *Archives of General Psychiatry, 49*, 881–887.

ONDCP. (1999). *National Drug Control Strategy: 1999*. Washington, DC: Office of National Drug Control Policy.

Osborn, L., Bristow, L., Hoffman, N., McClellan, T., & Love, C. (1998). *Physician Leadership on National Drug Policy*.

Payte, J. T. (1997) Methadone maintenance treatment: The first thirty years. *Journal of Psychoactive Drugs, 29*(2), 149–154.

Payte, J. T., & Zweben, J. E. (1998). Opioid maintenance therapies. In A. W. Graham & Schultz, T. K. (Eds.), *Principles of Addiction Medicine* (2nd ed., pp. 557–570). Chevy Chase, MD: American Society of Addiction Medicine, Inc.

Peele, S. (1995). Controlled Drinking Versus Abstinence. *Encyclopedia of Drugs and Alcohol* (Vol.1, pp. 92–97). New York: Simon & Schuster Macmillan.

Perez-Arce, P, Carr, K. D., & Sorensen, J. L. (1993). Cultural issues in an outpatient program for stimulant abusers. *Journal of Psychoactive Drugs, 25*(1), 35–44.

Pomeranz, B. (1987). Scientific basis of acupuncture. In *Acupuncture: Textbook and Atlas*. Berlin: Springer-Verlag.

PRO. (1999). A checklist of symptoms leading to relapse. *Pharmacists Rehabilitation Organization Newsletter, 3*(1).

Public Health Service. (1999). *Mental Health: A Report of the Surgeon*

General. http://www.surgeongeneral. gov/library/mentalhealth/home.html.

Raine, A., Phil, D., Lencz, T., Bihrle, S., LaCasse, L., & Colletti, P. (2000). Reduced prefrontal gray matter volume and reduced autonomic activity in anti-social personality disorder. *Archives of General Psychiatry, 57,* 119–127.

Regier, D., Narrow, W., & Rae, D. (1999). Personal communication based on *Epidemiologic Catchment Area Study* and the *National Comorbidity Study.*

Reid, M. S., Mickalian, J. D., Delucchi, K. L., Hall, S. M., & Berger, S. P. (1999). An acute dose of nicotine enhances cue-induced cocaine craving, *Drug and Alcohol Dependence, 49,* 95–104.

Ricaurte, G. A., Seiden, L. S., & Schuster, C. R. (1984). Further evidence that amphetamines produce long-lasting dopamine neurochemical deficits by destroying dopamine nerve fibers. *Brain Research, 303,* 359–364.

Rose, J. E., Behm, F. M., Westman, E. C., et al. (1994). Mecamylamine combined with nicotine skin patch facilitates smoking cessation beyond nicotine patch treatment alone. *Clinical Trials Therapy, 56,* 86–99.

Ruiz, P., & Langrod, J. G. (1997), Hispanic Americans. In J. H. Lowinson, P. Ruiz, R. B. Millman, & J. G. Langrod (Eds.), *Substance Abuse: A Comprehensive Textbook* (3rd ed., pp. 705–712). Baltimore: Williams & Wilkins.

Rustin, T. A. (1998). Management of nicotine withdrawal. In A. W. Graham & T. K. Schultz (Eds.), *Principles of Addiction Medicine* (2nd ed., pp. 571–582). Chevy Chase, MD: American Society of Addiction Medicine, Inc.

Saitz, R., Mulvey, K. P., Plough, A., & Samet, J. H. (1998). Physician unawareness of serious substance abuse. *American Journal of Drug and Alcohol Abuse, 23*(3), 343–354.

SAMHSA (Substance Abuse and Mental Health Services Administration). (1998, 1999). *Substance Abuse and Mental Health Statistics Source Book, 1998.* Rockville, MD: National Clearinghouse for Alcohol and Drug Information (NCADI). http://www.samhsa.gov.

SAMHSA/TEDS. (1999). *Treatment Episode Data Sets 1992–1997.* Office of Applied Studies. http://www.samhsa. gov.

Schnoll, S. (1993). Prescription medication in rehabilitation In A. W. Heineman (Ed.), *Substance Abuse & Physical Disability* (pp. 79–91), Binghamton, NY: The Haworth Press, Inc.

Schuckit, M. A. (1994). Goals of treatment. In M. Galanter, & H. D. Kleber, (Eds.), *Textbook of Substance Abuse Treatment,* (pp. 3–10). Washington, DC: American Psychiatric Press.

Senft, R. A. (1991). Experience with clonidine-naltrexone for rapid opiate detoxification. *Journal of Substance Abuse Treatment, 8*(4), 257–259.

Sher, K. J. (1997). Psychological characteristics of children of alcoholics. *Alcohol Health & Research World, Children of Alcoholics, 21*(3), 247–254.

Shulman, A., Jagoda, J., Laycock, G., & Kelly, H. (1998). Calcium channel blocking drugs in the management of drug dependence, withdrawal and craving. A clinical pilot study with nephedipidine and verapamil. *Australian Family Physician, Supplement 1*:S, 19–24.

Simpson, D. D., Joe, G. W., Fletcher, B. W., et al. (1999). A national evaluation of treatment outcomes for cocaine dependence. *Archives of General Psychiatry, 57*(6), 507–514.

Smith, D. E., Buxton, M. E., Bilal, R., & Seymour, R. B. (1993). Cultural points of resistance to the 12-step recovery process. *Journal of Psychoactive Drugs, 25*(1), 97–108.

Smith, M. O., Brewington, V., Culliton, P., Lorenz, K. Y. Ng., Wen, H. I., & Lowinson, J. H. Acupuncture. In J. H. Lowinson, P. Ruiz, R. B. Millman, & J. G. Langrod (Eds.), *Substance Abuse: A Comprehensive Textbook* (3rd ed., pp. 91–100). Baltimore: Williams & Wilkins.

Snyder, E. et al. (1999). Human neural stem cells advance distant prospect of reseeding damaged brain. *Nature Biotechnology, 1-25-99.*

Steiner, R. P., May, D. L., & Davis, A. W. (1982). Acupuncture therapy for the treatment of tobacco smoking addiction. *American Journal of Chinese Medicine, 10*(1–4), 107–121.

Stevens-Smith, P., & Smith, R. L. (1998). *Substance Abuse Counseling: Theory & Practice.* Upper Saddle River, NJ: Merrill.

Strain, E. C., Bigelow, G. E., Liebson, I. A., & Stitzer, M. L. (1999). Moderate vs.

high-dose methadone in the treatment of opioid dependence. *JAMA, 281,* 1000–1005.

Thompson, G. H., & Hunter, D. A. (1998). Nicotine replacement therapy. *Annals of Pharmacotherapy, 32*(10), 1067–1075.

Trice, H. M. (1995). Alcoholics Anonymous. In D. B. Heath (Ed.), *Encyclopedia of Drugs and Alcohol* (Vol.1, pp. 85–92). New York: Simon & Schuster Macmillan.

UFDS (1998). *Uniform Facility Data Set Survey, 1995–1997.* Bethesda, MD: SAMHSA.

Vaillant, G. E. (1995). *The Natural History of Alcoholism Revisited.* Cambridge: Harvard University Press.

Valenzuela, C. F., & Harris, R. A. (1997). Alcohol: Neurobiology. In J. H. Lowinson, P. Ruiz, R. B. Millman, & J. G. Langrod (Eds.), *Substance Abuse: A Comprehensive Textbook* (3rd ed., pp. 122–123). Baltimore: Williams & Wilkins.

Vocci, F. (1999). Medications in the pipeline. Presentation at CSAM Conference, *Addiction Medicine: State of the Art.* Marina Del Rey, CA, October, 1999.

Volpicelli, J. R., O'Brien , C., Alterman, A., & Hayashida, M. (1992). Naltrexone in the treatment of alcohol dependence. *Archives of General Psychiatry, 49,* 876.

Wen, H. L., & Cheung, S. Y. C. (1973). Treatment of drug addiction by acupuncture and electrical stimulation. *Asian Journal of Medicine, 9,* 23–24.

Westermeyer, J. (1997). Native Americans, Asians, and new immigrants. In J. H. Lowinson, P. Ruiz, R. B. Millman, & J. G. Langrod (Eds.), *Substance Abuse: A Comprehensive Textbook* (3rd ed., pp. 712–715). Baltimore: Williams & Wilkins.

White, W. L. (1998). *Slaying the Dragon: The History of Addiction Treatment and Recovery in America.* Bloomington, IL: Chestnut Health Systems/Lighthouse Institute.

Wiehl, W. O., Galloway, G., & Hayner, G. (1994). Haight-Ashbury Free Clinics' drug detoxification protocols, Part 4: Alcohol. *Journal of Psychoactive Drugs, 26*(1), 57–59.

Windle, Michael T. (1999). *Alcohol use among adolescents.* Thousand Oaks, CA: Sage Publications.

Mental/Emotional
Health & Drugs

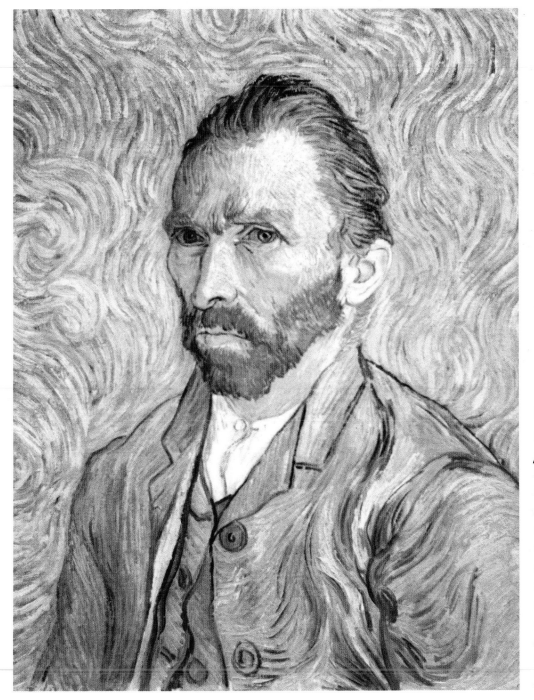

T he image of Vincent van Gogh was that of a person with mental illness and alcoholism who cut off his ear. Recently researchers at the University of California in Berkeley found that the liqueur absinthe, which contains the potent toxin alpha-thujone found in wormwood that can cause delirium, was partially responsible for his madness.
Musee D'Orsay, Paris. Courtesy of Simone Garlaund

MENTAL HEALTH & DRUGS

- **Introduction:** About 15% of adults with any mental disorder, such as depression, schizophrenia, bipolar disorder, or anxiety disorder, also have a co-occurring drug use disorder or drug-induced disorder.

  ◊ The neurotransmitters, receptor sites, and other brain mechanisms involved in mental and emotional problems and illnesses are the same ones affected by psychoactive drugs.

  ◊ Substance-related disorders are divided into substance use disorders and substance-induced disorders.

- **Determining Factors:** Heredity, environment, and the use of psychoactive drugs affect mental health in much the same way they affect drug use and addiction.

DUAL DIAGNOSIS OR THE MENTALLY ILL CHEMICAL ABUSER (MICA)

- **Definition:** The number of individuals suffering from both a substance abuse problem and a mental illness is growing. The decrease of inpatient mental facilities has magnified this problem.

- **Epidemiology:** There is a high incidence of mental imbalances among drug users and conversely many people with mental/emotional problems use drugs, often to self-medicate.

- **Patterns of Dual Diagnosis:** A mental illness can be preexisting, potential, or drug induced (temporary or permanent). Drug use can aggravate a mental illnesses or hide it.

- **Making the Diagnosis:** Because the direct effects as well as the withdrawal effects of drugs can mimic mental illnesses, diagnoses have to be initially tentative, i.e., "written in disappearing ink."

- **Mental Health (MH) vs. Chemical Dependency (CD):** The previous distrust between these two treatment communities has partly given way to cooperation and recognition of the duality of drug abuse and mental illness.

- **Psychiatric Disorders:** Major depression, schizophrenia, bipolar disorder (formerly called "manic-depression"), along with anxiety and personality disorders, are the most common psychiatric problems.

- **Treatment:** Mental illness and substance-related disorders have to be treated simultaneously or treatment will not be effective. Treatment can include individual therapy, group therapy, self-help groups, and psychiatric medications. Treatment takes place in a variety of facilities from outpatient to residential.

- **Psychiatric Medications:** Antidepressants, antipsychotics, bipolar medications, and antianxiety drugs are the principal medications used to control mental illnesses.

Drug, alcohol abusers likelier to suffer mental ills, study says

By Alison Bass
BOSTON GLOBE

BOSTON — Researchers said Wednesday that people who abuse alcohol or drugs are much more likely than nonabusers to suffer from pre-existing mental disorders, such as manic-depression, anxiety and schizophrenia.

"This study is one explanation for wh...

American Medical Association.

"If you get drug abusers detoxed and sober but fail to recognize their unde...-ing depression, they are much...
Good...
try t...
son...
ly us...
it. I...
...rs
ta...
...
...s
d...

an underlying psychiatric disorder.
For example, teen-agers who have a depressive or anxiety disorder are twi... ...kely to develop a ...r on.
...sting...
r tal...
...olof...
hile...
al i...
...een...
f p...
...ire...
su...
...l...
e...
...

Antidepressant use turns children into test subjects

By Tim Friend
USA TODAY

Children and adolescents are being widely prescribed new antidepressants by family physicians and pediatricians despite little scientific evidence that they are safe and effective for people under age 18, research suggests.

These new antidepressants, which include Prozac, are known as serotonin selective reuptake inhibitors, or SSRIs. The drugs are generally considered to be much more effective and safer than older types of antidepressants. But for treatment of depression, they are approved by the Food and Drug Administration only for adults because they have not been properly tested in children and adolescents.

Shrinks have high hopes for new drug

By LAURAN NEERGAARD
The Associated Press

WASHINGTON — The Food and Drug Administration approved a new drug for schizophrenia Tuesday that doctors say could help patients who don't respond to existing medicines.

Eli Lilly & Co.'s olanzapine, to be sold under the brand name Zyprexa, has not yet been adequately compared with existing medicines, so the FDA would not let the company advertise the drug as superior. But psychiatrists have high hopes for olanzapine because it is chemically similar to an older medicine that often proved best at controlling schizophrenia — except that many patients couldn't tolerate its side effects and thus had to take less effective drugs.

Federal study: Mentally ill inmates flood prison system

Cycle of poverty and incarceration touches many disturbed people who in the past would have been hospitalized

By FOX BUTTERFIELD
NEW YORK TIMES NEWS SERVICE

The first comprehensive study of the rapidly growing number of emotionally disturbed people in the nation's jails and prisons has found that there are 283,800 inmates with severe mental illnesses, about 16 percent of the total jail popula-

---

MENTAL HEALTH & DRUGS

INTRODUCTION

"I didn't think that I was a mentally ill person. I thought, 'Well, I'm a drug addict and I'm an alcoholic and if I don't drink and I don't use, then it should just be a simple matter of just changing my entire life; and I felt a little bit overwhelmed."

35-year-old man with major depression

Mental Health: A Report of the Surgeon General, released in December of 1999, states that of the 40 million Americans who experience any mental disorder such as schizophrenia, major depression, bipolar disorder, an anxiety disorder, or a personality disorder in the course of a year, about 15% (6 million) also experience a substance-related disorder (NIMH, 1999).

BRAIN CHEMISTRY

The interconnection between mental/emotional health and drug use is so pervasive that understanding this link gives us a valuable insight into the functioning of the human mind at all levels. The reason for the link is that the neurotransmitters affected by psychoactive drugs are the same ones involved in mental illness. Many people with mental problems are drawn to psychoactive drugs in an effort to rebalance their brain chemistry and control their agitation, depression, or other mental problems. The opposite is also true. For some people who abuse drugs, their chemistry becomes unbalanced enough to activate a preexisting mental illness, induce a new one, or mimic the symptoms of one (Barondes, 1993; Zimberg, 1999).

"I wound up preferring the heroin because I felt relaxed when I would snort it. I felt like I didn't have any troubles. I felt like I had some peace of mind and the drugs that were up, like 'speed' and cocaine, made me feel really anxious."

Recovering drug abuser with major depression

CLASSIFICATION OF SUBSTANCE-RELATED DISORDERS

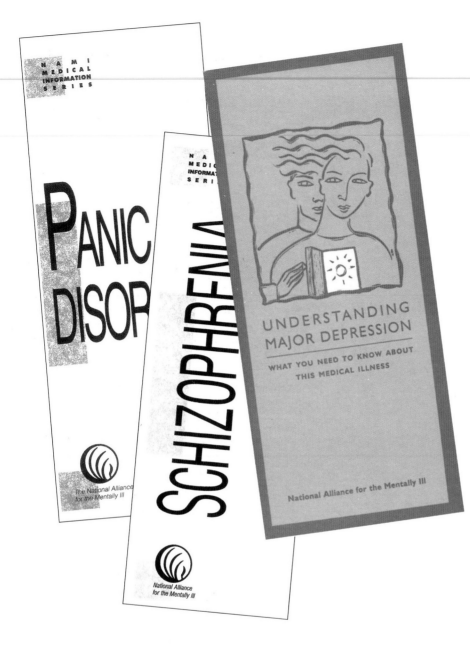

Substance-related disorders are classified in the *Diagnostic and Statistical Manual of Mental Disorders* (DSM-IV) as mental disorders. They are divided into two general categories: substance use disorders and substance-induced disorders (APA, 1994).

◇ **Substance use disorders** involve patterns of drug use and are divided into substance dependence and substance abuse. Note that the word "addiction" is not used.

Substance dependence is defined in the DSM-IV as "a maladaptive pattern of substance use, leading to clinically significant impairment or distress as manifested by tolerance, withdrawal, the need for larger amounts, unsuccessful efforts to cut down use, an expenditure of large amounts of time to get, use, and think about the drug, and continued use despite adverse consequences."

Substance abuse is defined as "recurrent substance use that results in disruption of work, school, or home obligations, recurrent use in physically hazardous situations, recurrent legal problems, and continued use despite adverse consequences."

◇ **Substance-induced disorders** include conditions that are caused by use of the specific substances. These conditions usually disappear after a period of abstinence, however, some of the damage can last weeks, months, years, and even a lifetime. Substance-induced disorders include intoxication, withdrawal, and certain mental disorders, e.g., delirium, dementia, amnestic disorder, psychotic disorder, mood disorder, anxiety disorder, sexual dysfunction, and sleep disorder. The substances specifically defined in the DSM-IV include alcohol, amphetamines, *Cannabis,* cocaine, hallucinogens, inhalants, opioids, PCP, and sedative-hypnotics.

This connection between mental health and drug use can be seen in the similarity between the symptoms of psychiatric disorders and the direct effects of psychoactive drugs or their withdrawal effects. For example,

◇ cocaine or amphetamine **intoxication** mimics mania, anxiety, or paranoid psychosis;

◇ cocaine or amphetamine **withdrawal** looks like major depression;

◇ excessive use of downers, including heroin, alcohol, or prescription sedative-hypnotics, mimics the depressed mood, lack of interest in surroundings, and excessive sleep characteristic of a major depression;

◇ psychedelic drugs, e.g., mescaline and LSD, mimic the delusional hallucinations associated with a major psychosis;

◇ the direct effects of the stronger stimulants, followed by the exhaustion of withdrawal, mimic a bipolar illness that includes manic delusions and then depression.

(Adapted from Goldsmith & Ries, 1998)

DETERMINING FACTORS

The three main factors that affect the central nervous system's balance and therefore a human being's susceptibility to mental illness as well as addiction are heredity, environment, and the use of psychoactive drugs (Brady, Myrick, & Sonne, 1998; Brehm & Khantzian, 1997). For example, nearly every neurochemical system involved in the onset and treatment of depression is also found to be abnormal in substance use and induced disorders (McDowell, 1999).

HEREDITY & MENTAL BALANCE

How does heredity affect our mental health? Research has already shown a close link between heredity and schizophrenia, bipolar disorder, depression, and even anxiety. For example, the risk of a child developing schizophrenia is somewhere between 0.5% to 1% if the child has no close-order relatives with schizophrenia. On the other hand, if the child has a close relative who has schizophrenia, the risk jumps, on average, to about 15% (Gottesman, 1991).

"My great uncle's got schizophrenia and my nephew's got schizophrenia. He's got it really bad because he can't control his fits. I didn't think about that growing up, only when I started hearing the voices. Then I thought, 'Hmm, just like my nephew.'"
28-year-old man with schizophrenia

Some individuals are born with a brain chemistry that gives them a susceptibility to certain mental illnesses. If the genetically susceptible brain chemistry is then stressed by a hostile environment or psychoactive drug use, then that person has an increased likelihood of developing mental illness. If there is a very heavy genetic susceptibility, it may not take as severe an environmental stress. If there's a low genetic susceptibility, it will take a much stronger environmental or chemical stress to trigger the illness.

Even if there is a high susceptibility with strong environmental stresses, mental illness may still not develop. In fact the statistics show that even if there is a close relative with major depression, five out of six children or siblings will not develop that illness (Goodwin & Jamison, 1990; Kendler & Diehl, 1993).

"In my family, my mom, my aunt, and my grandmother were diagnosed as manic-depressive. It runs in the family. It didn't have anything to do with drugs. It was just a lack of something in the brain."
16-year-old boy in treatment for bipolar illness

Genetic links for behavioral disorders, such as binge-eating disorder, compulsive gambling, and even attention deficit disorder, have been found in twin surveys. Identical twins raised by two different sets of foster parents often exhibit the same character traits and behaviors regardless of their different environments (Zickler, 1999).

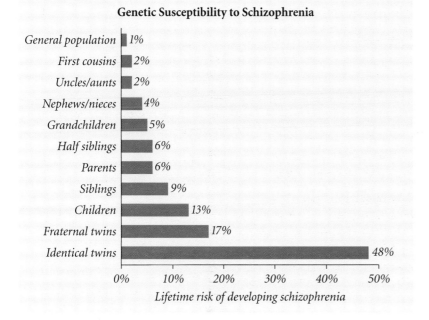

Genetic Susceptibility to Schizophrenia

General population	1%
First cousins	2%
Uncles/aunts	2%
Nephews/nieces	4%
Grandchildren	5%
Half siblings	6%
Parents	6%
Siblings	9%
Children	13%
Fraternal twins	17%
Identical twins	48%

Lifetime risk of developing schizophrenia

Figure 10-1 •

The risk of developing schizophrenia if a genetic relation has the disease varies with the number of shared genes. Second-degree relatives, such as nieces, only share 25% of one's genes, a parent shares 50% of the genes, and an identical twin shares 100% of the genes.

(Gottesman, 1991)

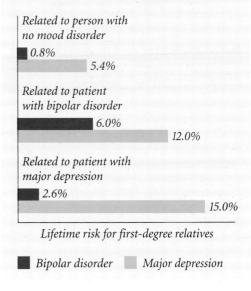

Genetic Susceptibility to Bipolar Disorder or Major Depression

Related to person with no mood disorder
0.8%
5.4%

Related to patient with bipolar disorder
6.0%
12.0%

Related to patient with major depression
2.6%
15.0%

Lifetime risk for first-degree relatives

■ *Bipolar disorder*　　■ *Major depression*

Figure 10-2 •

Risk of developing depression or bipolar disorder if a first-degree relative (parent, sibling, child) has the disease.

(Adapted from Goodwin & Jamison, 1990)

It is important to remember that heredity affects susceptibility to drug or behavioral addiction in much the same pattern that heredity affects susceptibility to mental illness. In other words, a high genetic susceptibility does not mean that that mental illness or addiction will occur, only that there is a greater chance that it will occur.

"Both my parents were alcoholics. My brother's an addict and alcoholic. I basically followed in my father's footsteps; the drinking, the running around, losing wives, kids, all that."
38-year-old recovering alcoholic with major depression

The relationship between heredity, mental illness, and psychoactive drugs can be seen by examining the connections between the neurotransmitter dopamine, the drug cocaine, and schizophrenia. Heredity can affect the formation of dopamine receptor sites and the ability of the brain to produce dopamine. Schizophrenia seems to be caused in part by the brain having too much dopamine. Cocaine stimulates the release of dopamine and so long-term use can induce a schizophrenic-like psychosis. With both the real psychosis and the drug-induced psychosis, excess dopamine seems to be a key element (Blum, Braverman, Cull, et al., 2000).

ENVIRONMENT & MENTAL BALANCE

The neurochemistry of persons subject to extreme stress can be disrupted and unbalanced to a point that their reactions to normal situations are different than those of most people. For example, continued stress depletes nor-epinephrine and that can cause depression. Such persons may react to stressful situations by running away, falling apart, becoming extremely angry, or using psychoactive drugs. The stressors they respond to don't even have to be dramatic. They can merely be normal family expectations. For such individuals, mother saying, "It's eleven o'clock, I wish you'd get out of bed," can result in extreme anger that further disrupts

the child's balance and, therefore, thought processes and, therefore, behavior (Barondes, 1993).

"My parents had a troubled marriage and they'd fight and argue and my mother would be beaten. I think maybe some of the rage and some of the anger manifested itself into the schizophrenia or just triggered it. After my schizophrenia became really prominent, I noticed that little things, like on-the-job stress, would get to me and I'd move on because it would trigger all sorts of problems."
28-year-old dually diagnosed client

Abuse and sexual molestation can be major negative environmental factors. Well over 50% of the young adults who are psychotic and have a problem with drugs experienced at least one form of abuse when they were children and the rate is much greater for women than for men. In addition over 75% of female addicts have suffered incest, molestation, or physical abuse as a child or adult (Zweben, 1996).

"My dad beat my mom when he was under the influence of alcohol. He was an alcoholic. He also beat my older sister and me. When he came home, I was always running and hiding. A few years after he left the family, I was molested. I was screwed up but when I went into the service, I found that the marijuana and the heroin I abused in 'Nam kept my emotions under control."
Vietnam veteran with posttraumatic stress disorder

The same environmental factors that can trigger a susceptibility to drug abuse can trigger mental/emotional problems.

PSYCHOACTIVE DRUGS & MENTAL BALANCE

Along with heredity and environment, the use of psychoactive drugs, the third factor that affects our mental balance, can deplete, increase, mimic,

or otherwise disrupt the neurochemistry of the brain. This disruption of brain chemistry can lead to drug addiction, mental illness, or both.

If a nervous system is impacted by enough psychoactive drugs, any individual may develop mental/emotional problems but it is the predisposed brain that is more likely to have prolonged and permanent difficulties. There is no set time for this to happen. The process may take years or, as in the case of psychedelic drugs, just one use can release an underlying psychopathology (Seymour & Smith, 1993). The brain that is not predisposed is the one most likely to return to its predrug functioning during abstinence.

"Apparently, through three generations of my family and our alcohol drinking or opium smoking, I inherited a tendency to manic-depression that wouldn't awaken under just alcohol abuse. It took a more exotic drug, one that was a little bit beyond the range of a northern European family to bring out my illness and that was marijuana."
45-year-old client with bipolar disorder

Every time a psychoactive substance enters the brain, it changes the equilibrium and the neurochemistry has to adjust. When exposure to that drug has ended, the brain does not always return to its original balance. For example, a brain predisposed to major depression can be pushed into activating that mental problem by heavy abuse of alcohol and sedative-hypnotics or withdrawal from stimulant drugs (Drake & Mueser, 1996). A brain predisposed toward schizophrenia can be activated by psychedelic abuse. One mental disorder, hallucinogen-persisting perception disorder, is marked by the transient recurrence of disturbances of perception (flashbacks) similar to those experienced while actually using an hallucinogen. The symptoms are disturbing and can cause impairment in everyday functioning. However, they may disappear in a few months or may last for years.

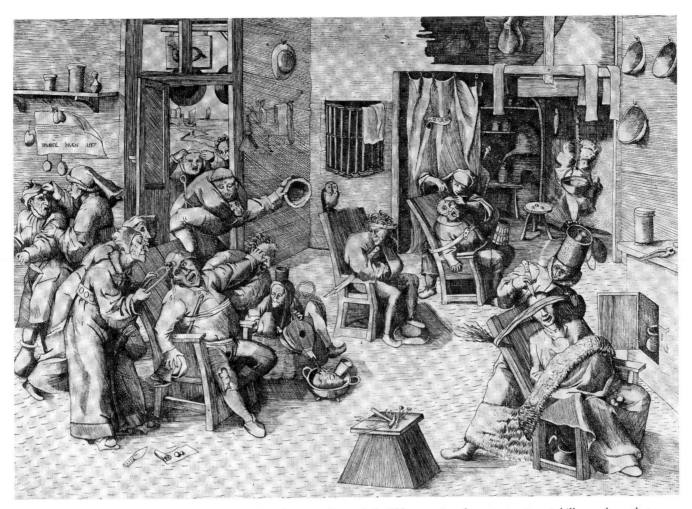

This illustration, The Extraction of the Stone of Madness *by Pieter Bruegal, the Elder, a satire of ways to treat mental illness, shows that even 300 years ago, people thought that mental illness was caused by something physical inside the brain. Compare this to the modern view of many clinicians that mental illness can be treated by changing the neurochemistry inside the brain through psychotropic medications.*

Courtesy of the National Library of Medicine, Bethesda

DUAL DIAGNOSIS OR THE MENTALLY ILL CHEMICAL ABUSER (MICA)

DEFINITION

A growing number of chemically dependent individuals are under treatment for dual diagnosis. This is usually defined as "a person having both a substance abuse problem and a diagnosable significant psychiatric problem." What this means is that a cocaine user might also have a psychosis or paranoia even when not using drugs. An alcoholic might have severe depression that persists even when clean and sober.

The term "dual diagnosis" is more common in the chemical dependency treatment community. The term "MICA" (mentally ill chemical abuser) is preferred in the mental health treatment community. Other terms like "comorbidity," "concurrent disorder," and "double trouble" have also been used to refer to this condition (Evans & Sullivan, 1990).

"After more than 30 years of use, when I gave up the codeine and the Valium® in treatment, I started to remember the pain. You know the first

thing that flashed through my mind was my uncle's face when he was hurting me real bad when I was 10. I hadn't remembered it for 32 years."
45-year-old woman with major depression

"This previous client is a case where so much is being revealed as she gets clearer and clearer [from the drugs]. Clearly she's had major depression at different times and there may be an underlying personality disorder but

there is also some posttraumatic stress disorder in the sense that she is discovering, as she is getting clean and sober, an incest background and severe physical abuse from many persons, which she was not even aware of while when she was using. She wasn't just anesthetizing her feelings, she didn't even recognize the beatings as beatings."
Marjorie Colvin, Haight-Ashbury Detox Clinic counselor

The psychiatric disorders most often used to define dual diagnosis when seen in combination with drug use disorders are

◇ schizophrenia (thought disorder),

◇ major depression (mood disorder),

◇ bipolar disorder (mood disorder).

Many treatment professionals also include other mental problems within the scope of dual diagnosis:

◇ anxiety disorders, e.g., panic disorders, obsessive-compulsive disorders, posttraumatic stress disorder;

◇ organic disorders;

◇ attention deficit/hyperactivity disorder (AD/HD);

◇ developmental disorders;

◇ somatoform disorders;

◇ rage disorders;

◇ personality disorders, especially borderline personality disorder and antisocial personality disorder;

◇ eating disorders;

◇ impulse control disorders such as compulsive gambling.

(Levin & Donovan, 1998; Lilenfield & Kaye, 1996; Lowenstein, 1991; McElroy, Soutullo, & Goldsmith, 1998; O'Conner & Ziedonis, 1998; Salloum & Daley, 1994; Schuckit, 1996)

"I have this illness, mental illness, with manic-depression and when I take the alcohol, my functioning isn't as clear cut, not as sharp as say the average person who isn't suffering any mental problems."
52-year-old client with dual diagnosis

It is important to distinguish between having symptoms and having a major psychiatric disorder. Everyone feels blue and sad sometimes. Everyone has the capacity for grief and loneliness but this does not mean that a person is medically depressed, requiring medication or psychiatric treatment. It's really a question of severity and persistence of these symptoms (Woody, 1996; Zimberg, 1999). The connection is real. One study found the chance of major depression and alcoholism in women was substantially higher and probably was mainly the result of genetic factors but environment still had an influence (Kendler, Heath, Neale, & Eaves, 1993).

EPIDEMIOLOGY

In a study published in *Journal of the American Medical Association* (*JAMA*), 44% of alcohol abusers and 64.4% of other substance abusers actually admitted for treatment had, in addition to their drug problem, at least one serious mental illness (Regier, Farmer, Rae, et al., 1990). Certain drugs increase the likelihood of mental illness. For example, 3/4 of cocaine abusers had a diagnosable mental disorder as did 1/2 of all compulsive marijuana users. Many were self-medicating their psychiatric disorders with street drugs (Kessler, McGonagle, Zhao, et al., 1994).

"I believe I had depression all along, even before I started using, and so through alcohol, marijuana, and even heroin, I was treating that depression."
Dual diagnosis client

Conversely 29% of all mentally ill people had a problem with either alcohol or other drugs (Merikangas, Stevens, & Fenton, 1996). The overlap is even greater with certain mental disorders. Sixty-one percent of people with manic-depressive illness and 47% of people with schizophrenia also had a problem with substance abuse. Finally, in prisons, the prevalence of a psychiatric illness when the prisoner had an addictive disorder was a remarkable 81% (Beeder & Millman, 1997).

PATTERNS OF DUAL DIAGNOSIS

Depending on which drug is used and how it is used, psychoactive substances can be related to four different patterns of dually diagnosed patients.

PREEXISTING MENTAL ILLNESS

One kind of dual diagnosis involves the person who has a clearly defined mental illness and then gets involved in drugs; for example, the teen with major depression who discovers amphetamines. Here the drugs are often used to self-medicate symptoms of the mental illness.

"My mom asked my little brother if he thought I'd been depressed a lot in my life and he said I'd been depressed ever since he could remember. The 'speed' got me out of it except when I was coming down."
16-year-old boy

POTENTIAL MENTAL ILLNESS

Another kind of dual diagnosis associated with the use of psychoactive drugs occurs when there might be an underlying psychiatric problem that isn't fully developed as yet. There is neither clear-cut depression nor clear-cut schizophrenia before drug use begins. There may be some unusual thought patterns but these are not significant enough to be recognized as a mental illness. When that person starts to use psychoactive drugs, the effects of those substances activate or accelerate the development of the underlying mental disturbance.

"I think it was about six years ago when I had a suspicion of being a manic-depressive but I was so drunk, I really didn't know what was wrong with me. And when I quit using drugs,

I just felt horrible, even worse than I had before, like I was dying."
38-year-old dual diagnosis client

PERMANENT DRUG-INDUCED MENTAL ILLNESS

The third kind of dual diagnosis happens when there isn't a preexisting problem. However, as a result of years of use or some extreme reaction to the drug, the user develops a chronic psychiatric problem because the toxic effects of the drug permanently disrupt the brain chemistry (Ziedonis & Wyatt, 1998; Drake & Mueser, 1996).

"My initial flip out was in 1986 after snorting 'crank' for six weeks straight, about a half gram a day. Three weeks later I had my first manic episode. Later they put me on Haldol® and then lithium. I have three diagnoses: amphetamine psychosis, psychotic depressive, and manic-depressive."
28-year-old client

TEMPORARY DRUG-INDUCED MENTAL ILLNESS

There is a fourth condition that is not really dual diagnosis that occurs when the drug itself or withdrawal from the drug causes a transient depression, temporary psychosis, or other apparent mental illness. The imbalance in the brain chemistry in this type of diagnosis is usually temporary and with abstinence the mental illness will disappear within a few weeks to a year. This is not true dual diagnosis but only a temporary condition resulting from the toxic effects of the drug on the central nervous system (Seymour & Smith, 1993; Walker, 1992).

"This 'speed' run's only been 13 days but I get these sores and I get paranoid and real crazy. After I come down it'll be weird. It will take weeks to get back into shape. And all that other crap will disappear."
43-year-old heavy IV methamphetamine addict

MAKING THE DIAGNOSIS

ASSESSMENT

When people see a relative or friend acting oddly and having trouble coping with everyday life over a prolonged period, they don't know whether they should ascribe that difficulty to relationship problems, trouble at home, drug use, or mental illness. Substance abuse and mental health professionals have the same problem, as is evident from the variations in diagnoses cited above. Thus when assessing mental illness in a substance abuser, a general rule used by both mental health and substance abuse treatment professionals is that the initial diagnosis should be tentative or as one psychiatrist said, "The diagnosis should be written in disappearing ink because as the drug clears, the symptoms may change."

"The doctor told me that a person who drank 25 years like me would probably take a year to clear. That was one reason that I never figured out that I was manic-depressive. I didn't notice it. I figured I was depressed because I was drunk all the time."
35-year-old man

Since many mental symptoms can be a temporary result of drug toxicity or drug withdrawal, an early diagnosis may merely be drug toxicity rather than dual diagnosis. Thus the prudent chemical dependency clinician treats all dangerous symptoms but holds off making a psychiatric diagnosis until the drug user has had time to get sober, out of a state of drug intoxication, and beyond drug withdrawal (Senay, 1997).

Other factors that may influence the diagnosis include:

◇ the expertise of the clinician doing the diagnosis;

◇ the severity of the psychiatric disorder;

◇ the perspective of the assessment team, whether from the mental health or the chemical dependency treatment community;

◇ the population studied, e.g., the prevalence of dual diagnosis in a homeless drug-abusing population is greater than that seen in a group of school teachers.

Reasons for Increased Diagnoses

There are several possible reasons why the numbers of dually diagnosed clients on the streets seem dramatically higher in the 1990s than during the '60s and '70s. These include

◇ the diminishing number of inpatient mental health facilities (Fig. 10-3) due to nationally decreasing mental health budgets, decreasing mental health coverage by HMOs

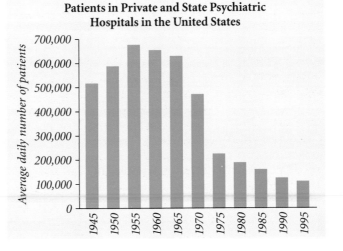

Patients in Private and State Psychiatric Hospitals in the United States

Average daily number of patients

Figure 10-3 •
The psychiatric hospital census has gone down while the overall numbers of people diagnosed with mental illnesses has gone up.

and other insurance programs, and misguided governmental policies on mental health support;

◊ increased prescribing of more effective medications for depression and psychosis, so more clients are treated on an outpatient basis;

◊ increased reliance, in general, on outpatient mental health facilities.

(Smith, Lawlor, & Seymour, 1996; Soderstrom, Smith, Dischinger, et al., 1997)

There are other somewhat less obvious reasons for the increase.

◊ The increasing numbers and greater expertise of licensed professionals working in the field of chemical dependency treatment have resulted in a greater recognition and documentation of dual diagnosis.

◊ Increased abuse of cocaine and amphetamines has also increased the numbers of patients with dual diagnosis. Since strong stimulants are more toxic to brain chemistry than most substances, except possibly inhalants and alcohol, those with fragile brain chemistry are more likely to be pushed over the edge into chronic neurochemical imbalance and mental illness (Keller & Dermatis, 1999).

◊ Finally, managed care and diagnosis-related group (DRG) payment for treatment services usually provide more financial incentives for the treatment of multiple medical and psychiatric problems than for just addiction treatment (Guydish & Muck, 1999). These payment structures can pressure some clinicians to over-diagnose mentally ill chemical abusers (MICA).

For these reasons an increasing number of people with psychiatric disorders have been forced to deal with their problems on an outpatient basis or on their own. Being detached from hospital supervision, clients are more likely to exhibit poor control of their prescribed medication, thus aggravating their mental problems and making them more likely to turn to street drugs for help. All of these factors have also

led to increases in mentally ill homeless people whose problems are exacerbated by the lack of a support system. The number of homeless in the United States in any given week is estimated at 500,000 to 600,000 and of those, about 85,000 have a mental illness and a substance abuse problem (Rahav, Rivera, Nuttbrock, et al., 1995). Many people with mental disorders self-medicate with alcohol, heroin, amphetamines, or dozens of other drugs in an attempt to control their symptoms. As a result, the incidence of dual diagnosis among compulsive drugs users and particularly among the homeless remains extremely high (Crome, 1999).

"I had used heroin to control my depression sort of as a mood stabilizer, and so withdrawing from it caused an even worse depression. When I came out of the sort of fog from the first five days of not having it, I felt better but the pink cloud feeling vanished quite quickly and was replaced with the depression that I was used to."
Patient with major depression in a halfway house

UNDERSTANDING THE DUALLY DIAGNOSED PATIENT

Understanding and adapting to the treatment complexities of the client with a mental health problem and a drug problem is a challenge for both drug treatment and mental health professionals.

"When I went into the hospital, I would tell them I had a problem, that I was on Valium® and codeine. The first thing they would then give me was a shot of Valium®. I told them that Valium® addiction was one of my problems. They still gave it to me."
40-year-old dually diagnosed woman

In the past, inability to treat a person who manifested both a drug and a mental problem, combined with an outright refusal to develop treatment strategies for the dually diagnosed client,

resulted in inappropriate and potentially dangerous interactions with clients. They were often shuffled aimlessly back and forth between the mental healthcare system and the chemical dependency system without receiving adequate treatment from either. Even though there's been an increase in facilities that address the dually diagnosed client, inappropriate care is all too often still the rule rather than the exception. Budget considerations and lack of expertise have much to do with this problem.

Substance abuse treatment facilities do not usually want these patients because they see them as too disorganized and too disruptive or, in many cases, too inattentive to participate in group therapy, which is frequently the core element of treatment. Psychiatric treatment centers also avoid these patients because they're perceived as chemically dependent, disruptive, and manipulative. They also frequently relapse into active substance abuse that interferes with medications used to treat mental illnesses (Wu, Kouzis, & Leaf, 1999).

MENTAL HEALTH (MH) VS. CHEMICAL DEPENDENCY (CD)

The following list contains eleven differences that have existed between the mental health treatment community and the chemical dependency treatment community. While certain differences continue, these two communities are moving toward a closer working relationship. An increasing number of facilities employ both mental health and chemical dependency staff employing a team approach to treatment. They offer on-site treatment for the dually diagnosed client or at least provide a cross-referral team approach to a separate mental health treatment provider.

1. Mental health (MH) used to say, "Control the underlying psychiatric problem and then the drug abuse will disappear." Chemical

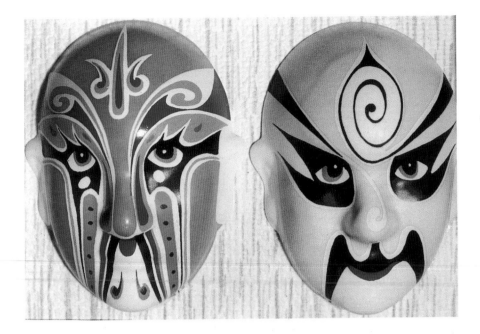

dependency (CD) used to say, "Get the patient clean and sober and the mental health problems will resolve themselves." While these statements might have been true in many cases, both disciplines are coming to recognize that perhaps 1/3 to 1/2 of their clients are legitimately dually diagnosed and require concurrent treatment of both the addiction and the underlying mental problems.

2. In the MH system, limited recovery from one's problems is more readily acceptable than in CD programs where most professionals believe that lifetime abstinence from all abused drugs, including alcohol and marijuana, along with a supporting program of recovery, are necessary to ongoing recovery.

3. Male dual diagnosis clients are more reluctant to seek help from the MH system than from CD treatment programs. This is probably because of the involuntary treatment aspects and the stigma of mental illness. Clients and their families hope that the problem is addiction from which they believe they can more fully recover than they can from mental illness. With women, the opposite is often the case. They experience greater

stigma about being an addict and will admit to an emotional or mental problem more readily than an addiction problem.

"I tell members of my family that I'm in a halfway house for drug addiction as opposed to mental health because it seems with drug addiction, I can get better but with mental health, people see it as a chronic, long-term problem."
19-year-old dually diagnosed male with major depression

4. MH relies more on medication to help the client function whereas CD programs tend to be divided between promoting a drug-free philosophy and substituting a less damaging drug such as methadone in a harm-reduction maintenance program. Alternatives to methadone, such as the opioid antagonist naltrexone that blocks the action of heroin and other opioids in the brain without producing psychoactive effects, provide a potentially viable alternative to drug maintenance that may be more acceptable to both drug-free adherents and the recovering community. Medically oriented programs, as opposed to drug-free CD programs, employ medications to help clients initially

detoxify before getting them into a long-term drug-free philosophy.

"I refused to take any psychiatric medication for a long time. I thought you had to be really crazy to take it and I thought that this was a big conflict that would limit my recovery. If I take medication, I'm a drug addict. But I'm glad I'm taking it now. I'm able to sleep and think better."
35-year-old client with major depression

5. MH uses case management, shepherding the client from one service to another whereas CD programs have traditionally emphasized self-reliance because they neither want to enable clients nor make clients transfer their dependence to the program. In spite of that, case management and an HMO approach to treatment are being adapted in many CD treatment programs. Cooperation may prove successful, with care providers availing themselves of services available from the other care providers. An addict can be referred to a psychiatrist while a client with depression and an addiction can be encouraged to go to 12-step groups to learn to live without drugs.

6. MH has a supportive philosophy whereas many CD programs will use confrontation techniques. A major conflict occurs when a patient is not responding to substance abuse treatment and has a severe psychiatric disorder or is HIV infected. One can't use the same threshold of bad behavior to terminate that patient from treatment as one would with a single diagnosis patient. In dual diagnosis programs, CD may put up with more drug-using behavior when a patient also has a psychiatric disorder and/or HIV infection. It is difficult to medically discharge patients being treated for mental illness or HIV when they relapse into drug addiction.

7. Both the MH system and the CD system have problems with sharing information because of confidentiality laws and regulations. In general, however, MH shares information with allied fields more readily than does CD.

8. In MH most of the treatment team is composed of professionals: social workers, psychiatrists, psychologists, and licensed counselors. In CD programs recovering addicts and professionals often work together. In 1940 in the United States, there were just 9,000 psychiatrists, social workers, and psychologists. Now there are more than 100,000 psychologists, 60,000 psychiatrists, and probably 150,000 social workers, not to mention those in allied mental health professions (Crome, 1999). The dual diagnosis clinics are likely to have staff from both disciplines.

9. MH relies heavily on scientific diagnosis and prognosis of an illness and is more process oriented. CD programs rely more heavily on the spiritual side of recovery and are more outcome oriented than process oriented. (Process oriented refers to a set of procedures that are implemented at specific times during the course of treatment to achieve positive benefits for the patient.) Cooperation is evident in recent years as MH has come to more actively utilize spiritual 12-step programs whereas CD has come to accept the neurochemical and psychiatric roots of addiction.

"All I can tell someone is, 'I have a problem. I don't know which way you're going to deal with it or tackle it but I have a problem, and I can't function, and I need help.'"
Dual diagnosis patient with major depression

10. MH pays a lot of attention to the idea of preventing the client from getting worse. In the past, CD programs, taking their cue from early 12-step fellowship beliefs, had more of a tendency to allow people to hit bottom in order to break through the denial of addiction. Most CD programs now see that approach as outmoded and dangerous. They rely more on intervention to break through denial and on diagnosis-driven treatment, using such criteria as those developed by the American Society of Addiction Medicine. Some clinics take both philosophies into account and recognize that both problems have to be treated. In particular, chemical dependency recognizes that relapse is a part of recovery and many centers allow more slips and relapses than they did in the past.

11. In MH, patient education and training are nonstructured and more individualized. In CD programs they are more standardized, concentrating on information about the drugs themselves, the progression of addiction, and the 12-step process. Presently, education techniques from both disciplines are used with the dually diagnosed client since both conditions need to be treated.

(Inaba, Cohen, & Holstein, 1996).

While the situation may be improving from the perspective of the MH treatment community, dual diagnosis has represented an almost insurmountable challenge to the clinical expertise of the staff of CD programs, especially to their assessment skills and even their underlying concept of recovery or sobriety. It can be difficult to differentiate an underlying psychiatric illness from a drug-induced mental illness. Often a diagnosis of mental illness is made too early in the treatment or assessment process, resulting in patients being referred to mental health programs that, all too often, then reject these individuals because of their drug abuse problems.

CD programs often lack or resist developing the expertise needed to diagnose and treat mental health problems. Fiscal and other limited resource problems prevent the expansion of their services to meet the needs of dually diagnosed clients, creating a tendency to establish mental health problems as an exclusionary criteria for treatment admission or continued treatment in many CD programs. Even CD programs with expertise in this area sometimes mistake psychoactive drug reaction symptoms for proof that there is an existing psychiatric diagnosis.

RECOMMENDATIONS

Research over the past decade recognizes that the dually diagnosed patient must be treated for both disorders and is best treated in a single program when appropriate resources are available (Kosten & Ziedonis, 1997). Where programs equipped to handle dual diagnosis cases are not available, CD programs need to establish linkages with MH service providers and vice versa, so that they can work together in providing the client with their combined treatment expertise. This is particularly important because when patients are admitted for treatment for psychiatric problems, they are more willing to acknowledge coexisting substance abuse problems and more receptive to facing the need for additional treatment (RachBeisel, Dixon, & Gearon, 1999). Each discipline needs to recognize that mental health and substance abuse treatment are both long-term propositions and therefore they need to establish both short-term and long-range services to address the problems of dual diagnosis (Minkoff & Regner, 1999). Recent research also suggests that incorporating behavioral (motivational) approaches to substance abuse treatment is more effective for the dually diagnosed client because the structure is better suited to overcoming cognitive difficulties that accompany schizophrenia and certain other mental illnesses (Drake, Mercer-McFadden, Mueser, McHugo, & Bond, 1998).

OTHER DIAGNOSES

Triple Diagnosis

"One of the biggest things that caused me the most anxiety is, you know, I'm HIV positive and I really started having problems with sleep. I found that out

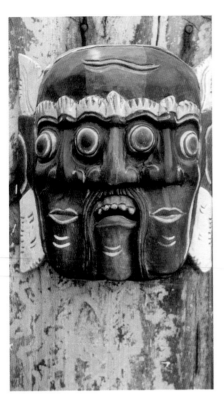

and I was really torn between cleaning up and staying clean or just going out and using. I felt like, 'Well, I'm going to die anyway, a nasty horrible death,' and I had nightmares and then my feelings surfaced to a point where a lot of other feelings came up about old stuff."

Recovering HIV-positive alcohol abuser with a general anxiety disorder

Triple diagnosis is defined as "the presence of an HIV infection in the dually diagnosed client." Persons with AIDS, an AIDS-related condition, an HIV-positive blood test, who are a partner of someone with AIDS require additional treatment expertise and specific services to effectively address their chemical dependency.

As the AIDS epidemic has progressed out of strictly gay and intravenous drug-using populations and into the cocaine- and other drug-using heterosexual populations, triple diagnosis is straining health department resources and further complicating treatment (Wechsberg, Desmond, Inciardi, et al., 1999).

"When we looked at the first 49 consecutive HIV-infected patients who came into our substance abuse services at San Francisco General Hospital, the bottom line was that 84% had some Axis I psychiatric diagnosis. A third had depressive disorders and another third had anxiety disorders. And 18% had organic brain syndromes, mild to moderate dementia, or organic psychosis."

Steven L. Batki, M.D., psychiatrist, Medical Director, SF General Hospital Substance Abuse Services (Batki, 1994)

Multiple Diagnoses

As the chemical dependency treatment community becomes more aware of other simultaneous disorders that complicate the treatment of addiction, it must be must willing to accept new challenges such as:

◇ multiple drug (polydrug) addiction;

◇ chronic pain in the chemically dependent individual;

◇ other medical disorders such as epilepsy, cancer, heart and kidney disease, diabetes, sickle cell anemia, and even sexual dysfunction.

Of special significance is the epidemic growth of hepatitis C and other severe liver diseases in chemically dependent patients. The prevalence of hepatitis C in IV drug users is now much greater than that of HIV.

In addition a variety of medical disabilities such as hearing or mobility impairment, social concerns including cultural attitudes toward chemical dependency and mental health treatment, and language barriers may also provide impediments to successful treatment.

Although not a disability issue, women, particularly those who are pregnant and/or parenting, have special treatment needs. For example, women process psychotropic medications differently than men and will have higher plasma levels for a given dose of a prescribed drug and therefore need lower doses (Zweben, 1996). In addition pro-

grams that treat the pregnant woman's addiction or her mental illness are usually organized separately, thus the pregnant addict with a mental illness can receive conflicting information (Grella, 1996). Finally the health risks to the fetus or newborn are greatly increased since both drug use and mental illness limit the normal nurturing qualities of the mother (Mallouh, 1996). These problems require the development of future drug programs that are holistic, use several modalities, and are multidisciplinary in order to meet the challenge of the evolving complicated clinical needs of the chemically dependent patient (Selwyn & Merino, 1997).

NOTE: The following sections will examine the different kinds of psychiatric disorders; discuss the relationship between heredity, environment, and psychoactive drugs as related to mental illness and drug addiction; then examine the various treatments available for the mentally ill substance-abusing patient, particularly the use of psychotropic medications in therapy.

PSYCHIATRIC DISORDERS

"A neurotic is the person who builds a castle in the air. A psychotic is the person who lives in it. And a psychiatrist is the person who collects the rent."

Anonymous

Overall about 21% of the U.S. population is affected by mental disorders during a given year (Table 10-1). Anxiety disorders are the most prevalent and then come mood disorders (especially depression). Schizophrenia is much scarcer but extremely debilitating (NIMH, 1999).

PRINCIPAL DUAL DIAGNOSIS DISORDERS

Although there are hundreds of mental illnesses as classified by the mental health community, the following are the principal ones that are most often associated with dual diagnosis.

TABLE 10–1   BRAIN DISORDERS IN ADULTS (1-YEAR PREVALENCE)

Diagnosis	Percent of U.S. Adults (18-54)	Percent of U.S. Adults (55 & Older)	Percent of Children & Adolescents
Schizophrenia	1.3%	0.6%	1.2%
Mood disorders	**7.1%**	**4.4%**	6.2%
Bipolar I disorder	1.1%	0.2%	
Major depressive episode	5.3%	3.8%	
Unipolar major depression	5.3%	3.7%	
Anxiety disorders	**16.4%**	**11.4%**	13.0%
Obsessive-compulsive disorder (OCD)	2.4%	1.5%	
Panic disorder	1.6%	0.5%	
Simple phobia	8.3%	7.3%	
Posttraumatic stress disorder (PTSD)	3.6%	—	
Agoraphobia	4.9%	4.1%	
Any brain disorder (one person might have multiple disorders)	**21.0%**	**19.8%**	**20.9%**

(NIMH, 1999; Shaffer, Fisher, Dulcan, et al., 1996)

Schizophrenia

Schizophrenia is a thought disorder believed to be mostly inherited. It is characterized by

◇ hallucinations (false visual, auditory, or tactile sensations and perceptions);

◇ delusions (false beliefs);

◇ an inappropriate affect (an illogical emotional response to any situation);

◇ autistic symptoms (a pronounced detachment from reality);

◇ ambivalence (difficulty in making even the simplest decisions);

◇ poor association (difficulty in connecting thoughts and ideas);

◇ poor job performance;

◇ strained social relations;

◇ an impaired ability to care for oneself.

The signs have to be present for at least six months for the diagnosis to be made (APA, 1994).

"I was hearing voices, and the voices wouldn't go away, and they followed me wherever I went. I got into creating scenarios as to who they were and what they were doing."

28-year-old man with schizophrenia

Schizophrenia usually strikes individuals in their late teens to early adulthood and can be with them for life, although occasionally there is spontaneous remission. Schizophrenia is extremely destructive to those with the illness as well as to their friends and families.

When diagnosing schizophrenia, clinicians try to determine which drugs are being used by the patient. When these are not taken into consideration, clinicians may end up with a false or incomplete diagnosis. Clinicians can accomplish this assessment by taking a thorough medical history, interviewing close friends and family, or by using urinalysis or hair analysis. Unfortun-

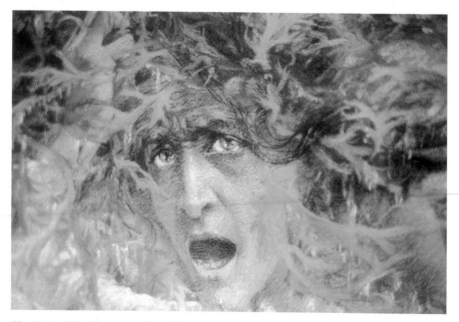

The Angry Wave *by Lucien-Lévy Dhurmer.*
Musee D'Orsay, Paris. Courtesy of Simone Garlaund

ately, a large percentage of drug and alcohol problems are still missed.

Several abused drugs mimic schizophrenia and psychosis, producing symptoms that can be easily misdiagnosed. Cocaine and amphetamines, especially when used to excess, will cause a toxic psychosis that is almost indistinguishable from a true paranoid psychosis. Steroids can also cause a psychosis. Drug-induced paranoia can be indistinguishable from true paranoia. Most drugs, but particularly the uppers, MDMA ("ecstasy") and related stimulant/hallucinogens, and even marijuana, can cause paranoia.

The psychedelics, such as LSD, peyote, psilocybin, and PCP, disassociate users from their surroundings, so all arounder abuse can also be mistaken for a thought disorder. Also withdrawal from downers can be mistaken for a thought disorder because of extreme

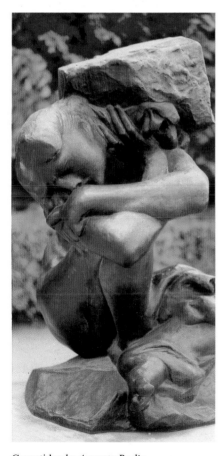

Caryatides *by Auguste Rodin*
Rodin Museum, Paris. Courtesy of Simone Garlaund

agitation. Many of the drug-induced psychiatric symptoms should disappear as the body's drug levels subside upon treatment and detoxification (Senay, 1997, 1998; Delgado & Mereno, 1998).

Major Depression

Major depression is classified as an affective disorder, along with bipolar affective disorder and dysthymia (mild depression). A major depression is likely to be experienced by 1 in 20 Americans during their lifetime. It is characterized by

◇ depressed mood,

◇ diminished interest and diminished pleasure in most activities,

◇ disturbances of sleep patterns and appetite,

◇ decreased ability to concentrate,

◇ feelings of worthlessness,

◇ suicidal thoughts.
(APA, 1994)

All of these symptoms may persist without any life situation to provoke them. For example, a patient with major depression may win a lot of money in a lottery and respond to it by being depressed.

For the diagnosis of major depression, these feelings have to occur every day, most of the day, for at least two weeks running. Organic causes, such as an illness or drug abuse, should rule out a diagnosis of major depression as should natural reactions to the death of a loved one, separation, or a strained relationship.

"The depression just came when it wanted to come. I just sat there and thought about something and I got depressed. The anger came because every male that has ever been in my life has beaten me or used me, you know, mentally and physically—not sexually thank goodness."
Severely depressed 17-year-old boy

The withdrawal symptoms that occur with most stimulant addictions (cocaine or amphetamine) and the

comedown or resolution phase of a psychedelic (LSD, "ecstasy") result in temporary drug-induced depression that is almost indistinguishable from that of major depression but will clear in time with the completion of withdrawal or comedown.

Bipolar Affective Disorder (formerly called "manic-depression")

This illness is characterized by alternating periods of depression, normalcy, and mania. The depression phase is described above. The depression is as severe as any depression seen in psychiatry. If untreated, many bipolar patients have frequent suicide attempts. The mania, on the other hand, is characterized by

◇ a persistently elevated, expansive, and irritated mood;

◇ inflated self-esteem or grandiosity;

◇ decreased need for sleep;

◇ the pressure to keep talking and being more talkative than usual;

◇ flight of ideas;

◇ distractibility;

◇ an increase in goal-directed activity or psychomotor agitation;

◇ excessive involvement in pleasurable activities that have a high potential for painful consequences (e.g., drug abuse, gambling, or inappropriate sexual advances often leading to unsafe sex).
(APA, 1994)

These symptoms can be severe enough to cause marked impairment in job, social activities, and relationships.

"The manic feeling is a real feeling of elation and euphoria. There's that grinding, angry sort of—I don't really get angry and violent, well I did in jail, but I don't really want to hurt anybody or anything. And as far as being depressed goes, I can really say I've only been depressed about three times, once to the point of being suicidal."
30-year-old man with a bipolar disorder

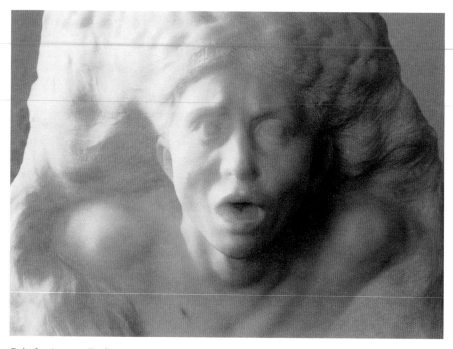

Pain *by Auguste Rodin.*
Rodin Museum, Paris. Courtesy of Simone Garlaund

Bipolar affective disorder usually begins in a person's 20s and affects men and women equally. Many researchers believe this disease is genetic in origin.

Toxic effects of stimulant or psychedelic abuse will often resemble a bipolar disorder. Users experience swings from mania to depression, depending upon the phase of the drug's action, the surroundings, and their own subconscious feelings and beliefs.

OTHER PSYCHIATRIC DISORDERS

Anxiety Disorders

Anxiety disorders are the most common psychiatric disturbances seen in medical offices. About 16% of adults (18–54 years of age) will experience an anxiety disorder in a given year (NIMH, 1999). There are a number of anxiety disorders.

1. **Panic disorder** with and without agoraphobia (fear of open spaces)

"I'd be waiting for my prescription at a drugstore and someone would just look at me and all of a sudden, my whole body just went inside itself and I started shaking. My heart was racing. I couldn't say anything. I crossed my arms in front of me and I was just in total panic. I couldn't move. All I did was shake inside like I was terrified. And my mind kept saying there's nothing to be scared of but I couldn't control it. I had no idea what really triggered it. My husband would come up and hold me and sit there and say, "Breathe." And after a couple of minutes I would be all right and I would use one of my pills for anxiety, Lorazepam®, a benzodiazepine. I think that my use of cocaine over a period of several years messed up my neurochemistry, particularly my adrenaline system. Then I was always afraid of being someplace where I would have an attack and not be able to get help."
50-year-old woman with a panic disorder

2. **Agoraphobia** without history of panic disorder (a generalized fear of open spaces)
3. **Social phobia** (fear of being seen by others acting in a humiliating or embarrassing way, e.g., fear of eating in public)
4. **Simple phobia** (irrational fear of a specific thing or place)
5. **Obsessive-compulsive disorder** (uncontrollable intrusive thoughts and irresistible often distressing actions, such as cutting one's hair or repeated hand washing)

"I had a number of obsessions. The obvious one right now is my hair. I cut my hair obsessively in a crew cut, constantly, by my own hand. The thought would just come into my mind. It was something I didn't really have control over. I would smoke marijuana almost as compulsively as I cut my hair."
Client with an obsessive-compulsive disorder

6. **Posttraumatic stress disorder (PTSD)** (persistent reexperiencing of the full memory of a stressful event outside usual human experience, e.g., combat, molestation, car crash). It is usually triggered by an environmental stimulus, e.g., a car backfires and the combat veteran's mind relives the stress and memory of combat. This disorder can last a lifetime and be very disabling (Reilly, Clark, Shopshire, Lewis, & Sorensen, 1994). One estimate is that 20% to 25% of those in treatment for substance use disorders may have PTSD (Brady, 1999)

"My father committed suicide—that I think was a lot. It left me angry and just the way people have abused me or they have used me. It's made me angry just the way I had to grow up. The way that I lived was dysfunctional—it was hard and when I'm on drugs and alcohol I don't care about myself. I don't care about anybody else."
22-year-old recovering polydrug abuser

7. **Generalized anxiety disorder** (unrealistic worry about several life situations that lasts for six months or longer)

8. **Other anxiety disorders** (e.g., acute stress disorder)

(APA, 1994)

Sometimes it is extremely difficult to differentiate the anxiety disorders. Many are defined more by symptoms than specific names. Some of the more common symptoms in anxiety disorders are shortness of breath, muscle tension, restlessness, stomach irritation, sweating, palpitations, hypervigilance, difficulty concentrating, and excessive worry. Often anxiety and depression are mixed together. Some physicians think that many anxiety disorders are really an outgrowth of depression (Gastfriend & Lillard, 1998).

Toxic effects of stimulant drugs and withdrawal from opioids, sedatives, and alcohol (downers) also cause symptoms similar to those described in anxiety disorders and can be easily misdiagnosed as such (Nunes, Donovan, Brady, & Guitkin, 1994). In one study of college students, the odds of having an anxiety disorder were much greater if alcohol abuse and dependence were present and the odds of having alcohol dependence were also greater if an anxiety disorder was present (Kushner, Sher, & Erickson, 1999).

Organic Mental Disorders

These are problems of brain dysfunction brought on by physical changes in the brain caused by aging, miscellaneous diseases, injury to the brain, or psychoactive drug toxicities. Alzheimer's disease, one example of an organic mental disorder, is where older people suffer the unusually rapid death of brain cells, resulting in memory loss, confusion, loss of emotions, and gradually the ability to care for themselves. Mental confusion from heavy marijuana use and various prescription drugs in an elderly patient may mimic symptoms of this disorder.

Developmental Disorders

These disorders, usually first diagnosed in infancy, childhood, or adolescence, include mental retardation, autism, communication disorders, and attention deficit/hyperactivity disorders. (*See Chapter 3 for more information on AD/HD.*) Heavy and frequent use of psychedelics like LSD or PCP can be mistaken for developmental disorders.

Somatoform Disorders

These disorders have physical symptoms without a known or discoverable physical cause and are likely to be psychologically caused, e.g., hypochondria (abnormal anxiety over one's health, accompanied by imaginary symptoms of illness). Cocaine, amphetamine, and other stimulant psychosis create a delusion that the user's skin is infested with bugs when no infection exists.

The Passive-Aggressive, Antisocial, Borderline, & Other Personality Disorders

These disorders are characterized by inflexible behavioral patterns that lead to substantial distress or functional impairment. Most of these personalities act out, that is, exhibit behavioral patterns that have an angry hostile tone, that violate social conventions, and that result in negative consequences. Anger is intrinsic to all three of these personality disorders, as are chronic feelings of unhappiness and alienation from others, conflicts with authority, and family discord. These disorders frequently coexist with substance abuse and are particularly hard to treat because of the acting out, which may include relapsing to drug use or creating a major disruption in their treatment setting (Smith & Seymour, 2000; Dimeoff, Comtois, & Linehan, 1998; Schuckit, 1986). One study found that close to 60% of those with substance use disorders had personality disorders, especially borderline personality disorder (Skodol, Oldham, & Gallaher, 1999).

Eating Disorders

These disorders, characterized by severe disturbances in eating behavior (*see Chapter 7*), include anorexia nervosa, bulimia nervosa, and binge-eating disorder. The roots of eating disorders are similar to those of drug use disorders and often coexist.

Other Disorders

There are dozens of other mental disorders including adjustment disorders, sleep disorders, sexual and gender identity disorders, and factitious disorders that can exist independently or in combination with other mental disorders and drug use disorders.

TREATMENT

The close association of unbalanced brain chemistry with the distorting effects of heredity, environment, and psychoactive drugs suggests that treatment of mental illness and/or addiction should be directed towards rebalancing the brain chemistry.

REBALANCING BRAIN CHEMISTRY

Heredity & Treatment

As of yet, we cannot alter a person's genetic code. As of yet, we can't change a person with alcoholic marker genes that signal a susceptibility to alcoholism, drug addiction, or other addictive behavior. As of yet, we can't decrease the genetic vulnerability of a teenager with a mother and grandmother who have schizophrenia. We can alert some people that they are more at risk for a certain mental illness, drug addiction, or other compulsive behavior (Blum et al., 2000). Hopefully current research in gene therapy that is aimed towards altering genetic factors will be a giant step in controlling hereditary factors.

Environment & Treatment

If we can't correct heredity, we can attempt to correct the environment that, in turn, can adjust brain chemistry. If people change where and how they live, they can avoid those stressors and environmental cues that keep them in a state

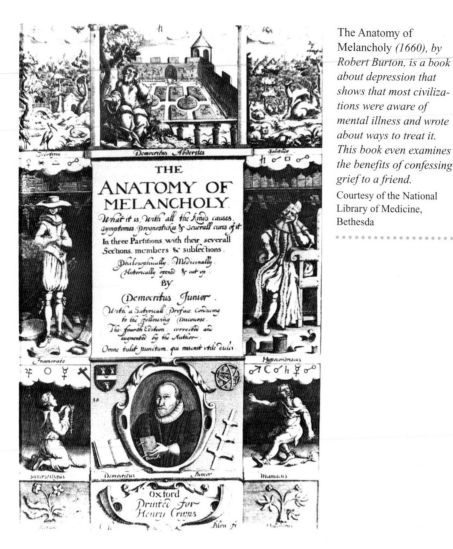

The Anatomy of Melancholy *(1660), by Robert Burton, is a book about depression that shows that most civilizations were aware of mental illness and wrote about ways to treat it. This book even examines the benefits of confessing grief to a friend.*
Courtesy of the National Library of Medicine, Bethesda

of turmoil, continually unbalance their neurochemistry, and make them more likely to abuse drugs, thereby intensifying their mental illness. For example, to help restore healthy ways of living, people can leave an abusive relationship, avoid their drug-using associates, get enough sleep, avoid situations that make them angry, seek out new friends in self-help groups to avoid isolation, and make sure they get good nutrition.

Hard as it might be, changing one's external environment is much easier than changing one's brain chemistry through manipulation of thoughts, feelings, or emotions (Seymour & Smith, 1987).

Psychotherapy, Individual Counseling, & Group Therapy

"Look into the depths of your own soul and learn first to know yourself, then you will understand why this illness was bound to come upon you and perhaps you will thenceforth avoid falling ill."
Sigmund Freud, 1924

Psychoanalysis and psychotherapy, which were originated by Sigmund Freud in the late 1800s, are a way of helping the dually diagnosed patient. They help clients explore their past to enable them to neutralize or minimize the emotional and neurochemical imbalance caused by heredity or the traumas and stresses of childhood, e.g., remembering sexual abuse that happened when they were young.

Individual or group therapy can also be effective but, by necessity, it has to be a long-term undertaking (even a lifetime project) to be truly effective in changing

individuals or at least in minimizing the damage they do to themselves (Davis, Klan, & Coyle, 1991; Zimberg, 1994).

"I go to Emotions Anonymous. I go there and it helps because I became a drug addict by not being able to deal with my emotions and my feelings."
25-year-old client

Psychoactive Drugs & Treatment

Finally, psychoactive drugs themselves can be used to treat mental illness. This form of treatment is attempted by both psychiatrists and by patients themselves who may self-medicate their condition with the use of abusable drugs. Of course there are dangers in self-medication. The uncontrolled use of street drugs, such as cocaine or some prescription medications like Ritalin®, can distort one's neurochemistry and thereby magnify or trigger mental problems.

"I took both alcohol and lithium for my manic-depression. The difference is that one is faster working. The alcohol works quickly, the lithium takes time to get there. But the alcohol caused other problems in my life in addition to my depression. I think I'll stick to the lithium."
50-year-old woman

There is an ever-expanding group of drugs called "psychotropic medications" (e.g., antidepressants, antipsychotics or neuroleptics, antianxiety drugs) that are prescribed by physicians to try to counteract neurochemical imbalance caused by mental illness or addiction and that help the dually diagnosed client lead a less destructive life. (The various psychotropic medications will be examined in detail later.)

The following Table 10-2 is a compilation of many of the ideas that have been covered in these pages regarding the relationship between brain chemistry, drug addiction, and mental illness.

Column 1 lists the neurotransmitters (the brain's messengers).

TABLE 10–2   THE RELATIONSHIP BETWEEN NEUROTRANSMITTERS, THEIR FUNCTIONS, STREET DRUGS, MENTAL ILLNESS, & PSYCHOTROPIC MEDICATIONS

COLUMN 1 Neurotransmitter	COLUMN 2 Normal Functions	COLUMN 3 Street Drugs That Disrupt the Neurotransmitter	COLUMN 4 Associated Mental Illnesses	COLUMN 5 Medications Used to Rebalance Neurotransmitters
Serotonin	Mood stability, appetite, sleep control, sexual activity aggression, self-esteem	Alcohol, nicotine, amphetamine, cocaine, PCP, LSD, MDMA ("ecstasy")	Anxiety, depression, bipolar disorder, obsessive-compulsive disorder	BuSpar®, tricyclic antidepressant, Prozac®, Zoloft®, tryptophan, Ritanserin®, Anafranil®, Paxil®
Dopamine	Muscle tone/control, motor behavior, energy, reward mech., attention span, pleasure, emotional stability, hunger/thirst/sexual satiation	Cocaine, nicotine, PCP, amphetamine caffeine, LSD, marijuana, alcohol, opioid	Schizophrenia, Parkinson's disease, attention deficit disorder	MAO inhibitors, Ritalin®, phenothiazine antipsychotics, thiazine antipsychotics, tyrosine, taurine, bromocryphine, amantadine, L-dopa
Norepinephrine and epinephrine	Energy, motivation, eating, attention span, pleasure, heart rate, blood pressure, dilation of bronchi, assertiveness, alertness, confidence	Cocaine, nicotine, amphetamine, caffeine, marijuana, MDMA, 2CB, CBR	Depression, bipolar disorder, anxiety, narcolepsy, sleep problems, attention deficit disorder	Tricyclic antidepressants, MAO inhibitors, phenothiazine, antipsychotics, prescription amphetamines, Ritalin®, clonidine, barbiturates, benzodiazepines, beta blockers (Propranelol®), tyrosine, d,l phenylalanine
Endorphin, enkephalin	Pain control, reward mechanism stress control (physical and emotional)	Heroin, other opioids, PCP, alcohol, marijuana	Schizophrenia, depression	Methadone, LAAM, Trexan®, buprenorphine, d,l phenylalanine
GABA (gamma aminobutyric acid)	Inhibitor of many neuro-transmitters, muscle relaxant, control of aggression, arousal	Alcohol, marijuana, barbiturates, PCP, benzodiazepines	Anxiety, sleep disorders, narcolepsy	Benzodiazepines, glutamine, modafinil (Provigil®, Cephalon®)
Acetylcholine	Memory, learning, muscular reflexes, aggression, attention, blood pressure, heart rate, sexual behavior, mental acuity, sleep, muscle control	Marijuana, nicotine, alcohol, PCP, cocaine, amphetamine, LSD	Alzheimer's disease, schizophrenia, tremors	Phenothiazine® antipsychotics, Artane®, Cogentin®, lecithin, choline
Cortisone, corticotrophin	Immune system, healing, stress	Heroin, cocaine	Schizophrenia, depression, insomnia, anxiety	Corticosteroids (Prednisone®, cortisone), ACTH, cortisol, metynapone
Histamine	Regulator of emotional behavior, sleep, inflammation of tissues, stomach acid, secretion, allergic response	Antihistamines, opioids	Depressive illness	Antihistamines, tricyclic antidepressants
Anandimide	Natural function is still unknown	Marijuana	Unknown	Marijuana antagonist

Column 2 describes the natural regulatory function of the neurotransmitters.

Column 3 lists the street drugs that strongly affect those neurotransmitters.

Column 4 describes the mental illnesses associated with the disrupted neurotransmitters.

Column 5 lists drugs used to correct the disruptions.

When studying the table, notice how many different neurotransmitters are affected by a single street drug, especially cocaine or alcohol. Also notice the physical and mental traits that are affected by a neurotransmitter and how a street drug affects those functions (Lavine, 1999).

Starting Treatment

With many dually diagnosed clients, it is hard to know where to start treatment. Do you start treating the mental illness or the addiction or do you treat them simultaneously right from the beginning?

Drug seems to help in treating PTSD

The Associated Press

NEW YORK — After watching one of his firemen die in the line of duty, fire Chief John Soave became withdrawn, had trouble sleeping and was bothered by flashbacks.

Doctors diagnosed him with post-traumatic stress disorder, a psychiatric condition once associated only with combat veterans but now

percent of Americans will suffer from post-traumatic stress at some point in their life.

As part of his treatment, Soave was prescribed Zoloft, a drug first approved in 1992 for depression

"It helped calm me down," s Soave, of Stoughton, Mass., who been taking Pfizer's once-a-day

Based on its early success, Zoloft later this year is expected to become the first prescription medication specifically approved by the federal government for post-traumatic stress.

Drug Administration

Jumpy mice give peek into anxiety

Scientists study brain chemistry

By JAMIE TALAN
Newsday

A strain of mice genetically bred to be nervous has been developed by a researcher who hopes the reticent rodents can provide answers about human anxiety.

Dr. Laurence Tecott, a psychiatrist at the University of California, San Francisco, created the anxious mice by blocking out a gene for a specific serotonin receptor.

Serotonin, a

> ❝❝We can't get into their heads to know what they are feeling. But this is pretty close to modeling the types

when in a new situation. Novelty is the last thing these animals want.

"We can't get into their heads to know what they are feeling," Tecott said. "But this is pretty close to modeling the types of symptoms we see in humans with these conditions."

The ultimate goal in creating animal models of anxiety is gaining the ability to design and test drugs that target this precise receptor system. Drugs that help alleviate symptoms of anxiety

Serotonin gene variant may cause depression

By JAMIE TALAN
Newsday

At a time when investigators are struggling to find genes for mental illness, Canadian scientists have uncovered the first evidence that people with a specific variant of the ene that manufactures serotonin ay be more vulnerable to depres-on and bulimia.

If this gene finding is replicated, ould lead to the first test to pre- who might be at risk for these avioral disorders. It may also er a hunt for medicines that d work directly on this gene he protein it makes.

Robert Levitan of the Center diction and Mental Health at iversity of Toronto has been ng for a biological explana-or depression and decided to look for clues in people with seasonal affective disorder (winter depression) and bulimia. He chose these disorders, because 12 percent

---

the booze or drugs, they should be able to engage in treatment but that's not always the case. A study of a number of dually diagnosed clients at a public hospital found that the majority were mildly to severely impaired and that they had difficulty participating in treatment. Reviewing screening exams on neurocognitive function at a veteran's hospital, researchers found that approximately 50% of the patients were mildly to severely impaired (Blume, Davis, & Schmaling, 1999).

For the treatment provider, what this means is the patient can repeat things but the information and therapy don't sink in. It takes from two weeks to six months after detoxification for reasoning, memory, and thinking to come back to a point where the dually diagnosed individual can begin to engage in treatment. Though the patient remains in treatment, treatment techniques have to be tailored to the person's ability to process the information that the doctor and staff are providing.

Developmental Arrest

Drug abuse and mental illness often result in the arresting of emotional development. Take the case of a young man in his late teens or early 20s who's fully grown and intelligent but has been using drugs since the age of 11 or 12 and has also had emotional and mental problems. This type of patient comes to treatment with all kinds of difficulties. One of the worst problems is that he's suffered developmental arrest at age 11 or 12, the point where most people begin to work through issues and stresses in their lives. Most people mature through all the struggles and go on to become adults but those who use drugs, who have avoided difficult emotions, and have not gone through that process of maturation will still experience all the emotions that they avoided five or six years ago.

"It's all those issues as a child that I seemed to take into my adulthood and they come out. I'd get my buttons

---

> *"I think that I start where the pain is. One patient, for example, couldn't talk about his marijuana use without talking about how depressed and suicidal he was. We addressed the pain, the pain being his massive depression, and then we enabled him, by doing that, to back off his marijuana use. In the case of another patient, she was in such a massively tormented state in terms of anxiety, panic, fear, and depression behind her use of benzodiazepines and codeine that we had to start detoxing immediately and we had to explain to her that we would be looking at the depression and the anxiety and probably medicating them as we detoxed her off her primary drugs of abuse."*
>
> Marjorie Colvin, Haight-Ashbury Detox Clinic counselor

A suicidal situation obviously needs to be attended to regardless of the cause. Similarly if patients are dangerous (homicidal or aggressive in some dangerous fashion) they have to be managed, often in an inpatient psychiatric facility. When the presentations are less malignant and less dangerous to self or others, then the treatment personnel generally ask, "What does it take to manage them?" The first rule of thumb is that the patient has to be somewhat cooperative and manageable. Patients in the midst of active drug abuse or a major psychiatric crisis are usually neither, so detoxification or emergency psychiatric treatment is often the first step.

Impaired Cognition

Unfortunately many clinicians involved in treatment believe that once dually diagnosed individuals put down

pressed. Someone gets me a little pissed off. You know, I really thought when I came into recovery I wouldn't be angry anymore. Well it took me almost three years in treatment to realize that anger is a legitimate feeling. It's how I deal with it today and how I used to deal with it. That's what I'm learning about."

30-year-old dually diagnosed client

What happens is that many dually diagnosed clients have the character traits that are normal in children but abnormal in adults, thus making treatment extremely difficult. Dr. Burt Pepper, a psychiatrist who treats young dually diagnosed clients, lists 11 of these characteristics.

1. They have a low frustration tolerance.

2. They can't work persistently for a goal without constant encouragement and guidance, partially because of their low tolerance for frustration.

3. They lie to avoid punishment.

4. They have mixed feelings about independence and dependence and then, feeling hostile about dependency, they test limits.

5. They test limits constantly because they haven't learned them yet or have rejected them.

6. Their feelings are expressed as behaviors. They cry, run away, and hit rather than talk, reason, explain, or apologize.

7. They have a shallow labile affect that means a shallowness of mood. Give a kid a toy, they laugh, take it away, they cry.

8. They have a fear of being rejected. Extreme rejection sensitivity can even be expressed as paranoid schizophrenia.

9. Some live in the present only but most of the older teens or young adults live in the past. Most dually diagnosed clients have no hope for the future, possibly because they remember the past too well or have trouble thinking.

10. Denial is a common characteristic in young children. One form is a refusal to deal with unpleasant but necessary duties. Another form is an unwillingness to stop something that's pleasurable, like kids playing roughhouse until one gets hurt badly.

11. They have the feeling that "Either you're for me or against me," a black and white approach to every judgment in life, with no modulation or moderation.

(Pepper, 1993)

These characteristics are also very common in those being treated solely for chemical dependency.

What these characteristics suggest is that any treatment program has to be highly structured. What the client needs to do is learn all those behaviors, ideas, and emotions that were not learned in youth or adolescence because of the drugs, the mental illness, or the turmoil of growing up.

The above difficulties are all chronic or even lifelong problems that cannot be treated with short-term therapy. These are problems of living, of living sober, and of living with the symptoms of the mental illness. The best treatment is inpatient care because it provides a great deal of monitoring and continuity over a fairly long period of time. Unfortunately resources (financial and professional) for long-term inpatient care do not usually exist.

PSYCHOPHARMACOLOGY

The field of medicine that addresses the use of medications to help correct or help control mental illnesses and drug addiction is called "psy-

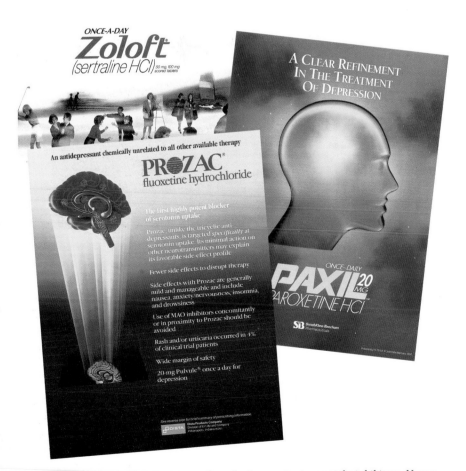

These three ads for antidepressants are for selective serotonin reuptake inhibitors. Newer ones are being constantly developed.

chopharmacology." The scope of this branch of medicine has grown rapidly in the last 10 years, producing hundreds of new medications and greatly expanding this approach to mental illness.

Quite often the dual diagnosis patient does need medication for the psychiatric disorder: tricyclic antidepressants for endogenous depression, lithium for a bipolar disorder, and antipsychotic (neuroleptic) medication for a thought disorder. These medications have to be handled carefully because the dual diagnosis individual has difficulty dealing with drugs. The clinician has to make sure the medication used for the psychiatric problem does not aggravate or complicate the substance abuse problem.

Medications are used on a short-term, medium-term, or even lifetime basis to try to rebalance the brain chemistry that has become unbalanced either through hereditary anomalies, environmental stress, and/or the use of psychoactive drugs and compulsive behaviors. These medications are used in conjunction with individual or group therapy and with lifestyle changes.

One of the biggest debates in treatment centers is about the level of medication that should be used. Some clinicians look at psychotropic medications as a last resort. Others feel that they should be the first step in treatment. However, there is no question that judicious use of these medications has freed many people suffering from mental illness from a life of misery (Zweben, 1998).

Pharmacology

The various psychiatric medications currently in use affect the manner in which neurotransmitters work in different ways.

◇ They can increase or inhibit the release of neurotransmitters and even block the receptor sites (phenothiazines).

◇ They can block the reuptake of neurotransmitters by the sending neuron, thus increasing the amount of neurotransmitter available in the synaptic gap (Prozac® and Zoloft® work this way on serotonin).

◇ They can speed up or inhibit the metabolism of neurotransmitters (Nardil® and MAO inhibitors), thereby enhancing the action of adrenaline or dopamine.

◇ They can enhance the effect of existing neurotransmitters (benzodiazepines such as Valium® increase the effects of GABA).

Besides manipulating brain chemistry, some drugs act directly to control symptoms. For example, beta blockers (Inderal®) calm the sympathetic nervous system that controls heart rate, blood pressure, and other functions that can go out of control in a panic attack or drug withdrawal state. They also calm the brain.

One problem with psychotropic medications is that it's very hard to design a drug that will only work on a certain neurotransmitter in a certain way. There are always side effects and since every patient and every illness is different, constant monitoring of each patient's reaction to the drug and the dosage is an absolute necessity. A careful explanation of the drug and a specific plan of use are necessary.

"The medication that we are talking about giving you in this treatment program is really designed to correct some of the damage that you did to your body and to your mind with the drugs or damage that had been happening as a result of some emotional or psychological problem. It does not mean you're sick, it does not mean you're defective, and it does not mean you're weak. It just means that your biochemistry has somehow got out of balance and the medications that we're recommending, especially the antidepressant medications, are to rebalance those chemicals and bring you to a point where you can fully and effectively function and then begin to work on your other problems."

Stanley Yantis, M.D., psychiatrist (consulting with a dual diagnosed client

Psychiatric Medications vs. Street Drugs

One of the advantages of physician-prescribed medications over street drugs is that generally, except for the benzodiazepines and stimulants, they are not addicting. In fact the treatment of anxiety, depression, and other mental problems through psychiatric medications can relieve many of the reasons and triggers for drug abuse. A study of the risk of substance use disorders in boys who were treated with methylphenidate and other AD/HD treatment drugs found a significant decrease in the risk of having drug use problems as adults compared to patients who were not treated (Biederman, Wilens, Mick, Spencer, & Farone, 1999).

Sometimes prescribing psychiatric medications for clients can cause problems for dually diagnosed clients because they are often taught to stay away from all drugs during recovery. The treatment profession has developed and distributed pamphlets to the various recovery fellowships explaining the need for psychiatric medications by many dual diagnosis patients in recovery. Nevertheless there are well-meaning members of these fellowships who insist that no one taking these medications is really recovering. The patient may be talked into flushing his or her medicine down the toilet with potentially adverse psychiatric results. Consequently it is essential that those responsible for treating dual diagnosis clients who are in recovery understand and support those clients through the potential problems of early recovery (Buxton, Smith, & Seymour, 1987, CSAT, 1995; AA, 1995).

When using street drugs, patients feel a great deal of control over which drugs they ingest, inject, or otherwise self-administer. The same patients, when receiving medication from a doctor, often express the feeling that they are not in control of their lives. Thus they are more apt to rely on street drugs rather than on psychiatric medications for relief of their emotional problems.

"Before I came to the clinic, I thought that using antidepressants was taboo.

I wanted to use street drugs but not any of these clinical ones. There's a stigma to it. I used marijuana to deal with my depression and I could take it when I felt I needed it, not a pill that I had to take every so often as prescribed by my psychiatrist."

35-year-old client with depression and a problem with marijuana

PSYCHIATRIC MEDICATIONS

Some of the major groups of psychotropic medications are tricyclic antidepressants, MAO inhibitors, serotonin reuptake inhibitors, antipsychotics (neuroleptics), anxiolytics (antianxiety drugs), lithium, and beta blockers. We will discuss the drugs under the heading of the mental illness that they are generally used to treat (Table 10-2). There is some overlap, for example, when a drug used for depression, such as Prozac®, is also used to treat obsessive-compulsive disorder or when an antidepressant is used also for bipolar disorder.

DRUGS USED TO TREAT DEPRESSION

Many in the psychiatric field feel that depression causes and, in turn, is caused by an abnormality in the production of the neurotransmitters norepinephrine (noradrenaline) and serotonin plus a few others. Antidepressants are meant to increase the amount of serotonin or norepinephrine available to the brain to correct this imbalance.

Tricyclic Antidepressants

Tricyclic antidepressants such as imipramine (Tofranil®) and desipramine (Norpramine®) are thought to block reabsorption of these neurotransmitters by the sending neuron, and so increase the activity of those biochemicals. This blocking effect, in turn, forces the synthesis of more receptor sites for these neurochemicals. The delay in the creation of new receptor sites may account for the lag time in effecting a change in the patient's mood. It usually takes two to six weeks for a patient to respond to the drug therapy.

The tricyclics are very effective in treating patients with chronic symptoms of depression. People without depression do not get a lift from tricyclic antidepressants as they do with a stimulant. In fact most of these medications actually cause drowsiness.

"The antidepressants did not get me high as far as what I could feel. It wasn't like feeling drunk or stoned. You don't get that sensation. The high I got is more like a lift, a mood lift. It's the difference between being lethargic and sad or active and happy."

41-year-old man with depression

The tricyclic antidepressants, available mainly as pills, can be dangerous if too many are taken, so careful monitoring of not only compliance by the patient with prescribed dosage but also constant feedback from the patient as to the effects and side effects is also necessary. Major side effects are dry mouth, blurred vision, inhibited urination, hypotension, and sleepiness (Zwillich, 1999).

"I went off antidepressants. And after a month, six weeks, I began getting depressed again but I had to be convinced that I was depressed again. And they said, 'You really should go back on medication,' and I didn't want to admit that I didn't want to be on medication. I wanted to exist without it."

35-year-old patient with major depression

These drugs are also dangerous to the heart, especially if they are taken with stimulants, depressants, or alcohol. Patients must abstain from abusing drugs while being treated with tricyclic antidepressants.

Monamine Oxidase (MAO) Inhibitors

MAO inhibitors such as phenelzine (Nardil®), tranylcypromine (Parnate®), and isocarboxazid (Marplan®) are also used to treat depression. These very strong drugs work by blocking an enzyme that metabolizes the neurotransmitters norepinephrine and serotonin. This, in essence, raises the level of these neurotransmitters. Unfortunately MAO inhibitors have several potentially dangerous side effects, so care and close monitoring are necessary in their use. They do give fairly quick relief from a major depression and panic disorder but the user has to be on a special diet and remain aware of the possibility of high blood pressure, headaches, and several other side effects. Combined use of MAO inhibitors with abused stimulants, depressants, and alcohol can be fatal. There are also a number of over-the-counter drugs that should not be taken with MAO inhibitors (PDR, 2000).

Newer Antidepressants

The newer antidepressants such as Prozac®, Deseryl®, Paxil®, Zoloft®, Welbutrin®, Remeron®, Serzone®, Depakote®, and Xanax® work through a variety of mechanisms.

Prozac®. Prozac® (fluoxetine) is the most popular of the newer antidepressants and has received a large amount of publicity both pro and con since its release in 1988. It seems quite effective in the treatment of depression with fewer side effects than tricyclic antidepressants or the MAO inhibitors. It is also used to treat obsessive-compulsive disorders and panic disorder.

Prozac® is classified as a selective serotonin reuptake inhibitor (SSRI) because it increases the amount of serotonin available to the nervous system. The amount needed to be effective varies widely from patient to patient and has to be adjusted. It generally takes two to four weeks for the full effect to be felt. The side effects are usually insomnia, nausea, diarrhea, headache, and nervousness. Most of the side effects are mild and will go away in a few weeks. Paxil® (paroxetine) and Zoloft® (sertraline) are also classified as SSRIs and work to block serotonin uptake and have similar side effects to Prozac®.

Xanax®. Alprazolam (Xanax®), a benzodiazepine sedative-hypnotic though not labeled as a treatment for depression, has been used clinically by several doctors to control mild depression or mixed depression and anxiety. If the patient also has a drug problem, benzodiazepines are only recommended for use in detoxification or immediate relief of acute psychedelic drug toxicity and not for long-term administration.

Stimulants

In the past, amphetamine or amphetamine congeners including Dexedrine®, Biphetamine®, Desoxyn®, Ritalin®, and Cylert® were used to treat depression. They work by increasing the amount of norepinephrine and epinephrine in the central nervous system. They are mood elevators when used in moderation but the problem was that since tolerance develops rapidly and the mood lift proved to be too alluring, misuse and addiction developed fairly rapidly. The overuse led to various physical and mental problems such as agitation, aggression, paranoia, and psychosis. Ritalin® is occasionally prescribed for patients with depression but usually for attention deficit disorder. But for a dually diagnosed client, these drugs should be used with utmost caution. In recognition of this potential problem, more psychiatrists are beginning to use nonstimulants like imipramine, desipramine, and bupropion to treat AD/HD.

DRUGS USED TO TREAT BIPOLAR DISORDER

Antidepressants, such as the tricyclics or bupropion (Welbutrin®) or fluoxetine (Prozac®), are initially used to treat severe depression in the bipolar patient and antipsychotics, including Thorazine® or Haldol®, are initially used to treat the severe manic phase. However, the main drug used for the treatment of bipolar illnesses over the last 30 years has been lithium.

Lithium

Lithium is started concurrently with an antidepressant or an antipsychotic. Lithium is a long-term medication taken for years, even a lifetime. Clinicians are careful when making the diagnosis since the patient might be in the manic phase that resembles schizophrenia or the depressive phase that resembles unipolar depression. Misdiagnosis can be dangerous since long-term treatment of these other conditions is quite different.

Lithium doesn't really prevent a person from having mood swings. The patients still have high and low swings. What it does is dampen them. Because the high swings aren't as high and the depressions aren't as low, lithium helps the bipolar patient function. About 80% of bipolar patients respond to lithium. Symptoms begin to change within 10 to 15 days after starting the drug.

"The way manic-depression works, at least for me, is the medicine can control about 20% of it. The other 80% is me. I have to learn how to control my moods with my mind because the medication is only a small part."

40 year old with bipolar disorder

Others

Tegretol® (carbamazepine) is used in patients who do not respond to lithium alone. It seems to help patients who have more rapid "cycling" of their highs and lows.

Depakene® (valproic acid) is used if the bipolar patient fails to respond to lithium and Tegretol®. Its use with the bipolar patient is still limited to cases resistant to other medications.

Depakote® (divalproex sodium) is used in bipolar and depressed patients who are nonresponsive to the other drugs.

DRUGS USED TO TREAT SCHIZOPHRENIA (ANTIPSYCHOTICS OR NEUROLEPTICS)

In the early 1950s, a new class of drugs, phenothiazines, was found to be effective in controlling the symptoms of schizophrenia. Some of the drugs such as Thorazine®, Mellaril®, Proloxin®, and Compazine® were initially referred to as major tranquilizers to differentiate them from barbiturates and benzodiazepines that were called "minor tranquilizers". More recently nonphenothiazines like Haldol®, Risperdal®, Zyprexa®, Clozaril®, Loxitane®, and Moban® have been developed. They act like phenothiazines and have similar side effects.

Researchers found that one of the major causes of schizophrenia is an excess of dopamine, a condition that is usually inherited. Most of the antipsychotic medications work by blocking the dopamine receptors in the brain, thereby inhibiting the effects of the excess dopamine. Generally antipsychotic drugs do work but they do not cure schizophrenia. They can also cause serious side effects. The difference in side effects is the main difference between many of the drugs.

The main side effects of antipsychotics have to do with the blockage of dopamine in the system. From Table 10-2, you can see that dopamine controls muscle tone and motor behavior. By blocking the dopamine, symptoms such as ticks, jumpiness, and the inability to sit still are common. Parkinsonian syndrome (mainly a tremor but also loss of facial expression and slowed movements), akathisia (agitation, jumpiness exhibited by 75% of patients), akinesia (temporary loss of movement and apathy), and even the more serious tardive dyskinesia (involuntary movements of the jaws, head, neck, trunk, and extremities) are the most common complications when using these medications. Often drugs such as Cogentin®, Artane®, Kemadrin®, or even Benadryl® are given to block side effects.

Patients on antipsychotics may seem drugged but for people suffering from schizophrenia who are agitated or violent, the sedative effect is very useful. These drugs are dangerous when used as a sleeping pill by patients who do not have schizophrenia or are not violent and agitated. The drugs can actu-

TABLE 10–3   MEDICATIONS USED TO HANDLE PSYCHIATRIC PROBLEMS

MAJOR DEPRESSION

Tricyclic antidepressants: imipramine (Tofranil®, Janimine®), desipramine (Norpramin®, Pertofrane®), amitriptyline, (Elavil®, Endep®), nortriptyline (Pamelor®), Doxepin® (Sinequan®, Adapin®), trimipramine (Surmontil®), protriptyline (Vivactil®), maprotiline (Ludiomil®)

Monoamine oxidase (MAO) inhibitors: phenelzine (Nardil®), tranylcypromine (Parnate®), isocarboxazid (Marplan®), pargyline (Eutonyl®), selegeline (formerly Deprenyl® now Eldepryl®)

New Antidepressants: fluoxetine (Prozac®), trazodone (Desyrel®), amoxapine (Asendin®), alprazolam (benzodiazepine, e.g., Xanax®), bupropion (Welbutrin®), sertraline (Zoloft®), Ritanserin®, paroxetine (Paxil®), mirtazapine (Remeron®), nefazodone (Serzone®), divalproex sodium (Depakote®), valproic acid (Depakene®)

Stimulants used as antidepressants: amphetamines, Dexadrine®, Biphetamine®, Desoxyn®, methylphenidate (Ritalin®), pemoline (Cylert®)

BIPOLAR AFFECTIVE DISORDER (formerly called "manic-depression")

Lithium: Eskalith®, Lithobid®

Others: carbamazepine (Tegretol®), valproic acid (Depakene®), divalproex sodium (Depakote®)

SCHIZOPHRENIA

Phenothiazines: trifluoperazine (Stelazine®), fluphenazine (Proloxin®, Permitil®),perphenazine (Trilafon®), chlorpromazine (Thorazine®), thioridazine (Mellaril®), mesoridazine (Serentil®), triflupromazine (Vesprin®), acetophenazine (Tindal®), piperacetazine (Quide®)

Others: halperidol (Haldol®), thiothixene (Navane®), loxapine (Loxitane®), molindone (Moban®, Lidone®), clozapine (Clozaril®), riperidone (Risperdal®, olanzapine (Zyprexa®), pimozide (Orap®), chlorprothixene (Taractan®)

GENERALIZED ANXIETY DISORDER

Benzodiazepines:
   Short-acting (2–4 hour duration of action): alprazolam (Xanax®), oxazepam (Serax®), lorazepam (Ativan®), triazolam (Halcion®), temazepam (Restoril®)
   Long-acting (6–24 hour duration of action): diazepam (Valium®), chlordiazepoxide (Librium®), clorazepate (Tranxene®), clonazepam (Klonopin®), prazepam (Centrax®), halazepam (Paxipam®)

Nonbenzodazepines: buspirone (BuSpar®)

OBSESSIVE-COMPULSIVE DISORDER (OCD)

Clomipramine (Anafranil®), sertraline (Zoloft®), fluoxetine (Prozac®)

PANIC DISORDER

First-line drugs (medications that should be tried first to control panic): imipramine (Tofranil®), desipramine (Norpramin® or Pertofrane®), alprazolam (Xanax®)

Second-line drugs: phenelzine (Nardil®), tranycypromine (Parnate®), clonazepam (Klonopin®)

Beta blockers: propranolol (Inderal®), atenolol (Tenormin®)

SOCIAL PHOBIA

Beta blockers: propranolol (Inderal®), atenolol (Tenormin®)

POSTTRAUMATIC STRESS DISORDER

First-line drugs: benzodiazepines and sedatives listed above under generalized anxiety disorder

Second-line drugs: antipsychotics listed above under treatment of schizophrenia

SLEEPING DISORDER

Sleeping pills: flurazepam (Dalmane®), triazolam (Halcion®), temazepam (Restoril®)

(Keltner & Folks, 1997; PDR, 2000)

ally cause symptoms of mental illness as well as severe side effects in patients who are not schizophrenic.

Antipsychotic drugs in general are also classified as high potency (Haldol®, Risperdal®, Zyprexa®, Clozaril®, Stelazine®, Prolixin®, Trilafon®, Navane®), and low potency (Thorazine® Mellaril®, Loxitrane®, Moban®).

In an emergency, patients are generally started on a high-potency antipsychotic. They are given several weeks to obtain a full response. If there is no response, either the dose can be raised or another drug tried. Most clinicians prefer to use low doses of these medications. The low-potency antipsychotics are used when patients also have problems sleeping. Manic patients are candidates for low-potency antipsychotic use.

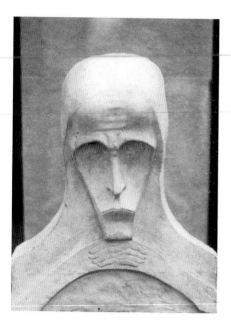

Since antipsychotics are so potent, attempts are made to stop or decrease the dose of these medications as soon as possible, i.e., when the symptoms subside. This approach is particularly important in treating elderly patients.

Recently atypical antipsychotic drugs have been tested. Clozaril® (clozapine) is effective in the 30% of patients who do not respond to standard antipsychotic drug therapy. Unfortunately weekly blood tests are necessary to monitor the side effects of Clozaril®, which make its use very expensive. The newer very potent antipsychotics, like Risperdal® and Zyprexa®, do not have this problem but are still more expensive than the older antipsychotics.

Patients who have been dually diagnosed with schizophrenia often self-medicate with heroin and other opioids to try to control their symptoms. Alcohol, other sedative-hypnotics, and even marijuana or inhalants are used as well. Since all of these street drugs have dangerous toxic effects when combined with antipsychotic drugs, pa-tients are exhorted to cease using them while under psychiatric treatment (Brier, Su, Saunders, et al., 1997).

DRUGS USED TO TREAT ANXIETY DISORDERS

For generalized anxiety disorder as well as some of the other anxiety disorders, the benzodiazepines are widely used. The most commonly used are Xanax®, Valium®, Librium®, and Tranxene®. Developed in the early 1960s, the benzodiazepines were considered safe substitutes for barbiturates and meprobamate (e.g., Miltown®). They act very quickly, particularly Valium®. The calming effects are apparent within 30 minutes. Some of the benzodiazepines are long acting (diazepam, chlordiazepoxide, clorazepate, clonazepam, prazepam, halazepam) and some are short acting (triazolam, lorazepam, temazepam). The main problem with these drugs is that they are habit forming, even at clinical dosages, and do have dangerous withdrawal symptoms, so they are almost always avoided with the dually diagnosed patient for whom they can retrigger drug abuse. If the drug must be used, dosages are kept as low as possible and the patient is monitored for addiction or relapse (Ikeda, 1994; PDR, 2000).

Buspirone (BuSpar®) is the only other drug labeled for generalized anxiety disorder. It is a serotonin modulator and will block the transmission of excess serotonin, one of the causes of the symptoms of many forms of anxiety. It also mimics serotonin, so it can also substitute for low levels of serotonin, a feature used by some doctors to treat depression. It takes several weeks to work and is not nearly as dramatic, initially, as the benzodiazepines. Consequently many patients are reluctant to use it. Its advantage however is that side effects are minimal and it is thought not to be habit forming.

Drugs for Obsessive-Compulsive Disorder (OCD)

For the obsessive-compulsive disorder, almost every type of psychotropic medication has been used in the past, usually with relatively poor results. Anafranil® (clomipramine) has recently been used with reasonable results. It is a serotonin reuptake inhibitor like Zoloft®, Paxil®, and Prozac®, which have also been used to treat OCD as well as depression.

Drugs for Panic Disorder

Several drugs are used to control panic disorder (as opposed to panic attacks). Panic attacks occur in someone who has panic disorder, in those on a bad LSD trip, in someone having an extreme reaction to a stimulant, in a heart patient experiencing rapid heart beating (tachycardia), and in reactions to various medications. Panic disorder consists of multiple panic attacks accompanied by fear and anxiety about having more panic attacks. Situations where a panic attack might occur and they would be without help are also to be avoided. It can be difficult to distinguish between a panic attack and a panic disorder.

Beta blockers calm the symptoms of a panic attack, including rapid heart rates, hypertension, and difficulty breathing, because they block excess muscular activity in the vascular system and lungs. Beta blockers also have a calming effect on the brain that is helpful in treating panic disorders. It takes about one hour for the medicine to work, so many people with a panic disorder or social phobia will take a dose one hour before entering a stressful situation.

CHAPTER SUMMARY

MENTAL HEALTH & DRUGS

Introduction

1. The neurotransmitters that are involved in mental illness are the same ones involved in drug abuse and addiction.

2. The direct effects of many psychoactive drugs as well as the withdrawal effects mimic many mental illnesses.

Determining Factors

3. Heredity, environment, and psychoactive drugs affect one's susceptibility to mental illness in much the same way they affect susceptibility to drug abuse.

4. The risk of developing a mental illness depends on heredity. The risk of a person developing schizophrenia if they have a close relative with schizophrenia jumps from 1% to 15%, for major depression, it jumps from 5% to 15%, and for a bipolar disorder, it jumps from 1% to 12%.

5. Environment can increase susceptibility to mental illness. Physical abuse in childhood is very common (50% to 75%) in those who are psychotic.

6. Psychoactive drugs can alter neurochemistry and aggravate preexisting mental illnesses, trigger latent ones, or create ones that never existed before.

DUAL DIAGNOSIS OR THE MENTALLY ILL CHEMICAL ABUSER (MICA)

Definition

7. Dual diagnosis is defined as "a condition in which a person has both a substance abuse problem and a diagnosable, significant, psychiatric problem."

8. The three main psychiatric disorders used to define dual diagnosis are schizophrenia (a thought disorder), major depression (a mood disorder), and bipolar disorder (mood disorder).

9. Other mental illnesses used by some to define dual diagnosis include anxiety disorders, such as panic disorder, phobia, obsessive-compulsive disorder, posttraumatic stress disorder, organic disorders, developmental disorders, somatoform disorders, attention deficit/hyperactivity disorders, and other personality disorders.

Epidemiology

10. About 37% of alcohol abusers and 53% of drug abusers also have a serious mental illness.

11. Up to 81% of those in prison with a drug problem also have a mental illness.

Patterns of Dual Diagnosis

12. The four different patterns of dual diagnosis are a preexisting mental illness that is aggravated by drug use, a potential mental illness that is triggered by drug use, a permanent mental illness induced by drug use, and a temporary mental illness that is induced by drug use.

Making the Diagnosis

13. A psychiatric diagnosis should always be conditional since abusable drugs can directly or indirectly mimic some mental illnesses.

14. The number of dually diagnosed patients has increased due to better diagnosis techniques, shrinking numbers of inpatient mental health facilities, greater numbers of drug abusers, and a reliance on psychiatric medications.

Mental Health (MH) vs. Chemical Dependency (CD)

15. Four main differences between the mental health (MH) treatment community and the chemical dependency (CD) treatment community are the following:

◇ MH says, control the psychiatric problem and the drug abuse will disappear. CD says, get the patient clean and sober and the mental health problem will disappear;

◇ in MH limited recovery is more acceptable whereas in CD most believe that lifetime abstinence is possible;

◇ MH often uses psychiatric drugs to treat the dual diagnosis patient whereas CD promotes a drug free philosophy;

◇ MH has a supportive philosophy whereas CD uses a confrontive philosophy.

16. Health professionals need to reconcile the two philosophies of treatment to develop programs that treat both illnesses (mental illness and addiction).

17. Triple diagnosis is usually the coexistence of a mental health problem, a drug addiction, and an HIV diagnosis.

Psychiatric Disorders

18. Schizophrenia, a thought disorder, is characterized by hallucinations, delusions, an inappropriate affect, poor association, impaired ability to care for oneself.

19. Major depression is characterized by a depressed mood, diminished interest and pleasure in most activities, sleep and appetite disturbances, feelings of worthlessness, and suicidal thoughts.

20. A bipolar affective disorder involves manic phases alternating with depressive phases.

21. Anxiety disorders include panic disorder, obsessive-compulsive disorder, posttraumatic stress disorder, and a generalized anxiety disorder.

22. Other mental illness include an organic mental disorder (e.g., Alzheimer's disease), developmental disorders (e.g., attention deficit/hyperactivity disorder), somato-

form disorders (e.g., hypochondria), and various personality disorders.

Treatment

23. Treatment for dual diagnosis can be done through psychotherapy, counseling, the group process, and/or with psychiatric medications.

24. Usually both the addiction and the mental problem need to be treated simultaneously.

25. Impaired cognition and developmental arrest make treatment of dual diagnosis difficult. Many people coming in for treatment are much younger emotionally than they are physically.

26. The major classes of psychiatric drugs are antidepressants, antipsychotics, anxyloitics, and drug used to treat bipolar disorder.

27. Psychiatric medications manipulate brain chemistry and relieve symptoms of mental illness. They can also cause undesirable and severe side effects.

28. Many with mental illnesses try to self-medicate with street drugs or alcohol.

Psychiatric Medications

29. Drugs used to treat depression are tricyclic antidepressants, MAO inhibitors, amphetamines, and newer SSRI antidepressants, such as Prozac®, Zoloft® and Paxil®.

30. Some of the drugs used to treat schizophrenia are the phenothiazines (e.g., Thorazine®), halperidol (Haldol®), clozapine (Clozaril®) risperidine (Risperdal®), and olanzapine (Zyprexa®).

31. The main drug used to treat a bipolar disorder is lithium.

32. The principal drugs used to treat anxiety are the benzodiazepines, such as Valium® and Xanax®, and the nonbenzodiazepine, BuSpar®.

REFERENCES

AA (Alcoholics Anonymous). (1995). *The AA Member—Medications and Other Drugs.* New York: AA Publications.

APA (American Psychiatric Association). (1994). *Diagnostic and Statistical Manual of Mental Disorders* (4th ed.). Washington, DC: Author.

Barondes, S. H. (1993). *Molecules and Mental Illness.* New York: Scientific American Library.

Batki, S. (1994). *Interview with authors at San Francisco General Hospital.*

Beeder, A. B., & Millman, R. B. (1997). Patients with psychopathology. In J. H. Lowenson, P. Ruiz, R. B. Millman, & J. G. Langrod (Eds.), *Substance Abuse, A Comprehensive Textbook* (3rd ed., pp. 551–562). Baltimore: Williams & Wilkins.

Biederman, J., Wilens, T., Mick, E., Spencer, T., & Faraone, S. V. (1999). Pharmacotherapy of attention deficit/hyperactivity disorder reduces risk for substance use disorder. *Pediatrics, 5.*

Blum, K., Braverman, E. R., Cull, J. G., Holder, J. M., Luck, R., Lubar, J., Miller, D., & Comings, D. E. (2000). "Reward deficiency syndrome" (RDS): A biogenetic model for the diagnosis and treatment of impulsive, addictive, and compulsive behaviors. *Journal of Psychoactive Drugs, 32*(supplement).

Blume, A. W., Davis, J. M., & Schmaling, K. B. (1999). Neurocognitive dysfunction in dually diagnosed patients: A potential roadblock to motivating behavior change. *Journal of Psychoactive Drugs, 31*(2), 111–115.

Brady, K. T. (1999). Treatment of PTSD and substance use disorders [23A]. *The American Psychiatric Association 152nd Annual Meeting,* Washington, DC.

Brady, K. T., Myrick, H., & Sonne, S. (1998). Comorbid addiction and affective disorders. In A. W. Graham & T. K. Schultz (Eds.), *Principles of Addiction Medicine* (2nd ed., pp. 983–992). Chevy Chase, MD: American Society of Addiction Medicine, Inc.

Brehm, N. M., & Khantzian, E. J. (1997). Psychodynamics. In J. H. Lowenson, P. Ruiz, R. B. Millman, & J. G. Langrod (Eds.), *Substance Abuse, A Comprehensive Textbook* (3rd ed., pp. 90–100). Baltimore: Williams & Wilkins.

Brier, A., Su, T. P., Saunders, R., Carson, R. E., Kolachana, B. S., De Bartolomeis, A., Weinberger, D. R., Weisenfeld, N., Malhotra, A. K., Eckelman, W. C., & Pickar, D. (1997). Schizophrenia is associated with elevated amphetamine-induced synaptic dopamine concentrations: Evidence from a novel positron emission tomography method. *Proceedings of the National Academy of Science, 94,* 2569–2574.

Buxton, M. E., Smith, D. E., & Seymour, R. B. (1987). Spirituality and other points of resistance to the 12-step process. *Journal of Psychoactive Drugs, 19*(3), 275–286.

Crome, I. B. (1999). Substance misuse and psychiatric comorbidity: Towards improved service provision. *Drugs: Education, Prevention and Policy, Source Id: 6*(2), 151–174.

CSAT (Center for Substance Abuse Treatment). (1995). *Assessment and Treatment of Patients with Coexisting Mental Illness and Alcohol and Other Drug Abuse.* Rockville, MD: DHHS Publication no. (SMA) 95-3061.

Davis, K., Klar, H., & Coyle, J. T. (1991). *Foundations of Psychiatry.* Philadelphia: Harcourt Brace Jovanovich, Inc.

Delgado, P. L., & Mereno, F. A. (1998). Hallucinogens, serotonin, and obsessive-compulsive disorder. *Journal of Psychoactive Drugs, 30*(4), 359–366,

Dimeoff, L. A., Comtois, K. A., & Linehan, M. M. (1998). Personality disorders. In A. W. Graham & T. K. Schultz (Eds.), *Principles of Addiction Medicine* (2nd ed., pp. 1062–1081). Chevy Chase, MD: American Society of Addiction Medicine, Inc.

Drake, R. E., Mercer-McFadden, C., Mueser, K. T., McHugo, G. J., & Bond, G. R. (1998). Review of integrated mental health and substance abuse treatment for patients with dual disorders. *Schizophrenia Bulletin, 24*, 589–608.

Drake, R. E., & Mueser, K. T. (1996). Alcohol-use disorder and severe mental illness. *Alcohol Health & Research World: Alcoholism and Co-Occurring Disorders, 20*(2), 87–93.

Evans, K., & Sullivan, J. M. (1990). *Dual Diagnosis: Counseling the Mentally Ill Substance Abuser.* New York: The Guilford Press.

Gastfriend, D. R., & Lillard, P. (1998). Anxiety disorders. In A. W. Graham & T. K. Schultz (Eds.), *Principles of Addiction Medicine* (2nd ed., pp. 983–1006). Chevy Chase, MD: American Society of Addiction Medicine, Inc.

Goldsmith, R. J., & Ries, R. K. (1998). Substance-induced mental disorders. In A. W. Graham & T. K. Schultz (Eds.), *Principles of Addiction Medicine* (2nd ed., pp. 969–982). Chevy Chase, MD: American Society of Addiction Medicine, Inc.

Goodwin, & Jamison. (1990). *Manic-Depressive Illness.* New York: W. H. Freeman and Co.

Gottesman, I. I. (1991). *Schizophrenia Genetics: The Origins of Madness.* New York: W. H. Freeman and Co.

Grella, C. (1996). Background and overview of mental health and substance abuse treatment systems: Meeting the needs of women who are pregnant and parenting. *Journal of Psychoactive Drugs, 28*(4), 319–344.

Guydish, J., & Muck, R. (1999). The challenge of managed care in drug abuse treatment. *Journal of Psychoactive Drugs, 31*(3), 193–195.

Ikeda, R. (1994). Prescribing for chronic anxiety disorders. *Journal of Psychoactive Drugs, 26*(1), 75–76.

Inaba, D., Cohen, W. E., & Holstein, M. E. (1996). *Uppers, Downers, All Arounders* (3rd ed.). Ashland, OR: CNS Productions, Inc.

Keller, D. S., & Dermatis, H. (1999). Current status of professional training in the addictions. *Substance Abuses: Journal of the Association for Medical Education and Research in Substance Abuse, 20*(3), 123–140.

Keltner, N. L., & Folks, D. G. (1997). *Psychotropic Drugs.* St. Louis: Mosby-Year Book, Inc.

Kendler, K. S., & Diehl, S. R. (1993). The genetics of schizophrenia: A current genetic-epidemiological perspective. *Schizophrenia Bulletin, 19*, 261–295.

Kendler, K. S., Heath, A. C., Neale, M. C., & Eaves, L. J. (1993). Alcoholism and major depression in women. A twin study of the causes of comorbidity. *Archives of General Psychiatry, 50*(9), 690–698.

Kessler, R. C., McGonagle, K. A., Zhao, S. Nelson, C. B., Hughes, M., Eshleman, S., Wittchen, H. U., & Kendler, K. S. (1994). Lifetime and 12-month prevalence of DSM-III-R psychiatric disorders in the United States. Results from the National Comorbidity Survey. *Archives of General Psychiatry, 51*, 8–19.

Kosten, T. R., & Ziedonis, D. M. (1997). Substance abuse and schizophrenia: Editors' introduction. *Schizophrenia Bulletin, 23*, 181–186.

Kushner, M. G., Sher, K. J., & Erickson, D. J. (1999). Prospective analysis of the relation between DSM-III anxiety disorders and alcohol use disorders. *American Journal of Psychiatry, 156*(5), 723–732.

Lavine, R. (1999). Roles of the psychiatrist and the addiction medicine specialist in the treatment of addiction. *San Francisco Medicine, 72*(4), 20–22.

Levin, F. R., & Donovan, S. J. (1998). Attention deficit/hyperactivity disorder, intermittent explosive disorder, and eating disorders. In A. W. Graham & T. K. Schultz (Eds.), *Principles of Addiction Medicine* (2nd ed., pp. 1029–1046). Chevy Chase, MD: American Society of Addiction Medicine, Inc.

Lilenfeld, L. R., & Kaye, W. H. (1996). The link between alcoholism and eating disorders. *Alcohol Health & Research World, 20*(2), 94–99.

Lowenstein, L. F. (1991). The relationship of psychiatric disorder and conduct disorders with substance abuse. *Journal of Psychoactive Drugs, 23*(3), 283–288.

Mallouh, C. (1996). The effects of dual diagnosis on pregnancy and parenting. *Journal of Psychoactive Drugs, 26*(4), 367–380.

McDowell, D. M. (1999). Evaluation of depression in substance abuse ([23B]. *The American Psychiatric Association 152nd Annual Meeting,* Washington, DC.

McElroy, S. L., Soutullo, C. A., & Goldsmith, R. J. (1998). Other Impulse control disorders. In A. W. Graham & T. K. Schultz (Eds.), *Principles of Addiction Medicine* (2nd ed., pp. 1047–1062). Chevy Chase, MD: American Society of Addiction Medicine, Inc.

Merikangas, K. R., Stevens, D., & Fenton, B. (1996). Comorbidity of alcoholism and anxiety disorders: The role of family Studies. *Alcohol Health & Research World, 20*(2), 100–106.

Minkoff, K., & Regner, J. (1999). Innovations in integrated dual diagnosis treatment in public managed care: The Choate Dual Diagnosis Case Rate Program. *Journal of Psychoactive Drugs, 31*(1), 3–12.

Morrison, M. A., Smith, D. E., Wilford, B. B., Ehrlich, P., & Seymour, R. B. (1994). Current perspectives on the nature and treatment of adolescent chemical dependency. *Journal of Psychoactive Drugs, 25*(4).

NIMH. (1999). *Mental Health: A Report of the Surgeon General.* Rockville, MD: National Institute of Mental Health.

Nunes, E. V., Donovan, S. J., Brady, R., & Guitkin, F. M. (1994). Evaluation and treatment of mood and anxiety disorders in opioid-dependent patients. *Journal of Psychoactive Drugs, 26*(2), 147–154.

O'Conner, P. G., & Ziedonis, D. M. (1998). Linkages of substance abuse with primary care and mental health treatment. In A. W. Graham & T. K. Schultz (Eds.), *Principles of Addiction Medicine* (2nd ed., pp. 353–362). Chevy Chase, MD: American Society of Addiction Medicine, Inc.

PDR. (2000). *Physicians Desk Reference (54th ed., 2000).* Montvale, NJ: Medical Economics Company, Inc.

Pepper, B. (1993). *Interview with psychiatrist Burt Pepper with authors in Eugene, Oregon.*

RachBeisel, J. Dixon, L., & Gearon, J. (1999). Awareness of substance abuse problems among dually diagnosed psychiatric inpatients. *Journal of Psychoactive Drugs, 31*(1), 53–7.

Rahav, M., Rivera, J. J., Nuttbrock, L., et al. (1995). Characteristics and treatment of homeless, mentally ill chemical-abusing men. *Journal of Psychoactive Drugs, 27*(1), 93–104.

Regier, D. A., Farmer, M. E., Rae, D. S., Locke, B. Z., Keith, S. J., Judd, L. L., & Goodwin, F. K. (1990). Comorbidity of mental disorders with alcohol and other drug abuse. *Journal of the American Medical Association, 264*(19), 2511–2518.

Reilly, P. M., Clark, H. W., Shopshire, M. S., Lewis, E. W., & Sorensen, D. J.

(1994). Anger management and temper control: Critical components of post-traumatic stress disorder and substance abuse treatment. *Journal of Psychoactive Drugs, 26*(4), 401–408.

Salloum, I. M., & Daley, D. C. (1994). *Understanding Major Anxiety Disorders and Addiction.* Center City, MN: Hazelden.

Schuckit, M. A. (1986). Alcoholism and affective disorders: Genetic and clinical implications. *American Journal of Psychiatry, 143,* 140–147.

Schuckit, M. A. (1996). Alcohol, anxiety, and depressive disorders. *Alcohol Health & Research World: Alcoholism and Co-Occurring Disorders, 20*(2), 81–85.

Selwyn, P. A., & Merino, F. L. (1997). Medical complications and treatment. In J. H. Lowenson, P. Ruiz, R. B. Millman, & J. G. Langrod (Eds.), *Substance Abuse, A Comprehensive Textbook* (3rd ed., pp. 597–682). Baltimore: Williams & Wilkins.

Senay, E. C. (1998). *Substance Abuse Disorders in Clinical Practice.* New York: W. W. Norton & Company.

Senay, E. C. (1997). Diagnostic interview and mental status examination. In J. H. Lowenson, P. Ruiz, R. B. Millman, & J. G. Langrod (Eds.), *Substance Abuse, A Comprehensive Textbook* (3rd ed., pp. 364–368). Baltimore: Williams & Wilkins.

Seymour, R. B., & Smith, D. E. (1993). *The Psychedelic Resurgence: Treatment, Support, and Recovery Options.* Center City, MN: Hazelden.

Seymour, R. B., & Smith, D. E. (1987). *Drugfree: A Unique, Positive Approach to Staying Off Alcohol and Other Drugs.* New York: Facts on File Publications.

Shaffer, D., Fisher, P., Dulcan, et al., (1996). The NIMH Diagnostic Interview Schedule for Children Version 2.3. *Journal of the American Academy of Child and Adolescent Psychiatry, 35,* 865–877.

Skodol, A. E., Oldham, J. M., & Gallaher, P. E. (1999). Axis II comorbidity of substance use disorders among patients referred for treatment of personality disorders. *American Journal of Psychiatry, 156*(5), 733–738.

Smith, D. E., Lawlor, B., & Seymour, R. B. (1996). Healthcare at the Crossroads. *San Francisco Medicine, 69*(6).

Smith, D. E., & Seymour, R. B. (2000). *The Clinician's Guide to Substance Abuse.* Center City, MN: Hazelden/McGraw Hill.

Soderstrom, C. A., Smith, G. S., Dischinger, P. C., McDuff, D. R., Hebel, J. R., Gorelick, D. A., Kerns, T. J, Ho, S. M., & Read, K. M. (1997). Psychoactive substance use disorders among seriously injured trauma center patients. *JAMA, 277*(22), 1769–1775.

Walker, R. (1992). Substance abuse and B-cluster disorders I & II: Understanding the dual diagnosis patient. *Journal of Psychoactive Drugs, 24*(3), 223–242.

Wechsberg, W. M., Desmond, D., Inciardi, J. A., Leukefeld, C. G., Cottler, L. B., & Hoffman, J. (1999). HIV prevention protocols: Adaptation to evolving trends in drug use. *Journal of Psychoactive Drugs, 30*(3), 291–298.

Woody, G. E. (1996). The challenge of dual; diagnosis. *Alcohol Health and Research World: Alcoholism and Co-Occurring Disorders, 20*(2), 76–80.

Wu, L., Kouzis, A. C., & Leaf, P. J. (1999). Influence of comorbid alcohol and psychiatric disorders on utilization of mental health services in the National Comorbidity Survey. *American Journal of Psychiatry, 156*(8), 1230–1243.

Zickler, P. (1999). Twin studies help define the role of genes in vulnerability to drug abuse. *NIDA Notes, 14*(4).

Ziedonis, D, & Wyatt, S. (1998). Psychotic disorders. In A. W. Graham & T. K. Schultz (Eds.), *Principles of Addiction Medicine* (2nd ed., pp. 353–362). Chevy Chase, MD: American Society of Addiction Medicine, Inc.

Zimberg, S. (1994). Individual psychotherapy: Alcohol. In M. Galanter & H. D. Kleber (Eds.), *The American Psychiatric Press Textbook of Substance Abuse Treatment* (pp. 263–273). Washington, DC: American Psychiatric Press, Inc.

Zimberg, S. (1999). A dual diagnosis typology to improve diagnosis and treatment of dual disorder patients. *Journal of Psychoactive Drugs. 31*(1), 47–51.

Zweben, J. E. (1998). Integrating psychotherapy and pharmacotherapies in addiction treatment. In A. W. Graham & T. K. Schultz (Eds.), *Principles of Addiction Medicine* (2nd ed., pp. 1081–1089). Chevy Chase, MD: American Society of Addiction Medicine, Inc.

Zweben, J. E. (1996). Psychiatric problems among alcohol and other drug-dependent women. *Journal of Psychoactive Drugs, 28*(4), 345–366.

Zwillich, T. (1999). Beware of long-term effects of antidepressants. *Clinical Psychiatry News, 27*(9), 16.

GLOSSARY

A

AA: *see Alcoholics Anonymous.*

abruptio placentae: premature separation of the fetus's placenta from the wall of the uterus often due to cocaine or amphetamine use during pregnancy.

abscess: a chronic, localized, pus-filled infection, common in injection drug users because of their use of infected needles, an inability to get the needle into a vein, or by the irritating effects of the drug on the skin and body tissues. They are often seen on the arms of IV drug users.

absinthe: a potent herb liquor containing wormwood, anise, and fennel that initially causes stimulation and euphoria but in large doses can be toxic.

absorption: the transfer of alcohol or other drug from the point of ingestion, injection, or inhalation until it enters the bloodstream.

abstinence: the act of refraining from the use of alcohol and any other drug. It also refers to stopping addictive behaviors, such as overeating and gambling.

abuse: the continued use of any drug or compulsive behavior despite adverse consequences; the step before addiction occurs.

academic model of addiction: a theory of addiction that says addiction is caused by the body's adaptation to continued use of psychoactive drugs.

"Acapulco gold": marijuana grown near Acapulco, Mexico that is usually gold in color.

acculturation: acceptance and adoption of customs and mores of one culture by another.

acetaminophen: a nonaspirin analgesic and antipyretic; often used in combination with opioids, such as codeine or hydrocodone; over-the-counter trade names include Tylenol and Datril .

acetone: a volatile solvent abused as an inhalant; minute traces are found naturally in the body.

acetylaldehyde: the first substance that is formed when alcohol is metabolized by the liver; it is more toxic than alcohol.

acetylcholine (ACH): the first neurotransmitter to be discovered, it works at the nerve-muscle interfaces. It also affects memory, learning, aggression, alertness, blood pressure, heart rate, sexual behavior, and mental acuity.

"acid": LSD (lysergic acid diethylamide).

ACoA (Adult Children of Alcoholics): a self-help, 12-step program to help adults whose parent or parents were alcoholic, to deal with the emotional turmoil caused by the addiction.

acquaintance rape: sexual assault by a person who is known to the victim, often a relative, neighbor, or even a date.

ACTH (adrenocorticotropic hormone): stimulates the adrenal cortex causing the secretion of cortisol (an anti-inflammatory substance) and other glucocorticoids.

acupuncture: a 3,000-year-old treatment modality that uses needle insertion at nerve intersections to help heal. Recently it has been used for heroin detoxification.

acute tolerance (tachyphylaxis): instant tolerance (adaptation of the body) to a toxic dose of a drug.

addiction: a progressive disease process characterized by loss of control over use, obsession with use, continued use despite adverse consequences, denial that there are problems, and a powerful tendency to relapse.

adenosine: an inhibitory neurotransmitter affected (blocked) by caffeine.

adenyl cyclase: enzyme, used by neurons and other cells to relay electrical signals from the exterior to the interior of the cell.

AD/HD (attention deficit/hyperactivity disorder): this disorder is characterized by inattention, impulsivity, and hyperactivity that begins in childhood and may extend into adulthood.

adrenaline: the principal stimulant neurohormone of most species; it stimulates heart rate and blood pressure, dilates bronchial muscles and alerts the senses; *see epinephrine.*

adulterant: a pharmacologically in-active substance used to dilute a drug.

adulteration: the dilution of a drug in order to increase its volume; used by street dealers to increase profits.

aerosol: liquid that is dispersed in the form of a fine mist.

affective disorder: any mood or emotional disorder, e.g., depression, bipolar affective disorder.

aftercare: the services that are provided recovering addicts after they leave a residential treatment program.

agonist: a drug that initiates an effect when it imitates a neurotransmitter rather than blocking it, e.g., morphine.

agoraphobia: a pervasive mental disorder that is characterized by an irrational fear of leaving home or a familiar setting and venturing outdoors or into a public place; often associated with panic attacks.

agua rica: a partially processed form of cocaine base in solution. Cocaine is often smuggled in this form.

AIDS (acquired immune deficiency syndrome): a disease/syndrome caused by the HIV virus and characterized by vulnerability to opportunistic infections.

Al-Anon: a 12-step organization to help the relatives and friends of alcoholics.

Alateen: a 12-step organization for teenagers affected by an alcoholic parent or friend. It helps them deal with the pain and disruption in their lives.

alcohol: an organic chemical created naturally by the fermentation of sugar, starch, or other carbohydrate. It can also be synthesized from ethylene or acetylene.

alcohol dehydrogenase: the principle enzyme in the liver that metabolizes alcohol.

alcoholic hepatitis: inflammation and impairment of liver function caused by excess use of alcohol.

alcohol-induced disorders: a diagnostic category in DSM-IV under alcohol-related disorders that describes a group of psychiatric symptoms caused by alcohol intoxication or alcohol withdrawal, including alcohol-induced withdrawal, amnesia, psychotic disorder, mood disorders, etc.

alcohol-related disorders: a diagnostic category in DSM-IV that includes alcohol use disorders and alcohol-induced disorders.

Alcoholics Anonymous: the first 12-step, self-help, alcoholism recovery group founded in 1934 by Bill Wilson and Dr. Bob (Robert Smith); tens-of-thousands of chapters exist worldwide.

alcoholism: addiction to alcohol; a progressive disease characterized by loss of control over use, obsession with use, continued use despite adverse consequences, denial that there is a problem, and a powerful tendency to relapse.

ale: a beer with a slightly more bitter taste and higher alcohol content that lager beer; uses the top fermentation process. The alehouse or pub and the use of ale rather than lager is a prominent feature of British life.

allele gene: a paired gene whose difference from a normal gene may be responsible for one of the 3,500 chromosomally linked human diseases. Normally, the alleles have the same function, e.g., two alleles control eye color but one is for blue eyes and the other for brown eyes. In terms of addiction, one allele may be responsible for normal alcohol metabolism while the other does the same job but does it poorly so the alcohol has a greater effect.

allergic reaction: an abnormal reaction to a substance; severe reactions such as anaphylactic shock caused by cocaine, can be fatal.

alkaloid: any nitrogen containing plant compound with pharmacological (often psychoactive) activity, e.g., morphine, cocaine, or nicotine.

alkanes: a class of hydrocarbons including methane, butane, and propane that can be inhaled.

alpha alcoholism: *see Jellinek.*

alveoli: tiny sacs at the end of the bronchioles in the lungs where inhaled air or vaporized drugs are transferred to blood in the capillaries.

Alzheimer's disease: the most widespread form of senile dementia, Alzheimer's is an organic disease marked by the progressive deterioration of mental functions.

Amanita muscaria **(fly agaric):** an hallucinogenic mushroom that is often prepared in liquid form and drunk.

amine: a nitrogen atomic group attached to a carbon molecule, i.e., amino acids, amphetamines.

amino acid precursor loading: a medical intervention technique to ingest protein supplements and amino acids to build up neurotransmitter supplies.

amino acids: organic nitrogen compounds that are the building blocks for proteins; some serve as neurotransmitters.

amotivational syndrome: a lack of desire to complete tasks or to succeed; sometimes attributed to the long-term effects of marijuana.

amphetamine: $C_6H_5CH_2CH(NH_2)$ CH_3; a nervous system stimulant that is closely related in structure and action to ephedrine and other sympathomimetic amines.

amphetamines: a class of powerful stimulants based on the amphetamine molecule that was first synthesized in 1887 and manufactured in the 1930s; the word is also used to include various methamphetamines. They are prescribed for narcolepsy, AD/HD, and until the early 1970s for obesity and depression.

amygdala: part of the limbic system or emotional center of the brain that coordinates the actions of the autonomic and endocrine systems and is involved in the basic emotions.

anabolic: anything that builds up the body, e.g., converting protein from amino acids to help build muscles.

anabolic-androgenic steroid: a steroid that builds muscles and strength; pharmacologically similar to testosterone; it also induces male sexual characteristics.

analeptic: any stimulant drug.

analgesic: a painkiller that works by changing the perception of the pain rather than truly deadening the nerves as an anesthetic would.

analog: a synthetic drug that is chemically slightly different from a controlled drug; *see designer drugs.*

anandamide: a recently discovered neurotransmitter whose effects are similar to the effects of marijuana.

anaphylactic reaction: a severe overreaction or even fatal shock due to the effects of a drug.

androstenedione: a natural hormone found in all animals and some plants. It is a metabolite of DHEA, a precursor of testosterone; used in sports to enhance recovery and growth from a workout.

androgenic: having a masculinizing effect.

anergia: a lack of energy and motivation; often caused by excess stimulant use.

anesthetic: a substance that causes the loss of the ability to feel pain or other sensory input, e.g., ether or halothane.

"angel dust": PCP.

anhedonia: the lack of the ability to feel pleasure; often caused by overuse of cocaine or amphetamines.

anorectic: a person with the eating disorder, anorexia nervosa; a substance that reduces appetite.

anorexia nervosa: an eating disorder marked by a refusal to eat and a fear of maintaining a minimum normal weight.

anorexic: *see anorectic.*

Antabuse (disulfuram): a drug that creates unpleasant side effects if alcohol is drunk; helps a recovering alcoholic to stay sober.

antagonist: a drug that blocks the normal transmission of messages between nerve cells by blocking the receptor sites that would normally be attached to certain neurotransmitters.

anterograde amnesia: amnesia cause by the use of drugs, such as Rohypnol , alcohol, or some benzodiazepines.

antianxiety drug: *see anxiolytics.*

anticholinergic drugs: a class of mild deliriant drugs found in certain hallucinogenic plants, e.g., belladonna, henbane, mandrake, datura. The active substances (scopolamine, atropine, and hyoscyamine) interfere with the action of acetylcholine, causing psychedelic reactions.

antidepressants: a series of drugs that are used to treat depression, mostly by boosting the levels of serotonin in the brain, e.g., tricyclic antidepressant, Prozac , and Zoloft .

antihistamines: any drug that stops the inflammatory actions of histamines; used for congestion, allergies, etc.

antihypertensive drugs: drugs used to reduce high blood pressure in order to prevent heart attacks or strokes.

anti-inflammatory: any substance, such as cortisone, that reduces inflammation.

antipriming: the use of medications to modulate or blunt the pleasurable reinforcing effects of psychoactive drugs.

antipsychotic (neuroleptic): a drug, especially a phenothiazine, that is used to treat schizophrenia or other psychosis. Others include haloperidol, clozapine, and loxapine.

antiretroviral therapy: the use of antiretroviral drugs in combination with others to control the replication of HIV, the virus responsible for AIDS.

antisocial personality disorder: a mental disorder in which the person disregards the rights and feelings of others, feels no remorse, needs instant gratification, cannot learn from mistakes, cannot form personal relationships and is often involved in risk taking, drug abuse, pathological lying, and criminality.

antitussive: any medication that relieves coughing, such as codeine.

anxiety: a state of intense fear and apprehension. Symptoms include higher pulse, respiration, and sweating. Long-term anxiety can increase one's susceptibility to drugs use since some drugs, e.g., alcohol, heroin, and prescription sedatives, can control the symptoms of anxiety.

anxiety disorders: a series of mental disorders marked by excessive anxiety, fear, worry, and avoidance, including panic attacks, panic disorder, agoraphobia, obsessive-compulsive disorder, posttraumatic stress disorder, and generalized anxiety disorder.

anxiolytics: drugs used to treat anxiety disorders including benzodiazepines and barbiturates.

AOD: alcohol and other drugs; an acronym used in the drug abuse prevention field.

aphrodisiac: a substance, such as Viagra , that increases sexual desire and/or performance.

aqua vitae: a medieval name for distilled liquor literally "water of life," when alcohol was thought to have unique medicinal and rejuvination properties.

arrhythmia: irregularity of heartbeat (loss of rhythm) that can be lethal; often caused by drug use.

ARRRT: acronym for **A**cceptance, **R**eduction of stimuli, **R**eassurance, **R**est, and **T**alk-down, steps for treatment of a bad psychedelic experience.

asthma medications: a series of respiratory medications that include anti-inflammatory agents, decongestants, and bronchodilators to control asthma. Their use is restricted in sports competition but medical use is allowed.

ataxia: inability to coordinate muscular activity, often caused by brain disorders or drug use.

atherosclerosis: fat and plaque deposits on the lining of blood vessels caused by high blood pressure, stress, smoking, and cocaine or methamphetamine use. It is often the cause of heart attacks, heart failure, and heart disease. It is also commonly known as hardening of the arteries.

atropine (hyoscyamine): an active ingredient of the belladonna plant; an anticholinergic alkaloid and hallucinogen that can cause tachycardia, pupil dilation, etc.

attention deficit/hyperactivity disorder: *see AD/HD.*

autonomic nervous system: part of the peripheral nervous system that controls involuntary functions, such as circulation, body temperature, and breathing.

autoreceptor: a specialized neurotransmitter receptor on the button of a sending neuron that signals the cell to produce more or less of the neurotransmitter.

aversion therapy: a form of therapy that inflicts pain as the client uses a substance; i.e., some stop-smoking programs shock clients (electrically) when they smoke.

axon: part of the nerve cell that conducts the impulse away from the cell body to the terminals; they can be 40–50 cm long.

ayahuasca: an hallucinogenic beverage brewed from the *Banisteriopsis caapi* bush by the Peruvian Chama Indians.

AZT (azidothymidine, zidovudine): HIV virus inhibitor, used for control of HIV disease and AIDS.

B

BAC (blood alcohol concentration): the concentration of alcohol in the blood; used legally to identify drunk drivers, i.e., 8 parts of alcohol per 10,000 parts of blood equals a BAC of .08, which is the legal limit in many states. The other states have a legal limit of .10.

Bacchus: Roman god of wine; same as Dionysus, the Greek god of wine.

"bad trip": an unpleasant or dangerous panic reaction to a psychedelic such as LSD.

"bagging": putting an inhalant, such as airplane glue, in a plastic baggie and inhaling the fumes.

barbiturates: a class of sedative-hypnotic drugs derived from the barbituric acid molecule, e.g., phenobarbital, Seconal .

basal ganglia: a group of gray-matter structures at the base of the cerebral hemispheres that help control involuntary muscle movement.

base: a form of cocaine that can be smoked. The cocaine in cocaine hydrochloride has been freed from the hydrochloride molecule. "Crack" is freebase cocaine.

basing: the process of transforming cocaine hydrochloride to smokable cocaine freebase and the practice of smoking cocaine base.

"basuco": a brownish, putty-like intermediate product of cocaine refinement that can be smoked (usually in cigarettes); popular in coca-growing countries.

bee pollen: a combination of plant pollen with nectar and bee saliva that is used to increase endurance; can cause severe allergic reactions.

beer: an alcoholic beverage that is brewed by fermenting malted grains (usually barley) and hops, an aromatic herb. Beer includes, ale, bock beer, pilsner beer, malt liquor, stout, porter, and lager.

behavioral tolerance: use of parts of the brain that are not affected by a drug to compensate for the other parts of the brain that are.

belladonna: a hallucinogenic plant, also called "nightshade," whose active ingredients (hyoscyamine, atropine, and scopolamine) cause intoxication, hallucinations, and drugged sleep.

benzodiazepines: a group of minor tranquilizers, such as Klonopin® and Xanax®, that calm anxiety, relax muscles, and induce sleep.

benzoylecgonine: one of the metabolites of cocaine that can be found in the urine long after cocaine is no longer present in the body.

beta alcoholism: *see Jellinek.*

beta blockers: a class of drugs that calm the body's heart rate, respiration, and tension by blocking epinephrine (adrenaline) at the heart and in the brain often used to control panic attacks; used illegally in sports such as riflery, diving, and archery.

betel nut: a nut from the areca palm tree that is chewed by 200 million people, particularly in Asia, for mild stimulant effects.

bhang: an Indian name for the leaves and stems of *Cannabis* (marijuana) plants; it is a mild form of marijuana that can be prepared for smoking, drinking, or ingestion.

Big Book: The main book of Alcoholics Anonymous containing the philosophy of AA and autobiographical stories of recovering alcoholics; used extensively in AA meetings.

binding site: *see receptor site.*

"bindle": a piece of paper folded like a miniature envelope to hold a small amount of a drug, like one gram of cocaine.

binge: using large amounts of a drug in a short period of time, e.g., cocaine binge.

binge drinking: drinking large amounts of alcohol at one sitting; artificially defined as five drinks or more for men and four or more for women in one drinking session at least once every two weeks but being abstinent in between these times.

binge-eating disorder: recurring episodes of binge eating without resorting to vomiting or other methods used by the bulimic or anorexic to avoid gaining weight.

bioavailability: the amount of a drug that can be absorbed into the body from a given dose.

biotransformation: metabolic transformation of drugs to metabolites.

Biphetamine®: a trade name for a capsule containing two forms of amphetamines, used mostly in the 1950s, '60s, and '70s.

bipolar affective disorder: a mental illness characterized by mood swings between excessive elation and severe depression with periods of normalcy; also known as "manic-depression."

"black tar" heroin: a black or brown form of heroin produced in Mexico. It varies from hard to sticky, has 20% to 80% purity, and is water-soluble.

blackout: loss of awareness and recall without unconsciousness due to intoxication by alcohol or other drugs (amnesia while under the influence of drugs).

blood alcohol concentration: *see BAC.*

blood-brain barrier: tightly sealed cells lining the blood vessel walls in the brain; prevents most toxins, bacteria, and pathogens from reaching the brain. Psychoactive drugs breach this barrier.

blood doping: transfusing extra blood before an endurance sporting event in order to increase the oxygen-carrying capacity of the circulatory system.

"blotter acid": a form of LSD; a drop of the drug is absorbed on a small piece of blotter paper and swallowed or placed on the tongue to be absorbed.

"blow": street term for cocaine hydrochloride.

bock beer: a stronger, darker, and sweeter variety of lager that has a shelf-life of six

weeks; a seasonal beer made from the residue in vats; traditionally ready for consumption with the coming of spring.

"body packer": a smuggler who swallows balloons or condoms, usually filled with heroin or cocaine, and then defecates the drugs after clearing Customs.

"bong": a water pipe used to smoke marijuana. The smoke is cooled and made less harsh as it passes through the water.

borderline personality disorder (BPD): characterized by sharp shifts in mood, impulsivity (often self-destructive), anger, alienation, and unstable self-image; BPDs are often drawn to drug use.

brain imaging techniques: methods to make images of the brain without dissection or death. Techniques include PET, SPECT, MRI, and beta scans.

brain stem: located at the top of the spinal cord, this section of the hindbrain is the sensory switchboard for the mind. It is often affected by hallucinogens. Contains the medulla and reticular formation.

breathalyzer: a machine that can measure the blood alcohol concentration by analyzing the exhaled air of a drinker.

bromide: hydrogen bromide salts formerly used (before barbiturates) as sedatives, hypnotics (sleeping pills), and anticonvulsants.

bromocryptine: medication that increases dopamine in the brain; helps initial detoxification from cocaine or amphetamines.

buccal: having to do with the cheek; absorption site for several drugs that are used orally, e.g., chewing tobacco, coca leaf.

Buerger's disease: circulatory disease that can be caused by smoking. It can result in amputation.

bufotenine: an hallucinogenic drug found in the skin secretions of several frogs and some plants.

bulimia nervosa: an eating disorder characterized by binge eating followed by weight control techniques including vomiting, excessive exercise, laxatives, and starvation.

buprenorphine: a drug that can help block both withdrawal symptoms and the effects of heroin; useful in detoxification.

buproprion: an antidepressant that raises levels of norepinephrine and dopamine.

"businessman's special": *see DMT.*

buspirone: an antianxiety drug that was created to avoid parts of the brain that can lead to addiction.

butanol (butyl alcohol): a synthetic alcohol used in many industrial processes.

"button": the round top of a peyote cactus that is harvested because of its psychoactive ingredient, mescaline.

butyl nitrite: an inhalant that causes a brief rush by dilating blood vessels in the heart and head, followed by dizziness, headaches, and giddiness.

C

caffeine: a stimulant alkaloid of the chemical class called "xanthines" found in coffee, tea, chocolate, and colas.

caffeinism: intoxication due to caffeine use characterized by restlessness, insomnia, nervousness, diuresis, and gastrointestinal problems.

CALDATA (California Alcohol and Drug Treatment Assessment): the most comprehensive study of treatment effectiveness done in California; showed that each dollar spent in treatment saves at least seven dollars in reduced costs, e.g., incarceration, missed work, burglaries.

CAMP (Campaign Against Marijuana Planting): a multi-jurisdictional law enforcement campaign to search out and destroy illegal marijuana fields and plants.

cAMP (cyclic adenosine monophosphate): a neurotransmitter involved in the development of opioid tolerance and tissue dependence.

cannabinols: major psychoactive cannabinoids of the *Cannabis* plant.

cannabinoids: any of the psychoactive chemicals found in *Cannabis* plants, including THC, the major psychoactive ingredient.

***Cannabis*:** the botanical genus of all plants that contain marijuana or hemp.

   ***C. indica*:** contains the most THC (psychoactive ingredient) of all the species; short shrub.

   ***C. ruderalis*:** low THC content species.

   ***C. sativa*:** most common species; can be high in hemp fiber content or THC content; often 10–20 feet tall.

capillary: the tiniest blood vessel in the circulatory system; absorbs drugs from mouth, gums, intestinal wall, nose, or other points of contact.

carbohydrates: the main plant energy source for animals and humans; found in many nutritional supplements.

carbon monoxide: a poisonous gas that is one of the toxic byproducts of smoking tobacco. Its chemical symbol is CO instead of the nontoxic CO_2 (carbon dioxide) that we exhale and breath every day.

carcinogen: any substance or pathogen that can cause cancer.

cardiovascular: relating to heart and blood vessels, e.g., the cardiovascular system.

catecholamine: a class of neurotransmitters that are particularly affected by psychoactive drugs, especially by stimulants, e.g., epinephrine, norepinephrine, dopamine.

cathinone: the active stimulant alkaloid ingredient, along with cathine in the plant stimulant called "khat."

central nervous system: the brain and spinal cord.

cerebellum: large part of the hindbrain. It affects motor systems and coordination.

cerebral cortex: outer part of the new brain (cerebrum) that enfolds the old brain. The gray matter is 1–4 mm thick. It processes sensory input, initiates voluntary movement, reasons, and thinks.

cerebral hemispheres: the two halves of the cerebrum that make up the cerebral cortex and the basal ganglia. Each half controls the sensory input and motor functions of the opposite half of the body.

cerebrum: largest part of the brain, it consists of the cerebral cortex (gray matter) and the thicker white matter that connects the cerebral cortex to the rest of the brain.

charas: Indian word for the resin of the *Cannabis* (marijuana) plant that is made into hashish.

"chasing the dragon": heating heroin on a piece of metal foil and inhaling the smoke through a straw.

chemical dependency (addiction): physical and/or psychological dependence on one or more psychoactive drugs; *also see addiction.*

chemotherapy: use of medications or chemicals to control disease, usually with cancer.

chewing tobacco: tobacco leaves that are processed to be chewed and the nicotine-laden tobacco juice absorbed by capillary blood vessels in the mouth, mostly in the gums. Chewing was the most common use of tobacco in the United States before 1900.

"chillum": a cone-shaped clay, wood, or stone pipe used to smoke bhang, ganja, or charas (various parts of a *Cannabis* plant); widely used in India.

"China white": 1. refined and unusually pure heroin from Southeast Asia, mostly from the Golden Triangle. 2. synthetic heroin (e.g., alpha-methylfentanyl).

"chipper": one who uses drugs occasionally; often applied to sporadic heroin user.

"chiva": Spanish street word for Mexican tar heroin.

chlamydia: the most common sexually transmitted disease in the United States; the presence of the infection is marked by a fluid discharge from the genitals or rectum.

cholinergic: pertaining to receptor sites and other neuronal structures involved in synthesis, production, storage, and function of the neurotransmitter acetylcholine.

chromatography: drug-testing process; gas chromatography and thin layer chromatography are the main uses.

chromosome: rod-shaped structures made of DNA and protein in the nuclei of cells. Each of the 46 chromosomes (in 23 pairs) in one cell contains more than 1000 genes (our genetic code).

"chronic": 1. slang for marijuana. 2. potent marijuana. 3. "crack" smoked with a marijuana cigarette.

chronic obstructive lung disease: progressive degeneration of the air sacs in the lungs, e.g., emphysema, chronic bronchitis; often caused by smoking tobacco or, less often, marijuana.

cirrhosis: a serious progressive liver disease that scars the liver; often caused by heavy chronic alcohol abuse.

clonidine: antihypertensive medication used to help block withdrawal symptoms from heroin, alcohol, sedatives, and even nicotine.

coca (*Erythroxylum coca*): the leaves of this shrub contain .5 to 1.5% cocaine; the leaves are chewed for a mild high; 95% of all coca is grown in South America.

cocaethylene: a toxic metabolite of cocaine formed by use of alcohol and cocaine; causes more severe cardiovascular effects and often more anger.

cocaine: the active ingredient of the coca bush. This alkaloid, first extracted by Albert Niemann in 1853, is a powerful fast-acting stimulant.

cocaine freebase: a smokable form of cocaine; made by releasing the hydrochloride molecule from cocaine hydrochloride; has a lower vaporization point than snorting cocaine.

cocaine hydrochloride: the refined extract from the coca bush. This white powder is used as a topical anesthetic for surgery and misused by addicts for snorting or injecting.

coca paste: the first extract of the refinement process that converts coca leaf to cocaine; often smoked (mostly in South America) but contains sulfuric acid and other impurities.

cocaine psychosis: a drug-induced mental illness; symptoms include extreme paranoia and hallucinations.

codeine: an extract of opium discovered in 1832. Between 0.5% and 2.5% of opium is codeine. This opiate analgesic is used for mild pain, cough suppression, and diarrhea control; also called "methyl morphine."

codependency: " . . . a pattern of painful dependence on another person's compulsive behaviors and on approval from others in an attempt to find safety, self-worth, and identity" (Scottsdale definition). Codependents judge their self-worth by relying on other's opinions of them, so they try too hard to please, have low self-esteem, are very impulsive, and are into denial.

cognition: accurate appraisal of one's surroundings; often disrupted during drug use, detoxification, and initial abstinence.

"cold turkey": detoxification from a drug, such as heroin, without the use of lower doses or other drugs to ease the withdrawal symptoms.

collapsed vein: a blood vessel that collapses on itself due to repeated injections or other traumas.

"coke": cocaine.

"coke bugs": imaginary insects a long-term cocaine abuser thinks are crawling under the skin. They often cause abusers to scratch themselves bloody.

compulsion: an uncontrolled need to perform certain acts, often repetitively, in order to forget painful thoughts or unacceptable ideas.

compulsive behaviors: compulsive gambling, anorexia, bulimia, overeating, sexual addiction, compulsive shopping, codependency, etc. Drug addiction is a compulsive behavior.

compulsive gambling: a progressive impulse control disorder characterized by a preoccupation with and a compulsion to bet increasing amounts of money on games of chance, continued gambling despite financial, work-related, and relationship problems, compulsion to chase losses, use of illegal acts or lying to get money with which to bet, and extreme denial that there is a problem.

computer games addiction: compulsion to play games, both online and through stand-alone systems.

computer relationship addiction: excessive searching through the Internet for relationships that can lead to cyberaffairs.

concurrent disorder: having a drug use disorder along with a mental disorder; also called "dual diagnosis" or "MICA."

confrontation: a counseling technique used individually or in a group that challenges the client's denial. This technique is crucial in treatment since most addicts are reluctant or afraid to change.

congeners: 1. a chemical relative of another drug. 2. by-products of fermentation (organic alcohols and salts) that add flavor and bite to alcoholic beverages.

contact high: 1. a nondrugged person emotionally experiencing a drug-like experience from being around or in contact with drug users. 2. getting high from skin absorption of a drug such as LSD. 3. actually inhaling enough drugs (marijuana, cocaine, heroin) to be affected by being in an environment where other people are smoking drugs.

controlled drinking: a controversial harm reduction technique that permits some drinking rather than abstinence as a way to limit alcohol abuse.

controlled drugs: psychoactive substances that are strictly regulated according to the Controlled Substances Act of 1970, e.g., cocaine, heroin, amphetamines, marijuana; there are five levels of controlled substances.

convulsions: involuntary muscle spasms, often severe, that can be caused by stimulant overdose or by depressant withdrawal.

coronary arteries: arteries that directly supply the heart with blood.

corpus callosum: the group of nerve fibers that connects the cerebral hemispheres.

cortex: the outer part of an organ, e.g., cerebral cortex.

corticosteroids: a class of drugs related to cortisol, a hormone normally produced by the body; helps control allergic reactions; relieves inflammation and pain

and can create a sense of physical well-being; different than anabolic steroids.

corticotropin: a neurotransmitter involved in the immune system, healing, and stress.

cortisol: *see hydrocortisone.*

cortisone: a steroid-like metabolite of hydrocortisone, a compound that reduces inflammation.

cotton fever: a blood poisoning or infection caused by injecting cotton fibers, pyrogens, or bacteria when using heroin, cocaine, or amphetamines intravenously. Symptoms include chills and fever.

countertransference: when a therapist or counselor lets personal feelings influence how he or she treats a client.

"crack": slang for cocaine that is made smokable by transforming cocaine hydrochloride to freebase cocaine using baking soda, heat, and water.

"crank": street term for methamphetamine sulfate but applied to any methamphetamine.

crash: the comedown from a high (usually a stimulant high) in which energy is depleted by the drug and by staying awake for days. Depression and anhedonia are common.

craving: the powerful desire to use a psychoactive drug or engage in a compulsive behavior. It is manifested in physiological changes, such as raised heart rate, sweating, anxiety, drop in body temperature, pupil dilation, and stomach muscle movements.

creatine: a nutritional supplement, this compound is synthesized in the body from amino acids or extracted from fish and meat; helps muscle energy metabolism, allowing someone who is working out to recover faster.

cross-dependence: occurs when an individual becomes addicted or tissue-dependent on one drug, resulting in biochemical and cellular changes that support an addiction to other drugs.

cross-tolerance: the development of tolerance to other drugs by the continued exposure to a drug that affects body mechanisms to tolerate other drugs, e.g., tolerance to heroin translates to tolerance to morphine, alcohol, and barbiturates.

"crystal meth": usually a street name for methamphetamine hydrochloride but now used to denote other amphetamines like dextromethamphetamine ("ice"), a smokable form of methamphetamine.

cue extinction: *see desensitization.*

cybersexual addiction: excessive use of online pornography or sex-related chat rooms to set up virtual or real sexual relationships.

cycling: using different steroids over set periods of time to minimize side effects and maximize desired strength- and muscle-enhancing effects.

cystic acne: an inflammation of oil glands in the skin, characterized by eruptions and scarring; often caused by prolonged use of anabolic-androgenic steroids.

D

DARE (Drug Abuse Resistance Education): a drug and violence prevention curriculum usually taught in fifth grade by police officers. The private organization is international.

date rape: sexual assault by a date rather than by a stranger. This and acquaintance rape are the most common types of rapes.

date-rape drug: drugs like Rohypnol (flunitrazepam), a strong sedative-hypnotic that can induce amnesia and GHB are slipped into a drink so that a date can be assaulted while in a stupor and not remember what happened. It is now banned in the United States.

DATOS: Drug Abuse Treatment Outcome Study done between 1991 and 1993 to study the effectiveness of treatment.

datura: hallucinogenic plant used throughout history that contains the alkaloids hyoscyamine and scopolamine. It disrupts the action of acetylcholine.

DAWN (Drug Abuse Warning Network): a federally funded data collection system that gathers information on drug fatalities, ER incidents, and use patterns from medical examiners and emergency rooms.

DEA: Drug Enforcement Administration, the federal agency charged with the job of policing drug abuse.

decriminalization: the elimination of criminal penalties for drug possession or use and replacing them with fines or other civil penalties.

dehydration: a deficiency of water in the body that can be aggravated by some drugs, particularly when exercising or dancing, e.g., GHB, creatine, MDMA and some stimulants.

delirium tremens: severe withdrawal symptoms from high-dose, chronic alcohol use; symptoms can include visual and auditory hallucinations, trembling, and convulsions; sometimes results in death.

deliriant: drugs that cause hallucinations, delusions, and confusion, e.g., ketamine, nutmeg, datura, belladonna, and deadly nightshade.

delta ( )-9-tetrahydrocannabinol: the main active ingredient in marijuana; also known as THC.

delusion: a mistaken idea that is not swayed by reason, often involving the senses.

demand reduction: a strategy to reduce drug use by lessening people's desire to begin use through prevention, treatment, and education.

dementia: intellectual impairment, found in some older people; includes loss of memory, abstract thinking, personality changes, and social skills; often found in those with Alzheimer's disease.

Demerol® (meperidine): an opioid analgesic like morphine, prescribed for moderate to severe pain.

dendrite: tiny fibers that branch out from nerve cells to receive messages from other nerve cells. Many drugs act on the ends of the dendrites and affect this transmission.

denial: the inability or the unwillingness to perceive one's addiction to a drug; a defense mechanism manifested by drug abusers and addicts.

dependence: 1. physiological adaptation to a psychoactive drug to the point where abstinence triggers withdrawal symptoms and readministration of the drug relieves those symptoms. 2. psychological need for a psychoactive drug to induce desired effects or avoid negative emotions or feelings. 3. reliance on a substance (or compulsive behavior).

depersonalization: a mental state when there is a loss of the feeling of reality or of one's self; can be caused by several psychoactive drugs, particularly hallucinogens.

depressant: a psychoactive drug, such as alcohol, a sedative-hypnotic, or an opiate, that decreases the actions in the brain resulting in depressed respiration, heart rate, muscle strength, and other functions; also called a "downer."

depression: a psychological mood disorder characterized by symptoms such as depressed mood, feelings of hopelessness, sleep disturbances, and even suicidal feelings.

depressive symptoms: feelings of sadness caused by grief, medical conditions, or

reactions to stress; they are usually short-lived compared to depressive disorders that can last for many months or years.

desensitization: a therapy technique that first exposes drug addicts to drug cues and drug-using situations that increase craving and then desensitizes them through education, biofeedback, or talk-down; also called "cue extinction."

designer drugs (analogues): drugs formulated by street chemists that are similar to controlled drugs. There are designer amphetamines that act partly like psychedelics, e.g., MDMA, MDA, and designer heroin, e.g. MPPP.

detection period: the time period in which a drug can be detected by drug testing.

detoxification: a drug therapy technique for eliminating a drug from the body. It can take a few hours to two weeks or more depending on length of use and the type of drug. It is the first step in most treatment protocols for addiction.

developmental arrest: the slowing or stopping of emotional development in a drug user, an abused child, or child with other psychological problems.

developmental disorders: mental disorders, such as mental retardation and AD/HD first diagnosed in childhood.

dextroamphetamine: a strong amphetamine stimulant sold as Dexedrine and Eskatrol .

DHEA (dehydroepiandrosterone): a hormone supplement used by some athletes to try and increase testosterone levels.

diacetylmorphine: chemical name for heroin.

Diathesis-Stress Theory of Addiction: a theory of addiction that says a predisposition to addiction, caused by hereditary and environmental factors is aggravated/triggered by stress and drug use.

diencephalon: an area of the brain located beneath the cerebral cortex consisting of the thalamus and hypothalamus.

diet pills: any substance that reduces appetite, most often amphetamine congeners, such as Redux® and Pondimin® or amphetamines, such as Desoxyn®.

diffusion: the tendency of drug molecules to spread from an area of high concentration to an area of low concentration.

diluent: usually a pharmacologically inactive substance used to dilute or bind together potent drug substances. Street drugs can contain active diluents like quinine or aspirin.

"dirty basing": a process of making smokable (freebase) cocaine using baking soda alone without ether, resulting in a product that contains many diluents and impurities.

disease concept: this model maintains that addiction is a chronic, progressive, relapsing, incurable, and potentially fatal condition that is mostly a consequence of genetic irregularities in brain chemicals. The addiction is set into motion by drug use in a susceptible host in an environment that is conducive to drug misuse. Loss of control and compulsive use quickly follow.

disinhibition: the loss of control over behavior, making the person more likely to perform formerly unthinkable or difficult actions, e.g., drinking alcohol makes them more likely to overcome shyness and talk to others.

dispositional tolerance: cellular and chemical changes in the body that speed up the metabolism of foreign substances, i.e., the creation of extra cytocells and mitochondria in the liver to handle larger and larger amounts of alcohol.

distillation: a chemical process that vaporizes the alcohol in fermented beverages and then collects the concentrated distillate. It can raise the percent of alcohol in a beverage from 12% (in wine) to 40% (in brandy).

distribution: the transportation of a drug through the circulatory system to other tissues and organs.

disulfuram (Antabuse®): a drug used to help prevent alcoholism relapse by triggering unpleasant side effects if alcohol is drunk.

"ditch weed": low-grade marijuana that is often found along the roadside in ditches. It was more plentiful when hemp was grown all over the United States.

diuresis: excess excretion of water due to excess intake or drug use.

diuretic: a drug that decreases the amount of water in the body by increasing the frequency and quantity of urination; often used to make one's competing weight in sports.

diversion: 1. diverting prescription drugs from legal sources into the illegal market, mostly opiates and sedative hypnotics. 2. putting a first-time drug offender in a treatment program rather than jail.

DMSO (dimethyl sulfoxide): a liquid that is easily absorbed through the skin and often used to transport other drugs, such as steroids, through the skin.

DMT (dimethyltryptamine): a short-acting hallucinogenic drug found in several plants (yopo beans, epena); also found in the skin secretions of some frogs, or synthesized in the laboratory as a white, yellow, or brown powder; a.k.a. "businessman's special" because of its short duration of action.

DNA (deoxyribonucleic acid): an organic substance found in the chromosomes of all living cells that stores and replicates hereditary information. The other type of nucleic acid is RNA, ribonucleic acid.

DOB (2,5-dimethoxy-4-bromoamphetamine): a synthetic, illegal stimulant/hallucinogen.

DOM (2,5-dimethoxy-4-bromo-amphetamine): a long-lasting synthetic hallucinogen; also known in the 1960s as "STP" and classified as a phenylalkylamine psychedelic.

dopamine: a major neurotransmitter often affected by psychoactive drugs; involved in euphoria and voluntary muscle movement and emotional states of mind.

dopinergic pathway: sometimes referred to as the drug-reward pathway through which a psychoactive drug triggers a rush and euphoria.

dose-response curve: a graph that shows the relationship between the amount of drug taken and the effects observed in the user.

double trouble: the existence of a substance use disorder and a mental disorder; also called "dual diagnosis."

drug distribution: the process by which a drug reaches the various organs and tissues of the body.

drug diversion: *see diversion.*

drug-diversion programs: programs such as drug courts used to treat first-time drug users and keep them from advancing to abuse and addiction.

drug hunger: a strong craving for a particular drug.

drug interaction: the alteration of the effect of one drug by the presence of another drug; *also see synergism.*

drug testing: examining the blood, breath, urine, or hair of people to determine if they are using drugs.

drug therapy: 1. the use of drugs to detoxify a drug abuser, to reduce craving, or to substitute a less damaging drug for a damaging one. 2. any medical treatment that involves the use of medication.

dry drunk: an alcoholic who has quit drinking but is not in recovery. They crave alcohol constantly and generally have alcoholic personality traits such as insensitivity to others, rigid outlook, dissatisfaction, and lack of insight or self-examination but they have learned to resist the impulse rather than change their lifestyle.

DSM-IV (Diagnostic and Statistical Manual of Mental Diseases): a publication of the American Psychiatric Association that classifies mental illnesses.

DTs: *see delirium tremens.*

dual diagnosis: a substance abuser with a coexisting mental illness; also referred to as comorbidity, MICA (mentally ill substance abuser), "double trouble," and concurrent disorders.

DUI (driving under the influence): drunk driving or driving under the influence of another psychoactive drug.

DWI (driving while intoxicated): drunk driving or driving under the influence of another psychoactive drug.

dysphoria: a general malaise marked by mild to moderate depression, restlessness, and anxiety; less severe than major depression.

dysthymia: a depressive mood disorder that is not as serious as major depression but can last for years (at least two years).

E

EAP (employee assistance program): a company-provided counseling service to help with substance abuse and any other personal problem. Usually these services are contracted to an external professional treatment group.

eating disorders: includes anorexia nervosa, bulimia nervosa, binge-eating disorder, and compulsive overeating.

"ecstasy" (MDMA, "X"): a synthetic analog of the methamphetamine molecule that causes some psychedelic effects; *see MDMA.*

edema: accumulation of excess water and other fluids in the tissues of the body.

EEG (electroencephalography): a technique that detects and measures patterns of electrical activity emanating from the brain by placing electrodes on the scalp.

effective dose: the dose of a drug that causes a desired effect 50% of the time. Twenty-five percent of the people tested require a higher dosage for the desired effect and 25% require a lower dosage.

EIA (enzyme immunoassay): in drug testing, the use of antibodies to seek out specific drugs.

"eight ball": 1/8 of an ounce of any drug, usually heroin, cocaine, or methamphetamine.

electroconvulsive therapy (shock therapy or ECT): the use of electric shocks to the brain approximately three times a week for two to six weeks to treat depression; developed in Italy in 1938.

elimination: the physiologic excretion of drugs and other substances from the body.

embalming fluid (formaldehyde): a chemical used to preserve dead bodies. It has been used as an inhalant and is also added to marijuana then smoked—known as "clickers" or "clickems" abuse. This material has also been used to help manufacture other illicit drugs including PCP.

embolism: blockage in a blood vessel caused by blood clots, additives in drugs, and other foreign matter associated with intravenous drug use such as cotton.

EMIT (enzyme multiplied immunoassay techniques): a sensitive urine drug test, rapidly and easily performed. Specific antigens are created for drugs that then react to them if they are present in the urine or blood sample.

emphysema: a lung disease, caused by smoking or by environmental pollutants, like asbestos, that gradually destroy the bronchioles of the lungs and their ability to take in air.

employee assistance program: *see EAP.*

EMT (emergency medical technician): a licensed medical technician who usually goes out on ambulance calls.

enabling: actions by anyone, especially relatives and friends, that allow addicts or abusers to continue their addictive behavior. It includes denial, codependence, paying off debts, lying to protect them, or providing money.

endocarditis: bacterial infection of heart valves that can be fatal; often induced by infected needles during IV drug use.

endogenous craving: craving for a drug caused by neurochemical changes in the brain such as depletion of dopamine resulting from cocaine abuse. The other craving is caused by environmental triggers (cue craving).

endogenous opioids: opioids that occur naturally in the body, including endorphins, enkephalins, and dynorphins;

antonym for exogenous opioids, e.g., heroin and opium.

endorphins: neurotransmitters that resemble opioids, They naturally suppress pain and induce euphoria. Heroin, morphine and other opioids mimic the effects of endorphins.

enkephalin: naturally occurring opioid peptides that are part of the endorphins and have shorter or less amino acids in their molecular structure.

environment: any external influence on a person, including relationships, school, work, living location, nutrition, availability of drugs, advertising, and kinds of friends. One of the three main factors most influential in forming a susceptibility to becoming an addict. The other two are heredity and the use of the drugs or the acting out of a compulsive behavior.

enzyme: a natural chemical that causes a chemical change in other substances (catalyst) without changing itself. Enzymes are often involved in the metabolism of drugs.

ephedra (ma huang): the natural source of the stimulant ephedrine.

ephedrine: an alkaloid stimulant extracted from the ephedra bush. It can also be synthesized in labs. It forces the release of norepinephrine, dopamine, and epinephrine in the brain's nerve cells. It can be used to manufacture methamphetamines and methcathinone. It is used as a bronchodilator in the lungs and a vasoconstrictor in the nose, so it is found in many OTC drugs, e.g., Sudafed®.

ephedrone: European street name for the stimulant methcathinone.

epinephrine: the body's own natural stimulant neurotransmitter (adrenaline); a catecholamine.

EPO (erythropoietin): a synthetic hormone that stimulates the production of oxygen-laden red blood cells; has potentially fatal side effects.

ergogenic drug: any drug that increases performance and strength in athletics or bodybuilding.

ergot: a toxic fungus found on rye, wheat, and other grasses that contains lysergic acid. It is used in the synthesis of LSD.

ergotism: poisoning by ergot often characterized by gangrene, numbness, and burning sensations.

Erythroxylum coca: the botanical name for the coca bush, the source of cocaine. It is grown mainly in South America but

some is grown in Indonesia. Other less prevalent plants include *Erythroxylum ipadu, Erythroxylum novotraterse,* and *Erythroxylum truxillense.*

estrogen: a hormone responsible for most feminine characteristics in women. Found in both men and women but in greater concentration in women, e.g., estradiol, formed by the ovary, placenta, testes, and possibly adrenal cortex; can be synthesized. Its production is often affected by drugs.

ethanol (ethyl alcohol, C_2H_6O): the main psychoactive ingredient in beer, wine, and distilled liquors; usually made from fermented grains, fruits, or carbohydrate based vegetables, such as potatoes and rice.

ether: a volatile liquid, it was the first anesthetic. It was discovered in 1730 and called "anodyne." It was used as a medicine, a drink, and an inhalant; often used for intoxication because it was thought to be less harmful than alcohol.

ethyl alcohol: *see ethanol.*

etiology: the study of the causes of a disease including addiction.

ETOH: a science data base on alcohol from the NIAAA (National Institute on Alcohol Abuse and Alcoholism).

euphoria: a feeling of well-being, extreme satiation, and satisfaction caused by many psychoactive drugs and certain behaviors, such as gambling and sex.

euphoriant: a substance that causes euphoria, e.g., cocaine, amphetamine, and heroin.

euthymia: a temporary elation; mental peace; less intense than euphoria.

excretion: the elimination of water and waste products, including drugs and their metabolites, due to metabolism through urination, sweating, exhalation, defecation, and lactation.

experimentation: the first stage of drug use where the person is curious but uses the drug only sporadically and there are no negative consequences.

F

facilitator: a professional intervention specialist or a knowledgeable chemical dependence treatment professional who arranges and participates in an intervention to break through an addict's denial and get him or her into treatment.

FAE (fetal alcohol effects): symptoms and physical defects in the fetus from alcohol use during pregnancy that are not as

severe as those found in fetal alcohol syndrome; *see FAS.*

false negative: a negative result on a drug test when the person should really test positive. It is often caused by operator error.

false positive: a positive result on a drug test when the person should test negative for drugs. False positives can be corrected through retesting and examination by a medical review officer.

family intervention: *see intervention.*

FAS (fetal alcohol syndrome): birth defects caused by excessive use of alcohol while pregnant. Signs of FAS include, retarded growth, facial deformities, and delayed mental development.

fat-soluble: capable of being absorbed by fat. Most psychoactive drugs are absorbed by the brain because the brain has a high fat content.

fen-phen (phen-fen): an acronym for the combination of dexfenfluramine and phentermine when prescribed for weight control.

fenfluramine: a drug that reduces appetite.

fentanyl: 1. a powerful synthetic opiate used to control severe pain and as an anesthetic in surgery. It is 100 times stronger than morphine; often abused in the medical community. 2. a street drug called "China white," used as a substitute for heroin, that uses the same basic formulation as pharmaceutical fentanyl.

fermentation: a chemical process that uses yeast to convert sugar usually found in grains, starches, and fruit, into alcohol.

fetal alcohol effects: *see FAE.*

fetal alcohol syndrome: *see FAS.*

fetus: an unborn yet formed human (from the eighth week to conception).

fight, flight, fright center: an area of the old brain and the peripheral nervous system that alerts us and helps us react to danger by increasing alertness, releasing adrenaline, and raising heart rate and respiration. It is initially triggered by emotional memories and instinctual drives in the amygdala and hippocampus.

FIPSE: Fund for the Improvement of Post-Secondary Education.

flashback: a remembrance of the intense effects of a drug, such as LSD or PCP, that is triggered by a memory, by encountering environmental cues, or by a residual amount of the drug being released, usually from fat cells.

fluoxetine: the chemical name for Prozac®, a popular antidepressant that acts by preventing the reabsorption of serotonin, a neurotransmitter.

fly agaric: a hallucinogenic mushroom named *Amanita muscaria.*

formaldehyde: *see embalming fluid.*

formication: a cocaine- or meth-amphetamine-induced sensation that makes users think that bugs are crawling under their skin.

fortified wine: wine whose alcohol concentration is raised to approximately 20% by adding pure alcohol or brandy.

freebase: cocaine that can be smoked as opposed to cocaine hydrochloride that is snorted or injected.

freebasing: transforming cocaine hydrochloride to cocaine freebase, using ether or other flammable solvent so it can be smoked. This method processes out impurities.

French Connection: a French heroin distribution syndicate, headed by Jean Jehan; it was the main supplier of refined heroin to the United States from the 1930s to 1973 when it was supposedly broken up by an international law enforcement coalition.

G

GABA (gamma-aminobutyric acid): this inhibitory neurotransmitter is one of the main neurochemicals in the brain.

gamma alcoholism: *see Jellinek.*

ganja (ghanga): Indian word for a preparation of the leaves and flowering tops of the *Cannabis* plant; less potent than charas, the resin, but more potent than bhang, the leaves and stems.

gas chromatography: *see GC/MS.*

gateway drug: any drug whose use supposedly leads to the use of stronger psychoactive drugs. The three most often mentioned are alcohol, tobacco, and marijuana.

GC/MS: gas chromatography/mass spectrometry; the most accurate method of drug testing. It can measure type of drug and amount. It is supposed to be 99.9% accurate.

generic name: the chemical name or description for a drug as opposed to the brand name, e.g., Valium® is the trade name while diazepam is the generic name.

genetic marker: any gene that makes a person more susceptible to the effects of a drug if they use that drug, e.g., a marker

gene for alcoholism that indicates slow metabolism for alcohol.

genetic predisposition: a genetic susceptibility to use drugs addictively that comes into play when that person starts using psychoactive drugs.

genetic susceptibility: *see genetic predisposition.*

genotype: the genetic make up of an individual; the totality of his or her inherited traits.

GHB (gamma hyhdroxybutyrate): synthetic version of a natural metabolite of the neurotransmitter GABA; used as a sleep inducer. It is popular among bodybuilders because it improves the muscle-to-fat ratio. It is also touted as a natural psychedelic and used as a party drug.

ginseng: a plant whose root has been used in Oriental herbal medicine for 4,000 years; advocates says it prolongs endurance, studies say it doesn't.

glaucoma: an eye disease that increases intraocular pressure. Marijuana is promoted as a medicine that can relieve the pressure.

glucose: a simple sugar found in fruits and plants that converts to alcohol when activated by yeast.

glutamine: an amino acid that is used as a nutritional supplement to rebalance neurochemistry and neurotransmitter formation.

glutethimide: a short-acting hypnotic that used to be a popular drug of abuse, usually in combination with codeine. It used to be sold as Doriden®.

Golden Crescent: an area of the Middle East that produces large amounts of opium   includes parts of Pakistan, Iran, and Afghanistan.

Golden Triangle: the major illicit opium-producing area in the world   includes parts of Burma, Thailand, and Laos.

gonorrhea: a common sexually transmitted infection usually marked by discharge from genitals or rectum and pain when urinating.

"goofballs": 1. street name for glutethimide (Doriden); a popular drug of abuse in the 1960s, '70s, and '80s. 2. the combination of "speed" and heroin.

gram: a metric unit of weight often used to measure drugs; 28.35 grams equals one ounce; 1,000 grams equals a kilogram or 2.2 pounds.

"grass": marijuana.

gray matter: the outer surface of the cerebral cortex and parts of the base of the cerebral hemispheres that consists mostly of dendrites and cell bodies.

group therapy: the use of several clients in a group to help each other break the isolation of addiction, increase knowledge, and practice recovery skills. There are different types of group therapy: facilitated, peer, 12-step, educational, topic-specific, and targeted.

growth hormone: *see HGH.*

gutkha: a mixture of betel nut, tobacco, lime, and flavorings sold mostly in India; it's chewed and the stimulant juice absorbed by the mucosa.

gynecomastia: enlargement of male breasts, often through the excess use of androgenic steroids that metabolize to an estrogen; steroid users often report this effect.

gyrus (gyri): ridges of convoluted, rounded brain tissue of the cerebral hemispheres

H

habit: a term for addiction, i.e., "he has a habit."

habituation: a level of drug use just before abuse where the substance (or behavior) is used on a regular habitual, basis but does not yet have regular serious consequences. There is some loss of control.

half life: the time it takes for half of a drug that has entered the bloodstream to be inactivated through metabolism and excretion.

halfway house: a treatment facility where the addict works and has outside contacts while being involved in a treatment program.

hallucination: a sensory experience that doesn't relate to reality, such as seeing a creature or object that doesn't exist. A common effect of mescaline, psilocybin, PCP, and occasionally LSD (illusions are more common with LSD).

hallucinogen: a substance that produces hallucinations; often used interchangeably with psychedelic, psychotomimetic, and psychotogenic, e.g., LSD, mescaline, peyote, DMT, psilocybin, and potent marijuana.

hangover: alcohol withdrawal symptoms that occur 8–12 hours after stopping drinking. They include headache, dizziness, nausea, thirst, and dry mouth. The causes are the direct effects of alcohol and its additives.

hard drugs: used in the past to refer to strong schedule I drugs, such as heroin, cocaine, and amphetamines.

harm reduction: a tertiary prevention and treatment technique that tries to minimize the medical and social problems associated with drug use rather than making abstinence the primary goal, e.g., needle exchange and methadone maintenance.

Harrison Narcotics Act: one of the first U.S. laws that controlled drug importation, manufacture, distribution, and sale of narcotics; enacted in 1914.

hash oil: an extract of marijuana (made using solvents) that is added to food or to marijuana cigarettes. Its THC content can be as high as 20% to 80%.

hashish: the potent sticky resin of the marijuana plant that is often pressed into cakes and sold or smuggled. The THC content is anywhere from 8% to 40%.

HCG (human chorionic gonadotropin): drug used to restart testosterone production in the body after long-term or high-dose anabolic steroid use. It can be toxic.

HCV: hepatitis C virus.

"head shop": a store that sells drug paraphernalia, including roach clips, water pipes, and "crack pipes."

hemp: a generic term often used to describe *Cannabis* plants that are high in fiber content and low in THC content.

henbane (*hyoscyamus niger*): an hallucinogenic plant containing the alkaloids scopolamine, hyoscyamine, and atropine.

hepatitis: liver disease that can inflame or kill liver cells. It is caused by a virus or by a toxic substance, such as alcohol. The most common strains of viral hepatitis are A, B, C, D, and E. Depending on the strain, they can be transmitted through contaminated needles, exchange of body fluids, or feces. Hepatitis B and C are the most common strains in injection drug users. *Also see alcoholic hepatitis.*

hepatitis B: a common form of hepatitis that is transmitted by contaminated blood, semen, vaginal secretions, and saliva. It is the ninth leading killer in the world. Often transmitted by high-risk sex and contaminated needles.

hepatitis C: a form of viral hepatitis found, in some studies, in 70% to 80% of injection drug users. It is a major cause of liver failure and liver cancer.

Herbal Ecstasy®: a commercial OTC stimulant that contains herbal ephedrine and herbal caffeine.

heredity: the transmission of physical and even mental characteristics through genes, chromosomes, and DNA .

heroin (diacetyl morphine): a powerful opiate analgesic, derived from morphine. It was discovered in 1874 and soon became the object of abuse and addiction.

herpes simplex: common sexually transmitted disease usually marked by intermittent painful blisters or sores on the genitals or mouth.

HGH (human growth hormone): a substance produced by the body that stimulates body growth and muscle size. It is used illicitly in sports but can have dangerous side effects; can now be synthesized rather than extracted from cadavers.

high-risk behavior: dangerous behavior, such as unprotected sex, violence, and risk taking, that can lead to injury or infection. It is often caused when drugs lower inhibitions or impair reasoning.

hippocampus: an area of the primitive midbrain in the temporal lobe that is responsible for emotional memories and converts short-term to long-term memory. It compares sensory input with experience to decide how to react.

histamine: a natural amine in the body that stimulates gastric secretions, constricts bronchi, and dilates capillaries, usually to bring healing to an injured area of the body.

"hit": a dose of a drug.

HIV (human immunodeficiency virus): the virus that causes AIDS symptoms and diseases.

homeostasis: the balance of functions and chemicals in the body as well as the process by which that balance is maintained; the process responsible for the development of tissue dependence, tolerance, and subsequent withdrawal from psychoactive drugs.

hops: an aromatic herb that comes from the dried cones of the *Humulus lupulus* vine, used in the brewing of virtually all beers; provides the bitter "hoppy" taste of beer.

hormone: a biochemical manufactured by an organ that can alter body function, e.g., pituitary gland.

"huffer": slang for an inhalant user or abuser.

human growth hormone: see *HGH.*

hydrocodone (Vicodin): a widely abused opiate based painkiller for moderate to severe pain.

hydromorphone (Dilaudid): a synthetic opiate analgesic prescribed for moderate to severe pain.

hyperplasia: precancerous changes in the bronchial tubes of the lungs characterized by abnormal and increased cell growth; often caused by smoking.

hypertension: high blood pressure. It can be caused by stimulant use (and sometimes psychedelics) or by withdrawal from depressants.

hypnotic: a drug that induces sleep, e.g., some benzodiazepines, barbiturates, bromides, and large amounts of alcohol.

hypodermic needle: a device for injecting a fluid into the body intramuscularly (in a muscle), intravenously (in a vein), or subcutaneously (under the skin).

hypoglycemia: a condition where an extremely low level of glucose is in the blood; often found in people with eating disorders. It causes symptoms of lethargy, lightheadedness, and hunger.

hypothalamus: part of the brain that controls the autonomic nervous system and maintains the body's balance. It also controls the hormonal system and is located near the top of the brain stem.

hypoxia: very low level of oxygen in the blood or tissues; can be caused by inhalant abuse.

I

iatrogenic addiction: addiction caused by medical treatment, i.e., liberal use of opiate analgesics in a hospital setting that leads to opiate addiction in a susceptible individual.

ibogaine: a long-acting psychedelic from the iboga shrub that, when used in high doses, acts like an hallucinogen; in low doses it acts as a stimulant; it is currently being researched as a treatment for heroin addiction.

ibuprofen: a nonopiate pain reliever that controls pain, fever, and inflammation.

"ice": street name for dextromethamphetamine, (actually dextro isomer methamphetamine base), a crystalline form of amphetamine that is smokable. It has slightly milder physical effects than methamphetamine hydrochloride but more severe mental effects.

illusion: a mistaken perception of a real stimulus, e.g., a rope is mistaken for a snake; a distortion of one's perceptions.

immune system: a complex system of white blood cells, macrophages, and other cellular and genetic components that defend the body against foreign organisms.

immunosuppression: a decrease in the effectiveness of the body's disease fighting mechanisms; can be caused by the use of certain drugs, by the HIV virus, or by other infectious agents.

immunoassay: testing for drugs using drug antigens, *see EMIT.*

impairment: physical and mental dysfunction due to psychoactive drugs or other addictive behaviors.

indica: a species of *Cannabis* that is high in THC content, *see* Cannabis.

individual counseling: one-on-one interaction between a therapist, counselor, or other treatment specialist and a client with emotional or mental problems to help him or her understand and cope with the illness.

indole psychedelics: a class of hallucinogens that includes LSD, psilocybin mushrooms, ibogaine, DMT, and yage.

information addiction: a form of Internet addiction that involves excessive surfing of the Web looking for data and information.

ingestion: taking food, liquid, drugs, or medications into the stomach by mouth.

inhalant: any substance that is vaporized, misted, or gaseous that is inhaled and absorbed through the capillaries in the alveoli of the lungs.

inhibition: controlling and restraining instinctual, unconscious, or conscious drives especially if they conflict with society's rules.

inhibitory neurotransmitter: a neurotransmitter, such as GABA or serotonin, that keeps a neurotransmitter from relaying a message.

injection: a method of rapid drug delivery that puts the substance directly in the bloodstream, in a muscle, or under the skin.

inpatient treatment: a 7–28 day program in a hospital or other residential facility that focuses on detoxification, therapy, and education.

insufflation: a term for snorting a drug, such as cocaine, heroin, or methamphetamine.

insulin: a hormone secreted by the pancreas to help control blood-sugar levels; diabetics need to use oral medications to force the pancreas to release more insulin or give themselves injections of insulin. Compulsive overeating can induce diabetes.

interdiction: a supply reduction, drug abuse prevention technique of intercepting drugs before they are distributed to dealers or users.

Internet addiction: a compulsion to overuse various services available on the Internet; it includes cybersexual addiction, computer-relationship addiction, net compulsions, information addiction, and computer games addiction.

intervention: a planned attempt to break through addicts' or abusers' denial and get them into treatment. Interventions most often occur when legal, workplace, health, relationship, or financial problems have become intolerable.

intoxication: functional impairment; loss of physical and mental processes due to substance use. It can be acute due to high-dose use or chronic due to continuous lower-dose use. In both cases it is most often caused by the drug's effect on the central nervous system.

intramuscular injection: injecting a drug into a muscle. It takes three to five minutes for the drug to reach the brain and have an effect.

intravenous injection: injecting a drug directly into a vein. It takes 15–30 seconds for the drug to reach the brain.

inverse tolerance (kindling or sensitization): continuous use changes brain chemistry to the point that the same dose suddenly starts causing a more intense reaction. The user becomes more sensitive to the drug's effects as use continues.

isopropyl alcohol: *see propanol.*

J

Jellinek, E. M. (1890-1963): famed researcher of alcoholism and founder of the Center of Alcohol Studies and co-founder of the National Council on Alcoholism. His well-known *The Disease Concept of Alcoholism* delineated five levels of alcoholism: alpha (problem drinking), beta (problem drinking with health problems), gamma (loss of control with severe health and social consequences), delta (long-term heavy drinking), and epsilon (periodic) alcoholism. These terms are not used nowadays but the descriptions are.

jimsonweed: an hallucinogenic plant of the *Datura* family; contains the anticholinergic substances hyoscyamine, scopolamine, and atropine.

"joint": slang for a marijuana cigarette.

"Jones": 1. withdrawal from chronic heroin use; symptoms include chills, sweating, and body agony. 2. term for any compulsive or addictive behavior, e.g., "Internet Jones."

"juice": street name for methadone, PCP, or steroids.

"junk": heroin or any psychoactive drug.

"junkie": someone who is addicted to a psychoactive drug, especially heroin.

K

Kaposi's sarcoma: a form of cancer that usually erupts as purple splotches on the skin. It is considered to be an opportunistic disease that is one of the signs of AIDS.

Keeley Institute: a series of 118 treatment centers in the United States that treated alcoholics, drug addicts, and tobacco smokers between 1880 and 1920.

ketamine: used as a recreational club drug, it is an anesthetic that produces catatonia and deep analgesia; side effects include excess saliva, dysphoria, and hallucinations. Its chemistry and effects are very similar to PCP.

khat: a 10–20 foot shrub whose active ingredient is cathinone, a mild to medium stimulant. It is brewed in a tea or the leaves can be chewed and the active ingredient absorbed. It is popular in Somalia, East Africa, Yemen, and other Middle Eastern countries.

kilogram: a metric unit of weight that equals 2.2 pounds.

kindling: see inverse tolerance.

Klonopin®: clonazepam; a popular benzodiazepine sedative. People in methadone maintenance use it to increase the high from methadone.

"knockout drops": old street term for chloral hydrate, a sedative hypnotic.

kola nut: the seeds of the *Cola nitida* tree found in Africa. It contains a high concentration of caffeine.

Korsakoff's psychosis: *see Korsakoff's syndrome.*

Korsakoff's syndrome: a disease that most often affects heavy, long-term drinkers; symptoms include short-term memory failure, confusion, emotional apathy and disorientation.

"krystal": street name for PCP; not to be confused with the street terms "crystal" or "crystal meth" that denote methamphetamine.

L

LAAM (levo-alpha-acetyl-methadol): a long acting opiate used as an alternative to methadone for heroin addiction treatment.

lag phase: the time between first use of a drug and the development of problematic use.

latency: delay between the time a person uses a drug and the time it appears in urine, blood, saliva, or other fluid.

laudanum: a popular opium preparation, first compounded by Paracelsus in the sixteenth century and popularized at the end of the nineteenth century.

laughing gas: nitrous oxide; an anesthetic that was originally used and abused in the nineteenth century for its intoxicating effect.

legal high: intoxication by a legal drug, such as alcohol or prescribed medication. Some include tobacco and caffeine use as legal highs.

legalization: a prevention concept that makes the cultivation, manufacture, distribution, possession, and use of drugs legal in order to reduce crime, drug dealing, and disease.

"lemon dope": slang for high-potency heroin. The name comes from the fact that lemon juice is sometimes added to heroin to make it ready for injection.

lethal dose: the amount of a drug that will kill the user. It can vary radically depending on purity, sensitivity of the user, tolerance, etc.

leukoplakia: white oral mucous that persists in the mouth and is sometimes a sign of HIV disease.

"lid": traditionally an ounce of marijuana; now any amount in a baggie is often called a lid.

ligand: a compound that binds to a receptor; the part of a neurotransmitter or peptide that slots into a receptor on a nerve cell's receiving dendrite.

limbic system: the emotional center in the CNS's midbrain. It includes the amygdala, hippocampus, thalamus, fornix, mammillary body, olfactory bulb, and supracallosal gyrus. It sets the emotional tone of the mind, stores intense emotional memories, alters moods and emotions, controls sleep, processes smells, and modulates the libido.

"line": a thin line of cocaine hydrochloride, about two inches long, that is snorted.

lipid solubility: the ability of a substance to be dissolved in a fatty substance. Many psychoactive drugs have a high lipid (fat) solubility.

lipophilic: a high lipid solubility.

lithium (carbonate): the main drug used to treat bipolar affective disorder.

liver: the largest gland in the body (2–4 pounds); metabolizes protein and carbohydrates and most psychoactive drugs that pass through the blood, especially alcohol.

lookalikes: legal drugs made with caffeine, ephedrine, or other legal substances to look like illegal sedatives or stimulants.

loss of control: the point in drug use where the user becomes unable to limit or stop use.

LSD (lysergic acid diethylamide): an extremely potent psychedelic (hallucinogen) discovered in 1943 that causes illusions, delusions, hallucinations, and stimulation. It was originally made from rye mold but is now made synthetically.

lysergic acid diethylamide: *see LSD.*

M

ma huang: an ancient Chinese tea that contains ephedra, a plant stimulant.

mace: the outer shell of nutmeg; has psychedelic qualities.

"magic mushrooms": hallucinogenic mushrooms, usually containing psilocybin or psilocyn.

"mainlining": using a drug, usually heroin, intravenously.

major depression: a mental illness characterized by a depressed mood and sleep disturbances without a life situation causing it.

major tranquilizer: antipsychotic drug.

malt: a grain, usually barley, that is sprouted in water, then dried and crushed; the resulting malt is used to brew beer; also used in many whiskeys as well as in many cereals.

malt liquor: a beer-like beverage with a slightly higher alcohol content than normal lager beer (6.5% to 7%).

mandrake (*Mandragora*): a bush found in Europe and Africa that contains anticholinergic psychedelics; popular in ancient and medieval times with shaman, witches, and medicine men.

mania: a period of hyperactivity, poor judgment, rapid thoughts, and speech; it can lead to a diagnosis of bipolar affective disorder (manic-depressive illness).

manic depression: *see bipolar affective disorder.*

MAO inhibitor: monoamine oxidase inhibitors; psychiatric drugs used to treat depression by raising the levels of norepinephrine and serotonin; can have severe side effects and has very dangerous cross reactions with other drugs and even foods.

marijuana: the common name for *Cannabis* plants that have high levels of psychoactive ingredients, especially THC. Also refers to the psychoactive portions of the *Cannabis* plant such as the flowering tops and resin.

Marinol®: brand name for dronabinol, a synthetic THC.

MDA (3,4-methylenedioxyamphetamine): a synthetic hallucinogen that became popular in the 1960s.

MDMA (3,4-methylenedioxymethamphetamine): commonly known as "X" or "ecstasy," a stimulant/hallucinogen first synthesized in the early 1900s and popularized in the '80s.

medial forebrain bundle: a nerve pathway involved in reward and satiation. It extends through the ventral tegmental area, the lateral hypothalamus, the nucleus accumbens, and the frontal cortex.

medical intervention: the use of medications to treat a substance-related or mental disorder. This is usually done in combination with group/individual therapy or other treatment techniques.

medical model: 1. using medications to treat addiction because addiction is caused by irregularities of brain cells and chemistry. 2. in mental health, the concept that mental illnesses are caused by a disease process and by changes in brain chemistry.

medical model detoxification program: use of medications and other medical therapies for detoxification, under the direction of medical professionals.

medical review officer (MRO): a physician who reviews positive drug test results to see if there is any other explanation or mitigating circumstances.

medulla: the part of the brain that controls heart rate, breathing, and other involuntary functions.

mentally ill chemical abuser (MICA): *see dual diagnosis.*

mescal: 1. toxic seed from the mescal tree that at nonpoisonous doses can cause hallucinations. 2. another word for peyote or mescaline as in mescal buttons.

mescaline: the hallucinogenic alkaloid of the peyote cactus; has also been found in other cacti (e.g., San Pedro cactus) and has also been synthesized.

mesolimbic dopinergic pathway: a nerve pathway in the limbic system of the brain that carries reward messages to the nucleus accumbens and frontal cortex; thought to play a crucial role in addiction.

metabolism: the body's mechanism for processing, using, inactivating, and eventually eliminating foreign substances, such as food or drugs, from the body.

metabolite: the byproduct of drug metabolism that can also have psychoactive effects on the brain; often used as markers in drug tests.

methadone: a long-acting synthetic opiate used orally to treat heroin addiction.

methadone maintenance: a treatment and harm reduction technique that keeps a heroin addict on methadone for long periods of time, even a lifetime. It helps them avoid infections from needle use, the need to break the law to support their habit, and the desire to return to the heroin lifestyle.

methamphetamine freebase: an altered form of methamphetamine called "snot." When methamphetamine is altered to the dextro isomer, methamphetamine base is called "glass," "batu," and "shabu." Both forms of methamphetamine base are smoked.

methamphetamine hydrochloride: also called "meth," "crystal meth," and "crystal;" an intense psychoactive stimulant based on the amphetamine molecule; used for injecting, ingesting, and snorting.

methamphetamine sulfate: a methamphetamine compound, sometimes called "crank," that is supposedly slightly harsher than methamphetamine hydrochloride.

methanol (methyl alcohol): wood alcohol; used a toxic industrial solvent; it can be synthesized.

methcathinone: a synthetic stimulant that is chemically related to the natural stimulant cathinone found in the khat bush.

methaqualone (Quaalude®): a sedative that was widely abused in the 1960s and '70s for its disinhibiting and intoxicating effects. It is now only available illegally and is usually counterfeited with a benzodiazepine or antihistamine.

methyl alcohol: *see methanol.*

methylphenidate (Ritalin®): an amphetamine congener stimulant used to treat attention deficit/hyperactivity disorder and narcolepsy. It has also been abused on the street; called "pellets" in street slang.

"Mexican brown": a heroin processed from poppies grown in Mexico; it is brown due to crude refining techniques.

MICA: mentally ill chemical abuser.

Mini Thins : small, thin tablets that contain pseudoephedrine and used by street chemists to make methamphetamine or methcathinone.

minor tranquilizers: antianxiety medications.

misuse: 1. an unusual or illegal use of a prescription, usually for drug diversion purposes. 2. any nonmedical use of a drug or substance.

monoamine oxidase inhibitors: *see MAO inhibitors.*

morning glory: a common garden plant that contains lysergic acid amide. The seeds are soaked and the liquid drunk, sometimes causing mild hallucinations.

morphine: a powerful analgesic that is extracted from opium sap that contains 10% morphine. Extracted and isolated in 1803, it set the stage for the refinement of other psychoactive substances present in many plant and even animal secretions.

MPPP & MPTP: MPPP is a chemical found in designer meperidine (Demerol®) whereas MPTP is the residue of the chemical used to make MPPP. The MPTP residue causes brain damage to dopamine producing neurons and produces the "frozen addict," an addict that can't move muscles voluntarily; similar to Parkinson's disease.

MRI (magnetic resonance imaging) scan: a technique of imaging the brain that relies on magnetic waves rather than x-rays. Its 3-D images have been used to visualize the neurological effects of psychoactive drugs.

MRO: *see medical review officer.*

mucous membranes: moist tissues lining various structures of the body including the bronchi, esophagus, stomach, gums, larynx, tongue, nasal passages, small intestine, vagina, rectum. Drugs can be absorbed on these tissues.

"mule": someone who smuggles drugs in their luggage, clothing, or body; *see body packing.*

multiple diagnosis: the presence of drug addiction in combination with two or more other ailments, e.g., polydrug diagnoses, diabetes.

"munchies": a strong desire to eat excessively that is caused by marijuana use.

muscarine: a neurologic toxin found in the *Amanita muscaria* mushroom that acts as a parasympathetic nervous system stimulant.

muscle relaxant: skeletal muscle relaxants; central nervous system depressants prescribed to treat muscle tension and pain.

muscling: injecting a drug into a muscle. This route takes three to five minutes for the drug to reach the central nervous system.

Muslims: followers of Islam who are forbidden alcohol and most other psychoactive drugs by their religion.

mutation: an alteration in a gene caused by radiation, chemicals, or medications.

N

NA (Narcotics Anonymous): a 12-step self-help group created in 1947 on the model of Alcoholics Anonymous.

naloxone (Narcan®) & naltrexone (Revia®): opioid antagonists that block the effects of heroin or other opiates; used to treat overdoses and to help prevent relapse during treatment.

Naproxen®: a pain reliever (analgesic): a drug that relieves pain and fever.

"narc": narcotics officer who sometimes works undercover.

narcolepsy: a sleep disorder characterized by sudden periods of sleep during the day and sleep paralysis or interrupted sleep at night; often treated with amphetamines.

narcotic: this term from the Greek *narkotikos*, meaning "benumbing"; originally used to describe any derivative of opium but came to refer to any drug that induced sleep or stupor. In 1914 it became a legal term for those drugs that were believed to be highly abused, like cocaine and opiates.

Narcotics Anonymous: a 12-step program developed along the lines of Alcoholics Anonymous but focusing on those addicted to drugs.

Native Americans: refers to indigenous people of North and South America who predated the colonizing European settlers of the fifteenth through nineteenth century. They are thought to have crossed over the Bering Strait from Asia 10,000 to 20,000 years ago.

Native American Church: a religious sect of about 250,000 Native Americans that uses the hallucinogenic peyote cactus as a sacrament for their rites that combine elements of Christianity and vision-quest ritual.

natural high: a feeling of elation and satisfaction that is induced without the use of psychoactive drugs, e.g., painting, sexual activity, or running.

"needle freak": an IV drug user who prefers the use of a syringe as a method of drug delivery; someone who has become addicted to using a needle to inject drugs.

negative reinforcement: a hypothesis about learning that says we learn an action when the response lets us avoid a negative stimulus or removes the negative circumstance, i.e., the threat of severe withdrawal from heroin reinforces the continued use of the drug.

neonatal: referring to the period immediately after birth and through the first 28 days of life; also referred to as a newborn.

neuroleptic: any drug used to treat a psychosis, particularly schizophrenia.

neuron: nerve cell made up of a cell body, axon, dendrites, and terminals.

neuroses: an older term that refers to any defensive behaviors that are used to control excess anxiety. These behaviors often impair the persons functioning.

nerve cell: the basic building block of the nervous system consisting of the cell body, the axon, the dendrites, and the terminals.

neuron: *see nerve cell.*

neuropathy: any condition that affects any segment of the nervous system.

neurotransmitters: chemicals that transmit messages between nerve cells. The activity of these chemicals are strongly affected by psychoactive drugs.

"nexus": 1. street name for 2CB, a hallucinogenic drug. 2. street name for methcathinone, a synthetic stimulant.

NIAAA: National Institute on Alcohol Abuse and Alcoholism.

"nickel bag" (now "dime bag"): five dollars worth of a drug, such as heroin; inflation has made it hard to find.

Nicotiana tabacum: the genus and species of plant that produces smoking and smokeless tobacco.

nicotine: the active stimulant alkaloid of the tobacco plant, it mainly affects the natural neurotransmitter acetylcholine.

nicotine replacement therapy: a treatment technique for smokers that supplies a smoker with lower and lower doses of nicotine (through patches, inhalers, and gum) to alleviate withdrawal symptoms.

nicotinic receptors: a type of cholinergic receptor that is affected by nicotine.

NIDA: National Institute on Drug Abuse.

NIH: National Institutes of Health.

nitrites: synthetic drugs (butyl, amyl, and isobutyl nitrite) that are used as inhalants; originally they used to treat heart pain (angina); the effects include a rush and mild euphoria followed by headaches, dizziness, and giddiness.

nitrosamines: chemicals found in tobacco that can cause cancer.

nitrous oxide: *see laughing gas.*

nonpurposive withdrawal: consists of objective physical signs that are directly observable during withdrawal; e.g., seizures, sweating, goose bumps, vomiting, diarrhea, and tremors.

nootropic drugs: so-called smart drugs that are supposed to improve mental ability, particularly for the elderly. They are often comprised of mild OTC stimulants, e.g., ephedrine and protein neurotransmitter precursors, like lecithin and d,l phenylalanine.

norepinephrine: a neurotransmitter that affects energy release, appetite, motivation, attention span, heart rate, blood pressure, dilation of bronchi, assertiveness, alertness, and confidence.

normative assessment: a prevention technique that teaches people that the true extent of drug use is less than they think; the idea is to lessen the pressure they might feel to use.

NORML: National Organization for the Reform of Marijuana Laws, the major political organization trying to legalize marijuana.

"nose candy": a street term for cocaine hydrochloride.

NSAIDs (nonsteroidal anti-inflammatory drugs): drugs used to control inflammation and lessen pain, e.g., Motrin, Advil.

nucleus accumbens septi: an area in the limbic system of the brain, sometimes called the "reward/pleasure/satiation center," that is activated by most psychoactive drugs; it produces a surge of pleasure or feeling of satiation when activated.

nutmeg: a spice that contains MDA and can therefore cause psychedelic and stimulant effects.

nutritional supplements: these substances include food extracts, vitamins, and minerals; used in treatment to build strength, neurotransmitters, and better athletic performance.

nystagmus: involuntary tics of the eye pupils as they move or even when they are not moving; often caused by drug use, especially PCP and alcohol.

O

obsessive-compulsive disorder: an anxiety disorder characterized by disturbing obsessive thoughts that can only be resolved by acting out some compulsive behavior, such as hand washing.

obsessive-compulsive personality disorder: a personality disorder marked by excessive neatness, rigid ways of relating to others, perfectionism, and lack of spontaneity.

occipital lobe: part of the cerebrum involved in vision; found at the rear of each hemisphere.

old brain: brain stem, cerebellum, and the mesocortex; these areas regulate physiologic functions and help the person experience basic emotions and cravings.

ololiqui: a variety of the morning glory plant; the seeds contain lysergic acid amide, a weak psychedelic.

ONDCP (Office of National Drug Control Policy): the cabinet level coordinating agency for drug control activities in the United States.

opiates: 1. any refined extract of the opium poppy, e.g., codeine, morphine, or semisynthetic derivatives of opium, e.g., heroin, hydromorphone. 2. a generic term that refers to any natural refinement, semisynthetic derivative, or synthetic drug that resembles the actions of opium extracts.

opioids: a term for synthetic opiates, e.g., fentanyl, Demerol, methadone, and Darvon.

opium: a drug that consists of the sap of the opium poppy; used legally for analgesia, cough suppression, and diarrhea control and illegally for euphoria or pain suppression.

oral gratification: satisfaction or pleasure obtained by placing something (tobacco, food) in the mouth.

organic mental disorders: mental illnesses caused by physical changes in the brain due to injury, diseases, or drugs and chemicals.

organic solvents: hydrocarbon-based compounds refined from petroleum that are used as fuels, aerosols, and solvents. They are often inhaled for the psychoactive effect. They include gasoline, paints, paint thinners, nail polish remover, and acetone.

OTC: *see over-the-counter.*

outpatient treatment: programs in which the client lives at home but receives therapy and support from a facility (such as a hospital), therapist, or therapy group.

outreach: programs in which therapists or community workers go into the community to identify and assist drug abusers and addicts rather than waiting for them to come into a treatment facility.

over-the-counter drugs: drugs and medications that can be obtained without a prescription and are legally sold in supermarkets and drugstores. These legal OTC medications include nonprescription drugs, such as NSAIDs, analgesics, aspirin, and nasal sprays.

overdose: the accidental or deliberate use of more of a drug than the body can handle; causes severe medical consequences, including coma and death.

P

P-300 waves: a brain wave involved in information processing that has been shown to be less active in alcoholics and in sons of alcoholics who have not begun to drink; it shows less responsiveness to sensory, particularly auditory stimuli.

panic attacks: short episodes (10–20 minutes) of intense anxiety, nervousness, heart palpitations, sweating, and shortness of breath due to anxiety, certain prescription medications, and use of stimulant drugs, including cocaine and amphetamines; withdrawal from depressant drugs can also induce an attack.

panic disorder: an anxiety disorder characterized by multiple panic attacks (sudden repeated episodes of intense anxiety, panic, and confusion).

Papaver somniferum: the botanical name for the opium poppy.

paranoia: irrational suspicions that someone or something is out to harm you; often induced by psychoactive drugs.

paranoid psychosis: irrational fears that someone or something is out to get you; the condition can be mimicked by drug use, particularly strong stimulant use.

paraphernalia: drug-using equipment such as syringes, glass pipes, and water pipe.

paraquat: an herbicide that has been used to destroy illegal marijuana crops.

parasympathetic nervous system: part of the autonomic nervous system that acts to balance the sympathetic nervous system, e.g., the sympathetic system speeds up heart rate and breathing while the parasympathetic system slows it down; the parasympathetic system mostly uses acetylcholine while the sympathetic system mostly uses norepinephrine.

paregoric: a tincture of opium and alcohol used since the early eighteenth century, mainly for diarrhea.

parenteral drug use: injecting a substance into a vein or muscle or under the skin.

parietal lobe: the area of the cerebral cortex that receives information from surface body receptors; found in the middle of the cerebral hemispheres.

Parkinson's disease: a disease caused by destruction of one of the dopamine-producing areas of the brain, the basal ganglia; symptoms include tremors, rigidity, and mask-like faces. The misformulation of a designer drug, MPTP induces a severe form of this disease.

passive smoking: inhaling secondhand smoke.

"pasta": Spanish for cocaine paste.

paste: an intermediate product of cocaine refinement that contains impurities, such as kerosene and sulfuric acid. This light-brown doughy substance can be smoked, often in countries that grow or refine the coca leaf.

patent medicines: medicines that were very popular in the eighteenth, nineteenth, and early twentieth centuries that promised cures for almost any ailment. They often contained opium, cocaine, *cannabis,* and alcohol. The unregulated distribution was responsible for the creation of thousands of opium, morphine, and cocaine abusers and addicts.

Paxil (paroxetine): an antidepressant that is a selective serotonin reuptake inhibitor

PCP (phencyclidine): a psychedelic drug first used as an anesthetic for people then for animals, but the side effects were too outlandish. It was smoked, snorted, swallowed, or injected as a street drug, starting in the 1960s, because it distorted sensory messages, deadened pain, and stifled inhibitions. It can cause catatonia, coma, or convulsions.

peer facilitator: a recovering addict and/or alcoholic who acts as a mentor, advisor, or confidante to help a drug abuser recover; also called a "sponsor."

peer group: a group of people with similar interests; peer pressure can encourage drug use.

"pep pills": an old street name for amphetamines.

peptides: a compound of two or more amino acids that can form into neurotransmitters.

performance-enhancing drugs: a broad category of drugs and substances used to increase energy, endurance, and strength, e.g., steroids.

periaqaueductal gray area: an area at the base of the brain that blocks or inhibits incoming pain messages.

perinatal: pertaining to the time before, during, or after birth.

peripheral nervous system: one of the two major divisions of the human nervous system (consists of the autonomic and somatic systems); the other part of the complete system is the central nervous system.

personality disorders: abnormal and rigid behavior patterns that begin in childhood, often last a lifetime, and are often self-defeating. They include paranoid, antisocial, narcissistic, borderline, and obsessive-compulsive personality disorders.

PET (positron emission tomography) scan: a brain imaging technique that uses the action of glucose to show brain activity.

peyote: a small cactus found in northern Mexico and the American Southwest that contains the hallucinogen mescaline.

peyotl: the Native American name for peyote.

phantasticants: a word once used for hallucinogens.

pharmacodynamic tolerance: a defense mechanism of the brain that causes neurons to become less sensitive to the effects of psychoactive drugs.

pharmacodynamics: the study of the effects of drugs on living organisms.

pharmacokinetics: the science that examines the movement of drugs within the body, including uptake, absorption, transportation, diffusion, and elimination.

pharmacology: the science of drug action in the body.

phencyclidine: *see PCP.*

phenothiazines: a class of psychiatric medications, developed in the early 1950s and used to treat schizophrenia; also called "neuroleptics" or "antipsychotics."

phenotype: the totality of a person as determined by genetic and environmental factors.

phenylalkylamine psychedelics: a class of psychedelics that is chemically related to adrenaline and amphetamine, e.g., peyote, MDMA.

phenylpropanolamine: a decongestant and mild appetite suppressant that is used in many over-the-counter medications to treat the symptoms of colds and allergies and in lookalike stimulants. This is also an active ingredient in lookalike stimulants.

pheromones: natural human hormones found in sweat that increase sexual desire and stimulation by their odor.

physical dependence: *see tissue dependence.*

PID (pelvic inflammatory disease): a common sexually transmitted disease; an infection of the uterus, fallopian tubes, and ovaries.

pilsner beer: any light lager beer; originated in Pilsen, Czechoslovakia, it has a high wheat content with the malted barley.

placebo: a nonactive substance, e.g., sugar pill, that is given to a patient to let him think he is getting a real medication. It's used as a control to test the effects of an active medication.

placebo effect: a symptomatic response to a nonactive substance caused by the user's emotional and mental response rather than by true pharmacological reactions.

placental barrier: a membrane between the mother's and the fetal blood supply that allows the absorption of nutrients by the embryo while trying to keep toxic substances out. Unfortunately, psychoactive drugs cross this barrier.

polydrug abuse: the use of several drugs either in succession or at one time that causes significant physical, mental, or social distress.

"poppers": street name for the inhalants amyl, butyl, and isobutyl nitrites.

postsynaptic: the end of the dendrite of a nerve cell that's on the receiving side of a neural message.

posttraumatic stress disorder (PTSD): persistent reexperiencing of the memory of a stressful event outside usual human experience, such as combat, molestation, or a car crash.

"pot": marijuana.

potentiation: an exaggerated effect caused by using two drugs together; a synergistic effect.

potency: the pharmacological activity of a given amount of drug.

potentiate: to increase the potency of a medication or brain chemical through the use of another drug.

"pothead": marijuana abuser or addict.

precursor: any physiologically inactive substance that is converted to an active enzyme, drug, hormone, neurotransmitter, or other precursor by chemical processes.

predisposition: a susceptibility to overreact to the use of a drug; heredity and environment along with drug use, can activate this tendency to abusive and addictive use of psychoactive drugs.

prefrontal cortex: the front tip of the brain. It is responsible for a person's emotional response to situations, e.g., despair, elation, ecstasy. It is also part of the reward pathway that helps determine a user's reaction to drugs.

prescription drugs: any medication that needs a doctor's permission to use.

prevention: a group of social, medical, psychological, economic, or legal measures used to lessen potential for or the actual impact of drug abuse and addiction.

primary prevention: a series of prevention techniques aimed at nonusers to promote abstinence, delay drug use, increase drug education, and promote healthy alternatives.

primitive brain: also referred to as the old brain, it is the area surrounded by the reasoning cerebrum. It therefore handles instincts, automatic body functions, and emotions. A version of it is found in all animals.

"primo": 1. marijuana and "crack" smoked together. 2. really potent drugs.

problem drinking: a pattern of drinking, similar to abuse, in which the drinker is experiencing serious life problems due to drinking but has not yet earned a definitive diagnosis of alcoholism.

prodrug: any drug that becomes active when metabolized by the body, e.g., the amino acid tyrosine is converted to the active neurotransmitter dopamine in the brain.

prohibition: a supply reduction prevention technique that prohibits the importation, sale, or use of a drug. It is carried out through laws and interdiction.

proof: a measure of the amount of pure alcohol in an alcoholic beverage. Generally in America, 100% pure alcohol equals 200 proof, so 50% alcohol equals 100 proof.

propanol (isopropyl alcohol): also called "rubbing alcohol," it is used in shaving lotion, shellac, antifreeze, and lacquer.

protease inhibitors: drugs that help repress HIV reproduction by inhibiting an HIV enzyme (protease). Drugs such as indinavir, nelfinavir, and ritonavir are use in combination with other drugs for antiretroviral therapy.

protracted withdrawal: experiencing craving, side effects, and withdrawal symptoms long after being detoxified from a psychoactive drug usually due to environmental cues that stimulate memories of withdrawal, release small amounts of the drug from fat storage, or release accumulated toxic metabolites in the body.

Prozac® (fluoxetine): an extremely popular antidepressant medication that is classified as a selective serotonin reuptake inhibitor (SSRI). It increases the action of serotonin in the brain by preventing its reabsorption.

pseudoephedrine: an isomer of ephedrine that is used in the illicit manufacture of methamphetamines; found in many over-the-counter products, such as bronchodilators.

psilocin: an active hallucinogenic ingredient of the *Psilocybe* mushroom.

Psilocybe: a genus of mushrooms that contain the hallucinogenic substances psilocybin and psilocin, e.g., *Psilocybe cubensis* and *Psilocybe cyanescens*.

psilocybin: an active hallucinogenic substance found in psilocybe mushrooms. It is converted to psilocin in the body.

psyche: the psychological makeup of a person; the soul.

psychedelic: a common term for any drug that can induce illusions or hallucinations, including LSD, MDMA, psilocybin, ketamine, PCP, and for some, marijuana.

psychoactive drug: any substance that directly alters the normal functioning of the central nervous system when it is injected, ingested, smoked, snorted, or absorbed into the blood.

psychological dependence (psychic dependence): drug-caused altered state of consciousness that reinforces dependence on the drug. This is different than tissue or physical dependence.

psychosis: a psychiatric disorder that grossly distorts a person's thinking and behavior making it difficult to recognize reality and cope with life. Schizophrenia, bipolar disorders, and organic brain disorders are the main divisions.

psychotherapy: a technique of treatment for emotional, behavioral, personality, and psychiatric disorders based principally on verbal communication and interventions with a patient as opposed to physical and chemical interventions.

psychotic: of or relating to psychosis or the behavior associated with psychosis.

psychotomimetic: a drug that can induce behavioral and psychological changes that mimic psychosis.

psychotropic drugs: drugs used to treat mental illnesses, e.g., antidepressants, antipsychotics, and anxiolytics.

PTSD: *see posttraumatic stress disorder.*

P₂P: phenyl-2-propanol, a chemical used to make methamphetamine.

pupillometer: a device for measuring the size of the pupil that is used to detect drug use.

purging: self-induced vomiting, often used by those with bulimia to maintain weight.

purity: a measure of the freedom from contaminants in a sample of a drug.

purposive withdrawal: withdrawal symptoms falsely reported by the addict to get drugs from a doctor or psychosomatic symptoms triggered by the expectation that symptoms will occur.

Q

Quaalude® (methaqualone): a sedative-hypnotic that is no longer available except through street chemists and illegal distribution channels. It was popular in the 1960s, '70s, and the early '80s. It was popular because of its strong disinhibition effect.

quid: a ball of chewed drug (coca leaf, tobacco) that is kept in the mouth to allow the active ingredient to be absorbed by the capillaries in the mouth; also called a "chaw" or a "plug."

R

random testing: a method of drug testing with unannounced or short notifications; used by many sports organizations.

rapid opioid detoxification: a technique to rapidly induce opioid withdrawal using naloxone or naltrexone and then mitigate the withdrawal symptoms with other medications.

Rational Recovery: a self-help recovery group that uses a cognitive-behavioral approach to treatment and recovery.

"rave": a music party (held in a rented warehouse, in the desert, in a nightclub, or even outdoors in a field) where drugs, particularly psychedelics like LSD, "ecstasy" (MDMA), "GHB," and ketamine, are readily available.

receptor: a protein found on the dendrites or cell body of neurons and other cells that receives and then binds specific neurotransmitters; this process of "slotting in" to the receptor causes nerve messages to be transmitted.

recovery: the final step in drug treatment, following abstention, initial abstinence, and long-term abstinence in which clients have changed their style of living and have overcome their major physical and mental dependence on psychoactive drugs or addictive behaviors and are committed to abstinence; acceptance of one's addictive disease and commitment to a continued drug-free lifestyle.

recreational drugs: also known as "social" or "street drugs," these legal and illegal drugs include alcohol, tobacco, marijuana, cocaine, methamphetamines, LSD, heroin, and even caffeine.

recreational (social) drug use: a level of drug use after experimentation where people seek out the drug to experience certain effects but there is no established pattern of use and it has a relatively small impact on their lives; use is sporadic, infrequent, and unplanned.

"reefer": a marijuana cigarette; also called a "joint."

rehabilitation: restoring an abuser or addict to an optimum state of physical and psychological health through therapy, social support, and medical care.

reinforcement: a learning process whereby a person receives a reward for a certain action. That reward, in turn, increases the likelihood that the person will repeat that action.

relapse: reoccurrence of drug use and addictive behavior after a period of abstinence or recovery.

relapse prevention: a treatment technique that focuses on preventing the recovering addict from using again.

resiliency: the ability of an individual to resist drug use and abuse. The resistance qualities are formed by hereditary and environmental influences at home, in school, and in the community.

resin: the psychoactive secretions of the *Cannabis* plant on the outer portions of the plant and on the flowering buds.

resistance skills training: a prevention technique that involves training an individual to resist the use of psychoactive drugs and peer pressure.

reticular activating system: the heart of the brain stem involved in maintaining consciousness; it can be blocked by several drugs, including anesthetics.

reuptake channels: sites on the axon terminals of neurons that reabsorb neurotransmitters that have been emitted, absorbed, and released in the synaptic gap.

reverse tolerance: a turnaround in the body's ability to handle greater and greater amounts of a drug, i.e., aging or excessive alcohol abuse reduces the liver's ability to handle alcohol, so a chronic alcoholic in his 40s or 50s might only be able to handle a few drinks instead of the case of beer he could 20 years earlier.

Revia : *see naltrexone.*

reward deficiency syndrome: a theory of addiction that proposes a common biological substrate and pathway for drug and behavioral addictions. It further proposes that a person's hereditary inability to experience reward due to a scarcity of dopamine receptor sites in the reward pathway makes the person more likely to search for intense experiences to trigger this pathway.

reward/pleasure center: *see mesolimbic dopinergic pathway.*

"roid": street name for an anabolic steroid.

RIA (radio immunoassay): a method of drug testing that uses antibodies to seek out drugs in biofluids.

risk factors: hereditary and environmental factors that put adolescents and adults at risk to abuse drugs; e.g., physical and mental abuse, a family history of drug abuse, living in poverty, and lack of self-esteem.

"rig": syringe or hypodermic needle.

Ritalin : *see methylphenidate.*

"rock": 1. a piece of "crack" cocaine. 2. slang for "crack."

Rohypnol (flunitrazepam): a potent sedative-hypnotic, currently banned in the United States, that can cause sleepiness, relaxation, and amnesia; sometimes used in cases of date rape.

"roid rage": sudden outbursts of anger caused by excess steroid use. The rage goes away when the drug is stopped.

"rush": a sense of elation or intense satisfaction caused by some psychoactive drugs. The sensations can be mimicked by natural highs, such as thrill seeking, meditation, and fasting.

S

sacrament: visible sign of an inward connection with a deity. Historically, a number of psychoactive drugs have been used sacramentally in religious services.

SAMHSA: Substance Abuse and Mental Health Services Administration.

scheduled drugs: drugs that are controlled by the Controlled Substances Act of 1971. Illegal drugs like cocaine, heroin, and methamphetamines are schedule I. Strong drugs used medicinally are schedule II, e.g., morphine, Demerol®, and Ritalin .

schizophrenia: a mental illness (psychosis) characterized by hallucinations, delusional and inappropriate behavior, poor contact with reality, hallucinations, and an inability to cope with life. Strong stimulants, including methamphetamine, can mimic the symptoms of schizophrenia.

scopolamine: an alkaloid found in certain plants, such as deadly night shade that can induce sleep. It has been called "truth serum."

second messenger: a neurotransmitter that attaches itself to another neuron to limit or increase the release of neurotransmitters, i.e., the release of endorphins to inhibit the release of substance "P," a pain transmitter.

secondhand drinking: the effect of heavy drinking on nondrinkers, e.g., unwanted sexual advances, vomit in the hallway.

secondhand smoke: cigarette or cigar smoke that is inhaled by a nonsmoker while they are in the presence of smokers.

secondary prevention: a strategy to identify those who are beginning to experiment with drugs and prevent them from using more drugs or having problems with drugs.

Secular Organization for Sobriety: (SOS): a 12-step group self-help group for agnostics and atheists.

sedative: a drug that eases anxiety and relaxes the body and mind; also called "tranquilizers" and "muscle relaxants."

sedative-hypnotic: any drug that either relaxes and soothes the body and mind, eases anxiety, or induces sleep. The two main categories are benzodiazepines, such as Xanax and Klonopin , and barbiturates, like phenobarbital.

selective tolerance: the variable development of tolerance for different effects of a drug. It means that as the user develops a tolerance for desired mental effects, he or she may be developing less tolerance to other lethal effects of that drug, thus making overdose more likely.

selective serotonin reuptake inhibitors: see SSRI.

Selective Severity Assessment Test: one of the main diagnostic tests for addiction; evaluates 11 physiologic signs of addiction.

sensitization: the development of susceptibility to the effects of a drug over a period of use in which the same amount can trigger a greater effect; see inverse tolerance.

serotonin: a neurotransmitter involved in mood stability, especially depression, anxiety, sleep control, self-esteem, aggression, and sexual activity.

set: the mood and mental state of a person when taking a drug.

setting: the location where a drug is taken; ambiance is important in determining the overall effect of a psychoactive drug, such as LSD, on a user.

sexual addiction: sexual behavior over which the addict has no control including excessive use of pornography, masturbation, serial affairs, phone sex, and the use of prostitutes.

"shabu": slang for smokable methamphetamine ("ice").

shaman: a medicine man or priest who uses magic or spiritual forces to cure illness, speak to the spirits and control the future. They often use psychoactive drugs to help them reach the desired mental state or trance.

"shoot up": to inject oneself with a drug.

"shooting gallery": a building or room where drugs are regularly injected.

SIDS (sudden infant death syndrome): a sudden and often unexplainable death of an otherwise healthy infant.

sildenfil citrate: Viagra .

simple phobia: irrational fear of a specific thing or place.

sinsemilla: a technique for growing high-potency marijuana that consists of keeping female marijuana plants from being pollinated by male ones, thus greatly increasing the THC content from a few percent to as high as 30% or more.

"skin popping": injecting a drug under the skin rather than into a vein or muscle.

"smack": slang for heroin.

smokeless tobacco: chewing tobacco or snuff; any tobacco that is not smoked.

snorting: inhaling a drug through the nose to let the capillaries in the mucosal membranes absorb the drug; it takes 5–10 minutes for a drug to reach the brain when it is snorted.

snuff: 1. powdered tobacco that is absorbed through nasal membranes when it is snorted. 2. a term for finely chopped tobacco leaves that are put into the buccal membrane of the mouth for absorption (e.g., Copenhagen , Skoll).

sobriety: a term for abstinence from drugs or alcohol (being sober); the concept is used mostly in Alcoholics Anonymous and other 12-step groups.

social drinking: a level of drinking between experimentation and habituation; drinking is sporadic, infrequent, and non patterned; i.e., moderate drinking at social occasions rather than by oneself.

social drug use: see recreational use.

social model recovery program: a non-medical outpatient drug treatment program that uses a number of therapies.

social phobia: fear of being seen by others acting in a humiliating or embarrassing way.

soda doping: ingesting sodium bicarbonate 30 minutes prior to exercise to supposedly delay fatigue.

sodium ion channel blockers: a class of medications that interferes with neuron transmission to mute cocaine's or other drug's effects.

soft drugs: a general vague term for drugs like marijuana, alcohol, and tobacco that are less intense than hard drugs, e.g., cocaine, heroin, and amphetamines. Soft drugs cause more social and public health problems than so-called hard drugs.

Soma : 1. an ancient term for *Amanita muscaria*, an hallucinogenic mushroom. 2. trade name for carisoprodol, a skeletal muscle relaxant drug.

somatic system: part of the peripheral nervous system that transmits sensory messages to the central nervous system and then transmits responses to muscles, organs, and other tissues.

somatoform disorders: mental illnesses in which psychological conflicts manifest themselves as physical symptoms.

somatotype: body type of a person; particularly influenced by genetics.

SPECT (single photon emission computer tomography) scan: a brain imaging technique that measures cerebral blood flow and brain metabolism; enables clinicians and researcher to study how a brain functions before, during, and after drug use; can also image brain function of people with neurological diseases or syndromes, such as Alzheimer's or AD/HD.

"speed": street name for any amphetamine or methamphetamine.

"speedball": a drug combination of an upper and downer, usually heroin and cocaine or heroin and methamphetamine, that is injected, snorted, eaten, or smoked in combination with each other.

"speedfreaks": an old street term for methamphetamine abusers.

spirituality: an individual's personal relationship with his or her higher power; awareness or acceptance that one is part of a greater purpose or existence than just their own worldly existence; a crucial part of 12-step groups.

spit tobacco: a term for smokeless tobacco, including chewing tobacco and snuff.

SSRI (selective serotonin reuptake inhibitor): a group of antidepressants that increase the levels of serotonin in the central nervous system, e.g., Prozac , Zoloft , Paxil , and Effexor .

stacking: using two or more steroids at one time to increase effectiveness.

St. Anthony's Fire: a name for ergot poisoning. Ergot is a rye or wheat fungus that contains lysergic acid amine, a hallucinogen. One of the symptoms is a burning sensation of the skin.

stash: 1. a hiding place for an illegal drug supply. 2. a supply of illegal drugs.

"step on": adulterating a drug with the addition of cheap or inactive substances to increase the amount available for sale.

steroids: *see anabolic steroids.*

stimulant: any substance, including cocaine, amphetamines, diet pills, coffee, khat, betel nuts, ephedra, and tobacco, that forces the release of epinephrine and norepinephrine, the body's own stimulants. They stimulate the nervous system by increasing the electrical and chemical activity of the brain.

stout: a top-fermented variety of ale that is very dark and sweet, mostly associated with Ireland.

street drugs: illegal psychoactive drugs, such as cocaine, heroin, and marijuana.

stress: the body's reaction to illness and environmental forces. It produces psychological strain and physiological changes, including the release of cortisol, rapid respiration and heart rate, constricted blood vessels, and release of hormones.

subcutaneous: under the skin.

sublingual: under the tongue; a route of drug administration where the drug is absorbed by mucous membranes.

substance abuse: continued use of a psychoactive drug despite adverse consequences.

substance dependence: maladaptive pattern of substance use, e.g., addiction.

substance P: the neurotransmitter that transmits pain from neuron to neuron.

substance-induced disorders: disorders caused by the actual use of psychoactive drugs.

substance-related disorders: the overall classification for drug disorders that is divided into substance use disorders and substance-induced disorders.

substance use disorder: a classification of substance-related disorders defined by the pattern of drug use, including substance dependence and substance abuse.

substantia nigra: part of the extrapyramidal system in the brain that helps control muscle movements.

substitution therapy: using a drug that is cross-tolerant with another to detoxify a user who has become physically dependent.

sudden infant death syndrome: *see SIDS.*

supply reduction: a prevention approach that uses techniques, such as interdiction of illegal drugs, drug use laws, legal penalties, and crop eradication, to reduce the supply of drugs available to users, abusers, and addicts.

susceptibility: a person's individual vulnerability to use drugs addictively or engage in compulsive behaviors; it is based on heredity, environment, and drug use or acting out. These factors make one more likely to use and another to resist use.

sympathetic nervous system: part of the autonomic nervous system; it helps control involuntary body functions, including digestion, blood circulation, and respiration; works with the parasympathetic nervous system to balance body functions.

synapse: the process of nerve cell communication through the release of neuro-

transmitter chemicals that cross the synaptic gap to transmit a message from one nerve cell to another.

synaptic gap: the tiny gap between the terminal of the sending nerve cell and the dendrites or body of the receiving cell.

synergism: an exaggerated effect that occurs when two or more drugs are used at the same time. One reason why this effect occurs is because the liver or body is busy metabolizing one drug while the other slips through unchanged.

synesthesia: an effect of hallucinogens that converts one sensory input to another, i.e., colors are heard, sounds are seen.

synthesis: the process of making drugs in the laboratory with chemicals and artificial techniques rather than extracting them from plants or animals.

syphilis: a sexually transmitted disease with three levels of infection severity; less common with the discovery of penicillin and other antibiotics.

syringe: a device for injecting drugs directly into the body.

T

T-cells: a type of white blood cell (lymphocyte) that helps fight infection. Low numbers of T-cells signal an impaired immune system, possibly caused by HIV infection.

tachycardia: rapid beating of the heart caused by cardiovascular disease or drugs, especially stimulants.

tar: a by-product of smoking that is carcinogenic.

"tar" heroin: a black or dark brown heroin originally grown and processed in Mexico. It contains many impurities but can be 20% to 80% pure. It is water soluble. Tar heroin is now processed in Africa and South America as well as Mexico.

tardive dyskinesia: a nerve disorder caused by a side effect of antipsychotic drugs; symptoms include involuntary facial tics and involuntary movements of the tongue.

temperance: a philosophy of light to moderate drinking that is an alternative to abstinence or prohibition.

temporal lobe: the sides of the cerebral cortex involved in emotions, language, sensory processing and short-term memory.

teratogen: a drug that produces a birth defect.

terminals: small buttons at the end of nerve cells that release neurotransmitters.

tertiary prevention: a prevention strategy aimed at drug abusers and addicts to reduce harm to themselves and to society. Intervention, treatment, and harm reduction techniques are used.

testosterone: the most potent male hormone, formed mainly in the male testes; the major naturally occurring anabolic steroid.

tetrahydrocannabinol: *see THC.*

"Texas shoeshine": spray paint containing toluene and abused as an inhalant.

Thai sticks: marijuana buds tied to bamboo shoots; a potent packaging of marijuana.

thalamus: part of the diencephalon that helps relay information to the cerebral cortex.

THC (tetrahydrocannabinol): the main psychoactive ingredient of marijuana; mimics the natural neurotransmitter anandamide.

theobromine: an alkaloid from the cacao plant that is similar to caffeine. It is used as a diuretic, heart stimulant, muscle relaxant, and vasodilator.

theophyline: an active alkaloid found in tea leaves along with caffeine; used as a diuretic, heart stimulant, muscle relaxant, and vasodilator.

therapeutic community: any long-term (one to three years) residential inpatient program that provides full rehabilitative and social services.

therapeutic drugs: drugs, including anti-inflammatories, painkillers, and muscle relaxants, that are used for specific medical problems.

therapeutic index: the effective dose of a drug vs. the lethal or dangerous side effects of that drug; the ratio of the lethal dose to the effective dose.

therapy: the treatment of addiction or other problem through a variety of methods, including counseling and group therapy, that is conducted by a licensed or credentialed professional.

theriac: an opium-based cure-all that was developed almost 2,000 years ago. It has undergone many changes in formulation but the opium remained.

thin layer chromatography (TLC): a moderately precise drug-testing method that tests the urine.

threshhold dose: the minimum amount of a drug that produces a desired effect.

tissue dependence: the biological adaptation of body cells and functions due to excessive drug use.

titration: adjusting the dose of a drug to achieve a desired effect.

toad secretion (bufotenine): an hallucinogenic substance that is found in the skin secretions of certain toads.

tobacco: the cured leaves of *Nicotinia tabacum* or other tobacco plant. It is the source of nicotine. It is smoked, chewed, or used as snuff.

tolerance: the increasing ability of the body to metabolize greater and greater amounts of a drug or other foreign substance to limit the impact on the body.

toluene: a liquid hydrocarbon solvent that is used as an intoxicating inhalant. It is found in many household products and glues.

topical anesthetic: a solution, ointment, or jelly containing a substance that deadens sensations in the skin, mucous membranes, or conjuctiva; e.g., cocaine, lidocaine, procaine.

tough love: a treatment approach that requires an addict's family to set strict limits on behavior to break through denial.

toxic: a substance that is poisonous when given in certain amounts. Many toxins are poisonous at lower doses.

toxicology: the study of toxic substances.

tracking: the ability of the eyes to follow a moving object.

tracks: needle mark scars on an IV drugs user's body, especially on the arms.

trade name: a drug company's name for their patented medication.

trailing phenomena: a drug-induced visual distortion (usually marijuana) in which the user sees a trail following a moving object.

tranquilizers: drugs that have antianxiety or antipsychotic properties but don't induce sleep; also prescribed as muscle relaxants.

transdermal: a method of drug delivery where a drug-laden patch is adhered to the skin so it can be absorbed through the skin.

treatment: the use of various techniques and therapies to change maladaptive patterns of behavior and restore the client to full health.

trichlorethylene (TCE): a commonly used organic solvent found in typewriter correction fluids, paints, and spot removers.

tricyclic antidepressants: a class of psychiatric medications that increase the activity of serotonin to elevate mood and counter depression.

triggers: any object or action that activates craving in a recovering drug user, e.g., the sight of white powder, money, a syringe, an old drug-using partner.

triple diagnosis: the coexistence of drug addiction, a major mental illness, and AIDS or another physical illness.

tryptophan: an amino acid that is a precursor for serotonin.

tuberculosis: a bacterial disease that can affect and damage any organ but most often the lungs.

"tweak": 1. a street name for methamphetamine. 2. unusual hyperactive behavior and emotions caused by excess amphetamine use.

twelve-step programs: self-help groups based on Alcoholics Anonymous and the 12 steps of recovery. Their purpose is to change addicts' thinking and behavior.

twin studies: long-term studies of adopted twins either raised together or separately to determine the influence of heredity on a person.

U

uppers: stimulants.

urethritis: inflammation of urinary tract often caused by excessive use of steroids.

urinalysis: analysis of urine to test for drug use.

U.S. Household Survey: a survey of drug use and attitudes in the United States done by the Substance Abuse and Mental Health Services Administration, Office of Applied Studies.

V

Valium (diazepam): the most popular benzodiazepine of the 1960s, '70s, and '80s. It is classified as a sedative-hypnotic.

vasodilation: dilation of blood vessels; can be caused by alcohol or other drug.

venereal disease: diseases, such as chlamydia and gonorrhea, that can be contracted by sexual contact with an infected person.

ventral tegmental area (VTA): the origin of a prominent dopamine pathway that ascends to various parts of the limbic system and is part of the reward pathway.

ventricles: a natural cavity in the brain, heart, or other organ. The brain's ventricles are filled with cerebrospinal fluid.

vesicle: the microscopic sacs in the terminals of nerve cells that store neurotransmitters until they are released into the synaptic gap.

Vicodin (hydrocodone): a semisynthetic opiate used for moderate pain. Hydrocodone is the most prescribed opiate.

Vitas vinifera: the most common species of grape used to make wine; comes in more than 5,000 types.

volatile nitrites: *see nitrites.*

volatile solvents: petroleum distillates that are abused as inhalants.

W

WCTU (Women's Christian Temperance Union): women's crusade to close saloons and promote temperance; founded in 1874, it had a peak membership of 500,000.

"weed": street name for marijuana.

Wernicke's encephalopathy: a central nervous system disease caused by excessive long-term drinking and linked to thiamine deficiency; symptoms include delirium, loss of balance, tremors, and visual impairment; often seen in combination with Korsakoff's syndrome.

whey: a protein supplement made from the watery portion of milk that remains after curdling; often used by athletes to help repair, rebuild, and grow muscles.

Whippets®: small metal canisters containing nitrous oxide (laughing gas). They are sold as whipped cream propellants but abused as an inhalant.

whiskey: a distilled alcoholic beverage made from a mash of fermented grains, including rye, barley, corn, oats, and wheat; usually contains about 40% alcohol (80 proof).

white matter: brain matter composed mostly of axons.

"whites": street name for Benzedrine (amphetamine sulfate) tablets, originally prescribed for weight control.

wine: an alcohol beverage made from the fermented juice of grapes; can be made from other fruits and vegetables, e.g., rice wine, plum wine, apple wine; alcohol content of wine is usually 10% to 14%.

"wired": intoxicated with stimulants, like cocaine or methamphetamine.

withdrawal: the body's attempt to rebalance itself after prolonged use of a psychoactive drug. The symptoms range from mild (caffeine withdrawal) to severe (heroin withdrawal). The onset and duration of symptoms are generally predictable.

Women for Sobriety (WFS): a self-help group therapy organization for female alcoholics.

"works": syringe, cotton, and other paraphernalia used to inject heroin or other drugs.

X

Xanax : (alprazolam): a popular benzodiazepine used to relieve anxiety.

xanthine: a class of alkaloids found in 60 plants, e.g., *Coffea Arabica, Thea sinensis, Theobroma cacao, Cola nitida*l. The most prominent xanthine is caffeine.

"XTC": *see "ecstasy."*

Y

yage: an hallucinogenic psychedelic drink made from the ayahuasca vine of South America.

yeast: a fungus that exists in fruits, some vegetables, soil, and animal excreta; used to ferment carbohydrates, especially sugars, into alcohol and to make bead rise.

yohimbe tree: the source of yohimbine, a stimulant brewed in water as a tea or used in tablet or liquid form as an aphrodisiac.

Z

zero tolerance: a prevention philosophy that allows no tolerance or second chances for drug use; often used in schools.

Zoloft : an SSRI antidepressant.

I N D E X